Y0-COU-114

Dynamics of Development: Euthenic Pediatrics

Dynamics of Development: Euthenic Pediatrics

DOROTHY V. WHIPPLE, M.D.

Clinical Associate Professor of Pediatrics,
Georgetown University School of Medicine

The Blakiston Division

McGRAW–HILL BOOK COMPANY

New York Toronto Sydney London

DYNAMICS OF DEVELOPMENT: EUTHENIC PEDIATRICS

Library of Congress Catalog Card Number: 65-19094

69525

Acknowledgments

I have a great debt to my many friends and colleagues who have given generously of their time, interest, and knowledge. They have eliminated many errors, but for those errors which remain and also for the basic philosophy of this book as a whole, I alone am responsible.

These friends and colleagues have read and criticized the parts of the book as noted.

The entire manuscript was read by:

Dr. Philip L. Calcagno, Professor of Pediatrics and Chairman of the Department of Pediatrics, Georgetown University School of Medicine, Washington, D.C.

Dr. Helen J. Ossofsky, Clinical Assistant Professor of Pediatrics, Georgetown University School of Medicine, Washington, D.C.

Dr. Charles H. Watson, Instructor in Pediatrics, Georgetown University School of Medicine, Washington, D.C.

Dr. Clarence H. Webb, Past President, American Academy of Pediatrics, Children's Clinic, Shreveport, Louisiana

Section I

Dr. Philip D. Lawrence, Chief, Health Interview Survey, U.S. Department of Health, Education and Welfare, Washington, D.C.

Dr. O. K. Sagen, Chief, National Vital Statistics Division, U.S. Department of Health, Education and Welfare, Washington, D.C.

Section II

Dr. Jorge Labbarraque (Obstetrician and Gynecologist) Clinical Instructor, Georgetown University School of Medicine, Washington, D.C.

Dr. N. C. Myrianthopoulos (Geneticist) George Washington University Hospital, Washington, D.C.

Dr. Josephine Renshaw (Obstetrician and Gynecologist) Attending Physician, Washington Hospital Center, Washington, D.C.

Section III

Dr. Nancy Bayley, Chief, Section on Early Development, Laboratory of Psychology, National Institutes of Health, Bethesda, Maryland

Section IV

Dr. Richmond S. Paine (Neurologist) Chairman, Department of Neurology, Children's Hospital, Washington, D.C.; Assistant Professor of Pediatrics, George Washington School of Medicine, Washington, D.C.

Dr. John Dolan (Pathologist) Director of Laboratories, Arlington Hospital, Arlington, Virginia

Dr. Bernard Walsh (Cardiologist) Clinical Professor of Medicine, Georgetown University School of Medicine, Washington, D.C.

Dr. Sanford Leikin (Hematologist) Chief, Department of Hematology, Children's Hospital, Washington, D.C.

Dr. Sidney Ross (Pediatrician) Chief, Microbiology Section, Research Foundation, Children's Hospital, Washington, D.C.; Clinical Associate Professor of Pediatrics, Georgetown University School of Medicine, Washington, D.C.

Dr. Dabney Jarman (Urologist) Chief, Department of Urology, Children's Hospital, Washington, D.C.

Dr. Wellington Hung (Endocrinologist) Assistant Professor of Pediatrics, George Washington School of Medicine, Washington, D.C.

Dr. Donald M. Pillsbury (Dermatologist) Professor and Chairman, Department of Dermatology, University Hospital, University of Pennsylvania, Philadelphia, Pennsylvania

Dr. June Shafer (Dermatologist) Clinical Assistant Professor of Medicine, Georgetown University School of Medicine, Washington, D.C.

Dr. Mervyn Elgart (Dermatologist) Captain, U.S.A.F.

Dr. James C. Beyer (Pathologist) Department of Pathology, Arlington Hospital, Arlington, Virginia

Dr. Alan Walker (Otolaryngologist) Chief, Speech and Hearing Clinic, Children's Hospital, Washington, D.C.

Dr. John Parrott (Pediatrician) Director of Medical Staff, Children's Hospital, Washington, D.C.

Section V

Dr. O. Lee Kline (Nutritionist) Assistant Commissioner for Science, Food and Drug Administration, U.S. Department of Agriculture, Washington, D.C.

Section VI

Dr. O. Wells Goodrich (Psychiatrist) Chief, Biosocial Growth Center, National Institutes of Mental Health, Bethesda, Maryland

Dr. Belinda Straight (Psychiatrist) Research and Faculty Advisor, Children's Hospital, Washington, D.C.

Dr. Erik H. Erikson (Psychoanalyst) Harvard University, Cambridge, Massachusetts

Dr. Asa Skard (Psychologist) Professor of Psychology, University of Oslo, Oslo, Norway

Dr. Robert Lado (Linguist) Director, School of Linguistics, Georgetown University, Washington, D.C.

Mrs. Constance Ackerson, Kindergarten Teacher, National Cathedral Schools, Washington, D.C.

Section VII

Dr. Preston McLendon (Pediatrician) Professor of Pediatrics, George Washington University School of Medicine, Washington, D.C.

Section VIII

Dr. Alice Rivlin, Economist and Sociologist, Brookings Institute, Washington, D.C.

In addition to these colleagues I wish to express my gratitude to Mr. Seymour Taine of the National Library of Medicine, whose help in the library was far beyond the call of duty.

To Donald Helm I am grateful for his skillful work on many of the illustrations.

Except where otherwise noted, all the photographs were taken by me, and almost all the children are my patients. To the children and their parents I wish to express my appreciation for their helpful cooperation.

There are two people without whose aid and support this book might never have come to completion. The first is my husband, Ewan Clague, who has not only read and criticized the manuscript but has sympathetically and cheerfully seen me through the many vicissitudes of its preparation. The second is my secretary, Esther M. Logtens, who has typed the entire manuscript not once but time after time as it was revised, reorganized, and polished. In her enthusiastic devotion she has shared the spectrum of emotions involved in this task.

Foreword

The present century has witnessed an acceleration and broadening of that interest in the biological sciences which was so exciting to the scientific world of the nineteenth century. The initial involvement with classification, morphology, and life cycles in the plant and animal kingdoms was given new dimensions with availability of the microscope. The world of microscopic organisms and of cellular structure was opened. Rapid advances in physicochemical and physiological studies followed in the early part of this century, with application of bacteriology to the study of human and animal pathology and disease entities.

In more recent years emphasis on this structural approach to the study of the living world, although expanded by refinements of techniques and availability of funds and people for research, has been supplanted by a primary interest in the functioning of life processes. This holistic approach has inevitably stimulated concern with the developmental aspect of living creatures, and especially of man. For recognition has always existed that man differed from the remainder of the animal world in the degree and quality of specialized development, reflected in the long evolution of his species and in the prolonged maturation period in the individual, which prepared his brain for abstract thought and reasoning powers, for symbolism, speech, intricate hand use, and the many other unique abilities which set him apart.

Expansion of news media, to the point of almost instant availability of knowledge to a wide segment of the public, and participation in higher education by large masses of the population have tremendously increased the numbers who are interested in the biological sciences. Studies of man, his physical attributes, his cultural elaboration, his ecological adaptations, and his relationship to other living creatures, have had high priority in this expression of scientific curiosity.

Interest in man's development probably had its greatest stimulus from the prolonged debate over Charles Darwin's thesis about origins, especially of the human species. The general idea of the development of structure and function, for species and individual, replaced the static ideas of fixed and predetermined structure and function which prevailed before Darwin's time. The natural consequence of this approach was a greater awareness of the significance of man's long developmental period through infancy, childhood, and adolescence.

Pediatrics has come into the forefront of this special interest during the past half century because it is the science of human growth and development, from conception to maturity, and of those influences which foster, modify, or impede this process. Its devotees are also those physicians who make practical application of this knowledge to the everyday care and nutrition of the child. This concept of pediatrics, always present, was given strong impetus by the White House Conference of 1930, the first nationwide and multidisciplinary study of human growth and development. Out of it came studies, publications, and plans which have permeated pediatric though with increasing force. Prior to 1930, nutrition and infection were paramount in pediatrics; now they are considered, along with many other factors, in relation to their effect on growth and development.

Like its subject, the child, pediatrics is a young, virile, and growing entity among the biological and medical sciences. It has had an expanding influence on medical thought, medical care, and public attention, largely because of accelerated awareness of the significant preadult period of development.

Paralleling these medical advances, other disciplines have expanded their interest in this segment of human life. The judiciary has established juvenile and family courts, consistent with Western civilization's concept that women and children no longer can be regarded as vassals of the dominant male but are individuals with their own rights and potentials. Authors, educators, psychologists, sociologists, anthropologists, and a host of other professional people have contributed time and thought to the child's development and maturation. Educational methods have been revised, and experimentation in the educational process has loosened its former rigidity; research in education seeks further improvement and adaptation to knowledge acquired through many approaches and in other fields.

The anthropologist and sociologist have studied children in diverse settings and societies, seeking new facts which might answer old questions, more often finding new questions, but always contributing to understanding of this life period and those influences which press upon it. The archeologist adds his knowledge of ancient societies and of human culture dynamics, demonstrating further parallels between the development of species, of cultures, and of individuals.

In this ferment of general awareness, the student of the human developmental period is no longer content with the dry bones of quantitating and categorizing pounds and inches, grams and centimeters, infant and child. He looks for a dynamic approach to the study of the constantly growing, incessantly learning and daily changing organism which is the child, possessed of thoughts, impulses and emotions, with his mind fixed on the present but his entire body attuned to the future. One welcomes, therefore, a volume on development which centers around the whole child, his present and his future, and not simply his component parts—a volume which seeks and suggests those factors which favorably influence this process. The intimate personal involvement of the author in the intricacies of human development, as observed in day-to-day personal experience, assures the reader that he will participate in the study of a vital, developing, and unfolding subject. For the human infant and child, worthy of attention in his own right and full of promise for the future, is the most exciting subject for study of all creatures in the universe.

Clarence H. Webb

Preface

Euthenic* pediatrics applies a name to the pediatrics that is being practiced more and more in the United States today. The objective of euthenic pediatrics is to help children reach their full stature physically, intellectually, emotionally, and culturally. It includes not only the care of sick children and the prevention of disease but also the cultivation of the positive elements, in the child himself and in his milieu, which foster the optimal development of his original potential.

Many children fail to achieve the promise that seemed apparent in their babyhood. Some bright healthy little children grow up into ordinary or subordinary adults. Other children whose handicaps—physical, intellectual, or environmental—augured badly for their ultimate well-being, become creative members of society.

There is much that is not known about how to nurture the human material so that the maximal potential is achieved. Yet much of what *is* known is not put to use.

This book is an outgrowth of a lifetime spent with the young, as a pediatrician, as a teacher of potential pediatricians in medical school, and as a parent in the modern society of the United States.

The book traces the path of development on many fronts. It discusses the forces from within the child that push him onward; it also discusses the forces from the milieu that aid or hinder that progression. Each organ system has its own timetable of development, an understanding of which is essential to appreciate behavior. Behavior of many kinds matures as the child is able to control his physical structure. The child's ego comes into being as he reacts to his body and to his environment. Many threads of development mature simultaneously but not independently. The fabric that is woven from these many threads is the total child.

In this book the individual threads are described "vertically." Some begin in early fetal life, others are not apparent until birth, and still others appear during childhood. Each thread is followed from its inception to maturity. Following the "vertical" descriptions is a "horizontal" summation in which the total child is described at selected ages.

The background which prompted the writing of this book is experience,

* Euthenics, from the Greek *euthenein*, to thrive. A science that deals with developing human well-being and efficient functioning through the improvement of environmental conditions. (*Webster's Third New International Dictionary, unabridged, G. & C. Merriam Company, Publishers, Springfield, Massachusetts, 1961.*)

but its actual preparation has led to long journeys into the literature of many fields. It is forever apparent that no one person can know in depth the many fields of knowledge that constitute the background for helping children achieve the best that is in them.

Early in this task the decision was faced as to whether to ask individual experts to write on each facet of development or whether to attempt the job single-handedly. Since the purpose of the book is to portray the protean manifestations of development that can, and must, be part of a pediatrician's armentarium, and since experts tend to write for other experts, I decided to undertake a single-authored volume and to ask experts to review sections pertaining to their special fields. The breadth of this presentation prohibits an exhaustive treatment of each topic. Condensation of material carries the hazard of a brevity that sometimes leads to oversimplification. While some of the discussions are inevitably cursory (especially in the eyes of experts), it is hoped that they are not only accurate but that the salient points for this presentation—the developmental changes—are clear.

It is hoped that this book will have value to the practicing pediatrician as he extends his care of children into the realm of euthenics. It is also hoped that it will be of value to the student obtaining his basic pediatric training. The book, however, is not a practical guide; rather it provides a philosophic background and a point of view for understanding what makes children tick. An appreciation of developmental forces in physical structure, in behavior, and in ego maturation is necessary in order to encourage the constructive aspects in a particular child's total environment. This appreciation also sharpens the ability to pick out deviant development when it is still possible to swing the onward stream into constructive channels.

The challenge of euthenic pediatrics is enormous, the rewards great, the heartaches many. The nurturing of maximum human potential is certainly one of the most significant tasks of modern society. Pediatricians are not the only professionals who play a significant role in this process. Nurses, teachers, social workers, psychologists, public health officials, and ministers all have an important impact on children and their parents. This book, or parts of it, may be useful to some of them, but it is the pediatrician, who, because of his continuing contact with children through all their growing years, has the opportunity to play a central role.

Contents

Acknowledgments v

Foreword ix

Preface xiii

Section I THE SCOPE OF PEDIATRICS

1 The Evolution of Pediatrics 3

2 Pediatrics in the United States Today 5

3 The Incidence of Illness and Disability 11

4 The Risk of Death 18

Section II BEGINNINGS

5 Heredity 33

6 Before Birth 56

7 Birth Itself 73

Section III INCREMENT IN POUNDS AND INCHES

8 Human Growth through the Ages 83

9 Assessment of Physical Growth 100

10 Tempo of Growth 115

11 Differential Growth Rates 120

12 Fringe Children 128

Section IV DEVELOPMENT OF ORGANIC STRUCTURE

13 The Nervous System 139

14 The Respiratory System 153

15 The Cardiovascular System 160

16 Formed Elements in the Blood 172

17 The Gastrointestinal Tract 185

18 The Reproductive System 198

19 The Urinary System 213

20 The Endocrine System 221

21 Connective, Adipose, Supportive, and Muscular Tissue 228

22 The Integumentary System 242

23 Organs of Special Sense 259

24 Immune Mechanisms 287

Section V LIFE PATTERNS OF SLEEP AND NUTRITION

25 Sleep 311

26 Nutrition 320

Section VI DEVELOPMENT OF BEHAVIOR

27 On Being Human 347

28 Eating through Life 365

29 Motor Behavior 386

30 Eliminative Function 407

31 Sexual Maturation and the Development of Loving 419

32 Communication and Language 451

33 Play and Discipline 489

34 Sensation, Learning, Cognition 504

Section VII HORIZONTAL PICTURES

35 The Premature and the Low-birth-weight Infant 527

36 The Infant 535

37 The Toddler 550

38 The Preschool Child 558

39 The School-age Child 563

40 The Adolescent 573

41 Age-portrait Summaries 592

Section VIII SOCIOLOGICAL CONSIDERATIONS

42 The Family 619

Index 633

Section I

THE SCOPE OF PEDIATRICS

1

The Evolution of Pediatrics

For most of man's history, children have been born, lived to grow up, or died along the way, without much heed from their adult society. Birth rates the world over were high, but in most societies less than half the children born grew to adulthood. About a century ago, man began to throw the searchlight of his growing knowledge on the problem of the waste of human life during infancy and childhood. In those early days of the emerging medical specialty of pediatrics, the mere fact of survival seemed a satisfactory goal. If a child had a club foot, a dislocated hip, or a warped personality, these mishaps seemed of minor importance compared with the miracle that he grew up at all.

Not only therapeutics but other sciences shed light on, first, the cause and, later, the prevention of many diseases. As a result death rates of infants dropped slowly from more than 500 per 1,000 live births a century ago to the present level of about 25. In the United States today, it is no longer a monumental task to raise a child to adult life. Clean milk, safe water, freedom from disease-carrying mosquitoes and flies are all taken for granted. Knowledge is available with which to calculate diets and administer immunizations. The skills of the surgeon and the biochemist can sometimes remedy developmental errors. When a child does become ill, the pediatrician in the United States has effective techniques at his command. His patients seldom die from dehydration or from malnutrition as they did in the years gone by. Of course there are still unsolved problems—plenty of them. Nevertheless in both the prevention and the treatment of childhood diseases enormous strides have been made in the past century.

Now that the problem of mere survival is under fairly good control, more and more attention is being focused on the quality of the human beings growing to maturity. Freedom from disease and buoyant health are still to be strived for, but the goal now includes stable emotions, intellects working at full capacity, children with a joy in life, with capacity for warm relations with their fellow men, with creative ability to see beyond their immediate needs, and the maturing of these children into adults who can use the full potential with which they were endowed. This goal may seem unattainable, but a reduction of mortality from 500 to 25 seemed unattainable a century ago. Much has been learned of how man's physical body develops; someday there may be greater understanding than at present of how his emotional, intellectual, and creative potentialities may be cultivated.

In the Middle Ages, it was generally believed that the sperm deposited by a man in a woman's womb contained a homunculus, a minute replica of the child-to-be, complete in all details, and that during pregnancy this tiny being merely expanded in size. It was thought that at birth he left his mother's body and continued his expansion until ultimately he reached his adult size.

It has taken man centuries to discover that growth is not just a process of expansion. The sperm, deposited by a man in a woman's womb, when combined with the ovum, makes the zygote. The zygote is but a single cell. It has neither the physical form of a human body nor a personality. It has only a blueprint of what is to come, with no guarantee that the plan will be fulfilled.

Many disciplines have contributed knowledge concerning the metamorphosis of the zygote into an adult. No one person can be an expert in physical medicine, psychology, anthropology, linguistics, sociology, to mention but a few of the many fields whose data impinge upon the maturing of the human child. And yet, unless all the accumulated wisdom is to remain in the ivory towers of the universities for the intellectual enjoyment of the experts, it must be gathered together and interpreted to the parents who do the actual job of bringing up children.

Pediatricians are accepting the challenge of supervision of the total child, since it is to them that families look for guidance in all matters concerning the well-being of their children. This challenge is accepted modestly, with the full realization of the impossibility of knowing in depth all the fields of special study concerning human development.

2

Pediatrics in the United States Today

In 1961 there were 11,317 pediatricians in the United States. Of these 8,593 were in private practice, and 1,243 were full-time pediatricians on the staffs of hospitals, members of medical school faculties, engaged in research, or in administration or preventive medicine (Stewart and Pennell, 1963). In addition, 1,481 young pediatricians were in training programs in hospitals as interns or residents. Thus over 85 per cent of all pediatricians who had finished their training were "out in practice."

THE HOSPITAL-BASED PEDIATRICIAN

Most children seen in a hospital are ill, and those admitted to the wards are either seriously ill or suffering from some disorder that requires hospital techniques for accurate diagnosis. The hospital-based pediatrician is in constant daily contact with serious pathologic conditions and becomes an expert in the diagnosis and treatment of disease. While he may be interested in the total child, he seldom sees his patients except during illness.

THE PEDIATRICIAN IN PRIVATE PRACTICE

The clinician "on the outside" spends his time, not with a selected group of ill children, but with a small segment of the entire child population. He will see the same children many times over the years, guide their development, protect them from preventable disease, cure them when they become ill. His interest is in the total child, which in addition to the child himself

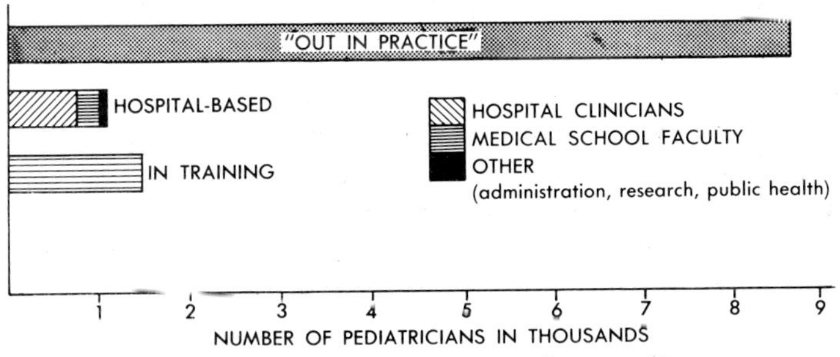

Fig. 2-1. Activities of pediatricians in the United States.

includes his parents, his home, and the community at large. Such a clinician practices *euthenic pediatrics.*

The private pediatrician in the United States goes frequently to the hospital to care for his own hospitalized patients and to attend ward rounds and clinical conferences. Many pediatricians have regular hospital assignments on the wards, in the outpatient department, in special clinics, or on the teaching staff. Thus the private pediatrician does not lose touch with hospital activities, and although he is not in as constant contact with seriously ill children as he was during his training as a resident, he has ample opportunity to maintain his diagnostic acumen.

Sick Children

The majority of the illnesses of childhood in the United States at present can be adequately treated by a well-trained pediatrician, either in his office or in the child's home. Laboratory procedures are often necessary, but relatively few children require the highly specialized techniques for diagnosis or treatment found only in the hospital. Some children will need the services of other specialists.

For every 1,000 patients under the care of a pediatrician the age distribution may be roughly about 100 under 1 year, 400 between 1 and 5 years, 300 between 5 and 10, and 200 over 10 years (Table 2-1).

TABLE 2-1

Pediatric Practice in USA: Nature of Visits per 1,000 Patients

Age in years	Number of children	Number of visits for health supervision per child per year	Total visits for health supervision per year	Number of acute illnesses per child per year	Total visits for acute illnesses per year	Total visits all reasons
0–1	100	12	1,200	3.7	377	1,570
1–5	400	2	800	3.7	1,480	2,280
5–10	300	1	300	1	300	600
10+	200	1	300	1	200	500
Totals	1,000		2,600		2,350	4,950

Virtually all children have numerous acute illnesses. If each of the 500 children under 5 have 3.7 acute illnesses per year (the countrywide average, p. 11), that means 1,850 cases of acute illness per year in these children. The 500 older children may not average more than 1 acute illness each per year. Altogether for every 1,000 children there will be 2,350 cases of acute illness. Some of these illnesses may be so mild that pediatric care is not needed; others may require several visits; and a few, probably between 10 and 20, will be so severe that hospitalization is necessary.

In addition to acute illness it can be expected that among the 1,000 patients, between 100 and 200 will have some chronic illness or organic handicap that warrants special treatment (p. 15). These chronic conditions will probably be detected during the course of health examinations, discussed below. Many will be mild conditions that the pediatrician can treat in the course of an office visit (e.g., posture problems); others will require referral to a specialist (e.g., poor vision). Some will require more elaborate procedures, and a few, 5 to 10, will require hospitalization for complete work-up. (This is in addition to children hospitalized for acute illness.)

Thus each year the private pediatrician will see roughly 2,500 cases of acute and chronic illness for each 1,000 children in his practice. He will probably hospitalize not more than 30 of these patients.

Well Children

In addition to seeing his patients when they are sick, the private pediatrician in the United States will see each of his patients for routine health supervision. The infants he will see on an average once a month; the toddlers, twice a year; and the older children, at least once a year. For the age distribution suggested, this adds up to a total of 2,600 visits per year for the routine health supervision of 1,000 children (Table 2-2). This is in

TABLE 2-2

Distribution of Total Visits to Pediatrician per 1,000 Patients per Year

	Number	%
For acute illness	2,350	47
For health supervision in which chronic illness or handicap detected (200 cases, 3.9%)	2,600	53
Total visits	4,950	100

addition to the 2,350 visits of these same children for acute illness. Some of these children may be seen more frequently when special problems arise.

During the routine health examination, the pediatrician will administer immunizations and will have the opportunity to ferret out any deviations from optimal physical health; he will discuss diet, sleep, exercise. But his obligation to his patient does not end here. His patient is growing not only a body but also a personality. There are, however, certain fundamental differences between the nurturing of the body and the nurturing of a personality.

THE NURTURING OF PHYSICAL HEALTH

The raw materials that build the physical body consist of food supplied through the maternal organism during uterine life and consumed by the child himself after birth. A physical body fails to grow adequately if some raw material is lacking, or sometimes if it is overabundant, or if some noxious agent interferes with optimal progression or if the original blueprint in the genes was defective. The raw materials out of which the physical body is constructed and the external agents which affect the growth of the body are concrete; they can be dealt with objectively. The microscope and laboratory can supply information useful to the physician in providing the growing human being with what he physically needs.

The time-honored technique of the doctor in dealing with physical health is to give orders. He prescribes diet, he orders medicine, he administers immunizations. The doctor is the authority, his knowledge is respected, his orders are followed. His authoritarian attitude instills confidence in his patients (or their parents) and relieves them of the anxiety of taking responsibility they do not feel competent to assume.

THE NURTURING OF PERSONALITY

A personality too must have raw materials out of which to develop, but the raw materials of ego development are not concrete; they cannot be seen, with or without a microscope; the biochemist cannot analyze them. It is reasonably well accepted that feelings are the raw materials out of which the ego develops.

Unlike physical structure, the ego does not begin to develop until after birth. During the early weeks of life the infant begins to respond to his mother. How the mother feels about her infant and how she expresses her feelings initiate the first phase of her child's ego development. Later, how the child feels about himself, his family, and his age-mates pushes his ego this way or that. Ultimately, the larger world of school and society modify the growing human being's feelings about himself and the outside world. His ego is a distillate of all these feelings.

The importance of feelings makes the approach to guidance of ego development quite different from that toward physical health. An authoritarian approach is useless. One cannot order a mother to feel this way or that way as one can order her to give a dose of medicine, nor can a child be told how to feel. Human feelings are not under the control of the will—either the will of the person doing the feeling or the will of the person trying to direct development. Feelings come willy-nilly. The human adult can exercise his will and control his actions; he can decide whether or not to beat up the neighbor who makes him angry, but he cannot decide whether or not to feel angry. While it is desirable for a mother to love her child, no amount of telling her that she must love him will alter her feeling.

While feelings cannot be ordered, there is much that a skillful pediatrician can do in a relatively brief time, as he conducts health examinations.

Parents worry about their child's development. Is he normal? He doesn't eat enough; he doesn't talk as early as the child down the street; he doesn't mind; he plays with his genitals; he tells lies; he is rude; and so on. Parents are irritated by troublesome behavior. The child won't go to bed; he is destructive; he talks constantly; or he is secretive. Parental worry and irritation cause anxiety, which all too often results in pressures on the child to make him conform to a pattern acceptable to the parent. Worry, anxiety, and pressures are apt to be interpreted by the child as lack of love and interfere with optimal development of his ego.

A great deal of parental worry can be alleviated or avoided completely by knowledge of normal developmental trends. Instructing parents before the appearance of worrisome behavior constitutes an essential part of euthenic care of the total child (Janeway, 1963). A mother who is told ahead of time that her child will eat less at a year than he did at 8 months is quite often able to accept with equanimity her child's decreased food consumption. Parents who know that it is normal for a 3-year-old to be interested in his genitals are not apt to worry about it.

For the pediatrician to allay anxieties, he must be thoroughly conversant with all the kaleidoscopic changes that take place as the zygote marches to adulthood.

In addition it is helpful for the pediatrician to have some understanding about the families of his children. Chamberlin has analyzed the attitudes of parents toward the whole concept of family life and child rearing. He has classified them into three categories which he calls "autocratic," "cooperative," and "indulgent–over protective." Using his criteria it is not difficult for the practicing physician to identify these ideologies in the families under his care. Depending somewhat on his own ideology he will find it easier to deal with some families than with others. Nevertheless understanding the nature of the family patterns will help him avoid attempting to change the unchangeable.

Occasionally, one hears a pediatrician say that he enjoys his child patients but that he cannot stand the mothers and all their silly questions. One can no more guide a 2-year-old youngster without considering his mother than one can fry an egg without a frying pan. One also hears adverse comments about mothers with college degrees who read about child development and then quiz their doctors. An important part of pediatric practice is that of educating parents (Webb, 1963). An intelligent young mother who wants to understand the job on which she is spending 24 hours a day, 365 days a year, needs encouragement and guidance and help with her bibliography, not ridicule.

Physical growth and ego development are intimately bound together. One must look always at a growing body, a maturing ego, and a milieu. While each thread of development must be understood in its own essence, the interrelationships must always be in the back of the mind.

BIBLIOGRAPHY

CHAMBERLIN, ROBERT W., JR.: Approaches to Child Rearing: Their Identification and Classification, *Clin. Pediat.*, **4**:150, 1965.

JANEWAY, CHARLES A.: Pediatrics in 1984—An Attempt to Look into the Crystal Ball, *Clin. Proc. Child. Hosp.*, **19**:33, 1963.

STEWART, WILLIAM H., and MARYLAND Y. PENNELL: Pediatric Manpower in the United States and Its Implications, *Pediatrics*, **31**:311, 1963.

WEBB, CLARENCE H.: Pediatric Practice. A. The Pediatrician as a Specialist, *Pediatrics*, **31**:151, 1963. B. The Pediatrician as a Family Medical Advisor, *Pediatrics*, **31**:509, 1963. C. The Pediatrician as a Teacher, *Pediatrics*, **31**:876, 1963.

3

The Incidence of Illness and Disability

Morbidity is more difficult to evaluate than mortality. Every death is recorded on a death certificate which gives information concerning the cause of death and the individual's age, sex, and residence. Mortality statistics provide accurate and detailed information on a countrywide basis. There is, however, no sickness certificate, no central place from which data on all illnesses can be compiled. Certain communicable diseases are reported, and some information is thus provided on the incidence of these diseases; these diseases, however, represent but a small fraction of all illness. Since 1957 the National Health Survey has collected data annually on certain aspects of illness, based on interviews of a sample population.

All disability (Fig. 3-1), that from conditions severe enough to require confinement to bed and that from conditions which only restrict activity, remains relatively constant until middle age, when all forms of disability increase. At all ages and even in childhood disability is higher in the female than in the male. This is a surprising finding in view of the greater mortality of the male throughout life (p. 19).

The data from the National Health Survey are divided into acute and chronic conditions. Three months is used as the definitive time for an acute illness. A chronic illness is one which has lasted more than 3 months or one due to an uncorrectable impairment. The amount of disability from acute illness is amazingly constant throughout the life span; that from chronic illness is low in childhood and mounts as life advances (Fig. 3-2).

ACUTE ILLNESS

After the neonatal period and throughout infancy and childhood, an overwhelming number of illnesses are acute (Fig. 3-3). The incidence per child under 5 in 1960–1961 was 3.7, or a total of more than 77 million cases of acute illness per year in children under 5 in the nation. Eighty-two million people under 25 years of age suffered from 235 million acute illnesses each year (Schiffer and Hunt, 1963).

Respiratory Diseases

Diseases of the respiratory tract constitute the bulk of acute illnesses not only in the early years but throughout life. Fifty-seven per cent of all acute

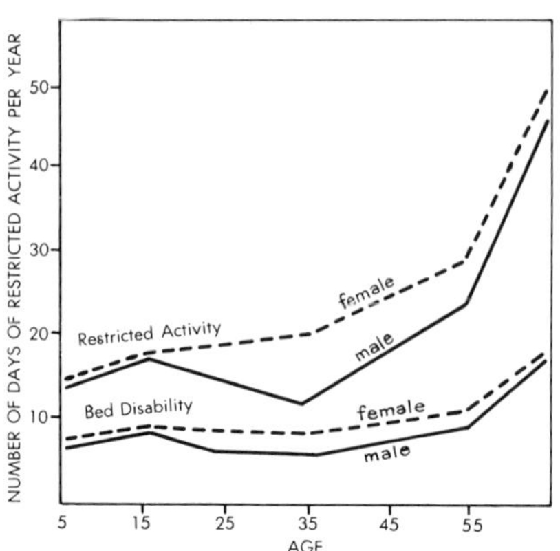

Fig. 3.1. Disability from all causes, U.S., July, 1957 to June, 1958. (*From Health Statistics, U.S. National Health Survey Series B-6 and B-10.*)

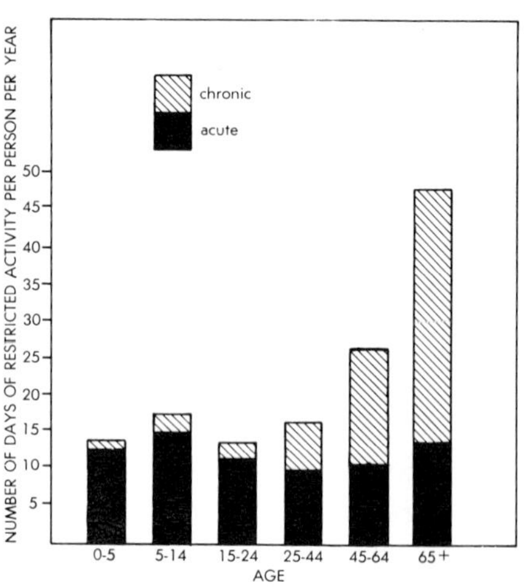

Fig. 3-2. Disability from acute and chronic diseases, U.S., July, 1957 to June, 1960. (*From Health Statistics, U.S. National Health Survey Series B-6 and B-10.*)

illness is respiratory, according to the National Health Survey. In childhood, since acute illness accounts for most illness, the respiratory diseases loom larger in the total sickness picture than later in life when chronic disease is a more important factor than acute illness (compare Figs. 3-3

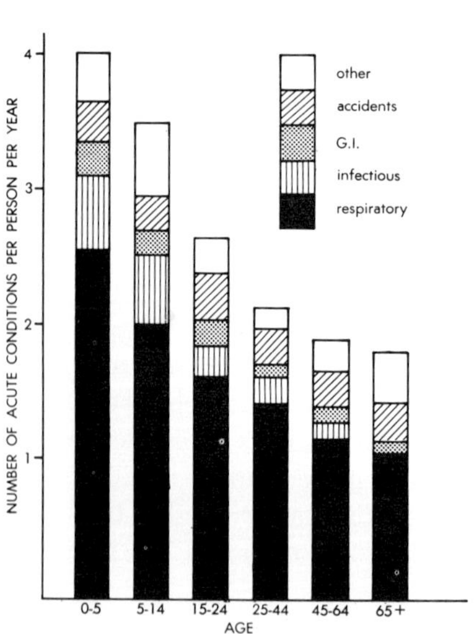

Fig. 3-3. Acute conditions per person per year, U.S., July, 1961 to July, 1962. (*From Health Statistics, U.S. National Health Survey Series C 502.*)

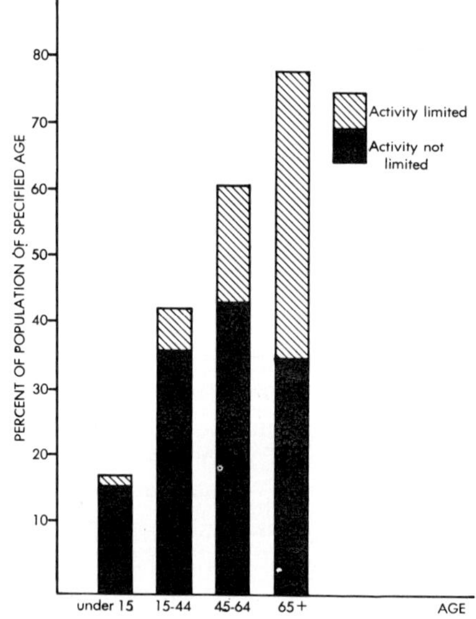

Fig. 3-4. Chronic conditions in specified age groups, U.S., July, 1961 to July, 1962. (*From Health Statistics, U.S. National Health Survey Series B-10.*)

and 3-4). While ailments of the respiratory tract are frequent, very few of these diseases are sufficiently severe to threaten life. Under the age of 5, when deaths from respiratory diseases constitute a larger percentage of total deaths than those from any other organ system (p. 27), the actual number of respiratory deaths per 1,000 children in 1961 was but 1.07, whereas the *incidence* of respiratory disease was 2,060.

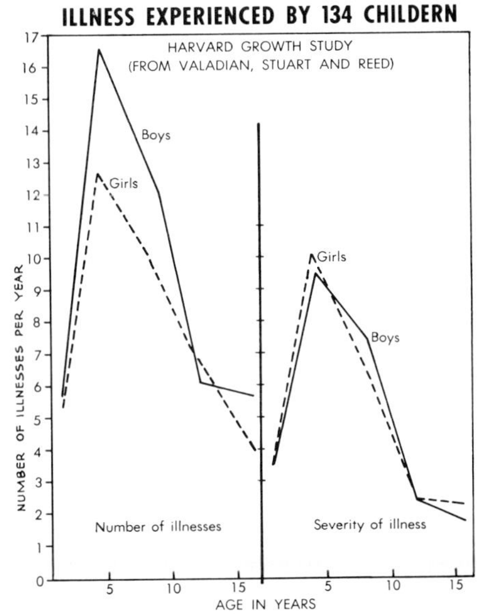

An investigation of the illness record of the children followed in the Harvard Growth Study from birth to 18 years of age confirms the cross-sectional data of the National Health Survey. In the Harvard Study it was found that the period from 2 to 6 years of age was the time of greatest vulnerability to disease, both in incidence and in severity (Fig. 3-5). Throughout the period of the Harvard Study (18 years) respiratory illness constituted 83 per cent of all illness. In this study, accidents were not classed as acute illness, which doubtless partly explains the difference between the two studies in incidence of respiratory disease (roughly 60 per cent as against 80 per cent).

Fig. 3-5. Illnesses experienced by 134 children. (*From Valadian, Stuart, and Reed, Patterns of Illness Experiences, Pediatrics, 24:940, supp., Nov., 1959.*)

Colds, pharyngitis, tonsillitis, sinusitis, otitis media, croup, bronchitis, and pneumonia are the diseases children suffer from most frequently.

Infectious and Parasitic Diseases

After respiratory disease, the specific infectious diseases have the next highest incidence in children (Fig. 3-3). Since one attack of most of these diseases produces a relatively permanent immunity, it is not surprising that their incidence declines sharply after childhood.

In the families studied by the National Health Survey, it was found that the incidence of specific infectious disease was lower among those children growing up on farms than those growing up in cities. However, as the farm children grew to adult life, they succumbed to these diseases in greater numbers than their more exposed urban age peers (Fig. 3-6).

Prevention of those diseases for which a specific immunization is available has been most spectacular. Smallpox has been virtually wiped out. Diphtheria is a rare disease. Whooping cough has been greatly decreased, although there were a total of 36,000 cases of this disease in 1962 in chil-

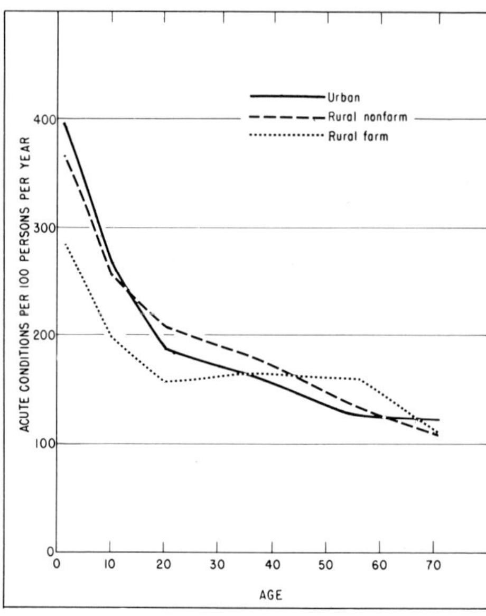

Fig. 3-6. Incidence of acute conditions per 100 persons per year by residence and age, July, 1960 to June, 1963. (*From Health Statistics, U.S. National Survey.*)

dren under 16. Poliomyelitis has been reduced from about 40,000 cases annually to about 5,000. Measles is still a problem of considerable magnitude. Prior to 1963, hardly a child grew up without having an attack of measles (6,848,000 cases in children under 16 in 1962). Serious complications from measles, while relatively rare (about 1:500), nevertheless involved many children every year. The measles vaccine, it is hoped, will soon make this disease as rare as smallpox and diphtheria. Scarlet fever is not preventable with present techniques and caused illness in 190,000 children in 1962. Chickenpox and mumps had an incidence in children under 16 in 1962 of 4,800,000 and 2,600,000, respectively.

Gastrointestinal Tract Diseases

Acute diseases of the gastrointestinal tract are a small proportion of all illnesses throughout life. They are more frequent in infants than in older children or adults. Incidence is again many times higher than mortality—200 cases of gastrointestinal illness per 1,000 children under 5 compared with but 0.4 deaths in the same group in 1962. Incidence of gastrointestinal disease has decreased greatly since water and milk supplies have been improved. In addition, treatment of severe gastrointestinal disease, especially in young children, has improved so enormously in the last two decades, since fluid balances have been understood, that mortality from these diseases has dropped precipitously.

ACCIDENTS

Sixty-nine children out of every hundred under the age of 16 had an accidental injury during 1960. This amounted to more than twelve million accidents in the entire country. While this is an appreciably lower incidence than that of acute illness, the mortality from accidents presents a grim picture (p. 26).

Accidents constitute an unsolved public health problem. The epidemiologic approach has proved fruitful (MacFarland and Moore, 1961). As with the epidemiology of a disease, three factors are significant: (1) the host, (2) the agent, and (3) the environment.

The *age of the host* is significant. Little children do not have sufficient maturity to assume responsibility for avoiding the dangerous. A toddler cannot be kept safe by explanations, prohibitions, punishments; he can only be protected by prevention of contact with the dangerous object or situation. As he matures, protection slowly gives way as education provides the tools for assuming responsibility. Dietrich has emphasized the timetable of this developmental progression.

In a study of families of children who repeatedly ingested poisonous substances Sobel and Margolis found that behavior problems in the child (especially hyperactivity and negativism) and distant child-parent relationships were highly correlated with repetitive episodes of poisoning. They suggest that repeated childhood poisoning may indicate family psychopathology which may require treatment (Johnson, 1961).

While all little children and some adults appear more likely to be involved in accidents than older children and other adults, there are temporary factors that can operate in anyone. Among such factors can be mentioned fatigue, certain emotional states, illness, and drugs (especially alcohol). It is probably true that some people (including children) are more susceptible than others to precipitating an accident under stress. However, *all* people are more likely to have an accident at one time than at another.

The time of highest incidence of accidents to preschool children was found to be between 3 and 6 P.M., when the children were tired and hungry; the highest incidence in school-age and adolescent children came later in the day and in the early evening. Highway accidents are most frequent and most severe after midnight.

Innumerable campaigns have been carried out to reduce the hazards—the *agents producing the accidents*—of modern living in the home, in the factory, on the highways. Specific suggestions concerning the prevention of hazards to children have been compiled by the American Academy of Pediatrics.

Awareness that accidents are amenable to control is a significant *environmental factor* in reducing our present accident toll, since it assigns responsibility instead of accepting accidents as inevitable and as "nobody's fault." Dietrich (1965) makes an impassioned plea to doctors, and especially pediatricians, to inform and educate all their families.

CHRONIC ORGANIC ILLNESS AND HANDICAPPING CONDITIONS

According to the National Health Survey, the incidence of chronic illness and the amount of disability caused by chronic impairment are low in childhood but increase later in life. The National Health Survey found that 17.5 per cent of children under 15 years of age had some chronic impairment

Relatively few (1.5 per cent) were restricted in activity during childhood because of their impairments (Fig. 3-4).

Harper compiled statistics from many sources on the incidence of selected handicaps in children (Table 3-1). Harper's data are for selected handicaps and thus do not attempt to give incidence on all handicaps. Nevertheless, if his figures are added together, the data suggest that about 10 per cent of all people under 21 years of age suffer from one of the listed handicaps.

TABLE 3-1

Estimated Prevalence of Selected Handicaps Among Children Under 21 Years of Age

Handicap	*Incidence per 1,000 children*
Sensory loss:	
Vision	
Blind (visual acuity less than 20/200 in better eye after correction or visual field of less than 20 degrees)	0.2
Partially seeing (visual acuity 20/70 to 20/200 in better eye after correction)	2.0
Hearing	
Deaf (75 or more decibel loss)	1.0
Hard of hearing (30–75 decibel loss)	7.0
Speech—major handicaps only	17.0
Orthopedic—including foot defects	17.0
Cerebral palsy	5.0
Epilepsy	5.0
Cleft palate or lip or both	1.3
Cardiac—all grades of handicap	10.0
Mental retardation—all grades	30.0
Total:	98.9

SOURCE: Paul A. Harper, "Preventive Pediatrics," Appleton-Century Crofts, New York, 1962.

Harper did not include the atopic diseases in his list of handicapping conditions. It has been variously estimated that about 10 per cent of children possess the hypersensitive state. Inclusion of children with allergies would therefore increase the incidence of handicapping conditions to about 20 per cent. This figure is doubtless not valid statistically, since the handicapping conditions are not mutually exclusive (e.g., a child who is hard of hearing or a child with an orthopedic handicap is just as likely to have an allergy as a child with normal hearing). The figure (17.5 per cent) given by the National Health Survey may be a more valid estimate of the amount of chronic impairment in the child population.

ABERRATIONS OF BEHAVIOR

While seldom considered chronic illness, emotional disturbances are probably the most important obstacle to optimal functioning of the human being. School problems such as truancy, academic failure of youngsters with adequate mental endowment, disruptive behavior in the classroom, school dropouts—all these are more often than not due to emotional disturbance. The problem of delinquency is laid at the door of emotional inadequacy. Alcoholism and drug addiction are almost always frankly emotional diseases.

The foundation of stable emotions begins in the cradle, and the adequate nurturing of this aspect of the developing child poses a great challenge to anyone who would work for the improvement of total child (and adult) health.

BIBLIOGRAPHY

"Bulletin on Accident Prevention," American Academy of Pediatrics, Evanston, Ill., 1965.

DIETRICH, HARRY F.: The Role of Education in Accident Prevention, *Pediatrics,* **17**:297, 1951.

———: Preventing Childhood Accidents. What Doctors Must Do, *Clin. Pediat.,* **4**:1, 1965.

HARPER, PAUL A.: "Preventive Pediatrics," Appleton-Century-Crofts, Inc., New York, 1962.

JOHNSON, WILLIAM C.: The Family Approach, in Maxwell H. Halsey (ed.), "Accident Prevention," McGraw-Hill Book Company, New York, 1961.

MACFARLAND, ROSS A., and ROLAND C. MOORE: The Epidemology of Accidents, in Maxwell H. Halsey (ed.), "Accident Prevention," McGraw-Hill Book Company, New York, 1961.

SCHIFFER, CLARA G., and ELEANOR P. HUNT: "Illness among Children," Department of Health, Education, and Welfare, U.S. Children's Bureau, 1963.

SOBEL, RAYMOND, and JAMES A. MARGOLIS: Repetitive Poisoning in Children: Psychosocial Study, *Pediatrics,* **35**:641, 1965.

Health Statistics from United States National Health Survey. Statistics on illness, accidental injuries, disability, use of hospital, medical, dental and other health related topics based on data collected in the continuing National Health Survey, Series 10, July, 1961–June, 1962.

———: Earlier reports similar to those in Series 10, Series B, July 1957–June 1958.

———: Children and Youth Selected Health Characteristics, U.S., Public Health Service Publication 584cl. Series C, July, 1957–June, 1958.

VALADIAN, ISABELLE, HAROLD C. STUART, and ROBERT B. REED: Patterns of Illness Experience, *Pediatrics,* Nov. suppl., p. 940, 1959.

4

The Risk of Death

Death comes because some vital structure fails. In the very beginning of life, death is most often due to structure formed inadequately for the job it must perform. Either the original genetic material was at fault (p. 42), or some early hazard prevented adequate maturation (p. 61). Death from profound malformations occurs during fetal life; less serious malformation may cause death soon after birth, or in infancy, or even later in life. In addition to being the result of structural inadequacy, neonatal death may also be due to prematurity—the organism is pushed out of the uterus before it is ready to perform the functions required of it. Later, the vicissitudes of life may overwhelm vital structure. Both genetic constitution and life experiences influence the capacity to withstand stress.

The death rate in the United States has been reduced by almost half since the beginning of the century. This impressive reduction has come about through increasingly effective controls over environmental hazards and through improved medical skills. In parts of the world where public health measures have not as yet been effectively put into operation and where adequate medical care is not available, people die early in life from causes no longer a major hazard in the United States—malaria, whooping cough, gastritis (Fig. 4-1).

SEX AND DEATH

There is a greater risk in being a male than a female. From the early weeks after conception until the eighth decade of life more males die than females. More males are conceived than females. The exact proportion is difficult to determine, but from what evidence exists, there may be as many as 140 males conceived for every 100 females (Eastman and Hillman, 1961). Why more males than females are conceived is in the realm of speculation. Whatever the reason, this fact, taken together with the greater fragility of the male, results in producing populations of relatively equal numbers of the two sexes during the reproductive life of the female.

During the entire period of intrauterine life about 50 per cent more males succumb than females (Eastman and Hillman, 1961); at birth, the ratio between the sexes in the white population is 105 males to 100 females.

The ratio of male to female deaths varies at different times in life (Table

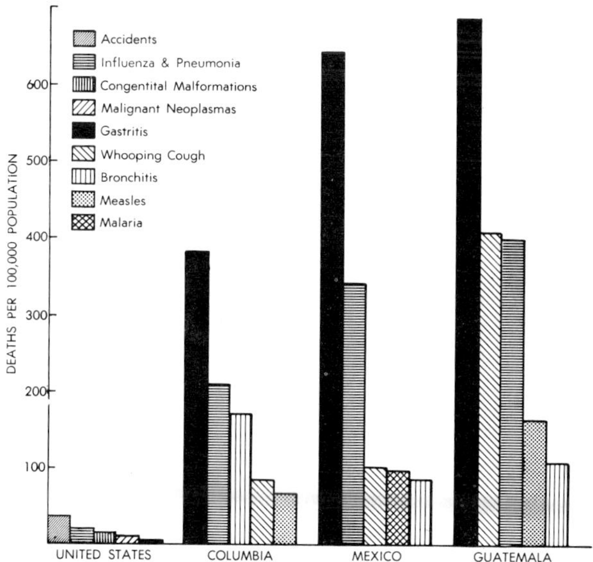

Fig. 4-1. Five principal causes of death in children, ages 1 to 4, in four countries of the Americas. *(From Pan American Health Organization Publication no. 64, 1964.)*

4-1). In the first 24 hours of life—the most lethal period in all of life—135.7 males died in 1960 for every 100 females.

In the age period between 15 and 24 the mortality of males is extraordinarily high. In 1960 for each 100 females who died 244.8 males died. This disparity is often attributed to the hazardous activities of young males. If all accidents are subtracted, the ratio of male to female deaths in this age group dropped (142:100). These are the years when females are subjected to the hazards of childbirth. If deaths from this cause are subtracted, the ratio of male to female deaths is increased. From causes not related to either accidents or childbearing 153 males died in 1960 for each 100 females. Thus while young men do die more frequently than young women from accidents, nevertheless the frailty of the young male cannot be attributed solely to his hazardous occupations (Washburn et al., 1963).

A study (Washburn, Medearis, and Childs, 1965) of sex differences in mortality from bacterial meningitis covering the period from 1933 to 1962 has demonstrated a significant male preponderance in death at all ages and especially during infancy. The advent of antibiotic therapy, while reducing the total number of deaths, actually increased the ratio of male to female deaths. Females with a greater capacity to combat infection appear to benefit more from specific therapy than the more vulnerable males.

The incidence (rather than mortality) of staphylococcal infections in the neonatal period in an underdeveloped area was found to occur four times more frequently among males than females (Simon, Allwood-Paredes, and Trejas, 1965).

From almost every category of disease, males die more frequently than females. Of the 36 major categories of diseases listed in the vital statistics data there were only 4 in which the female rate was higher in 1961 than

TABLE 4-1

Deaths of Males per 100 Female Deaths by Age Groups

Age	Male deaths per 100 female deaths
0–24 hours*	135.7
1–28 days*	155.4
1 month–1 year*	130.8
1–4 years	123.4
5–9 years	139.6
10–14 years	176.3
15–19 years	239.8
20–24 years	249.8
25–29 years	187.3
30–34 years	156.8
35–39 years	150.6
40–44 years	161.0
45–49 years	171.1
50–54 years	185.3
55–59 years	192.4
60–64 years	175.6
65–69 years	161.6
70–74 years	136.3
75–79 years	114.2
80–84 years	92.1
85–89 years	77.0
90–94 years	63.2
95–99 years	54.3
100+ years	46.2
All ages	131.6

* 1960 data.

SOURCE: "Vital Statistics of the U.S. 1961, Mortality from Selected Causes by Age, Race, and Sex," Tables 5 to 12, 1961.

the male rate. These are benign neoplasms, diabetes, cholelithiasis, and childbirth disorders (Table 4-2).

The males, it would seem, have a more tenuous hold on life than the females. A plausible speculation concerning this fact is related to the female's possession of two X chromosomes and the male's possession of but one (p. 44).

AGE AND DEATH

The beginning of life and old age are the times in life when death is most imminent (Fig. 4-2). Death in the earliest period is due, in the main, to the fact that structures were not put together in a fashion compatible with life. But early deaths also reflect the fact that the very young and immature organism is in a delicate state of balance and unable to withstand even small amounts of stress.

Death in extreme old age is brought about by the wearing out of previously adequate structures. This wearing out renders the very old, like the very young, in a shaky equilibrium, easily thrown out of balance by minor environmental hazards. Stress and strain which can successfully be coped

TABLE 4-2

Death Rates of Males and Females from Disease, per 100,000 U.S. Population

Cause	Male	Female
All causes	1073.8	790.8
Tuberculosis, all forms	8.1	2.9
Syphilis & its sequelae	2.3	0.9
Dysentery, all forms	0.2	0.1
Scarlet fever and strep throat	0.1	0.1
Diphtheria	0.0	0.0
Whooping cough	0.0	0.0
Meningococcal infections	0.4	0.3
Acute poliomyelitis	0.1	0.0
Measles	0.2	0.2
Other infective and parasitic diseases	3.4	2.8
Malignant neoplasms	163.4	136.0
Benign neoplasms	2.4	2.8
Asthma	3.5	1.9
Diabetes mellitus	13.5	19.4
Anemias	1.8	1.8
Meningitis (except meningococcal and tubercular)	1.5	1.0
Major cardiovascular-renal disease	578.9	448.7
Influenza and pneumonia	34.6	25.8
Bronchitis	3.2	1.3
Ulcer of stomach	9.4	3.3
Appendicitis	1.2	0.8
Hernia and intestinal obstructions	5.0	5.0
Gastritis and enteritis	4.5	4.1
Cirrhosis of liver	15.1	7.6
Cholelithiasis	2.2	3.0
Acute nephritis	1.0	0.7
Infection of kidney	4.5	4.3
Hyperplasia of prostate	4.6	. . .
Pregnancy	. . .	0.9
Congenital malformations	13.2	10.8
Certain diseases of early infancy	42.6	29.4
Ill-defined conditions	12.4	8.6
All others	47.3	29.0
Accidents	70.3	31.1
Suicides	16.1	4.9
Homicides	7.0	2.8

SOURCE: "Vital Statistics of the U.S. 1961, Mortality from Selected Causes by Age, Race, and Sex," Tables 5 to 12.

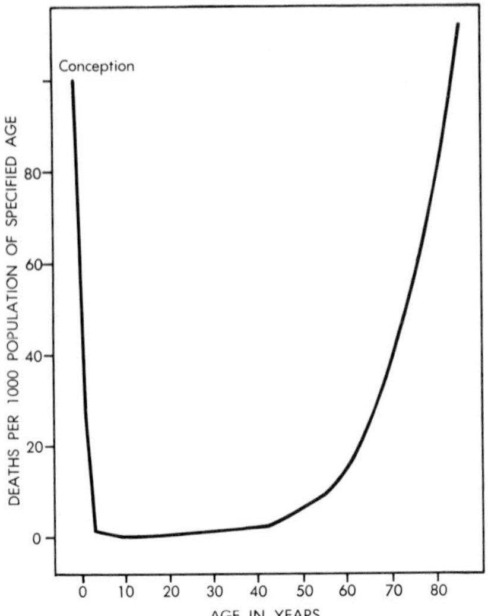

Fig. 4-2. Death rate by age in the United States, 1961. (*From Shapiro, Jones, and Densen, Fetal Mortality, Milbank Mem. Fund Quart., 40:9, 1962. Postnatal mortality from Vital Statistics of U.S., 1961.*)

with during the in-between years cause death in the very young and the very old.

FETAL DEATH

Eastman and Hillman have estimated that about 10 per cent of all infants conceived die in utero and that two-thirds of these deaths occur prior to 20 weeks of gestation. Shapiro, Jones, and Densen found, in a study of 6,844 pregnancies, that 14.17 per cent ended in fetal death. Almost half of these deaths took place before 12 weeks of gestational age, and 88 per cent before 20 weeks (Figs. 4-3 and 4-4). These figures suggest a fetal mortality of between 100 and 150 per 1,000 of the specified population, a rate not exceeded until after the age of 80 years.

Fetal deaths are caused in part by faulty germ plasm, which is incapable of directing development of a viable organism, and in part by unsatisfactory intrauterine environment. Carr has reported that 6 out of 25 previable fetuses showed chromosomal aberrations (24 per cent). Chromosomal ab-

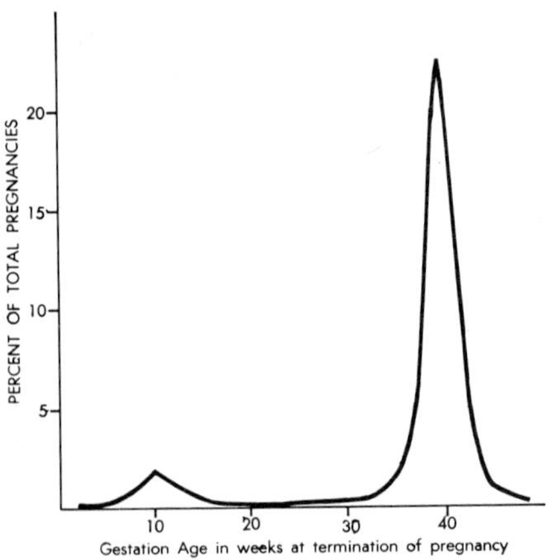

Fig. 4-3. Percent of total pregnancies terminating at specified gestation age. (*From Shapiro, Jones and Densen, A Life Table of Pregnancy Terminations and Correlates of Fetal Loss, Milbank Mem. Fund Quart., 40:9, 1962.*)

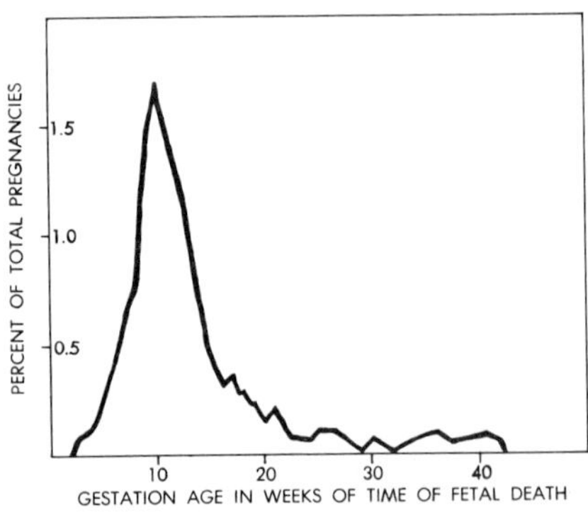

Fig. 4-4. Percent of total pregnancies terminating in fetal death by gestation age. (*From Shapiro, Jones, and Densen, A Life Table of Pregnancy Terminations and Correlates of Fetal Loss, Milbank Mem. Fund Quart., 40:9, 1962.*)

normalities are but a gross estimate of genetic mistakes. With present techniques there is no way of knowing whether other errors in the genetic material were responsible for the deaths of previable fetuses. It is possible that fetal loss, especially in the early weeks of pregnancy, may increase over the years as the number of mutated genes in the human genetic pool increases (p. 52).

Shapiro et al. found that the age of the mother and the number of previous pregnancies were each correlated with fetal death. The fewest fetal deaths were found in the women between 20 and 30 years of age having their first pregnancy. Nokes, Thornton, and King found that very young mothers (under 14) constituted almost as high a risk group as mothers over 40 (Fig. 4-5).

Fetal mortality as recorded in the vital statistics data of most of the states of the United States is defined as fetal death after 20 weeks of gestation. As shown above this represents but a small fraction of all fetal loss and is probably related more to adverse intrauterine conditions than to biologic defects in the embryo. This fraction of the fetal mortality has dropped slowly in the United States over the past 50 years (Fig. 4-6). The decrease is due primarily to improvement in the health of the pregnant woman.

INFANT DEATH

Mortality is highest in the first hour after birth. It then drops rapidly during the rest of the neonatal period and continues its downward trend throughout the first year (Fig. 4-2).

When all deaths during the first year are considered together, the death rate as recorded in the 1960 vital statistics data was 26.04 deaths per 1,000 live-born infants. This figure is, by definition, infant mortality. However,

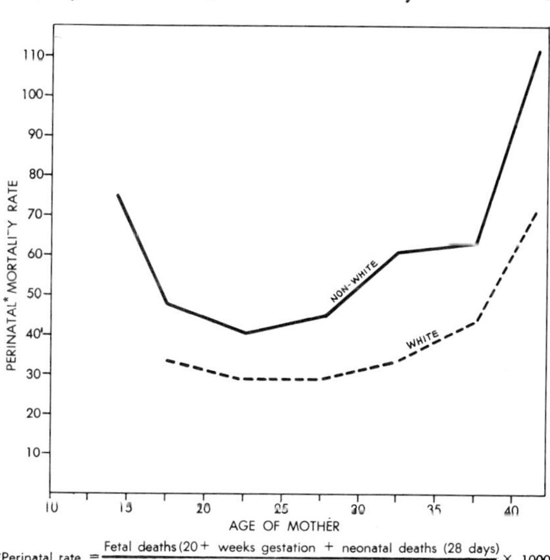

Fig. 4-5. Perinatal mortality by maternal age and race, Baltimore City, 1960. (*From Battaglia, Frazier, and Hellegers, Obstetric and Pediatric Complications of Juvenile Pregnancy, Pediatrics, 32:902, 1963.*)

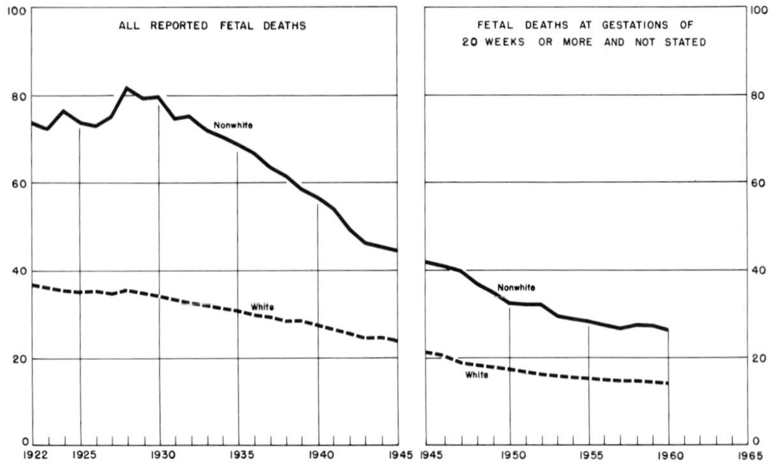

Fig. 4-6. Fetal death ratios by color in the United States, 1922 to 1960. (*From Vital Statistics of U.S., Fetal Mortality, vol. 2, section 4, 1960.*)

71.9 per cent of these deaths took place during the first month of life (neonatal mortality) (Fig. 4-7).

Neonatal deaths do not take place at a uniform rate throughout the first month. If death rates for the entire first year are calculated on a basis of deaths per hour, the enormity of the immediate postnatal loss becomes startlingly clear (Table 4-3).

Immaturity, asphyxia, birth injuries, and malformations are responsible for 87 per cent of the deaths during the first day of life (Fig. 4-8).

Despite the decrease in infants' deaths that has come about because of reduction in birth injuries, improved techniques of resuscitation, and better care of, and a reduction in the number of, prematurely born infants the

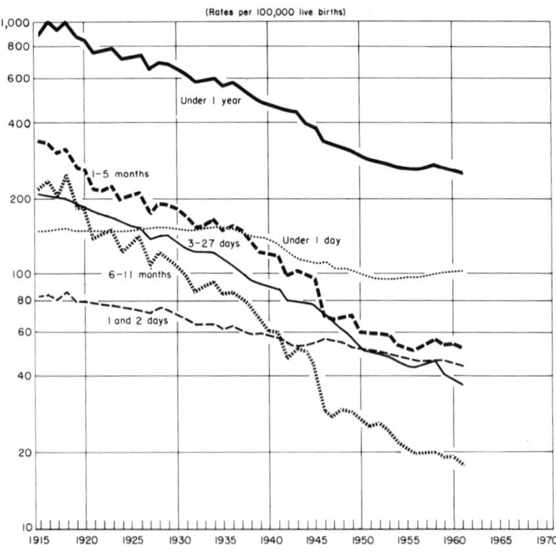

Fig. 4-7. Infant mortality rates in the U.S. by age, 1915 to 1961. (*From Vital Statistics of U.S., Infant Mortality, vol. 2, section 3, 1962.*)

TABLE 4-3

Infant Deaths per Hour at Ages Specified

	Total deaths	Deaths per hour
Under 1 hour	8,223	8,223.0
1–23 hours	35,810	1,557.0
1–28 days	35,702	58.5
28 days to 1 year	31,138	3.87

SOURCE: "Vital Statistics of the U.S. 1961, Infant Mortality," vol. II, sec. 3, Table 3-1.

mortality of infants under 24 hours of age has shown only a slight decrease in the past 50 years (Fig. 4-7). As of now, the vast majority of infants who die within the first 24 hours of life die because they were not equipped to live; their deaths are not preventable by currently known techniques.

After the first 24 hours of life the infants with gross abnormalities have been eliminated, and the surviving ones have demonstrated a capacity for independent existence. Some of them will succumb during the latter part of the neonatal period because of abnormalities which, though not severe enough to cause immediate death, are nevertheless sufficiently detrimental to prevent the maintenance of vital function. However, as the days pass, an increasing percentage of deaths is due to the vicissitudes of life imposed by the environment rather than inherent defects within the infant.

Infection is the great killer of those infants equipped at birth with organs capable of maintaining life. Infections begin to take their toll in the late neonatal period and continue through childhood.

After his initial period of establishing his viability the factors which help an infant survive are more and more within the realm of human knowledge. The infant must have food and warmth and freedom from infection. Infant mortality after the first 24 hours of life has dropped steadily as im-

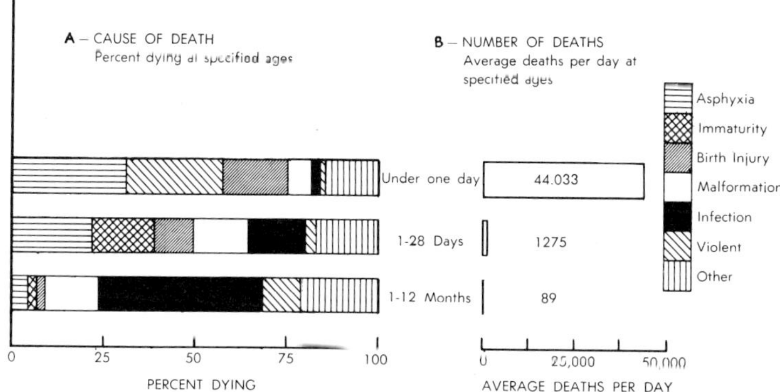

Fig. 4-8. Death in first year of life, U.S., 1960. (*Calculated from data in Vital Statistics of U.S., Infant Mortality, vol. 2, section 3, 1961.*)

proved techniques for providing these essentials have become known and utilized on a wider and wider scale (Fig. 4-8).

CHILDHOOD DEATH

After the age of 1 year death rates are low and remain low for the first two decades of life (Fig. 4-2). However, many children do die during these two decades. In 1961 there were 16,629 deaths between 1 and 4 years of age, 8,784 between 5 and 9, 7,484 between 10 and 14, and 12,024 between 15 and 19. This makes a total of 44,921 deaths between the ages of 1 and 20 years in the United States.

Why did these children die? The vital statistics data can be analyzed in several ways. One way is to classify deaths by cause; another is to classify deaths by the organ system primarily involved in the fatal illness.

DEATH BY CAUSE

All deaths can be attributed to one of the following primary causes: infection, neoplasm, violence, and inherent inadequacies. Infections include deaths due to bacterial, viral, parasitic diseases; neoplasms are primarily malignant, although a few benign growths are listed as a cause of death. Violence includes accidents, homicides, and suicides. Inherent inadequacies are malformations, metabolic errors, structural defects, and diseases not in the above categories for which no known external agent is causative. Figure 4-9 shows these data.

The enormous toll accidents take in the child population is strikingly clear. Between the ages of five and nine 30.2 per cent of all deaths were due to violence; this figure rises to 43.6 per cent between 10 and 14 and 56.2 per cent between 15 and 19. During these ages only about 1 child per 1,000 dies, but of those who do die an enormous percentage succumb to some kind of violence, more than from any other cause. Of the 44,921 deaths between 1 and 19 years of age, 18,406 were due to violence. Almost all these deaths are preventable (p. 14).

Inherent defects in the organism are the next most frequent cause of death. These diseases take a great toll immediately after birth. Although the most seriously defective individuals have been eliminated after the first year, nevertheless, throughout childhood, the inadequate organism is less able to cope with life. As age advances, a larger and larger proportion of deaths is due to inherent defects as compared to external factors. The organism wears out, until finally some vital structure can no longer function. External factors may, of course, speed this wearing-out process.

Infections loom large in the earliest years but gradually decrease as a cause of death as the individual builds up immunity (p. 296). Later in life infections are an insignificant factor in the total number of deaths. It is only within the last half century, in this country, that deaths from

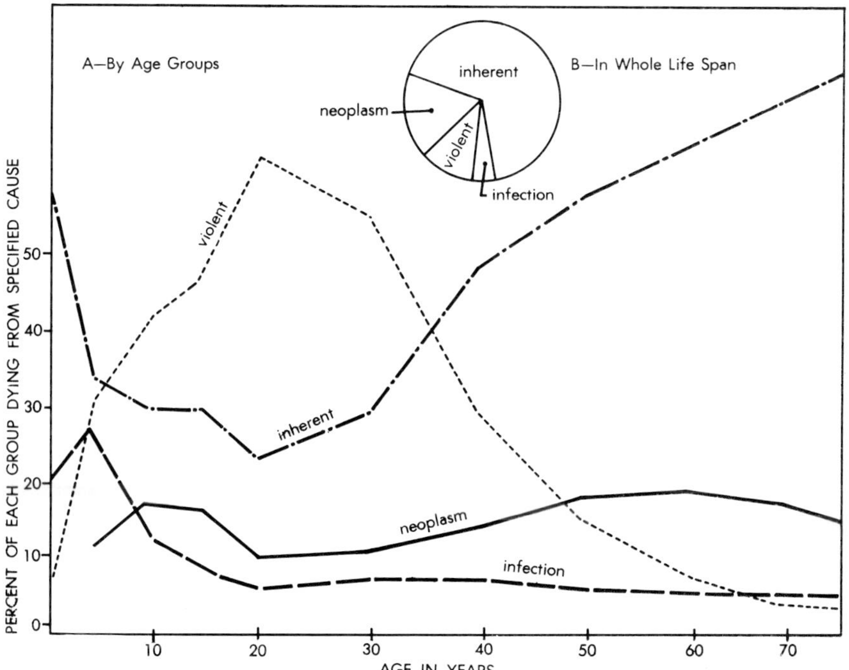

Fig. 4-9. Deaths from specified causes, U.S., 1961. (*Calculated from data in Vital Statistics of U.S., Deaths from 59 Selected Causes by Age, Color and Sex, 1962.*)

infection have been reduced to this low level. Of the total deaths in 1900 at all ages 64.8 per cent were due to the common infections as compared to 0.53 per cent in 1961 (Historical Statistics of the United States, 1957).

It is of interest to compare the cause of death of children in the United States with the cause of death of children in less developed parts of the world. Not only do more children die in underdeveloped areas, but those who do die succumb to the communicable diseases which have been, for the most part, eliminated in this country (Fig. 4-1).

After the age of 10 years in the United States there are more deaths from neoplasms than from infection. The childhood deaths from neoplasms are predominantly those due to leukemia.

DEATH BY ORGAN SYSTEM

Deaths as reported in the vital statistics data can shed some light on what part of the human organism is most likely to fail. The vital statistics data were regrouped, putting together deaths, regardless of cause, that affected primarily one or another organ system. Deaths due to violence were kept as a separate category. In the first decade, the respiratory system is more vulnerable than any other part of the body (Fig. 4-10). In the second decade, it gives way to the hematopoietic system, which reflects

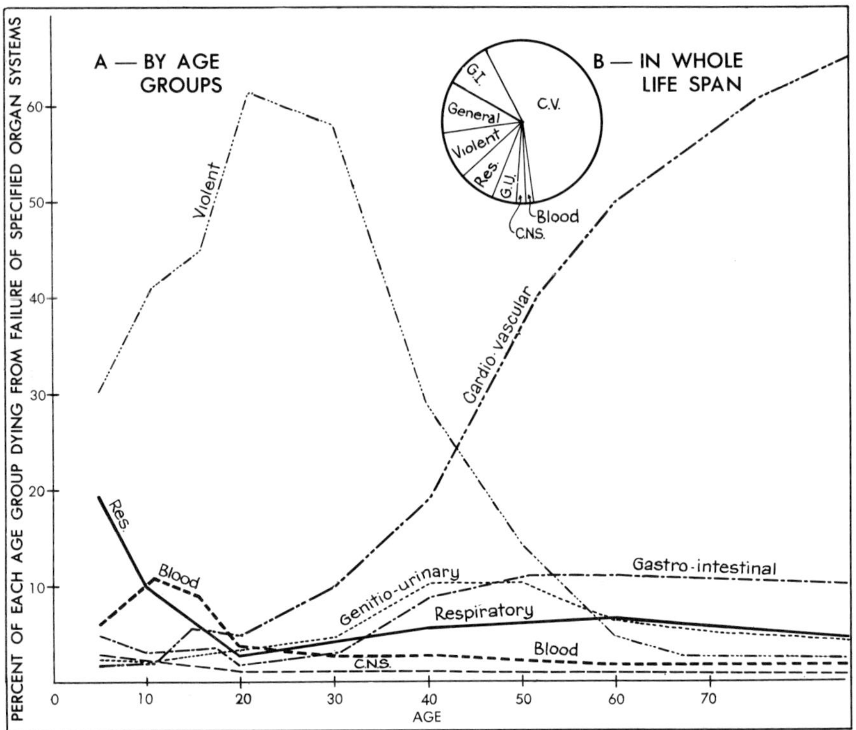

Fig. 4-10. Deaths classified by organ systems, U.S., 1961. (*Calculated from data in Vital Statistics of U.S., Deaths from 59 Selected Causes by Age, Color and Sex, 1962.*)

the high place that leukemia occupies as a cause of childhood deaths. The other organ systems are about equally susceptible to failure in the first decade. In the second decade, death due to disease of the cardiovascular system begins its upward trend. After the age of 20, deaths due to cardiovascular disease rise abruptly; by the age of 50 they are responsible for 40 per cent of all deaths and by the age of 80, almost 70 per cent. It is the cardiovascular system which apparently wears out more frequently than any other part of the body. Future research in cardiovascular disease may some day disclose controllable environmental factors, applicable early in life, that can reduce the vulnerability of this part of man's organism.

Certain aspects of longevity are doubtless inherent in the genetic code. Even in times and places where death rates were high, some individuals managed to live to old age. Those people who survived the hazards of early life lived as long as people of today. In 1850 in Massachusetts, while the life expectancy at birth for a male child was but 38.3 years, those males who survived to age 60 had virtually the same number of years of life to look forward to as men of 60 today (15.6 years for the 60-year-old man in 1850 compared with 15.9 years for the man of the same age in 1960). The possible length of life has hardly been altered, but the number of people achieving the human potential has more than trebled during the century. Only 4 per cent of the population was 60 years old or more in 1850; in 1960, however, 13.2 per cent achieved 60 years of life. It is probable that this figure will increase in the years to come.

BIBLIOGRAPHY

BATTAGLIA, FREDERICK G., TODD F. FRAZIER, and ANDRE E. HELLEGERS: Obstetric and Pediatric Complications of Juvenile Pregnancy, *Pediatrics,* **32:**902, 1963.

CARR, D. H.: Chromosome Studies in Aborted Fetuses and Stillborn Children, paper presented at the American Society of Human Genetics Meeting, New York, July, 1963.

CHILDS, BARTON: Genetic Origins of Some Sex Differences among Human Beings, *Pediatrics,* **35:**798, 1965.

EASTMAN, NICHOLSON J., and LOUIS M. HILLMAN: "Williams Obstetrics," 12th ed., Appleton-Century-Crofts, Inc., New York, 1961.

Historical Statistics of the United States: Colonial Times to 1957, U.S. Bureau of the Census, Washington, D.C., 1960.

NOKES, J. M., W. N. THORNTON, and T. C. KING: A Critical Analysis of the Young and Elderly Primiparas, *South. M. J.,* **45:**266, 1952.

Pan-American Health Organization Publication 64, 1962.

SHAPIRO, SAM, ELLEN W. JONES, and PAUL M. DENSEN: A Life Table of Pregnancy Terminations and Correlates of Fetal Loss, *Milbank Mem. Fund Quart.,* **40:**7, 1962.

SIMON, HAROLD J., JUAN ALLWOOD-PAREDES, and ALFONSO TREJAS: Neonatal Staphylococcal Infection, *Pediatrics,* **35:**254, 1965.

Vital Statistics of the United States: "1960 Infant Mortality," vol. II, sec. 3; "1960 Fetal Mortality," vol. II, sec. 4; "1961 Deaths from 59 Selected Causes by Age, Color and Sex;" "1960 Life Tables," vol. II, sec. 2, Table 2-2.

WASHBURN, THOMAS C., DONALD N. MEDEARIS, and BARTON CHILDS: Sex Differences in Susceptibility to Infection, *Pediatrics,* **35:**57, 1965.

Section II

BEGINNINGS

5

Heredity

Beginning at conception and extending throughout the whole life span, the drama of development unfolds. To understand as completely as possible the plot of this drama the prologue must be read.

At conception gamete *A* from the mother and gamete *B* from the father join together to make zygote *AB*. At this moment a new person comes into being, different from every other member of the species (except his identical twin, if he has one) and yet sufficiently like all others to be called human.

The zygote carries the potential for the mature adult. To what extent that potential will be realized depends both upon the protection from harm this new individual receives and upon the opportunities for fulfillment met on the journey from zygotehood to adulthood. The zygote carries the potential for a certain kind and amount of development; it carries no assurance that genetic goals will be reached.

HEREDITY AND EVOLUTION

Throughout the entire living world, from single-cell structures to man, the chemical substance that carries the genetic information is fundamentally the same.

It is conceivable that billions of years ago, when the first "living molecule" appeared on the planet, it consisted of a tiny fragment of genetic material. The new power of this molecule lay in its ability to direct synthesis of more like itself. This living molecule, Beadle (1957) suggests, may be thought of as the bridge between the inorganic world that preceded it and the organic world that ultimately followed.

This microscopically small particle had, in addition to its power of replication, the ability to undergo change—mutation. Once mutated the genetic material of the living molecule repeated its new form with the same exactness with which it duplicated its original self. The power of replication and the ability to undergo mutation inherent in the genetic material are responsible for the drama of evolution. This genetic material has persisted since the beginning of life on this planet and gives evidence that it will continue as long as life continues (Dobzhansky, 1955).

CONTINUITY OF THE GENETIC MATERIAL

Since every living animal shares with every other animal the same basic directing mechanisms, it is not surprising that there is a continuity of structure in all living forms, including the human. In the human embryo a yolk sac is developed, and the tiny embryo sprawls across it with wide-open gut in what looks like an attempt to absorb nourishment. But since human beings are mammals, the yolk sac is empty of yolk, and the developing embryo must find an alternative method of nourishment. It does so by transforming the useless yolk sac into a passageway to a new organ, the placenta. But every human embryo goes through the circuitous path of first forming and then discarding a yolk sac. This is gene-directed activity.

Many examples of this sort of phenomenon can be given. The embryo grows gill slits and then transforms them into thyroid, parathyroid, and thymus glands. It builds a skeleton out of cartilage, adequate for water-living forms whose bodies are buoyed up by their environment but inadequate for weight-bearing in air; then the embryo destroys the useless cartilage and replaces it by bone. Not only does structure show the imprint of the ancestral genes, but so do functions. The newborn exhibits the Moro reflex (p. 387), a vestigial reaction, no longer useful to the human being, which fades out as development proceeds. Young infants show clinging reactions, and slightly older ones show following reactions, both of which have overtones of ancestral patterns (see p. 395).

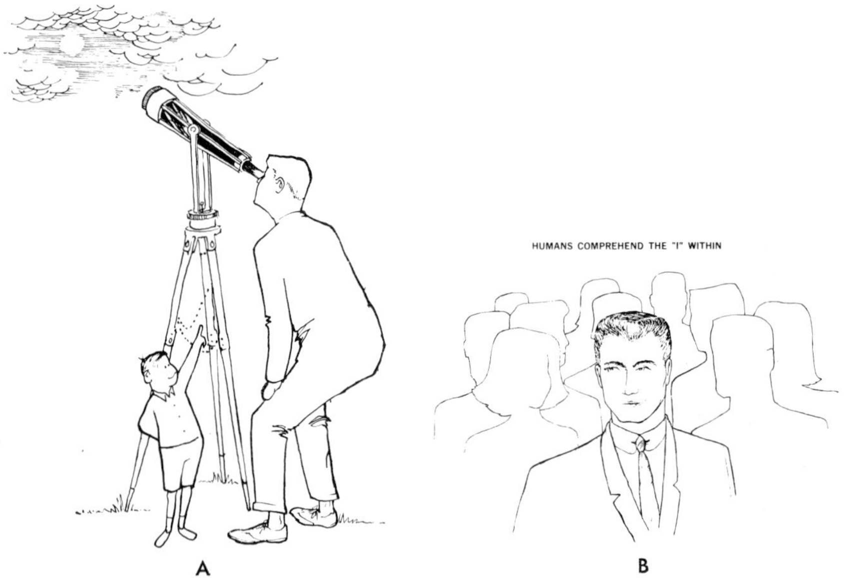

Fig. 5-1. Humans have species-specific genes. *A*, Only man speculates on the nature of the universe. *B*, Only man comprehends the "I" within.

In addition to the structural and functional attributes that show the human being's emergence from the ancestral past, man also has in his germinal material certain genes that direct development into uniquely human channels. These too show their ancestral origins. Man alone has developed the capacity to use speech, but glimmerings of the ability to symbolize are evident in the primates (p. 452).[1]

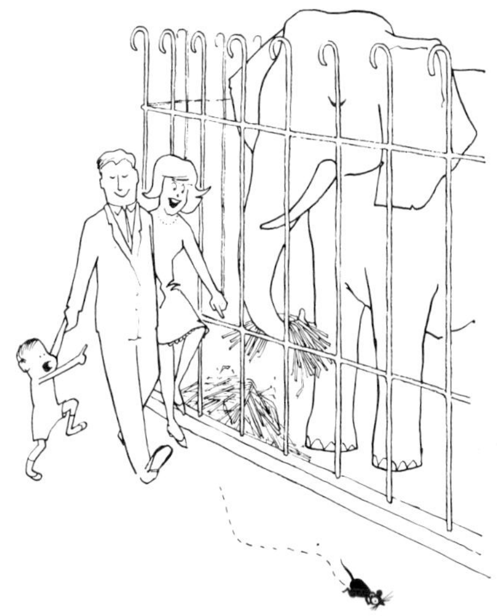

Fig. 5-2. The human being is kept within the limits of his species—all are bigger than mice; none is as big as an elephant.

Human structure, physiology, and even personality can be illuminated by tracing their origins through the laboriously slow changes in the genetic material that have brought them about. An understanding of the path each human being *must* travel is the tool needed for providing him with opportunities for optimal development. It is no more desirable to attempt to thwart, say, the following reaction in a toddler than it would be to try to prevent the embryo from reaching out to a nonexistent yolk.

VARIATION AND SOME OF ITS SIGNIFICANCE

While in every human being the structure, the functions, and the attributes that are characteristic of his species develop, no two people are exactly alike. The limits of variability are fairly narrow; all human beings are bigger than mice, and no human being is as big as an elephant. The human being must stay within the limits of his species.

But once these outside limits are accepted, there is within them considerable variability. The human genetic pool contains many alleles of the same gene (see The Basic Tenets of Heredity, below). Whenever people are measured—whether the measurements are of height and weight, of some physiologic component like pulse rate, blood count, chemical analyses of body fluids, or of intellectual capacity—there is a range of values. When such measurements are plotted, the figures usually fall into a bell-shaped curve. The individuals whose measurements fall near the center of the distribution usually have little difficulty adjusting to their environment—physically or emotionally. But people, especially children, who deviate considerably from the median may need help to accept themselves as adequate.

[1] Recent work on the dolphin has raised the question as to whether or not these animals possess a true language (p. 455).

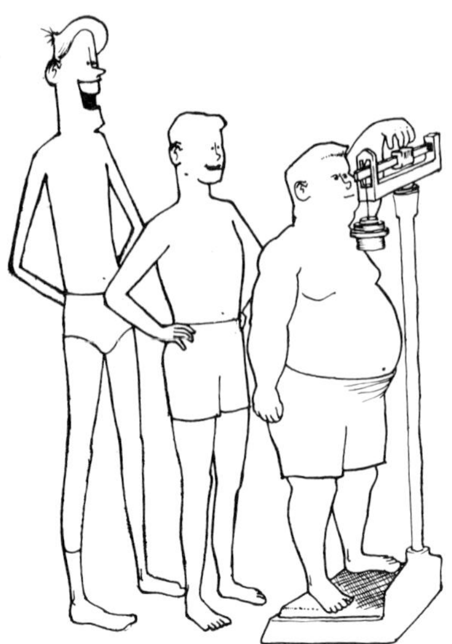

Fig. 5-3. Within species limitations there is much variation.

Life is different for a girl whose menarche comes at 10½ years of age compared to one in whom this event does not take place until the age of 16. Both girls may be "normal" in that neither has a disease which has influenced the time of appearance of the menarche, but they cannot be squeezed into the same mold and treated in the same fashion. The genes of these two girls are different and have made them unique individuals whose differences must be accepted and respected.

The child who is very short or very tall often needs a sensitive adult to help him accept himself as an adequate person. Awareness of these individual differences, many of which are inherent in the very stuff out of which a person is made, is essential in understanding what happens to any one human being during his whole life span.

While there are still gaps in our understanding of how the genetic material functions, nevertheless much is known of the basic mechanism whereby genetic information is passed from generation to generation.

In the present chapter only the broad outlines of genetics will be sketched. For more complete discussion the reader is referred to Srb and Owen, Auerbach, Beadle, Singleton, Stern, and Childs and Sidbury, and Boyd.

THE BASIC TENETS OF HEREDITY

Over the centuries, people have been interested in the resemblance between parents and their children, but the main concern in earlier times was with such major aspects of humanity as strength or beauty or intelligence or health. These qualities are so complex and so altered by environment that it was next to impossible to deduce basic principles of heredity from the occurrence of such composite qualities in a population.

It was Gregor Mendel, a nineteenth century Austrian monk, who conceived the idea that the enigma of heredity could be elucidated only by studying, in rapidly multiplying forms, the transmission of single, easily identifiable traits. From his studies on the garden pea Mendel postulated that certain hereditary traits are dependent upon basic elementary particles. Mendel called the hereditary particles *elements;* they were later named *genes* by Johansen.

Every individual (in sexually reproducing forms) receives two genes for each hereditary property, one from its father, one from its mother. If both these genes are identical in all members of a species, the property for which they are responsible cannot be identified. However, if two or more forms of the gene exist, individuals will show different characteristics depending upon which form of the gene they possess (the various forms of a gene are termed *alleles*).

When two forms of a gene exist, one allele is often dominant over the other, and the individual shows the property manifest by the parent contributing the dominant gene.

In Mendel's famous experiments a purple sweet pea was crossed with a white one. In the first generation (F_1) all the progeny had purple flowers. The gene for purple was dominant over the gene for white. In the second generation (F_2) Mendel found that three-fourths of the flowers were purple and one-fourth white. The allele for purple and the allele for white existed side by side in the F_1 generation, and the allele for white apparently did not participate in development; nevertheless it neither blended with the dominant allele nor died out.

The Law of Segregation

From these experiments Mendel formulated the law of segregation, a law which has been confirmed by later generations of geneticists. This law states that alleles do not blend but exist independently and at the time of gamete formation enter into the mature germ cells in their original form uninfluenced by their association with other alleles of the same gene.

An example in human genetics comparable to Mendel's purple and white garden peas is found in albinism. Two alleles exist in the human genetic pool—one, the dominant, which directs development of pigment in skin, hair, and iris of the eye, the other, a recessive allele, which prevents the development of this pigment. Individuals heterozygous for these two alleles have normal pigment; only when the two recessive alleles occur together does the individual develop into an albino.

While alleles maintain their unique integrity and are passed to the next generation in their original form, recessive alleles in some cases do influence development. The heterozygous individual may show a blending of traits—a white and a red flower producing a pink one. The blending, however, is only in the *expression* of the gene. The genes themselves are not blended; there is no gene for pink. When the pink flower forms gametes, it transmits to its progeny either an allele for red or an allele for white. Where this blending of the expression of two alleles exists, in some cases it provides means of identifying individuals who carry a recessive gene (see below).

A heredity trait or character is an observable feature of the individual. Some traits are the result of the action of many genes—polygenic traits.

Some genes influence more than one trait—pleiotropic genes. The function of genes will be discussed below.

The Inviolability of Genetic Material

The genetic material is not influenced by the vicissitudes of the individual life. An individual may have genetic material (possibly numerous genes) that can direct his height to 6 ft, but because of faulty nutrition or illness he may never achieve his might-have-been stature. Nevertheless the genetic material he transmits to his offspring has not lost its original potential. Thwarting of potential development does not weaken the genes transmitted, nor does giving a gene the maximum opportunity for development increase its power.

In the past there have been many advocates of the theory of the inheritance of acquired characteristics; however, this theory has been abandoned by modern geneticists. The one exception is the Russian school represented by Lysenko, who claims that ". . . the evolution of living nature is unthinkable without recognition of the inheritance of individual characteristics acquired by the organism under the conditions of its life." It is the consensus of Western geneticists that this view is supported more because of political ideology than scientific truth.

Any change in the genetic material comes about not by alteration in its *expression* but by an alteration within the genetic material itself. While the genetic material is extraordinarily immune to alteration, its immunity is not absolute. It can be altered by the process of mutation (p. 42). The essential point is that mutation is not brought about through anything that happens in the somatic cells during an individual life; it is a spontaneous change in the germinal material itself.

THE GENETIC MATERIAL ITSELF

The genetic material lies within the nucleus and is part of the chromosomes of all living cells. Chromosomes are most clearly seen during mitosis, when they appear as rodlike structures. The number of chromosomes is species-specific. It is the same in every cell of every individual of a given species (with a few exceptions mentioned below) but varies from species to species. In the human being the characteristic number is 46 (Tijo and Levan, 1956; Ford, et al., 1958; Hsu, 1952).

The 46 chromosomes of man consist of pairs. In the female there are 23 pairs; in the male, 22 pairs plus two heteromorphic chromosomes. The pairs of chromosomes differ morphologically one from the other to a sufficient degree that each pair can be identified and numbered. In each human chromosome there is a constriction which divides it into two arms. This constriction, called the *kinetochore,* varies in position in different chromosomes. In some it is in the center, in others almost at the tip, but its position remains constant for the individual chromosome. The kinetochore is thought to control the movement of the chromosome during cell division and is therefore of fundamental significance (McLeish, 1958).

Based on the position of the kinetochore, the length of the arms, and the total size of the chromosome, a system of nomenclature has been devised. The 22 pairs of chromosomes common to both males and females are called *autosomes.* They are numbered from 1 to 22 in descending order of length. In the female the twenty-third pair consists of two chromosomes called the X chromosomes (Fig. 5-4). In the male there is one X chromosome and one Y chromosome (Fig. 5-5).

The basic chemical structure of the genetic material in the chromosome has now been identified as deoxyribonucleic acid (DNA) (Watson and Crick, 1953). DNA is an extraordinarily complex molecule. Its molecular weight has not yet been determined, but in the human being it is probably of the order of 100 million. Structurally it consists of enormously long, thin fibers coiled around each other in two helical chains. The stretched

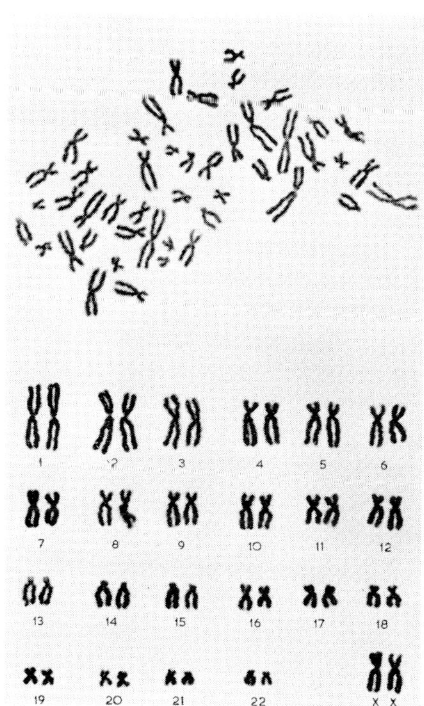

Fig. 5-4. Ideogram of human female chromosomes. (*From L. S. Penrose, Recent Advances in Human Genetics, J. A. Churchill Ltd., London, 1958.*)

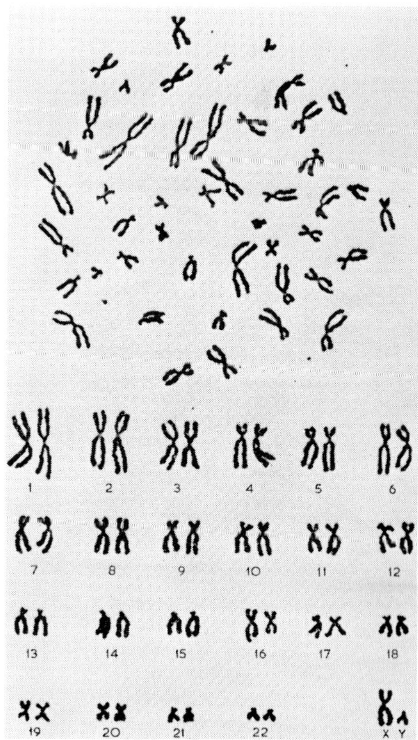

Fig. 5-5. Ideogram of human male chromosomes. (*From L. S. Penrose, Recent Advances in Human Genetics, J. A. Churchill Ltd., London, 1958.*)

out chromosome is probably no more than 50 μ long and no more than 2.5 μ wide. Models of this molecule have been built using a scale of 2 cm equal to 1 A. On such a scale a single chromosome would exceed 5,000 miles (Fig. 5-6).

Within this long DNA fiber are alternate groups of phosphate and sugar molecules linked together by nitrogenous compounds. This group—phosphate, sugar, and nitrogenous base—constitute a nucleotide. The phosphate and sugar units of the molecule are all alike. There are four different nitrogenous bases, two purines (adenine and guanine) and two pyrimidines (thymine and cytosine).

These four base pairs are so arranged that adenine and thymine are always opposite each other, and guanine and cytosine are likewise opposite each other.

These base pairs are thought to be responsible for the two fundamental properties of the genetic material, (1) its capacity to transmit genetic information and (2) its capacity to reproduce itself identically.

A single gene is thought to consist of a sequence of 1,000 to 10,000 nucleotides.

The mechanism by which the nucleotides transmit information is still in the realm of speculation, but the speculations assume that the sequence of the nucleotides in the DNA fiber is of ultimate importance; variation in this sequence transmits specific codes.

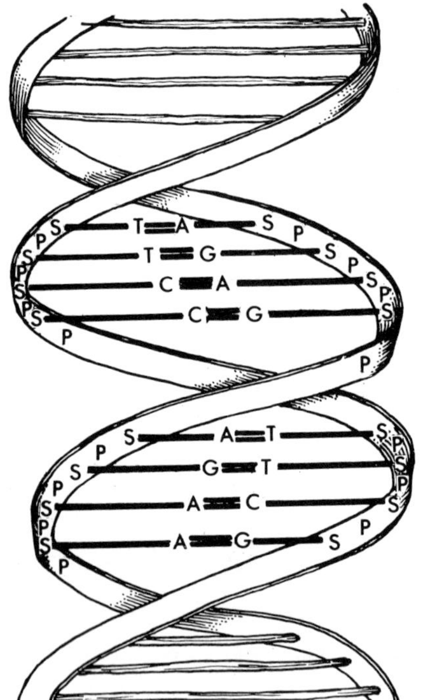

Fig. 5-6. Structure of DNA fiber. (*From Watson and Crick, Molecular Structure of Nucleic Acids, Nature, 171:737, 1953.*)

A four-letter code may seem too skimpy to transmit the huge number of genetic messages. However, when it is realized how many premutations and combinations of a four-letter code are possible within a single gene consisting of a minimum of, say, 1,000 nucleotides, namely, $4^{1,000}$, it becomes apparent that the four-letter code is entirely adequate for the transmission of an almost limitless series of genetic messages.

Replication of the DNA fiber is assumed to take place by the synthesis of a complementary copy of each strand of the fiber (Fig. 5-7).

THE FUNCTION OF GENES

The currently held hypothesis of the function of the gene was first sug-

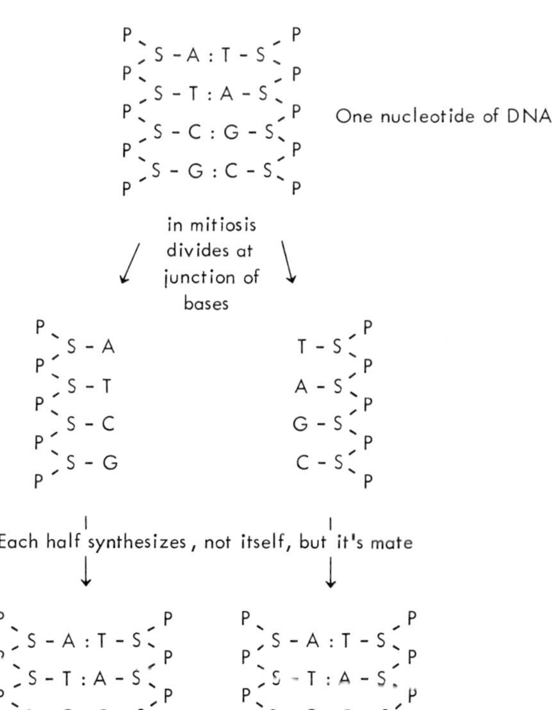

Fig. 5-7. Replication of DNA.

gested by Garrod in 1908 in his work on alkaptonuria. He hypothesized that certain diseases of a hereditary nature were due to failure of an enzyme governing a single metabolic process. Beadle formulated the one-gene–one-enzyme hypothesis. All biochemical processes are under genetic control, and these processes are accomplished a step at a time, each step directed by a single gene.

The manufacture of protein is the basis of development. There are only 22 different amino acids, but a protein molecule is composed of thousands of these 22 amino acids arranged in varying combinations and permutations. For normal development not only each gene but each nucleotide must exert its influence at the exact moment that certain linkages in the protein molecules are being formed. To do this each locus of each nucleotide within the DNA molecule must be maintained.

The mechanism of gene action has been described by Sutton. The gene remains within the nucleus of the cell, where it directs the manufacture of ribonucleic acid (RNA), which then migrates out of the nucleus into the cytoplasm. It is RNA which imprints the pattern on the nutrient molecules within the cytoplasm, selecting this, rejecting that, and combining the chosen ones into a specific pattern predetermined by the gene to form a protein molecule. Patterns are thus transmitted from the gene in the DNA (which remains in the nucleus) to RNA (which is found in both nucleus and cytoplasm) and then to the specific protein being synthesized.

MUTATION

A mutation is a spontaneous change at some locus within the DNA fiber. Theoretically, four types of changes could take place within the structure of the gene: (1) substitution of one nucleotide for another, (2) transposition of two nucleotides, (3) omission, or (4) duplication of a nucleotide. In each type of change one or more base pairs could be involved (Beadle, 1957).

One faulty gene can have profound effects on total development (Stanbury, Wyngaarden, and Fredrickson, 1960). All enzymatic defects are basically abnormalities in protein synthesis; however, the end product that becomes deranged as a result of a single mutated gene can be a protein, a carbohydrate, a lipid, or a hormone. Inborn errors of metabolism may be lethal early in life; on the other hand they may not become manifest until much later in life. Symptoms appear at any time that accumulated faulty products of metabolism interfere with normal function (Table 5-1).

The same mutations of some genes seem to occur over and over, which would indicate that there may be greater instability of the DNA molecule at some loci than at others.

Haldane (1932) has estimated that the normal gene mutates to the hemophilic gene about once in 50,000 gametes. He produced some evidence that this particular mutation from normal to hemophiliac took place in the ovary of Queen Victoria, who then transmitted the hemophilic gene to her descendants.

Mutation frequencies of from 1 per 100 million to 1 per 10,000 per generation are within the known range (Beadle, 1957). While it is impossible to know the mutation rate of each gene, Muller (1950) has estimated that the total mutation rate for all the ten thousand or more genes assumed to exist in the human chromosomes is such that there is, on the average, one new mutation in every 10 or fewer gametes. Muller also estimates that each individual carries about eight defective alleles.

Spontaneous mutations occur at intervals in any population for reasons which are quite unknown. It is known, however, that radiation increases the mutation rate (Russell and Russell, 1952).

Defective alleles become a problem only when two individuals heterozygous for the same defective allele mate and produce a homozygous offspring. However, the more defective alleles present in one person, the greater are his chances of selecting a mate who carries one of his defective alleles.

In order to detect carriers of defective alleles, techniques for the detec-

TABLE 5-1

Some Known Inborn Errors of Metabolism

Disorders of carbohydrate metabolism
Diabetes mellitus
Pentosuria
Fructosuria
Glycogen deposition diseases
Galactosemia
Hyperbilirubinemia
Disorders of amino acid metabolism
Familial goiter
Phenylketonuria
Tyrosinosis
Alkaptonuria
Albinism
Maple syrup urine disease
Diseases of abnormal lipid metabolism
Infantile amaurotic family idiocy
Niemann-Pick disease
Gaucher's disease
Disease of steroid metabolism
Adrenogenital syndrome
Diseases of purine and pyrimidine metabolism
Gout
Xanthinuria
Diseases of metal metabolism
Wilson's disease
Hemochromatosis
Diseases in blood and blood-forming tissue
Hereditary sperocytosis
Hereditary methemoglobinemias
Blood-clotting factors

SOURCE: John B. Stanbury, James B. Wyngaarden, and Donald S. Fredrickson (eds.), The Metabolic Basis of Inherited Disease, McGraw-Hill Book Company, New York, 1960.

tion of the heterozygous state are needed. In a few morbid conditions *loading tests* have been successfully applied. An individual with but one allele capable of performing a biochemical reaction can function adequately under usual conditions, but if subject to unusual need for this particular enzyme, his inadequacy becomes measurable. For example, the heterozygote carrying the phenylketonuria allele will produce a urine with detectable amounts of phenylalanine when given a large dose of this amino acid. A few other such loading tests have been worked out. The method has proved useful only for the detection of a handful of heterozygous conditions (Stanbury, Wyngaarden, and Fredrickson, 1960).

New methods are urgently needed. Some progress is being made by electrophoretic studies of biochemical fluids. Cook (1955) discusses the future possibilities of some of the work.

THE FORMATION OF GAMETES

An essential part of the hereditary mechanism in sexually reproducing forms is the formation of gametes (meiosis), during which two important events take place. The first is crossing over. This is a cell division in which homologous autosomal chromosomes wind around each other in such a way that some of their chains of nucleotides pass from one chromosome to the other. At the end of this cell division, each maturing germinal cell has its full quota of DNA, but it may have a configuration of genes different from that in the chromosomes of the somatic cells of the individual in which they lie (Fig. 5-8).

The second event in the maturing of a gamete is the reduction division, in which the newly arranged chromosomes do not replicate themselves but form daughter cells with one-half the number of chromosomes of the somatic cells. The mature human gamete thus has 23 *single,* not paired, chromosomes, and each chromosome may have a configuration of genes different from that of the chromosomes in the body of the adult in whom they lie. At fertilization, the union of two gametes, each with 23 *single* chromosomes, produces a zygote with 23 *paired* chromosomes, the full quota of the human being.

THE X AND Y CHROMOSOMES

As stated above the female carries two X chromosomes; the male has a heteromorphic pair of chromosomes, one X and one Y. Thus XX individuals are female and XY male. The chain of events following fertilization and the genetic decision concerning sex which leads to the full differentiation into male and female is discussed on p. 199.

The large X chromosome has been shown to carry genes not present in the small Y chromosome—genes which apparently have actions other than those of sex determination (Childs, 1965). Thus the female with her two X chromosomes is diploid with respect to all loci on the X chromosome, while the male with but one X chromosome must always be haploid with respect to these loci. This fact confers a certain biologic advantage on the female. Should an X chromosome contain a mutated gene, the female has the protection of a normal allele on her second X chromosome—a protection denied the haploid male.

While the female is known to have a biologic superiority to the male as evidenced by lower mortality rates (p. 18), this superiority has been modified by the evolution of a mechanism which tends to render the XX female more or less equal to the XY state of the male. This mechanism, known at present as the *Lyon hypothesis*, postulates an inactivation of one of the two X chromosomes in the female. This inactivation takes place early in embryogenesis. The choice of which of the two X chromosomes is selected for inactivation is apparently a random one, but once the choice is made, all descendants of that cell carry the same active and the inactive X chromosome (Lyon, 1962). The inactivated X chromosome, which takes a deeper stain than the active one, is pushed to the periphery of the nucleus (Barr, 1964). This chromatin mass is called the *Barr body*, and its presence in somatic cells is evidence of the genetic sex of the individual.

Because of the random selection of one or the other X chromosome for inactivation, the female somatic cells are a mosaic, some containing one X, others containing the other X, as the genetically active chromosome. Thus

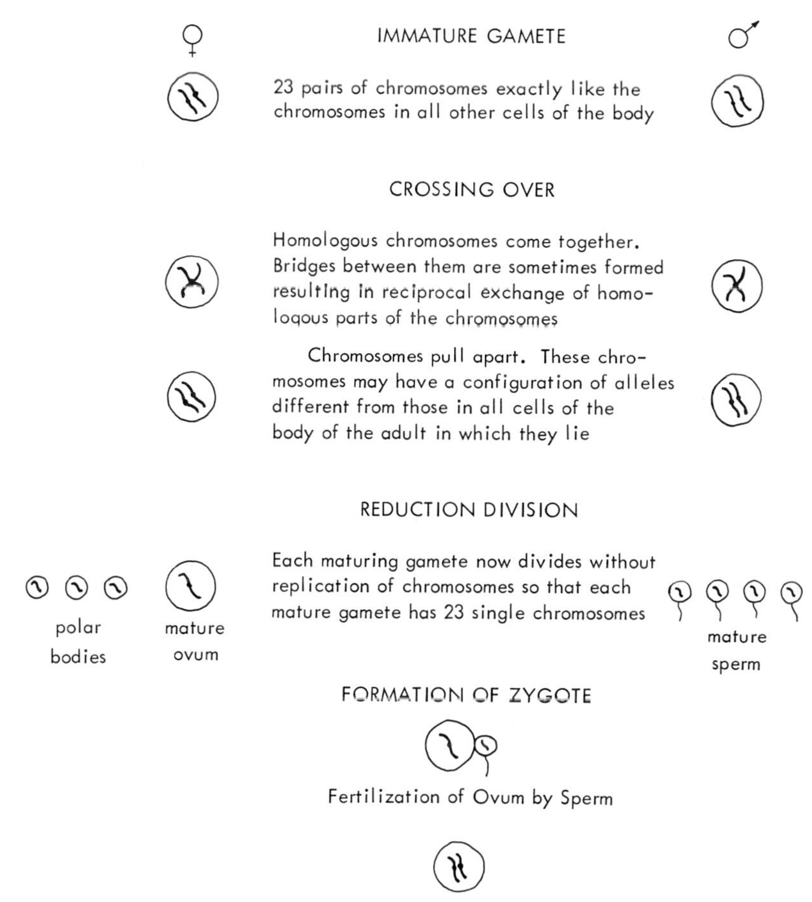

Fig. 5-8. Maturation of gametes and formation of zygote.

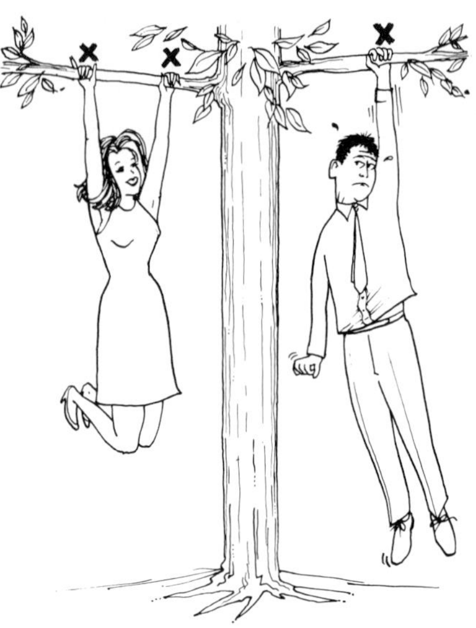

Fig. 5-9. The male's and the female's hold on life: Could it be that the female's two X chromosomes give her a firmer hold than the male's single X chromosome?

the female may show the phenotype of both alleles of a gene carried in the X chromosome. In the male, on the other hand, all somatic cells carry the same X chromosome, since the male is haploid for this chromosome.

Much recent work has been done on this theory of inactivation (reviewed by McKusick, 1962, and also by Davidson, 1964) and the consequences of the mosaic quality of the female somatic cells. It seems reasonable to assume that the female gains an advantage in biologic stamina by the possession of two X chromosomes even though some of the advantage is compensated for by mechanisms not completely understood at the present time.

A few human diseases known to be carried by defective genes on the X chromosome are:

Albinism of the eyes
Alopecia congenitalis
Anhidrotic ectodermal dysplasia
Colorblindness
Ichthyosis
Agammaglobulinemia
Hemophilia

CHROMOSOME ABERRATIONS

It appears that the episode of the reduction division in the maturation of either sperm or ovum is a hazardous moment. The mature gamete ends up with 23 chromosomes in the vast majority of cases, but rarely the phenomenon of nondysjunction takes place, whereby the separation of a pair of homologous chromosomes fails and both go into the same gamete. This leads to the production of some gametes with an extra chromosome and others with a missing chromosome. When such a gamete enters into the formation of a zygote, the resulting chromosomal pattern will contain 45 or 47 chromosomes instead of the normal 46. The presence or absence of one chromosome alters the genetic balance, and development is distorted.

Possible aberrations of the arrangement of the X and Y chromosomes are given in Table 5-2 (Rappoport and Kaplan, 1961). A zygote with the configuration XO develops into an individual with Turner's syndrome. At

TABLE 5-2

Possible Aberrations of X and Y Chromosomes

	Egg		Sperm	Zygote	Phenotype
a	X	a	X	XX	Normal female
	X		Y	XY	Normal male
b	No X	a	X	X	Turner's syndrome
	No X		Y	Y	Presumed lethal
	XX		X	XXX	Triple X
	XX		Y	XXY	Klinefelter's syndrome (chromatin positive)
a	X	c	XY	XXY	Klinefelter's syndrome (chromatin positive)
	X		Neither X nor Y	X	Turner's syndrome
a	X	d	XX	XXX	Triple X
	X		YY	XYY	Unknown
	X		Neither X nor Y	X	Turner's syndrome

a. Products of normal meiosis in male and female
b. Products of nondysjunction in female; meiosis 1 or 11
c. Products of nondysjunction in male meiosis 1
d. Products of nondysjunction in male meiosis 11

SOURCE: Rappoport and Kaplan, *Chromosomal Aberrations in Man, J. Pediat.*, **59**:415, 1961.

birth the infant looks like a female, but she never develops secondary sexual characteristics (Barr, 1959). If instead of XO the abnormality is YO, the zygote fails to develop. The complete absence of all X chromosome material is a lethal condition. The XXX configuration has been identified by Jacobs et al. (1959). This might be expected to produce the so-called "hyper-female"; however, individuals with this chromosomal pattern are mental defectives and nonfunctional females. The XXY configuration produces individuals with Klinefelter's syndrome. At birth such an individual appears to be male, but he fails to develop functional gonads and becomes a mental defective, as well. A few cases of Klinefelter's syndrome have been discovered with three or even four X chromosomes. The degree of mental deficiency seems to increase as the number of X chromosomes increases (Tjio, 1962).

Some aberrations of the autosomal chromosomes thought to be the result of nondysjunction have been identified in Table 5-3 (Rappoport and Kaplan, 1961). Down's syndrome (mongolism) has been identified with an extra chromosome 21 (Jacobs et al., 1959). Smith et al. have described six cases of multiple deformities associated with an extra chromosome, probably chromosome 18. Clinical syndromes have been described associated with trisomy of chromosomes 13 to 15 and 17 to 19 (Rappoport and Kaplan, 1961). No cases have so far been detected in which an autosomal chromosome is absent. Presumably such an error produces a nonviable zygote.

TABLE 5-3

Autosomal Aberrations and Clinical Syndromes

Number of chromosomes	Abnormality	Chromosome involved	Clinical findings
47	Trisomy	21	Mongolism (Down's syndrome)
46	Translocation	21–22	
		21 (13–15)	Mongolism (Down's syndrome)
45	Translocation	22 (13–15)	Mental retardation, dwarfism, multiple osseous malformations
47	Trisomy	13–15	Cerebral defect, anophthalmia, cleft palate and harelip, polydactyly and trigger thumbs, capillary hemangioma, heart defect
47	Trisomy	17	Dwarfism, webbed neck micrognathia, odd-shaped head with lowset ears, webbed fingers and toes, hypermobility of shoulders, shield chest, intraventricular defect
47	Trisomy	18	Retardation, micrognathia, lowset ears, finger deformities, intraventricular defect
47	Trisomy	22	Sturge-Weber syndrome
47	Enlarged Satellites	13–15 21	Marfan-like syndrome, nonspecific congenital anomalies

SOURCE: Rappoport and Kaplan, *Chromosomal Aberrations in Man, J. Pediat.*, **59**:415, 1961.

The Y chromosome is the only chromosome known which is not necessary for viability.

Nondysjunction appears to occur more frequently in gametes from older mothers. There is a positive correlation between advancing age in the mother and Down's syndrome, Klinefelter's syndrome, and some of the trisomies. For Turner's syndrome, on the other hand, maternal age is similar to that of controls. This suggests that nondysjunction may occur more frequently in oogenesis than in spermatogenesis (Rappoport and Kaplan, 1961).

Nondysjunction is not the only chromosomal aberration that can occur. A piece of one chromosome can break away and become attached to another chromosome, a phenomenon called *translocation* (Nowell and Hungerford, 1960; Baike et al., 1960). Chromosomes so altered are transmitted to subsequent generations. Translocation may account for some of the children with Down's syndrome born to young mothers in which this condition has been found familial (Polani, 1960).

In all the chromosomal variations discussed above, the vast majority of the cells of a given individual have the same chromosomal pattern. Tjio (1962) has reported individuals whose chromosomes were not all alike, a phenomenon he calls *mosaicism*. He found patients with Klinefelter's syndrome who possessed some cells with XXY configuration and others with XXXY. To account for this aberration, Tjio postulates an error similar to nondysjunction which takes place, not during gametogenesis, but in the zygote after fertilization. If the error occurs at the time of the division of the zygote, half the cells will contain 45 chromosomes and half 47 chromosomes. The same error at a subsequent division might produce a chromosome mosaic with 45, 46, and 47 chromosomes in various cells. The stage of development at which the error occurs determines the varying chromosomal patterns.

The discovery that chromosomal changes are associated with clinical syndromes is a milestone in the unraveling of many congenital abnormalities. Warkany et al. (1964) have published the results of the first 3 years of operation of the cytogenetic laboratory in Cincinnati.

GENETIC COUNSELING

When a defect, thought to be hereditary, occurs in a family, prospective parents are often anxious to find out what is the likelihood that a child of theirs will show the defect. This question is sometimes asked by a young couple before they have had any children; it is more frequently asked after one abnormal child has been born.

A true genetic defect must be distinguished from environmental maldevelopment. A cataract of genetic origin may appear indistinguishable from a cataract that is the result of a developmental accident induced by German measles during the first trimester of pregnancy.

A dominant gene, with complete pentration, produces its effect in every individual carrying it. One-half of the children of a carrier of such a gene will demonstrate the condition. Such conditions are extremely rare. Huntington's chorea and retinoblastoma are examples.

The great majority of harmful genes are recessive and thus only make themselves manifest in the homozygous state. The number of heterozygous carriers of a specific harmful allele varies with the frequency of the disease in the population. Study of the genealogy of families in which serious genetic disease has occurred can sometimes offer a statistical probability of the occurrence of the disease in a given mating.

Rates of recurrence are statistical averages occurring in families in which a case of the disease has occurred. Many diseases are partly genetic and partly environmental, but the influence of these two aspects is apt to differ in different families; therefore an average figure of risk may be quite inaccurate with respect to the actual risk for the family under consideration.

Fraser has calculated the risk figures for a few common pediatric diseases by culling the literature for reported series and combining them with those from his own clinic. Risk figures for hereditary diseases have not been compiled in any one source, but even if they were, the data are so tentative and so subject to change that published material would become out of date almost before publication.

In a specific case it would be wise to refer a couple to one of the specialists in the field of genetics and let him study the family background and make a prediction based, as far as possible, on their genetic makeup and the current knowledge of the defect under consideration. Reed has listed the clinics in this country and Canada in which competent genetic advice can be given (Table 5-4).

The role of the genetic counselor is to give the couple the facts from which they make their own decisions, but in addition he can sometimes help them to accept their own genetic makeup without shame or guilt. All people carry some defective genes, and it is only an accident of fate that both partners in a marriage happen to carry the same defective gene.

TABLE 5-4

Genetic Counselors

Location	Institution	Counselor
Berkeley, Calif.	University of California	Dr. Curt Stern
Los Angeles, Calif.	Los Angeles Medical Center	Dr. Stanley Wright
Seattle, Wash.	Department of Medicine, University of Washington	Dr. Arno Motulsky
Edmonton, Alberta	Heredity Counseling Service, University of Alberta	Dr. Margaret W. Thompson
Tempe, Ariz.	Arizona State University	Dr. C. M. Woolf
Austin, Texas	The Genetics Foundation, University of Texas	Dr. C. P. Oliver
Norman, Okla.	Dept. of Zoological Sciences, University of Oklahoma	Dr. P. R. David
Winnipeg, Manitoba	Hospital for Sick Children	Dr. Irene Uchida
Minneapolis, Minn.	University of Minnesota	Dr. S. C. Reed
Minneapolis, Minn.	Human Genetics Unit, State Board of Health	Dr. L. E. Schacht
Rochester, Minn.	Mayo Clinic	Dr. J. S. Pearson
New Orleans, La.	Genetic Counseling Service, Tulane University	Dr. H. W. Kloepfer
Madison, Wisc.	Dept. of Medical Genetics, University of Wisconsin	Dr. J. F. Crow
Chicago, Ill.	Children's Memorial Hospital	Dr. David Y-Y. Hsia
Ann Arbor, Mich.	The Heredity Clinic, University of Michigan	Dr. J. V. Neel
East Lansing, Mich.	Dept. of Zoology, Michigan State University	Dr. J. V. Higgins
Cleveland, Ohio	Department of Biology, Western Reserve University	Dr. A. G. Steinberg
Winston-Salem, N.C.	Bowman Gray School of Medicine	Dr. C. N. Herndon
Toronto, Canada	Hospital for Sick Children	Dr. N. F. Walker
Charlottesville, Va.	School of Medicine, University of Virginia	Dr. R. F. Shaw
Washington, D.C.	Genetics Counseling Research Center, George Washington University Hospital	Dr. N. C. Myrianthopoulos
Baltimore, Md.	Johns Hopkins Hospital	Dr. V. A. McKusick
New York, N.Y.	Albert Einstein College of Medicine, Yeshiva University	Dr. S. G. Waelsch
New York, N.Y.	New York State Psychiatric Institute	Dr. F. J. Kallman
New York, N.Y.	Rockefeller Institute	Dr. A. G. Bearn
Montreal, Quebec	Children's Memorial Hospital	Dr. F. C. Fraser
Providence, R.I.	Department of Biology, Brown University	Dr. G. W. Hagy
Boston, Mass.	Dept. of Immunochemistry, Boston University Medical School	Dr. W. C. Boyd

SOURCE. Sheldon C. Reed, Counseling in Medical Genetics, 2d ed., W. B. Saunders Company, Philadelphia, 1963.

SUMMARY AND IMPLICATIONS

Each individual is a unique experiment of nature. The moment of fertilization is crucial for subsequent development.

The objective of euthenic care is the nurturing of the given potential to the best interest of the individual. It includes fostering the development of some potential and circumventing the development of potential which is deleterious.

In nurturing potential one must be ever alert to an appreciation of what the potential really is. A child ultimately *must* accept himself as his genes decree. He can often be helped to reach his own heights, but he cannot be pushed beyond his inherent capacity. If he is destined to be deviant—bigger, smaller, brighter, stupider than the mean—the earlier in life he can be helped to accept himself as he is, the greater is the chance that his development will not be hampered by his degree of deviation. No dietary regime will get a small, slender boy on the football team; no educational plan will make a Ph.D. out of a child with an IQ of 100. The child who is pushed in any area beyond his capacities grows up with a sense of failure that may hamper him in the achievement of otherwise possible goals.

Circumventing deleterious potential consists, first, in detecting it before irreversible changes have taken place. An important step in detecting a pathologic condition is being alert to the possibility that it might exist. In the consideration of inherited diseases a carefully taken family history of the patient (or of the prospective infant) can sometimes bring to light genetic material that might carry deleterious genes. The cause of death of forebears, the occurrence and reasons for deaths in childhood, the presence of consanguineous marriages are all significant data (Morton et al., 1956).

The initial appraisal of the newborn needs to be complete and thorough. Routine blood and urine tests (p. 535) should be done during the first days of life and repeated at intervals. Microscopic study of chromosomes is helpful in some cases.

Unfortunately there are still many hereditary ailments for which there are, at the present time, neither tests for early detection nor means of circumventing the action of an abnormal genetic code.

One of the objectives of medical care is the preservation of the life of the individual and the making of that life as rewarding as possible. Innumerable disciplines have contributed to this goal; the low mortality rate in the United States today is indicative of the success of these efforts. The science of genetics has aided this total effort by providing means of distinguishing in early life some of those individuals whose genetic errors are amenable to therapy.

Muller (1950) has estimated that it takes a mortality of 20 per cent prior to the age of reproduction to maintain the human population with its current average of eight defective genes per person. Prior to the last century far more than 20 per cent of children born failed to survive, but in the United States at present, 95 per cent of infants born alive reach 25 years of age.

Deaths of infants in past centuries and in underdeveloped areas of the world today are not necessarily selective in the genetic sense. Children die from infections, from malnutrition, from injuries that may attack, indiscriminately, the genetically strong and the genetically weak. While infant mortality rates have, over the centuries, been so high that they have probably kept the proportion of defective genes at a relatively low level, civilized man will no longer tolerate this extravagant waste of human life.

Reduction of mortality permits survival of some individuals with defective genetic material. Insofar as such people live to reproduce, the human genetic pool is slowly accumulating an increased number of defective genes. Cook has emphasized the need for careful consideration of what is happening to the genetic pool of the race.

Further work in genetics and in biochemistry may before too long provide tools with which individuals harboring serious genetic mistakes may be identified. Mating between two people each carrying the same defective allele might then be discouraged.

It is to be fervently hoped that the human race will voluntarily accept a technique of *birth selection* which offers infinitely greater humanitarianism than the *death selection* by means of which the law of natural selection has operated. By voluntary controls it might be possible to keep mutated genes down to a level no higher than the spontaneous mutation rate.

BIBLIOGRAPHY

AUERBACH, CHARLOTTE: "The Science of Genetics," Harper & Row, Publishers, Incorporated, New York, 1961.

BAIKE, A. G., W. N. COURT-BROWN, E. BUCKTON, D. E. HARNDEN, P. A. JACOBS, and I. M. TOUGH: A Possible Specific Chromosome Abnormality in Human Chronic Myeloid Leukemia, *Nature*, **188**:1165, 1960.

BARR, MURRAY L.: Sex Chromatin and Phenotypes in Man, *Science*, **130**:679, 1959.

———: Some Properties of the Sex Chromosomes and Their Bearing on Normal and Abnormal Development, *Proceedings of the 2nd International Conference on Congenital Malformations*, The International Medical Congress, 1964, p. 11.

BEADLE, GEORGE W.: Genes and Chemical Reactions in Neurospora, *Science*, **129**:1715, 1959.

———: The Physical and Chemical Base of Inheritance, Condon Lecture, Oregon State System of Higher Education, Eugene, Oregon, 1957.

BOYD, WILLIAM C.: "Genetics and the Races of Man," Little, Brown and Company, Boston, 1950.

CHILDS, BARTON, and JAMES B. SIDBURY: A Survey of Genetics As It Applies to Problems in Medicine, *Pediatrics*, **20**:177 (suppl.), 1957.

———: Genetic Origin of Some Sex Differences among Human Beings, *Pediatrics,* **35**:798, 1965.

COOK, ROBERT C.: Detection of Carriers of Recessive Genes, *J. Hered.,* **46**:161, 1955.

———: Changing Patterns of Selection, *Acta genet. statist. med.,* **6**:349, 1956–1957.

———: Lethal Genes, A Factor in Fertility, *Eugenical News,* **38**:49, 153.

CROW, JAMES F.: Possible Consequences of an Increased Mutation Rate, *Eugenics Quart.,* **4**:67, 1957.

DAVIDSON, R. C.: The Lyon Hypothesis, *J. Pediat.,* **65**:765, 1964.

DOBZHANSKY, THEODOSIUS: "Evolution, Genetics and Man," John Wiley & Sons, Inc., New York, 1955.

FORD, C. E., P. A. JACOBS, and L. G. LAITHA: Human Somatic Chromosomes, *Nature,* **181**:1565, 1958.

FRASER, F. CLARK: Genetic Counseling in Some Common Pediatric Diseases, *Pediat. Clin. North America,* **475**, May, 1958.

GARROD, ARCHIBALD E.: Inborn Errors of Metabolism, Lecture 1, *Lancet,* **2**:1, 1908; Lecture 2, *Lancet,* **2**:73, 1908; Lecture 3, *Lancet,* **2**:42, 1908; Lecture 4, *Lancet,* **2**:214, 1908.

HALDANE, J. B. S.: "New Paths in Genetics," George Allen & Unwin, Ltd., London, 1941.

———: "Causes of Evolution," Longmans, Green & Co., Ltd., London, 1932.

HARDIN, GARRETT: "Nature and Man's Fate," Rinehart & Company, Inc., New York, 1959.

HSIA, DAVID Y.: "Inborn Errors in Metabolism," The Yearbook Medical Publishers, Inc., Chicago, 1959.

HSU, T. C.: Mammalian Chromosomes in Vitro, *J. Hered.,* **45**:167, 1952.

JACOBS, P. A., A. G. BAIKIE, W. M. COURT-BROWN, T. N. MACGREGOR, N. MACLEAN, and D. G. HORNDEN: Evidence of the Existence of the Human "Super Female," *Lancet,* **2**:2423, 1959.

———, ———, ———, and J. A. STRONG: The Somatic Chromosomes in Mongolism, *Lancet,* **1**:710, 1959.

KALLMAN, FRANZ J.: Psychiatric Aspects of Genetics Counseling, *Am. J. Human Genet.,* **8**:97, 1956.

LYON, M. F.: Sex Chromatin and Gene Action in the Mammalian X Chromosome, *Am. J. Human Genet.,* **14**:135, 1962.

LYSENKO, TROFIN, quoted in Ashley Montagu, "Human Heredity," Mentor Books, The New American Library of World Literature, Inc., New York, 1960.

MCKUSICK, VICTOR A.: "Heritable Disorders of Connective Tissue," The C. V. Mosby Company, St. Louis, 1960.

———: On the X Chromosome of Man, *Quart. Rev. Biol.,* **37**:69, 1962.

MCLEISH, JOHN, and BRIAN SNOAD: "Looking at Chromosomes," St. Martin's Press, Inc., New York, 1958.

MENDEL, GREGOR: "Experiments in Plant Hybridization," translation by Royal Horticultural Society of London, Harvard University Press, Cambridge, Mass., 1948.

MONTAGU, ASHLEY: "Human Heredity," Mentor Books, The New American Library of World Literature, Inc., New York, 1960.

Morton, Newton E., James F. Crow, and H. J. Muller: An Estimate of the Mutational Damage in Man from Data on Consanguineous Marriages, *Proc. Nat. Acad. Sc.*, **42**:855, 1956.

Muller, H. J.: Our Load of Mutations, *Am. J. Human Genet.* **2**:111, 1950.

———: The Production of Mutations, *J. Hered.*, **38**:259, 1947.

Neel, James V., and William Schull: "Human Heredity," The University of Chicago Press, Chicago, 1954.

Nowell, Peter C., and David A. Hungerford: A Minute Chromosome in Human Chronic Granulocytic Leukemia, *Science*, **132**:1497, 1960.

Penrose, L. S.: Maternal Age, Order of Birth and Developmental Abnormalities, *J. Ment. Sc.*, **85**:1141, 1939.

———: "Recent Advances in Human Genetics," J. A. Churchill Ltd., London, 1958.

Polani, P. E., J. H. Briggs, C. E. Ford, C. M. Clarke, and J. M. Berg: A Mongol Girl with 46 Chromosomes, *Lancet*, **1**:721, 1960.

Rappoport, Stanley, and W. D. Kaplan: Chromosomal Aberration in Man, *J. Pediat.*, **59**:415, 1961.

Reed, Sheldon C.: "Counseling in Medical Genetics," 2d ed., W. B. Saunders Company, Philadelphia, 1963.

Russell, W. L., and L. B. Russell: Radiation Hazards to the Embryo and Fetus, *Radiology*, **58**:369, 1952.

Schubert, Jack, and Ralph E. Lapp: "Radiation—What It is and How It Affects You," Viking Press, New York, 1957.

Shettles, L. B.: Nuclear Morphology of Human Spermatozoa, *Nature*, **186**:648, London, 1960.

Singleton, W. Ralph: "Elementary Genetics," D. Van Nostrand Company, Inc., Princeton, N.J., 1962.

Smith, David W., Klaus Patau, Beva Therman, and Stanley L. Inhorn: A New Autosomomal Trisomy Syndrome: Multiple Congenital Anomalies Caused by an Extra Chromosome, *J. Pediat.*, **57**:338, 1960.

Srb, Adrian M., and Ray D. Owen: "General Genetics," W. H. Freeman and Company, San Francisco, 1952.

Stanbury, John B., James B. Wyngaarden, and Donald S. Fredrickson (eds): "Metabolic Basis of Inherited Disease," McGraw-Hill Book Company, New York, 1960.

Stern, Curt: "Principles of Human Genetics," 2d ed., W. H. Freeman and Company, San Francisco, 1960.

Sutton, H. E.: Human Heredity and Its Biochemical Basis, in John B. Stanbury, James B. Wyngaarden, and Donald S. Fredrickson (eds.), "The Metabolic Basis of Inherited Disease," McGraw-Hill Book Company, New York, 1960.

Tjio, Joe Hin, and Albert Levan: The Chromosome Number of Man, *Heredita*, **42**:1, 1956.

———: Congenital Disorders of Chromosomes, Scientific Meeting on Mental Retardation, Washington, D.C., Dec. 6, 1962.

———, and T. T. Puck: Somatic Chromosomes of Man, *Proc. Nat. Acad. Sc.*, **44**:1229, 1958.

Wagner, R. P., and H. K. Mitchell: "Genetics and Metabolism," John Wiley & Sons, Inc., New York, 1955.

Warkany, Josef E., David Weinstien, Shirley W. Soukup, Jack D. Rubin-

STEIN, and M. C. CURLESS: Chromosome Analyses in a Children's Hospital, *Pediatrics,* **33**:290, 1964, and **33**:454, 1964.

WASHBURN, T. C., D. N. MEDEASIS, and BARTON CHILDS: Sex Differences in Susceptibility to Infection, *Pediatrics,* **35**:57, 1965.

WATSON, J. D., and F. H. C. CRICK: Molecular Structure of Nucleic Acids, A Structure of Deoxyribose Nucleic Acid, *Nature,* **171**:737, 1953.

WILKINS, LAWSON: Embryonic Sex Differentiation, Controlling Factors and Abnormalities, Diagnosis and Treatment, *Clin. Proc. Child. Hosp.,* **20**:1, 1964.

———, and HOWARD W. JONES, JR.: Masculinization of the Female Fetus, *Obstet. Gynecol.,* **11**:355, 1958.

———, M. M.. GRUMBACH, and J. J. VAN WYK: Chromosomal Sex in Ovarian Agenesis, *J. Clin. Endocrinol.,* **14**:1270, 1954.

WILLIAMS, ROGER J.: "Biochemical Individuality," John Wiley & Sons, Inc., New York, 1956.

6

Before Birth

Once again the zygote is the starting point for discussion. In the last chapter the glance was backward to see how the zygote came to be what it was. In this chapter, the glance is forward to see how the zygote becomes a baby.

NORMAL DEVELOPMENT WITHIN THE UTERUS

The time from conception to birth can be thought of in several phases: first cellular multiplication, then chemical differentiation, then tissue and organ formation, and finally organization and practice of function.

Cell Multiplication

The single-cell zygote is composed of a nucleus embedded in cytoplasm. In the nucleus are the chromosomes and all their multitude of genes which are about to initiate and direct the drama of life. What sort of human being will develop depends not only upon the start given by the genes but also upon the total environment.

The zygote begins to divide soon after conception. The nucleus elongates, the 46 chromosomes line up and split themselves into two parts, the cell membrane pinches together, and two cells exist where but one existed a moment before. In each cell is a full quota of all the genes present in the original cell. Each new cell repeats the process. Several hours elapse between each stage of cleavage. The early stages take place while the recently fertilized egg is drifting down the fallopian tube on its way to the uterus. This is a journey of 4 to 5 in. and takes about as many days. Once in the uterus, the egg floats freely for a few days and then becomes embedded in the wall of the uterus. At the time of the implantation of the embryo, the fetal membranes begin their formation. The first to appear is the amnion, which surrounds the primitive embryo and attaches it, through the body stalk, to the chorion. It is through the chorion that the embryo will ultimately receive maternal nutrients.

Differentiation

Simultaneously with the appearance of the fetal membranes tremendous changes take place within the embryo. The once homogeneous mass of cells begins to differentiate. The mass becomes a hollow sphere; a flattened group of cells, the embryonic disk, forms at one side. The inner layer of cells of this disk, the endoderm, spreads out and lines the inner margin of the sphere forming the primary yolk sac. At the opposite side of the embryonic disk another layer of cells, the ectoderm, envelops the embryo on the outside. A third group of cells, the mesoderm, pushes in between the ectoderm and the endoderm (Patten, 1953; Hamilton, Boyd, and Mossman, 1947).

Thus by the time the embryo is 2 weeks old, it has attached itself to the uterine wall, developed protective and nutrient membranes, and organized the three fundamental germinal layers.

How and why all this takes place is one of the many mysteries. As far as can be detected the cells formed in the early cleavage stages are exactly like the zygote from which they came. The assumption is made that each cell acts on all the others and in some way alters the environment sufficiently so that interaction of genes and cytoplasm produces cells with qualities that vary from the parent cell.

Wilson (1959) has suggested a schematic representation of the events taking place in the maturing embryo (Fig. 6-1). Beginning with the genes in the zygote, RNA is formed (p. 41) which seeps into the cytoplasm, where it directs the synthesis of enzymes. These enzymes act upon each other, creating a chemical differentiation within the cytoplasm of the newly created cells. From these cells (now distinct from each other chemically) cellular differentiation becomes apparent, and ultimately morphologically distinct cells form themselves into aggregates. Wilson sees the entire process as an increasingly elaborate set of chemical reactions all of which originate from the genes in the zygote.

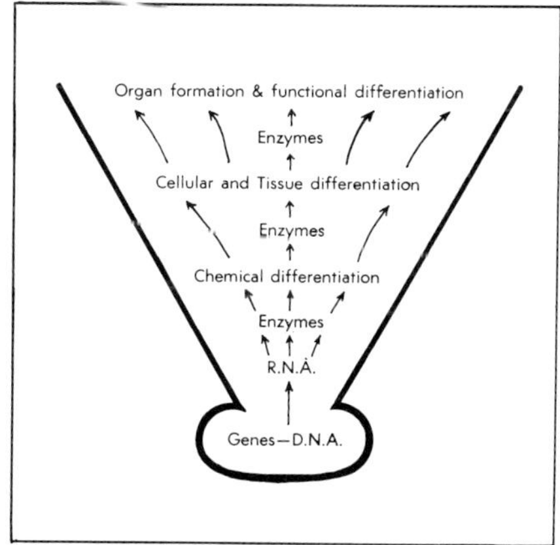

Fig. 6-1. The growing embryo. (*From Wilson, Experimental Studies on Congenital Malformations, J. Chronic Dis., 10:111, 1959.*)

The original division into the three germinal layers foreshadows future development. From the endoderm there will develop the gastrointestinal tract and its appendages, and most of the respiratory apparatus. From the mesoderm will develop the epithelium of the gonads and their ducts, the kidneys and their ducts, the cortex of the adrenal gland, and the lining of the abdominal cavities. The mesenchyme is a diffusely cellular substance derived from the mesoderm, which differentiates into all the connective, vascular, skeletal, muscular, and hematopoietic tissues. From the ectoderm the brain, nervous tissue, sense organs, and skin and its appendages will develop.

This original division into the three germinal layers is not equal and undoubtedly varies from embryo to embryo, depending probably partly upon the genetic code and partly on the intrauterine conditions. Slight differences—a few cells more or less thrown into one germinal layer or the other—may make vast differences in the ultimate man. It is possible to speculate that a little more endoderm may mean a greater proportion of the body substance destined to be part of the gastrointestinal system. This may mean the formation of an endomorphic body type with its long intestinal tract and its biologic orientation toward alimentation. In the same way a few cells directed toward the mesoderm may from this early embryonic age predispose toward the development of the muscular, skeletal child and adult. Or if the slight edge is given to the ectoderm, from this age on the structure will develop in the path of the linear adult with large surface area and dominant nervous system. The type of body constitution does not spring full-blown at birth; the structures have possibly been headed in the direction of their particular character since the early separation of the germinal layers.

Emergence of Organ Systems

The tiny already differentiated embryo now between 2 and 3 weeks old is only ⅕ in. long and is supplied with nutrients through its already formed fetal membranes. Up to this time it has been completely parasitic, but now it is ready to take its first step in establishing its own independence. The initiation of the drive for self-sufficiency is shown in the manner by which the embryo obtains the raw material needed for further development. The maternal circulation does not flow through the embryo; the mother's blood comes up to the placenta, spreads out into the basic units of the placenta—the villi which consist of tiny projecting spikes of chorion each bathed in maternal blood. Here, as it were, the maternal organism offers itself to the embryo. To use this proffered nutriment the embryo must build blood channels of its own and a heart with which to pump the needed material to its own growing structure. When the embryo is 3 weeks of age the heart makes its appearance, and within a week it has started its lifelong rhythmic contractions. Simultaneously vascular channels appear in the yolk sac, and tiny capillaries penetrate into the center of each spike-like villus of the chorion, where they make osmotic contact with the mother's capillaries on the maternal side of the villus. Blood cells appear in the embryonic vascular channels, and by the fourth week a primitive circulation is in operation within the embryo.

Once the circulation is established, creation of new cells and differentiation of these cells, slowed while arrangements for adequate nutrition were being established, proceeds at a rapid pace. The ground plan of the new individual can now be distinguished. There is a longitudinal axis, a right and left side, a head and tail differentiation. The ectoderm forms a long cylindrical tube from which the brain and spinal cord develop. The endoderm shapes itself into another tubelike structure with a wide-open area communicating with the yolk sac. From this tube the gastrointestinal tract and all its glands emerge. From the same tube, buds of rapidly growing tissues form the respiratory apparatus. Between these two tubes paired streaks of mesoderm are beginning to develop into muscles. By the end of the second month of uterine life the organism has graduated from embryo to fetus. The fetal heart is beating at a regular rhythm; the fetal circulation is pushing its own blood cells through the main blood vessels. The deep skeletal muscles are present, and muscles to the extremities are pushing their way to the rapidly forming arms and legs, hands and feet. Viscera are formed and are beginning to function; the diaphragm is in place; face, tongue, mouth, eyes, and ears are in the process of organization. The fetus at this stage is hardly more than 1 in. in length, and yet, tiny as he is, he is capable of considerable independent activity. He has been pumping his own blood for almost a month; the skeletal muscles can contract and rotate the rump; the extremities twitch spasmodically.

During the third month the fetus trebles his 2-month size and reaches about 3 in. in length. Refinements in the already present structures have taken place. The neuromuscular system is developing rapidly, and as new connections between neurons and muscle fibers develop, the fetus acquires new capability for action which he immediately puts to use.

During the first 3 months after conception, the basic structure of the new human being is formed. This is a time of rapid creation of new material. Development is not equally rapid in all areas at the same time; first one area, then another is in the forefront of creation.

The oldest parts of the organism phylogenetically, the most vital organs for maintaining life, are formed first; the refinements of human structure, late to appear on the evolutionary scale, make their appearance late in fetal life. Some of the human refinements do not develop until well after the infant has left the uterus.

Practice of Function

By the fifth month the fetus is large enough and his muscular strength and activity are strong enough so that the mother is able to feel him move. At first these movements are but slight flutterings, but they gradually increase until the end of pregnancy. Doubtless the fetus has much individuality by this time if he could be seen.

Feeding patterns are beginning to emerge. The mouth opens and closes, the lips protrude; the fetus is beginning to get his mouth ready for the all important sucking. Movements of the facial muscles are practiced by midfetal life.

By the beginning of the sixth month, the fetus has reached about 1 lb in weight and 1 ft in length and is a presentable picture of what he will soon become. Should he be born prematurely now, he might make an effort to keep himself going. His chances of staying alive, however, are not too good, because of the immaturity of his respiratory apparatus.

From the sixth to the ninth months final refinements of structure and function will be added which will make survival almost automatic. The respiratory tract will complete its intricate development of the myriad muscles required to open and close the alveoli, and each will be supplied with its neural connections and its association fibers which make the whole structure sensitive to the ever-changing oxygen needs of all the tissues. The nostrils reopen, the eyelids become unsealed, the anus becomes perforate. The skin becomes cornified, a layer of adipose tissue is laid down under the skin, more adipose tissue surrounds and cushions the internal organs. Special fat pads form in the cheeks which aid the sucking mechanism.

The fetus is now ready for birth.

THE PLACENTA

Nourishment and protection of the fetus takes place by means of the placenta. The placenta is a metabolically active organ which does far more than act as a sieve. It functions for the fetus as a lung, alimentary tract, excretory organ, and endocrine gland (Avery, 1964). It also has barrier qualities.

Some substances pass through the placenta by simple diffusion (oxygen, carbon dioxide, water, urea). Other substances produced in the body of the normal pregnant woman (thyroxin, cholesterol, bilirubin, insulin, progesterone, estrogen) pass the placenta in such a way that the concentration in the infant's blood is always less than that in the mother's. Thyroxin (Schultz et al., 1965) and insulin (Gitlin, Kumate, and Morales, 1965) and certain other hormones (Wilkins et al., 1958) are manufactured in the fetal organism.

Still other substances are actively transported across the placenta and appear in the fetal blood in higher concentration than in maternal blood. These substances are in general the essential nutrients for fetal tissue—amino acids, glucose, glycerol, fatty acids, vitamins, minerals.

Finally the placenta acts as a barrier and holds back from the fetus most proteins, including thyroid-stimulating hormone and growth hormone, nucleic acids, neutral fats, and many bacteria and viruses. The barrier action of the placenta is more efficient against the normal products of the mother's metabolism than it is against bacteria and viruses or their products or against drugs administered to the pregnant woman. (Nyhan, 1961; Willner, 1965; Baker, 1960).

ABERRATIONS OF DEVELOPMENT

Congenital malformations have been with man since the dawn of history. Warkany (1959) has described the history of the study of this fascinating subject and detailed some of the incredible folklore surrounding the birth of an abnormal child.

Incidence

The number of infants with developmental defects has been variously estimated. Considering only major malformations detected during the neonatal period or observed anatomically in stillborn infants, Lamy and Frézal (1961) estimated that the incidence was from 1 to 1.5 per cent. McIntosh and his coworkers (1954) found an appreciably higher incidence. They detected major anomalies in 3.6 per cent of newborns during the neonatal period and in 7.5 per cent of these same children when reevaluated 5 years later.

Marden and Smith (1964) found an incidence of 14.7 per cent of minor anomalies among 4,412 newborns. These investigators discovered that a single minor anomaly had little significance but that the presence of two or more such defects was found frequently in infants with major

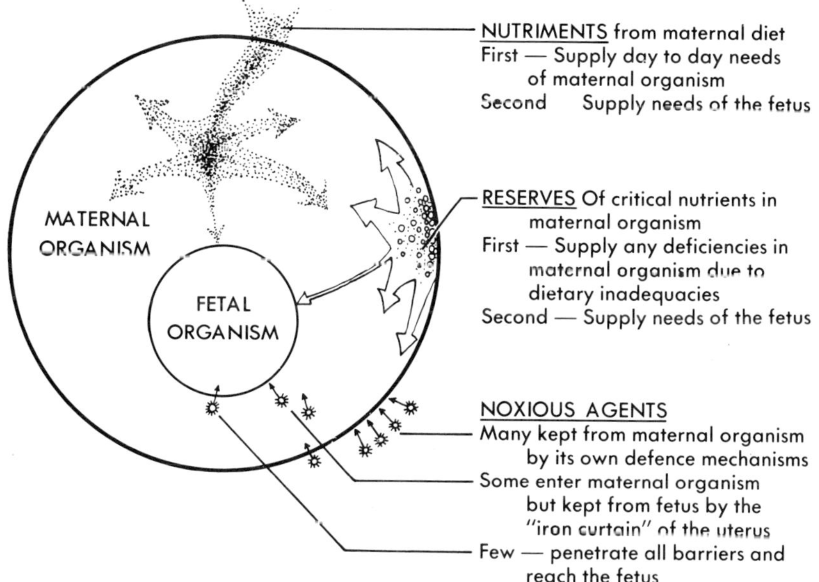

Fig. 6-2. Nutrition and protection of the fetus.

anomalies. They suggest that multiple minor defects are an alerting sign of possible serious embryonic defect.

Aberrations of development can come about either from faulty genes (see Chap. 5) or from faulty intrauterine environment. Sometimes both factors are involved. Fraser (1959) has estimated that less than 10 per cent of all malformations have a clear-cut genetic basis.

Critical Stages in Development

While there are many different hazards to which the developing organism may be subjected, the time when an adverse condition occurs determines to a great extent the amount and kind of damage suffered. Stockard found that different disturbances applied at the same stage of development would produce the same effect and that the same disturbing factor introduced at another phase would produce a different effect.

If the environment is unsuitable before chemical differentiation (Fig. 6-1) has taken place, the growth of all cells is slowed. At this early phase all cells are so similar that an injurious agent has a total overall effect. If the injury is sufficiently grave, the cells die, but if the injury is less severe, the recuperative powers of the embryo restore the slowed-down cells, and development proceeds. The organism injured at this early stage may show abnormalities of great degree and variety, including double monsters.

Later in development, after differentiation has taken place and the fetal membranes have formed, a noxious agent does the most damage to those cells which are growing fastest. The time when a structure is forming, the time when creation is at a maximum, is a crucial moment for that structure. During the brief moment given it for creation each organ in turn must grab its opportunity and fashion itself as best it can. Organ formation takes place during early embryonic life, so it is then that environmental hazards cause more damage than later.

The Qualities of the Embryo

In addition to the specific noxious agents and the time they exert their influence, the embryo itself is a factor in the amount of damage done. It is possible that the genetic code in some embryos is stronger than in others and more able to withstand environmental hazards. At all events only a portion of embryos show failures in development when all are subjected to apparently the same experimental noxious agent (Fraser, 1959).

Some failures in development may have their origin in the quality of the ovum or sperm from which the zygote developed. Willis (1958) suggests that overripeness of the ovum due to delayed fertilization may be a non-genetic cause of developmental failure or that other defects in ova may be due to maternal health, nutrition, or hormone state. It is also possible that conditions known to produce sterility in the male may occasionally result, not in complete sterility, but in less viable sperm. The age of the mother is known to be correlated with certain genetic defects in the ovum, but there is little evidence at the present time that maternal age is related to nongenetic loss of viability.

ENVIRONMENT OF THE DEVELOPING ORGANISM

The environment is the mother's genital tract, the fallopian tube for the zygote, and the uterus, over which the placenta stands guard, for the embryo and the fetus. While the developing organism is well protected, he is not completely immune to the events of the mother's life. He can be affected by her age, by her general state of health and nutrition, by certain drugs she may take, by some diseases she may contract, by physical agents impinging upon her, by her emotional state, and possibly by other factors as well. He is not affected directly by any acts of will on the mother's part. The woman cannot decide how the development of her unborn child will proceed. She can, however, cooperate or fail to cooperate in maintaining her own health, nutrition, and emotional composure.

ADEQUACY OF INTRAUTERINE CONDITIONS

The adequacy of the environment provided by the mother has two aspects: a positive one, whereby she provides needs, and a negative one, whereby she protects against harm.

Maternal competence in supplying needs, which are the raw materials out of which structure is built, depends upon (1) the availability at the right moment of each needed substance within the mother's body and (2) the ability of these substances to cross the placenta. Maternal protection depends upon (1) freedom of the mother's body from noxious agents and (2) imperviousness of the placenta to any such agents that happen to be present in her body.

The Supply of Raw Materials

The maternal organism, like most organisms, often has a supply of critical substances which can be drawn upon in case their day-to-day intake is not adequate. These maternal reserves, however, are not always immediately available for placental transport. In general, raw materials for development of the embryo come from the mother's diet and not from her bodily reserves. Thus, temporary deficiencies in the mother's diet which cause no manifest symptoms in her may cause devastating inadequacies within the uterus. In experimental dietary deficiencies the pregnant animal almost always fared better than the embryo (Warkany, 1942 and 1944; Burke et al., 1943). These findings refute the time-honored belief that the embryo draws on the mother's body even to her detriment. It appears that the embryo is not as favored a parasite as legend would have us believe.

The effect of maternal diet on the well-being of the offspring has been extensively studied in both animals and man. Warkany (1942 and 1944) has shown that specific maternal dietary deficiencies caused skeletal defects in rats. Vitamin A, various components of the B complex, vitamin D, and vitamin E have all been correlated with specific abnormalities in animals. Folic acid deficiency was particularly disastrous, causing aberrations in almost every organ and system in the body, varying of course with the stage of differentiation of the embryo when the deficiency was acute (Thiersch, 1952).

Inadequate dietaries in man are associated with greater than normal fetal loss and a generally higher incidence of congenital abnormalities. Burke's study at Harvard (1943) and Murphy's study in Philadelphia (1947) showed a high correlation between inadequate maternal diets and the incidence of stillbirth, neonatal death, and congenital malformations in the offspring. Specific nutritional requirements during pregnancy are discussed in Chapter 26.

Protection from Deleterious Agents

The placenta holds back most normal products of metabolism which are deleterious to the fetus. The substances the placenta is unable to restrain are some bacteria and viruses or their soluble toxins, some antibodies, and many drugs.

Maternal Infectious Disease

The surprising finding concerning infection in a pregnant woman is that the *severity* of the illness in the mother is not the factor most closely correlated with damage to the embryo or the fetus. Some disease conditions which are trivial and inconsequential in the mother can be disastrous for the developing embryo; other conditions which produce profound illness in the mother appear to do little damage within the uterus (Desmond, 1961).

German measles (rubella) was first suspected of being tetragenic by Gregg in Australia in 1941. A carefully controlled prospective study of the relation of rubella and fetal hazards was reported in 1960 by Manson, Logan, and Loy. They found that 15 per cent of infants born to mothers who contracted rubella prior to the twelfth week of gestation had major malformations at birth, as contrasted with 2.8 per cent of infants born to mothers who did not have the infection. After the twelfth week there was little difference between the control and the rubella groups. There was also a higher incidence of abortion and stillbirth in the rubella group. Sixteen per cent of the infants born after 36 weeks of gestation in the rubella group weighed 5½ lb or less compared with 3.8 per cent in the control.

The chief defects in the rubella group were heart disease, cataracts, and deafness. The overall impairment of hearing in the rubella group was 19 per cent.

These same investigators (Manson, Logan, and Loy, 1960) found no correlation between fetal hazards and infection with either mumps or chickenpox contracted by the mother at any time during pregnancy. They did find, however, that the fetal death rate, and the rate of malformation (11.1 per cent), was higher among infants whose mothers contracted measles (rubeola) than among the controls. In the instances of measles the fetal damage was not confined to early pregnancy. Poliomyelitis caused a higher death rate, but not a higher malformation rate. Toxoplasmosis has been incriminated as the cause of certain central nervous system defects (Feldman, 1958).

Question has been raised over the possible deleterious effect of vaccinating pregnant women with live virus vaccines (Connelly, 1964). Aborted fetuses born to mothers who have been vaccinated against smallpox have been found to have widespread visceral and skin vaccinial lesions (Naidon and Hirsch, 1963). A possible relation between congenital anomalies and the Sabin polio vaccine has been discussed by Katz (1964). McKay (1965), however, is convinced that the Sabin vaccine does not cause fetal loss. Question concerning live measles vaccine has been raised though to date no reports of cases incriminating this vaccine have been published. It would seem a safe policy to withhold from pregnant women all vaccinations with live virus vaccine until further knowledge is available.

Other Pathologic Conditions in the Pregnant Woman

High blood pressure in a pregnant woman is correlated with an increased loss of fetal life. Chesley and Annetto (1947) reported a fetal loss of 38 per cent in 301 pregnancies in which the mother's blood pressure was significantly higher than normal.

There is some evidence that maternal smoking may be related to prematurity or small size of the infant at birth.

The toxemias of pregnancy, hyperthyroidism, hypothyroidism, diabetes (Gaspar, 1945) are all associated with a higher incidence of fetal death than is found in women without these dysfunctions.

Antibody Transfer

Antibodies of low molecular weight—the 7 S gamma globulins—apparently pass the placenta by active transfer and appear frequently in higher concentration in fetal than in maternal blood. These antibodies provide the newborn with a passive immunity (p. 292). Antibodies of high molecular weight—the 17 S gamma globulins—do not normally pass the placenta.

In some instances antibodies transferred to the fetus are deleterious. The most outstanding example is in erythroblastosis foetalis, in which there is an incompatibility of blood between mother and fetus. The infant sensitizes his mother and induces in her the production of antibodies against his blood which is incompatible with hers. When these antibodies are transferred back to the infant, they cause hemolysis of fetal red cells.

Enormous strides have been made in the last few years in the understanding of erythroblastosis. Bowman and Pollock (1965) have developed a technique for removing amniotic fluid from the mother, examining it spectrophotometrically, and thereby determining accurately the severity of the disease in the fetus. If the disease has reached the danger point and the fetus has reached viability, early termination of the pregnancy followed by one or more exchange transfusions may save him. Liley (1965) has gone one step further in the management of this disease. He has devised a method of combating fetal anemia by a peritoneal transfusion of the fetus in utero. Sometimes one, sometimes several transfusions in utero are necessary to save a severely affected fetus until such time as he may be delivered with safety.

Drugs Administered to the Pregnant Woman

The placenta evolved as a mechanism for supplying nutrients and also of protecting the fetus from "normal" hazards. While the efficiency of the organ fails on occasion, the intricate mechanisms are amazingly effective. However, the placenta all too often fails as a barrier when subjected to man-imposed loads. Within recent years, especially since the advent of many new drugs, the effect on the fetus of drugs administered to the mother has received increased attention. Many of the mechanisms within the placenta both for active transport and for impenetrability are unknown (Willner, 1965). Research is hampered by the fact that species differences apparently exist, making data accumulated on animals difficult to apply to the human being (Wilson, 1962).

The disastrous epidemic of phocomelia in Europe in 1961 and 1962 was traced to the ingestion by pregnant women of thalidomide. Taussig (1962) estimates that there may have been as many as 5,000 deformed infants born before the relation of thalidomide and phocomelia was clearly established and the drug taken off the market. The critical period during which thalidomide produces its devastating effects has been narrowed down to between the twenty-eighth and forty-second day after conception. Not all infants are equally affected. In some cases a single dose caused severe malformation; in others, repeated doses caused only minor deformities (Taussig, 1962). Phocomelia has increased in frequency in the United States in the last few years. It is possible that other drugs besides thalidomide may be responsible (Webb, 1965; Jost, 1953).

Interest in tetragenic drugs crescendoed after the thalidomide experience. McKay and Lucey (1964) have summarized current knowledge on the subject and the American Academy of Pediatrics has published a report, a summary of which appears in Table 6-1.

TABLE 6-1

Placental Transmission of Drugs

Drug	Placental transmission	Action	Effects on fetus
Iodides	+++	Excess iodide may trap elemental iodine Iodides may block the di-iodinating enzyme	Goitrous cretinism
Thiouracil	+++	Blocks production of fetal hormone by fetal thyroid	Goitrogenic, respiratory obstruction
Thyroxin	+	Stimulates cellular metabolism	Slow and incomplete crossing with no definite adverse effects
Progestins Androgens Estrogens	++++ ++++ ++++	End organ effect	Masculinization of newborn female
Adrenal corticoid	+	End organ effect	Rarely causes adverse effects
Salicylates	++++	Hepatic damage	Bleeding tendency, amino aciduria (incidence of adverse effects not known)
Reserpine	+	Central	Nasal congestion, drowsiness, depressed respirations
Sulfisoxazole (Gantrisin) Long-acting sulfas	+++ +++	Competes with bilirubin for protein linkage	Rapidly excreted; no adverse effects Very slowly excreted by fetus; may cause kernicterus
Demethylchlortetracycline (Declomycin)	+++	Antimicrobial	None known
Tetracycline	+++	Antimicrobial	Noted to be deposited in bones and teeth of some infants. Questionable growth retardation
Terramycin	+++	Antimicrobial	Noted to be deposited in bones and teeth in some infants. No known adverse effects
Streptomycin	++++	Antimicrobial	VIII nerve damage
Chloramphenicol	++++	Antimicrobial	Bone marrow depression
Phenothiazine	++++	Central nervous depressant	Potentiates depressant action of narcotics, barbiturates, etc.
Barbiturates	++++ Significant transfer within seconds of I.V. administration	Sedation-hypnotic depression of CNS	Respiratory depression; potentiated by narcotics and tranquilizers; interference with early feeding efforts and breast feeding

TABLE 6-1 (Cont.)

Placental Transmission of Drugs

Drug	Placental transmission	Action	Effects on fetus
Meperidine (Demerol)	++++	Respiratory depressant narcotic	CNS depression and respiratory depression in excessive doses or with fetal anoxia; potentiated by barbiturates and tranquilizers
Menadione	++++	Interference with glucuronyl transference	Jaundice, kernicterus

SOURCE: "Effect of Drugs upon the Fetus and the Infant," American Academy of Pediatrics, Committee on Fetus and Newborn, 1961.

Physical Agents

Among the physical agents, x-rays, hypothermia, hypoxia, and elevated CO_2 level have all been found deleterious in animals. In man, massive doses of x-ray within the first 2 months of pregnancy have been found to cause abortion in a considerable proportion of cases, and when abortion does not occur, the incidence of malformed children is high. Murphy (1947) reported a series of 75 infants whose mothers received *therapeutic* x-ray over the pelvic organs during early pregnancy. Of the children resulting from these pregnancies 50.7 per cent were abnormal! (Murphy did not report the nature of the maternal conditions necessitating x-ray treatment.)

Loud noises, mechanical shaking, fever may produce increased activity of the fetus, but there is no evidence that these physical agents produce deleterious effects on development—nor is there any evidence that they do not.

Maternal Emotions

Emotional states in the mother may affect the uterine environment. There is a correlation between states of anxiety and fear and circulating hormones. Increased activity of the adrenals is known to occur in some emotional states, and increased epinephrine causes increased hydrocortisone (Fraser, 1957), which is known to pass the placenta. Experimentally, hydrocortisone (Fraser, 1957) injected into mice results in a large proportion of young with cleft palates. It is conceivable that a similar mechanism functions in man. Montagu has reported evidence suggesting that emotional disturbances during the first 10 weeks of pregnancy may be related to the production of cleft palates.

Other correlations between the mother's emotional state during pregnancy and psychologic and psychosomatic irritability after birth in the infant have been suggested, although at the present time there are no convincing data on the subject.

Summary

Thus, in attempting to provide an optimal environment for the developing new individual, the mother's well-being must be scrutinized with infinite care. It is not sufficient to assume that because she seems well, she is able to provide a satisfactory uterine environment. She needs a diet not only adequate for her own needs but adequate also for the fetus, and at the same time it is desirable that she not gain weight excessively. The pregnant woman needs to be protected against extreme fatigue and from emotional turmoil. It is certainly desirable that she not contract some of the infectious diseases. The greatest dilemma for the obstetrician of today is the management of the pregnant woman who becomes ill. The list of drugs which have been suspected of tetragenic effects is constantly growing. Probably the safest rule is to use as few drugs as possible and to avoid all drugs unless the need for them is unequivocal.

FETAL GROWTH IN THE LIFE SPAN

During fetal life, processes are initiated which continue according to a developmental plan throughout the life span. Interference with these processes at any time in life may result in malformation, its exact nature depending both on the noxious agent and on the time it exercises its actions. It is convenient to think of intrauterine environment as a thing apart, but it must be remembered that postnatal environment is also significant in the development or maldevelopment of structure.

Cell multiplication, rapid and extensive in every part of the embryo, continues in the gonad until the end of reproductive activity. X-ray and radiation are known to interfere with normal development in germinal cells during adult life.

Cell differentiation and the formation of organs, rapid in many structures in the embryo, continues in the long bones until all the epiphyses have united and in the jaw until the permanent teeth have erupted. The ossification of the epiphysis in adolescence is essentially the same process as the endochondral ossification in the embryo. New blood vessels form by capillary sprouting as long as new parts continue to grow. Myelinization of nerve fibers takes place during the first year of life and is essentially the same process as the myelinization within the uterus.

Failure of the environment to supply what is needed, or to protect against harmful agents can result in developmental malformations, not only during intrauterine life, but at least to puberty, and in the gonads to the end of reproductive life.

During fetal life not only is structure formed, but there are initiated basic drives that are carried through life. The drive for independent existence can be thought of as beginning in the embryo with the formation of the fetal heart. Independence develops rapidly as each of the fetal organs begins its function. Birth is an enormous step in independence when the infant takes over the responsibility for all his vital functions. Independence will continue to mature as the child slowly breaks away from maternal care and life within his family. In the maturation of independence there are critical stages in development, similar to those elaborated in relation to fetal development. Thus fetal life can be thought of not as an entity by itself but as part of a continuum.

TABLE 6-2

Summary of Intrauterine Development

1st week	Cell multiplication as zygote passes down the fallopian tube.
2nd week	Beginning chemical differentiation and formation of germinal layers as embryo floats freely in the uterus.
3rd week	Formation of fetal membranes.
4th week	First evidence of independence as heart and vascular tissues are established. Embryo accepts maternally offered nutrients but circulates them around its own body by means of its own organs.
2nd month	Embryo establishes its ground plan. Creation of new tissue is rapid.
3rd month	Basic structure for the most part now formed. Creation of new tissue slows down.
4th–9th month	Organization of function.

BIBLIOGRAPHY

AVERY, GORDON B.: A Brief Review of Placental Function, *Clin. Proc. Child. Hosp.*, **20**:111, 1964.

BAKER, J. B. E.: The Effects of Drugs on the Foetus, *Pharmacol. Rev.*, **12**:37, 1960.

BOWMAN, JOHN M., and J. M. POLLOCK: Amniotic Fluid Spectrophotometry and Early Delivery in the Management of Erythroblastosis Fetalis, *Pediatrics*, **35**:815, 1965.

BURKE, B. S., V. A. BEAL, S. B. KIRKWOOD, and H. C. STUART: Nutrition Studies During Pregnancy, *Am. J. Obstet. Gynecol.*, **46**:38, 1943.

CHESLEY, L. C., and J. E. ANNETTO: Pregnancy in the Patient with Hypertensive Disease, *Am. J. Obstet. Gynecol.*, **53**:372, 1947.

CONNELLY, JOHN P.: Viral and Drug Hazards in Pregnancy, *Clin. Pediat.*, **3**:587, 1964.

DESMOND, MURDINA M., ROBERT R. FRANKLIN, RUSSELL J. BLATTNER, and REBA M. HILL: The Relation of Maternal Disease to Fetal and Neonatal Morbidity and Mortality, *Pediat. Clin. North America*, **8**:421, 1961.

EBERT, JAMES D.: The First International Conference on Congenital Malformations, *J. Chronic Dis.*, **13**:91, 1961.

"Effect of Drugs upon the Fetus and the Infant," American Academy of Pediatrics, Committee on Fetus and Newborn, Evanston, Ill., 1961.

FELDMAN, H. A.: Toxoplasmosis, *Pediatrics,* **22**:559, 1958.

FRASER, F. CLARKE: Causes of Congenital Malformations in Human Beings, *J. Chronic Dis.,* **10**:97, 1959.

———, B. E. WALKER, and D. C. TRASLER: Experimental Production of Congenital Cleft Palate: Genetic and Environmental Factors, *Pediatrics,* **19**:782, 1957.

———: Medical Genetics in Pediatrics, *J. Pediat.,* **44**:85, 1954.

———: Genetic Counseling in Some Common Pediatric Diseases, *Pediat. Clin. North America,* p. 475, May, 1958.

GASPAR, J. L.: Diabetes Mellitus in Pregnancy, *West. J. Surg.,* **53**:21, 1945.

GITLIN, DAVID, JESUS KUMATE, CARLOS MORALES: On the Transport of Insulin Across the Human Placenta, *Pediatrics,* **35**:65, 1965.

GREGG, N. M.: Congenital Cataract Following German Measles in the Mother, *Tr. Ophth. Soc. Australia,* **3**:35, 1942.

HAMILTON, W. J., J. D. BOYD, and W. H. MOSSMAN: "Human Embryology," W. Heffer & Sons, Ltd., Cambridge, England, 1945.

JOST, A.: Degeneration of the Extremities of Fat Fetuses by the Action of Hormones, *Arch. franc. pediat.,* **10**:865, 1953.

KATZ, S.: Efficacy and Hazards of Vaccines, *New England J. Med.,* **17**:884, 1964.

LAMY, M., and J. FRÉZAL: The Frequency of Congenital Malformations, Proceedings of the First International Conference on Congenital Malformations, J. B. Lippincott Company, Philadelphia, 1961.

LILEY, A. W.: The Use of Amniocentesis and Fetal Transfusion in Erythroblastosis Fetalis, *Pediatrics,* **35**:836, 1965.

LUCEY, JEROLD F.: Hazards to the Newborn Infant from Drugs Administered to the Mother, *Pediat. Clin North America,* **8**:413, 1961.

MANSON, M. M., W. P. D. LOGAN, and R. M. LOY: "Rubella and Other Virus Infections During Pregnancy," Reports on Public Health and Medical Subjects, no. 101, Her Majesty's Stationery Office, London, 1960.

MARDEN, PHILIP M., and DAVID W. SMITH: Congenital Anomalies in the Newborn Infant, Including Minor Variations, *J. Pediat.,* **64**:357, 1964.

MCINTOSH, R., K. K. MERRITT, M. R. RICHARDS, M. H. SAMUELS, and M. T. BELLOWS: The Incidence of Congenital Malformations: A Study of 5,964 Pregnancies, *Pediatrics,* **14**:505, 1961.

MCKAY, R. JAMES, and JEROLD F. LUCEY: Neonatology, *New England J. Med.,* **270**:1231, 1964.

MCKAY, R. J., JR., Personal communication, 1965.

MONTAGU, ASHLEY: "Human Heredity," Mentor Books, The New American Library of World Literature, Inc., New York, 1960.

MURPHY, DOUGLAS P.: "Congenital Malformations, A Study of Parental Characteristics with Special Reference to the Reproductive Process," 2d ed., J. P. Lippincott Company, Philadelphia, 1947.

———: Ovarian Radiation and the Health of the Subsequent Child, *Surg. Gynec. & Obst.,* **43**:766, 1929.

NAIDON, P., and H. HIRSCH: Prenatal Vaccinia, *Lancet,* **1**:196, 1963.

NYHAN, WILLIAM L.: "Toxicity of Drugs" in the Neonatal Period, *J. Pediat.,* **59**:1, 1961.

PATTEN, BRADLEY M.: "Human Embryology," 2d ed., McGraw-Hill Book Company, New York, 1953.

POTTER, EDITH L.: "Pathology of the Fetus and the Newborn," The Year Book Medical Publishers, Inc., Chicago, 1952.

REED, SHELTON C.: "Counseling in Medical Genetics," 2d ed., W. B. Saunders Company, Philadelphia, 1963.

SCANLON, ROBERT T.: Placental Transmission of Drugs, *Clin. Proc. Child. Hosp.*, **20**:116, 1964.

SCHULTZ, MARVIN A., JEAN B. FORSANDER, RONALD A. CHEZ, DONALD H. HUTCHINSON: The Bi-directional Placental Transfer of 1¹³¹3:3′ Triiodothyronine in Rhesus Monkey, *Pediatrics*, **35**:743, 1965.

STOCKARD, C. R.: Developmental Rate and Structure Expression, *Am. J. Anat.*, **28**:115, 1921.

SWAN, C., A. L. TOSTEIN, and G. H. B. BLOCK: Final Observation on Congenital Defects in Infants Following Infectious Diseases during Pregnancy with Special Reference to Rubella, *Med. J. Aust.*, **2**:889, 1946.

TAUSSIG, HELEN B.: Thalidomide and Phocomelia, *Pediatrics*, **30**:654, 1962.

THIERSCH, J. B.: Therapeutic Abortions with Folic Acid Antagonist, *Am. J. Obstet. Gynec.* **63**:1298, 1952.

WARKANY, JOSEF: Congenital Malformations in the Past, *J. Chronic Dis.*, **10**:84, 1959.

———: Congenital Malformations Induced in Rats by Maternal Nutritional Deficiencies, *J. Nutrition*, **23**:321, 1942, and **27**:477, 1944.

WEBB, CLARENCE H.: Personal communication, 1965.

WILKINS, L., H. W. JONES, G. H. HOLMAN, and R. S. STEMPFEL, JR.: Masculinization of Female Fetus Associated with Administration of Oral and Intramuscular Progestins during Gestation: Nonadrenal Female Pseudohermaphroditism, *J. Clin. Endocrinol.*, **18**:559, 1958.

WILLIS, R. H.: "The Borderland of Embryology and Pathology," Butterworth & Co. (Publishers), London, 1958.

WILLNER, MILTON M.: Maturational Deficiencies of the Fetus and Newborn: Relationships to Drug Effects, *Clin. Pediat.*, **4**:3, 1965.

WILSON, JAMES G.: Experimental Studies on Congenital Malformations, *J. Chronic Dis.*, **10**:111, 1959.

WILSON, MIRIAM C.: The Effect of Maternal Medications upon the Fetus and the Newborn Infant, *Am. J. Obstet. & Gynec.*, **83**:818, 1962.

7

Birth Itself

After approximately 40 weeks of intrauterine life, the human zygote has become a fetus and has reached a degree of maturity such that independent life is possible. At this point, parturition takes place.

THE PROCESS OF NORMAL LABOR

The factors that initiate labor are not clearly understood at the present time. The muscular action of the uterus expels the baby, but what it is that changes the mild, painless contractions of this organ into the forceful and painful contractions of labor is still an enigma.

The nervous mechanism of the uterus is under control of the autonomic nervous system. At the time of labor, the uterus gradually becomes differentiated into two segments with diametrically opposed, though coordinated, functions. The upper segment of the uterus is the active, contracting, working part of the organ; the lower segment and cervix are the passive parts, the function of which is to relax and dilate. There is no quick reflex that dilates the muscle fibers of the lower segment and opens the cervix. Labor consists of a contest between the forces of expulsion and those of resistance, and its duration depends upon the balance between these forces. The expulsive forces depend upon the intensity, duration, and frequency of the contractions of the upper segment. The resistive forces depend primarily upon the tenseness of the circular muscle of the cervix.

For purposes of description, labor is divided into three stages: the first consists of the dilation and effacement of the cervix; the second, the descent and actual expulsion of the infant; and the third, the expulsion of the placenta (Greenhill, 1965).

The first stage is a uterine phenomenon. The second stage, the actual birth of the infant, is brought about by a combination of uterine and total body action. Once the cervix is dilated and the passageway is clear, the uterus is emptied in somewhat the same way as the rectum is emptied of its contents. The glottis is closed, the abdominal muscles contract, and the diaphragm is forced downward at the height of the uterine contraction. Thus the entire visceral mass pushes on the contracted uterus. The accessory body action, known as *bearing down*, is initiated automatically. There are striated as well as unstriated muscles involved in bearing down, so that the woman is able to cooperate and to bear down voluntarily. Bearing down has no function in the first stage of labor but is essential in the second stage. While the cervix of a woman under spinal block anesthesia is able to dilate, the infant cannot be expelled automatically, since the nervous connection between the sacral and upper segments of the mother's spinal cord are blocked off. However, if an attendant, palpating her abdomen, tells her when to bear down, she can perform this act voluntarily. Under normal circumstances the expulsion of the placenta is accomplished in the same fashion.

The Pain of Labor

Unlike all other smooth muscle action in health, the contractions of the uterus in normal, healthy parturition are painful. In no other mammalian species is the expulsion of the fetus at birth a painful ordeal. The pain of labor seems to serve no useful purpose, and yet it has existed in the human species as far back as records go.

Much of the pain of childbirth is due to the stretching of the lower uterine segment and especially of the cervix. If the cervix offers relatively little resistance, it dilates quickly, and the pain is slight or nonexistent, as in all mammalian species except man. However, if the cervix is kept rigidly firm, the uterine contractions must forcibly dilate it; it is this pushing and pulling at the cervix which causes the ordeal of childbirth. Eastman suggests that the pain of labor, like angina pectoris, is accentuated by anoxia in the compressed muscle tissue.

Grantly Dick Read's contention is that the cervix is kept tense and tight through fear. All fear, he points out, causes muscle tension; the specific nature of the fear determines what muscles will be tensed. Since time immemorial, women have talked to young girls about the ordeal of childbirth. Young women look forward with dread and fear to the inevitable termination of their first pregnancy. This fear causes increased tension in the circular muscle fibers of the cervix and prevents easy dilation. Read also believes that fear interferes with the circulation of the blood and accentuates the pain due to tension by the pain of muscle ischemia.

Whether or not Read's fear-tension-pain syndrome is the full explanation of the discomforts of childbirth is debatable. There is, however, no doubt that the emotional state of the parturient woman is a potent factor in the ease with which she delivers her baby.

Drugs during Labor

When properly cared for, instructed, and encouraged, some women will need no drugs; some actually will feel relatively little pain, and others will find what pain they experience quite bearable. Other women, however, even when handled well, will experience pain of sufficient intensity that some relief is urgently needed.

Drugs for relief of pain during labor are fraught with greater hazards than drugs used for surgical anesthesia. In the surgical patient muscular relaxation is desirable, but during labor, the drugs selected must not interfere with uterine contractions. During labor two patients must be considered: the parturient woman and her infant. Drugs which are relatively harmless to the mother may cause serious trouble to the infant. Degrees of anoxia so slight that they cause the mother no embarrassment may be fatal to the fetus, whose blood, even under the best of conditions, has a low oxygen tension. Drugs which reduce the mother's blood pressure again may do her little harm but have serious consequences for the fetus, whose systolic pressure is low at the moment of change from fetal to postfetal circulation. Sedative drugs, especially those of the morphine series, have an effect on the fetal respiratory center and may induce sluggish initiation of breathing.

Relieving severe pain is one of the duties of the physician, and certainly every woman in labor needs reassurance that if she needs relief, she will be given it. Obstetric analgesia in the first stage of labor may relieve the fear induced by pain so that the cervix actually will dilate more easily. Analgesia also avoids pressure on the obstetrician to rush into operative termination of a labor that, if given a little more time, would terminate normally. Details of the various drugs and techniques, including blocking of the sacral nerves, available for relief of pain during parturition are discussed by Eastman and Hillman, who emphasize the fact that no medication should be given before there is evidence that the cervix is dilating.

MATERNAL ATTITUDES AND MEDICAL CARE IN CHILDBEARING

All women share certain needs for basic medical care during pregnancy. They all need instruction in dietary requirements, in ways of avoiding illness, and in how to treat it promptly should it occur. They need to be warned against the promiscuous use of drugs. They need to learn about exercise and fatigue, about work, play, trips, and about many of the details of life that may have an effect upon their child. They need to be relieved of fear in relation to their forthcoming delivery.

Each woman reacts to pregnancy in her own individual way. Some women are casual about their pregnancy; others are elated, depressed, vindictive, anxious, guilty. The way a woman feels about her pregnancy reflects her entire personality. Her feelings are influenced by the circumstances under which she conceived her child as well as by the environment in which she is currently living.

The good obstetrician takes into consideration the total woman and not only treats her physical needs but tailors his care to meet her individual emotional outlook. One woman carrying a hard-to-conceive and much wanted baby may become fearful that she might do something that will harm her baby. She will need reassurance that the normal vicissitudes of life will not affect her child. Another woman carrying a child she views as an unwelcome burden may deliberately (or perhaps unconsciously) refuse to cooperate on matters of diet and hygiene. She needs very different medical counsel (Thomas, 1955).

The obstetrician who takes time with his patient, ferrets out what her feelings really are and talks occasionally with the husband, if this seems indicated, succeeds more often than not in building up a rapport with his patient by means of which he obtains her cooperation. Some patients are, of course, much easier to deal with than others, but the vast majority of women do respond to care from an understanding doctor.

A woman with respect for, and confidence in, her obstetrician approaches labor with a minimum of fear. She may want to know that her obstetrician will relieve her of most, if not all, of the pain of childbirth. Other women want to "be there" when their baby is born. They want to take part in what, to them, is a profoundly emotional experience. Such a woman wants to hear her child's birth cry, to fondle him as soon as he breathes. She is willing to bear some pain for the satisfaction of feeling that she has consciously produced her baby. A woman who has made up her mind during pregnancy that she wants to get along with the minimum of analgesia may discover during her actual labor that the pain is more than she bargained for and cry out for relief. Her initial decision need not be irrevocable.

Within the last decade, much more attention has been given to the psychic factors of pregnancy and labor than previously. Grantly Dick Read introduced the concept of natural childbirth. This is a broad concept and takes cognizance of the physiology of pregnancy and labor as well as the emotional orientation of the woman. Read includes prenatal education designed to eliminate fear, combined with exercises in relaxation and control of breathing. It well may be that the exercises have their most profound effect on the psyche rather than the physiology. The interest of the obstetrician in the patient's well-being and his conviction that he can help her impart confidence in him and in herself. It is this confidence that allays fear. Natural childbirth does not mean no drugs and no pain. It means an adroit management of all aspects of pregnancy and labor.

Read says, "Women demand of all things complete confidence in the physician who is caring for them during labor. They do not want soft words and sob stuff, but explanations, instructions and encouragement. They want to hear that all is going well, that the baby is all right and that they are conducting their job in an admirable manner."

Speck says that there is no routine method for caring for women in labor, because there is no routine woman. Having a baby is one of life's richest experiences, and this fact needs to be appreciated by the obstetrician.

When a woman is in pain, she needs the skillful reassurance of someone in whom she has absolute confidence. The presence of the obstetrician, says Speck, is worth many grams of analgesic.

Eastman and Hillman express the same thought this way: "The attitude we have in mind comes only as the result of long nights in the labor room and then only to those of an understanding heart. It is the stuff of which good doctors are made and is at once the safest and most welcome of obstetric anodynes."

Occasionally a father is permitted to be with his wife during labor, and he, like his wife, may feel an emotional exhilaration over the miracle of childbirth which may have lasting effects upon his relation with his wife and child. Many husbands, however, find the spectacle of childbirth disturbing. Such a man and his wife (to say nothing of the obstretrician) are better off if he leaves his wife entirely in the hands of the medical staff during labor.

RESUSCITATION

Failure to establish respiration is the most frequent cause of death in the perinatal period. A delay of 1 or 2 minutes suggests some interference with the breathing mechanisms. Unless breathing is soon established, the infant dies. A delay of more than 5 minutes in the initiation of breathing may subject the brain to a degree of anoxia such that permanent damage is done.

Criteria of adequate condition after birth has been formalized by Apgar (1953). One minute after complete birth the five Apgar tests can be evaluated and each given a score of 0, 1, or 2. A score of 10 indicates an infant in optimal condition. A score of 5 to 10 usually means the infant will be all right, needs careful watching, but needs no immediate treatment. Approximately 90 per cent of normal infants score 7 or better 1 minute after birth. An infant whose Apgar score is 4 or less at the end of his first 2

TABLE 7-1

Apgar Tests

Sign	0	1	2
Heart rate	Absent	Slow (below 100)	Rapid (over 100)
Respiratory effort	Absent	Slow, irregular	Good; crying
Reflex irritability (response to catheter in nostril)	No response	Grimace	Cough or sneeze
Color	Blue Pale	Body pink, extremities blue	Completely pink
Muscle tone	Flaccid	Weak	Strong

SOURCE: Apgar, A Proposal for a New Method of Evaluation of the Newborn Infant, *Current Res. Anesth. & Analg.*, 32: 260, 1953.

minutes of extrauterine life needs resuscitative measures. *Resuscitation in the Newborn,* a manual of the American Academy of Pediatrics, gives details of techniques which may be used.

BIRTH INJURIES

While injuries to the fetus during the process of birth may be of many kinds, for practical purposes they are divided into those occurring in the central nervous system and those occurring in the peripheral parts of the organism.

Central nervous system injuries involve hemorrhage or laceration of brain tissue and are frequently accompanied by delayed establishment of respiration—asphyxia neonatorum (p. 529). If the trauma is severe, respiration is never established, and the fetus dies—i.e., the birth is a stillbirth. While less severe trauma may delay respiration, it may not prevent its ultimate establishment. The prognosis in such a case depends upon the degree and duration of the cerebral anoxia, as well as the location and extent of the hemorrhage. Not infrequently the symptoms at birth are forgotten. The infant may appear normal during the early months, but ultimately abnormal development may become manifest. Such symptoms as convulsions, hyperactivity, mental retardation, spastic paralysis, ataxia, speech disorders, sensory disturbances, or combinations of any of these symptoms may occur in the brain-damaged child.

Cephalhematoma is relatively common, occurring in 1 to 2 per cent of all normal births. It is a subperiosteal accumulation of blood usually occurring over the parietal bone. The swelling becomes obvious between the first and fourth days of life as a soft fluctuating mass which does not pulsate and does not increase with crying. Slowly the margins become firm as new bone is laid down by the detached periosteum. Eventually the whole area is covered by bone and slowly disappears, a process often taking several months.

Injury to peripheral nerves occurs occasionally. The most frequent injury is to the nerves of the brachial plexus because of traction on the head in order to ease a shoulder through the birth canal. If the injury is slight, it may be only a stretching of the nerves, in which case full recovery of function can be expected. More severe injury may result in actual tearing of nerves and paralysis of the associated muscles. The muscles most often involved are the deltoid, biceps brachii, brachialis, and supinator. The arm hangs limp by the side. Lack of symmetry in the Moro reflex is suggestive of injury to the brachial plexus.

Injury to the facial nerve occurs once in a while as a result of pressure, usually from forceps. Usually this injury is slight and ultimate recovery takes place, although it is always possible that permanent damage has been done.

Fractures of various bones sometimes take place even during relatively easy labors. The clavicle and the bones of the extremities are the most frequently injured. They heal readily with proper care.

Soft tissue injuries and forceps marks are a frequent occurrence. While they may look ugly for a few days and distress the baby's parents, they are seldom serious and usually disappear within a matter of days.

Problems of the neonatal period will be discussed below (see Chaps. 36 and 37).

BIBLIOGRAPHY

APGAR, VIRGINIA, and L. S. JAMES, M.D.: Further Observations on the Newborn Scoring System, *Am. J. Dis. Child.*, **104**:419, 1962.

———: "Anesthesia for Obstetrics," J. P. Lippincott Company, Philadelphia, 1956.

———: A Proposal for a New Method of Evaluation of the Newborn Infant, *Current Res. Anesth. & Analg.*, **32**:260, 1953.

———: Correlation of Physical and Emotional Phenomena of Natural Labor, *J. Obst. & Gynaec. Brit. Comm.*, **53**:55, 1946.

EASTMAN, NICHOLSON J., and LOUIS M. HILLMAN: "Williams Obstetrics," 12th ed., Appleton-Century-Crofts, Inc., New York, 1961.

GREENHILL, J. P.: "Obstetrics," from the original text by Joseph B. DeLee, 13th ed., W. B. Saunders Company, Philadelphia, 1965.

READ, G.: "Childbirth Without Fear," Harper & Row, Publishers, Incorporated, New York, 1955.

"Resuscitation of the Newborn," manual prepared by the Committee on the Fetus and the Newborn, American Academy of Pediatrics, Evanston, Ill., 1958.

SPECK, G.: Childbirth with Dignity, *Obstet. & Gynec.*, **2**:544, 1953.

THOMAS, H.: The Preparation for Childbirth Program, *Obst. & Gynec. Surv.*, **10**:1, 1955.

Section III

INCREMENT IN POUNDS AND INCHES

8

Human Growth through the Ages

A human being starts being himself as a single cell. In 9 months he becomes a 6- or 7-lb baby; in less than 20 years he achieves 5 to 6 ft in height and 100 to 200 lb in weight. During this time there is a great temptation to evaluate how well he is doing by how big he has become. While in general there *is* a correlation between his size at any given time and his general well-being, the use of height/weight data as a measure of health is fraught with danger. However, although it is not possible to construct absolute standards of growth, enough is known to justify the cautious use of height/weight data.

THE NATURE OF GROWTH

Each animal species has a growth pattern characteristic of itself. Birds do not grow as do cows, but all birds follow a bird pattern. A hummingbird and an eagle follow similar patterns, even though the absolute values of their weights at any age are very different. In the same way a Jersey cow and a Holstein cow have in common a cow pattern (Fig. 8-1). This is as true of the human species as it is of the other animal species. A pigmy baby in Africa grows in the same way as a baby in Scandinavia or a baby in a Park Avenue apartment in New York (Fig. 8-2).

Mammals below the human being (except the primate group to which human beings belong biologically) grow rapidly in early life and soon reach their mature size. They do not pass through the long, slow growing period of middle childhood, nor do they show a pubescent spurt in growth. In most mammals puberty comes soon after weaning and is not accompanied by an increase in the rate of somatic growth.

The long postponement of puberty in the human being is an evolutionary trait. The development of the brain is the distinguishing factor that separates man from lower species, and it takes time for this elaborate mechanism to complete its development. The hypothalamus controls the onset of puberty. When this part of the brain reaches maturity, it triggers an endocrine mechanism that initiates the maturation of reproductive function. The long childhood of the human being allows time not only for somatic growth but also for the development of the qualities of humanness. During the early years the child is prepared for adulthood in all areas of development; his body increases in size and develops increasingly intricate motor capacities, his personality emerges, he absorbs his culture. Under optimal conditions he becomes not only a full-sized adult competent in motor activities but an adult mature on the human level. The changes are so profound that it is not surprising that optimal development on all fronts is not always achieved. While development takes place in all areas simultaneously, the rate of development varies from area to area. Somatic growth and development will be considered in this section.

The greatest increments in human growth take place prior to birth; in children in the United States this is roughly 20 in. During the first year another 10 in. is added, and during the second year another 5 in. The human child achieves approximately half his ultimate height by the age of 2 years. During the third year the annual increment slows down to 3 to 4 in. and thereafter to 2 to 3 in. per year, until the growth spurt of puberty begins to makes its appearance.

During intrauterine life nourishment is absorbed and body substances that did not exist before are created. The increase in size of the fetus is due to creation of nervous tissue, of bone, of muscle, of connective tissue, and of all the multitudinous tissues which compose the animal organism. Later in life, new-cell creation slows down in most tissues, and most of the further increase in size is due to enlargement of the already created cells.

The early growth of the fetus and the infant appears to be primarily

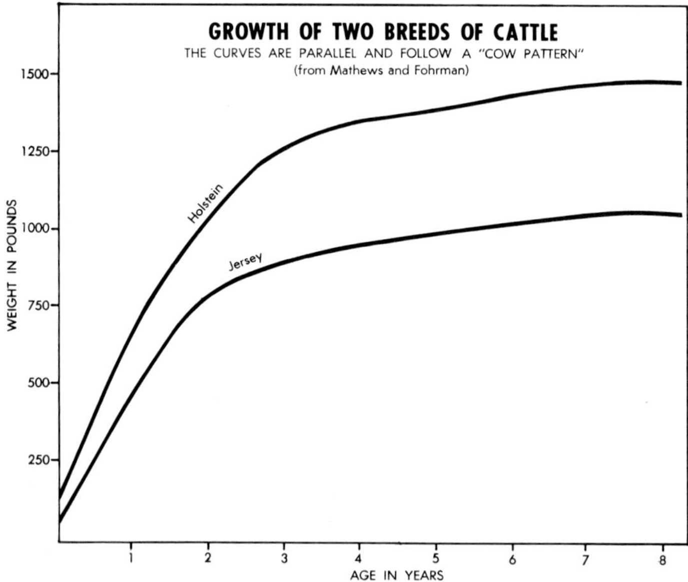

Fig. 8-1. Growth of two breeds of cattle. (*From Matthews and Fohrman, Bletsville Standards for Growth of Jersey and Holstein Cattle, U.S. Dept. Agric. Tech. Bull., 1098 and 1099, 1954.*)

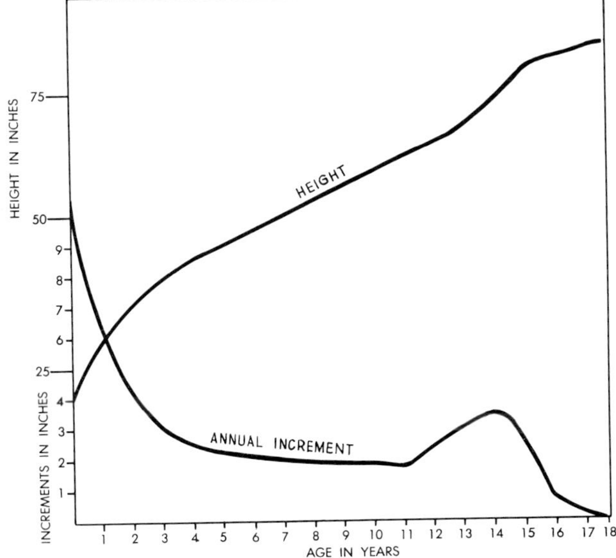

Fig. 8-2. Human growth pattern.

under control of the genes (Goldberg, 1955).[1] Retardation of growth prior to the age of 2 years is usually attributed to primordial dwarfism (Kogut et al., 1963) or intrauterine growth retardation (Szalay, 1964). The anterior pituitary hormones, especially the growth hormone, are thought to be responsible for the steady growth through the years of middle childhood. Thyroxin initiates the development of centers of ossification in the long bones. In the period immediately preceding puberty, androgens from the adrenal cortex and the testes and estrogens from the ovary begin to make their appearance, stimulated probably by gonadotropins from the hypophysis.

In the girl, the estrogens stimulate both the growth of the long bones and finally maturational changes in the epiphyses followed by their closure; simultaneously the estrogens stimulate reproductive maturing. In the boy, androgens stimulate growth of the long bones more than estrogen does in the girl, both in duration of effect and in magnitude of increments. Ultimately androgens bring about closure of the epiphyses in the male, and growth in height comes to an end. It is the androgens which are responsible for maturation of the male reproductive system and the male secondary sexual characteristics.

The controlling factors of human growth inherent in the organism are thus seen to be the genes and the endocrines. Since it is, in the last analysis, the genes which control the endocrines, the growth potential of any individual human being can be thought of as lying within his genes. The

[1] References cited in this chapter and in Chaps. 9 to 12 are listed in the Bibliography at the end of Chap. 12.

actual growth of an individual, however, is determined both by his genetic potential and by the environmental stresses and strains to which he is subjected. The assumption that there is an optima growth for each individual predetermined in his genes leads logically to a second assumption, namely, that deviants from this optimum reflect environmental hazards.

There are mountains of figures on human growth; nevertheless, what is optimum for any individual is still difficult to determine. It is possible, however, to cull from the available data some information that is useful in helping children attain their maximum well-being.

All growth studies fall into one of two categories: cross-sectional and longitudinal. Confusion between these categories is responsible for much of the prevalent misinformation about growth.

CROSS–SECTIONAL STUDIES

In a cross-sectional study all the children are measured once. Data are obtained, for example, from a school population of children varying in age from 6 to 18 years. The end result of such a study gives information on a group of 6-year-olds, a group of 7-year-olds, and so on for each age group. When all the data on the 6-year-olds are averaged, a figure of what the "average 6-year-old" has accomplished in 6 years is obtained. The meaning of this figure depends upon how homogeneous the group of 6-year-olds is. Size at age 6 varies with genetic background, with socioeconomic level, with physical and emotional health, and probably with other factors as well. If the population measured contains children who fall in many of these different categories, the average figure is not of much value as a standard against which to compare the accomplishments of any given child in 6 years. Average figures from a cross-sectional study are useful in comparing groups. The average size of 6-year-olds in a New York City public school can be compared with the average size of the 6-year-olds in a Japanese school or a French school or a Mississippi school or in an English school in 1850.

In a cross-sectional study the figures represent a static phenomenon. They are not a continuum, because no child moved from one group to the next. In many cross-sectional "growth" studies the data are used as though they were a continuum. The average figures of distance attained at the various ages are put together, and the resulting curve is called a "growth" curve (though nothing grew—all was static). In using cross-sectional data in this way the assumption is made that all children of age 6, when the study was made, will be of the same size 1 year hence as those age 7 at the time of measurement. This assumption is not valid; children do not progress at the same rate at different ages. Differences in the rate of progression exist at all ages, but during the spurt of growth at puberty the differences are very marked indeed. Each child grows rapidly for 1 or 2 years during his period of sexual maturation. However, there is about an 8-year span during which individual children pass through this growth spurt. Girls mature earlier than boys, but even within the same sex there is a range of several years during which maturation may take place.

A girl who has not started to mature may grow 1 in. in height between 11 and 12 years of age; another girl in early puberty at this age may grow 5 in. in this same chronological time. The difference obtained in a cross-sectional study of height between the average 11-year-old girl and the average 12-year-old girl gives a figure which distorts the amount of gain of the early- and late-maturing girls.

In Fig. 8-3*a* are plotted in individual increments in growth of girls maturing at different ages. The dotted line represents the average figure, which bears little resemblance to the individual curves. In Fig. 8-3*b* these data are replotted in such a way that peak growth in height of all the girls is placed at a single point. Again the dotted lines represent the average, which comes much closer to demonstrating the magnitude of the pubertal growth spurt than did the first average.

Valuable information can be obtained from cross-sectional studies, but such studies are of relatively little value in studying the velocity of growth —the increment per unit of time.

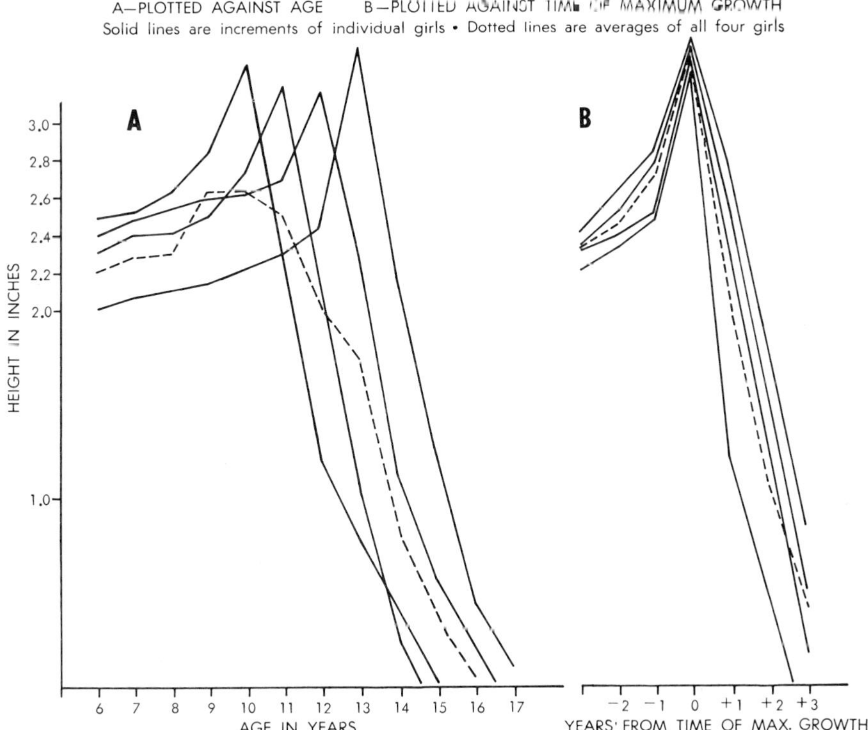

Fig. 8-3. Height increments of girls maturing at different ages.

LONGITUDINAL STUDIES

In a longitudinal study a group of children is followed over a period of time. The same children are measured at successive periods. *Growing*, not merely growth accomplishment, is measured. Data from individual children can be combined and recombined in many ways. For example all the girls who reach the menarche at age 12 can be put in one group and their growth compared with girls who reach the menarche at age 13. It is soon seen that age of menarche has far more significance for growth than chronological age.

Longitudinal studies are more difficult to conduct than cross-sectional ones. It takes years to complete a study in which the investigator is waiting for his subjects to grow up; families move about, so it is difficult to maintain a group of children for a long span of years; longitudinal studies are expensive; and investigators as well as children grow older with the years!

At the present time in the United States there are a number of large-scale longitudinal studies, some under way, others completed. The Brush Foundation Study of Child Health and Development in Cleveland, the Fels Research Institute Study of Prenatal and Postnatal Environment at Antioch, Longitudinal Studies of Child Health and Development of the Harvard School of Public Health in Boston, Studies of the Institute of Human Development in Berkeley, California, are some of the most outstanding studies.

GENETIC INFLUENCES

There are many genes which influence growth. Since it is of course impossible to identify them individually, the problem is to relate observable and measurable qualities of a child with his growth potential. Growth in childhood is correlated with (1) size at birth, (2) sex, (3) speed of maturation, and (4) body build, and perhaps with other factors, too.

Of these four factors sex, with only rare exceptions, is readily observable at birth. It is certainly genetically determined, and there is no conceivable environmental factor which can change this basic fact about the individual.[2]

Birth weight is information easy enough to come by, but by itself it does not offer enough information to warrant prediction of growth.

Body build and rate of maturing are probably genetically determined. Rate of maturing, while not determinable at birth, shows itself during the early years (p. 115). Combined with sex and birth weight, it offers the best information for predicting what a given child should accomplish under good conditions.

There is considerable evidence to suggest that although both body build

[2] Some of the new work on chromosomal patterns has cast doubt upon the absolute quality of sex. However, even for these infinitesimally few individuals with atypical chromosomal patterns, sex can still be considered a gene-determined absolute.

and rate of maturing are genetically determined, they, unlike sex, may both be subject to change by environmental forces (see below).

Size at Birth

The size at birth after full-term pregnancy is an index, although a rough one, of the ultimate size of the mature man. While dependent upon the genetic growth potential operating since conception, birth weight is influenced by many other factors. It is only a first step in estimating the growth potential of any given child.

First-born infants are usually smaller by some ounces than later-born infants (Meredith, 1950). Why this should be so is unknown, and there seems to be no correlation between this small difference and growth potential.

Infants born to small women and fathered by large men are often smaller at birth than would be expected as judged by their ultimate growth (Tanner, 1956). Apparently some dampening effect from the mother keeps an infant in utero from becoming too large to pass through her small birth canal.

Birth weight is related to duration of gestation. Lubchenco, Hansman, Dressler, and Boyd related birth weight to gestational age in a large series of premature and full-term infants. Their data suggest that infants destined to be large are already large by the end of 24 weeks of gestational age (p. 109).

Sex

Boys and girls have different growth patterns. At birth boys are slightly bigger (between 1 and 4 per cent) than girls in both height and weight. During the first year of life boys grow slightly faster than girls, but between the ages of 1 and 9 the growth rate differences between boys and girls are almost nonexistent.

At puberty the first significant differences in height and weight between the sexes becomes evident. It is at this time that the different endocrines exercise their effects—androgens in the male and estrogens in the female. Girls mature earlier than boys, so that for a few years the girls in any population group are larger

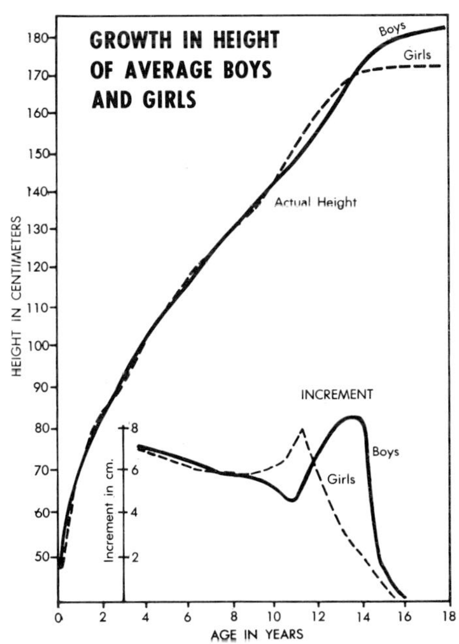

Fig. 8-4. Growth of average boys and girls.

than the boys in almost all dimensions. Then the boys begin their pubertal spurt; they catch up and pass the girls and end up roughly 10 per cent bigger (Fig. 8-4).

Speed of Maturing

Some children progress along their predetermined growth pattern at a faster rate than others. The age at which a child matures sexually is a milestone that is convenient to use as a peg. Some girls accomplish sexual maturity in eleven years from birth; others take 16 or even 17 years to reach the same level of maturity. Boys are not so speedy as girls. The speediest can reach manhood in 12 years; the slow ones may take 18 years.

Early maturers are early in all their physiologic accomplishments (Reed and Stuart, 1959). In general, during childhood they are taller and heavier than later maturers. Their skeletons grow faster, they get their teeth earlier, they develop muscular capacity and coordination a little sooner than the late maturers. The speed of maturation is a gene-determined phenomenon. The early maturers become adults who have more weight for height than late maturers (see Chap. 10).

Body Build

Adult human bodies vary in all their external dimensions. Almost all classifications consist of two extreme types and one intermediate one. At one extreme human beings are tall and thin, the typical Uncle Sam; at the other extreme they are short and fat, the John Bull. In between there is the strong muscular athlete, the Hercules (Fig. 8-5).

Sheldon uses the terms *endomorph, mesomorph,* and *ectomorph* to describe the three types (Fig. 8-6). The endomorph has a round head and large, fat abdomen predominating over his thorax. His arms and legs are short, with considerable fat in the upper arm and thigh but with slender wrists and ankles. He has a great deal of subcutaneous fat. His body is thick, his skeleton large. The endomorph is plump as a child and tends to put on weight as he gets older.

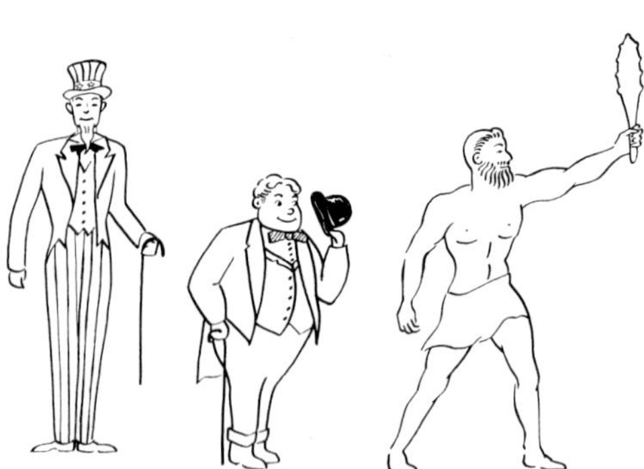

Fig. 8-5. Classic body builds: Uncle Sam, John Bull, and Hercules.

The mesomorph is the strong athlete. Bone and muscle predominate, but he has much less fat than the endomorph. He has broad shoulders and chest and heavily muscled arms and legs with the lower segment strong in relation to the upper.

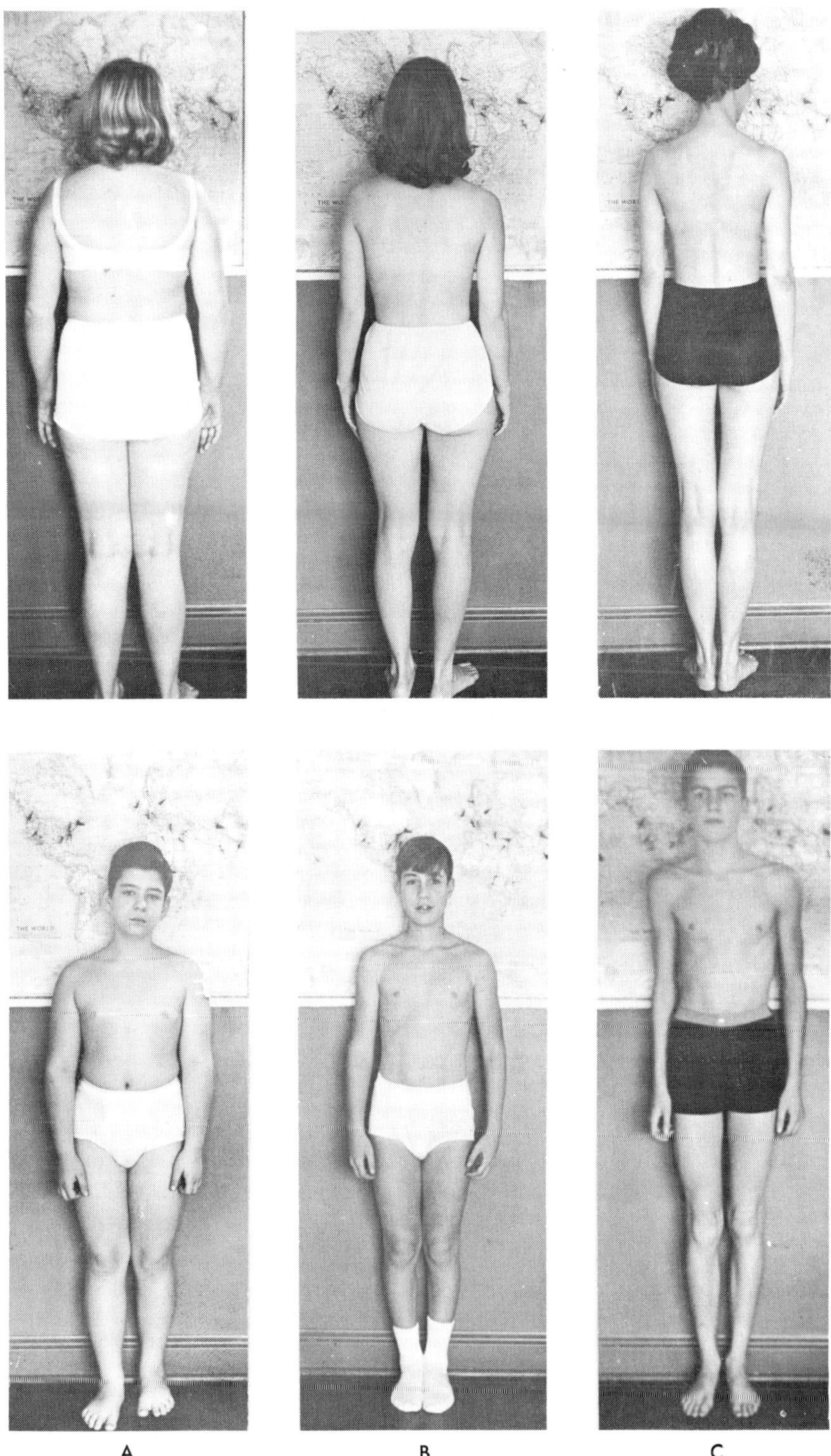

A B C

Fig. 8-6. Somatypes: A. endomorph, B. mesomorph, C. ectomorph.

The ectomorph is the linear man; he has a thin, peaked face with a receding forehead, a thin, narrow chest and abdomen, spindly arms and legs. His muscles are neither large nor strong. He has very little subcutaneous fat. He seldom becomes obese.

The majority of people have a moderate amount of each component in their somatotype. Virtually all somatotyping has been done on adults. In the Brush Foundation Growth Study a group that had been followed since childhood was somatotyped in early adult life. With the knowledge of their adult somatotypes their growth records were sorted out and recombined into groups of homogeneous somatotypes. The ectomorphs were taller than the mesomorphs at all ages from 4 onward, but the mesomorphs were heavier from age 2 onward. From the age of 2 the mesomorphs had more weight for height than the ecomorphs. (Figure 8-7 shows the growth of two boys, one high in ectomorphy, the other high in mesomorphy.)

Unfortunately somatotyping at the early ages has not at present been worked out. From longitudinal growth studies it was obvious, after the subjects reached adult size and could be somatotyped, that their growth in childhood varied according to the body build they finally achieved. This is important, but at present data are lacking with which to predict growth based on somatotype at birth (Dupertuis and Michael).

Bayley and Bayer (1946) have suggested another way of classifying body builds. They describe androgyny, the degree of masculinity in the female and femininity in the male. Androgyny emphasizes the fact that every individual has some characteristics of the opposite sex. Bayley and Bayer describe an undifferentiated pattern of body build characteristic of the neuter gender quality of early childhood. At puberty the pattern fans out either toward the hyperfeminine or the hypermasculine or remains intermediate (asexual). Some individuals travel all the way to the extreme of their sex; others stop part way, retaining elements of the undifferentiated pattern of childhood (Fig. 8-8).

While the final measurement of androgyny cannot be made until maturity is reached, nevertheless, like the somatotypes of Sheldon, the androgyny type is, Bayley and Bayer believe, an innate trait uniquely characteristic of the individual and possessed by him all his life. By means of certain anthropometric measurements during childhood these investigators have been able, at least roughly, to categorize children before puberty with respect to their androgyny scores.

In the androgyny score considerable emphasis is placed on the distribution of subcutaneous fat and muscles. Women on the whole deposit more fat than men, and men develop larger muscle mass than women. Amount of muscle and of fat are also factors in the somatotyping system of Sheldon.

These two different methods of describing body build overlap. The mesomorph of Sheldon is the muscular type and is closely related to the hypermasculine on the androgyny scale. As a male this type tends to mature

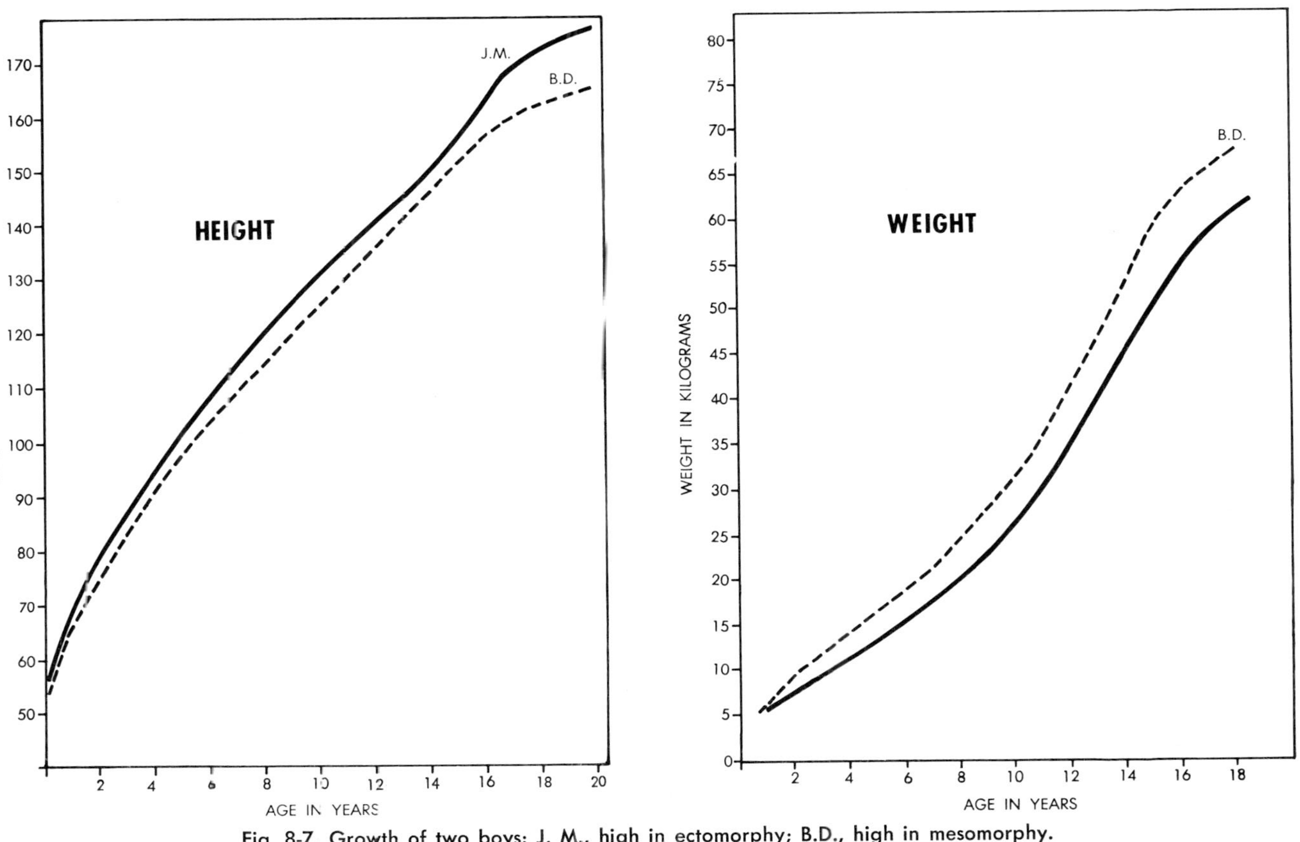

Fig. 8-7. Growth of two boys: J. M., high in ectomorphy; B.D., high in mesomorphy.

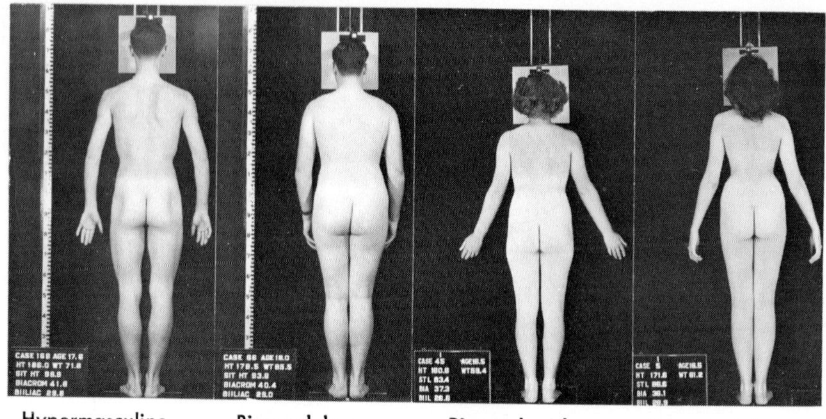

Hypermasculine Bisexual boy Bisexual girl Hyperfeminine

Fig. 8-8. Androgynic patterns. (*From Bayley and Bayer, Photos of Cases 5, 45, 66 and 168 in The Assessment of Somatic Androgyny, Am. J. Phy. Anthrop. 4:433, 1946. Courtesy of the Wistar Institute of Anatomy and Biology, Philadelphia.*)

early. The endomorph deposits an abundance of fat and is related to the hyperfeminine on the scale of Bayley and Bayer. As a female this type tends to mature early. The ectomorph of Sheldon, the linear person, is the asexual person of Bayley and Bayer; in both sexes they are late maturers. The muscular girl is high in mesomorphy on Sheldon's scale, high in masculinity on that of Bayley and Bayer. Unlike the muscular boy, she tends to be a later maturer. The fat boy is high in endomorphy and high in femininity. He does not follow the early-maturing pattern of the endomorphic girl, he tends to be a late maturer (Bayer, 1940).

Brozek raises the question of how stable the body type of an individual remains through the life span. He feels that while there are stable (genetic) aspects to body build, the variable (environmental) aspects have been confused in most of the attempts to categorize body build.

It is doubtless true that body build is not a simple, single, gene-directed characteristic. Body build is the result of the growth and development of the skeletal structure, the muscles, and the adipose tissue. Each of these parts of the organism is acted upon by many things, both intrinsic and extrinsic. Nevertheless there are measurable tendencies toward one or another of the recognized body types which are useful clinically.

ENVIRONMENTAL INFLUENCES

There is good reason to believe that nutrition is a factor not only in the rate of growth but also in the speed of growth and the ultimate stature achieved. Children known to be on poor diets can be stimulated to grow at a more rapid rate by improvements in their diets. Where the optimum is reached in relation to diet is not so clear. Can children on adequate diets (adequate to the best of our present-day knowledge) be stimulated to grow more by supplements of protein, minerals, vitamins, or anything else? Opinion is divided on this matter. There is also this question, by no means answerable at present: Is more necessarily better?

It is also obvious that physical health has an effect on growth. Children with serious organic disease such as congenital heart disease, nephritis, or some of the inborn errors of metabolism do not grow as do normal children. The decreased incidence of serious acute disease in children since the introduction of antibiotics and improved immunization procedures may play a role in the larger size of today's children. Emotional factors also affect growth. Infants deprived of maternal care fail to gain weight adequately even on excellent diets. But here, as in so many places in human development, the resultant growth depends not only upon the amount and kind of emotional deprivation but also upon the inherent traits of the child reacting to the deprivation.

An interesting trend in growth over the last hundred years is thought probably to be related to nutrition. The data on heights and weights of school children indicate that the whole process of growth has been undergoing a speeding-up process. Children born in the 1930s are appreciably larger at age 5 (and probably before) than children born at the beginning of the century (Meredith, 1941). The amount of this secular change is quite considerable. Figure 8-9 gives data from Sweden dating back to 1883 (Broman, Dahlberg, and Lichtenstein, 1942). This is one of the earliest cross-sectional studies. Unfortunately the youngest children measured were 7 years old, but at this age the data from 1938 show that the increased size of the twentieth-century children was clearly apparent at age 7 and continued to adult life.

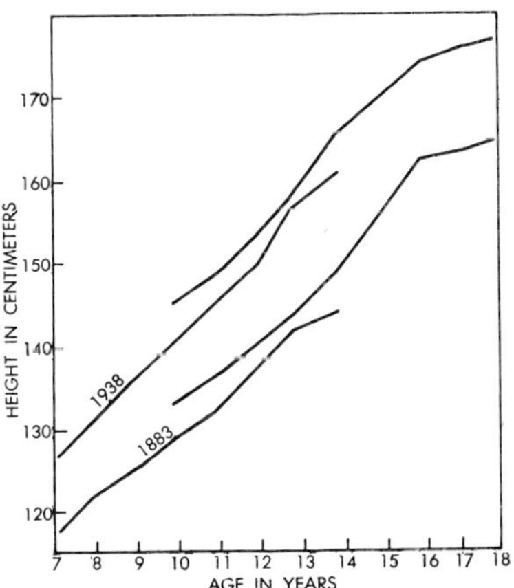

Fig. 8-9. Secular trend in height: Swedish children measured in 1883 and 1938. (*From Browman, Dahlberg, and Lichtenstein, Heights and Weights During Growth, Acta Paediat, Upsala, 30:1, 1942.*)

American (Meredith, 1941), British (Clements, 1953) and Swedish (Broman et al., 1942) data all give similar trends. The average gain between 1880 and 1950 is about 1½ cm and ½ kg per decade at ages 5 to 7 and about 2 cm and ½ kg per decade during puberty. The fully grown adult (Tanner, 1956) has increased in height about 1 cm per decade for the past century.

Hathaway compared the figures obtained by various American investigators from 1902 to 1952 (Fig. 8-10). The data from Hathaway's compilations are averages based on cross-sectional studies. Data from Bayley's longitudinal study of California children showed a similar increase

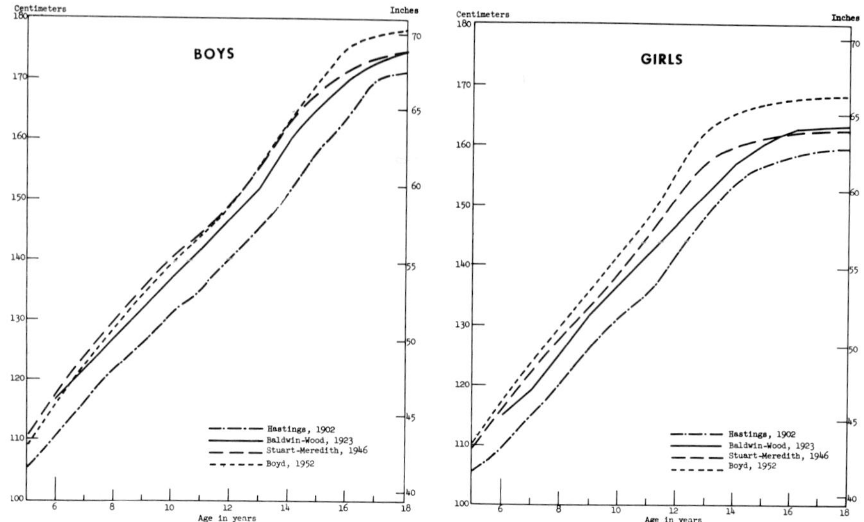

Fig. 8-10. Average heights of American children by various investigators. (*From Hathaway, Height and Weights in Children and Youths in the U.S., U.S. Dept. Agric., 1957.*)

in size of the children over their parents. The range of heights and weights at all ages has been unaffected over the years. There have been, and still are, big children and adults and little ones. But big and little alike are all a little bigger than they used to be.

How long has the secular trend been in operation? There is very little reliable data before 1880; however, Robert, in 1876 made a significant comment in discussing the physical requirements of factory children: "A factory child of the present day at the age of 7 years weighs as much as one of 8 did in 1833—each age has gained one year in 40 years" (Tanner, 1955); and Clements comments on the small size of the armor worn in the Middle Ages.

In this connection it should be pointed out that uniformly a high socioeconomic level is reflected in greater weight gains. Every study made the world over has shown that those children from the more privileged groups gain more and gain it sooner than the less privileged in any society. This class differential can be seen in overlapping data on Swedish children in Fig. 8-8. The children of the younger ages (7 to 14) came from the elementary school; their parents were in general of a lower economic level than the children of 10 to 18, who were drawn from the secondary schools. The class differential is apparent both in the early data and in the twentieth-century data.

The effect of socioeconomic levels has been demonstrated in many studies (Meredith, 1941). Chinese girls of upper class in Hong Kong grow larger and mature earlier than girls of similar genetic background but of a less favored economic level (Lee, Chang, and Chan, 1963). That economic level makes a difference is a clearly established fact. Why it should be so is not so clear. Probably, like the secular trend, nutrition is a factor, but so too may be other factors, like regularity of sleep and meals, more outdoor exercise, better medical care—factors that go along with a higher level of education and greater ease of life in the more prosperous groups in any society.

Does climate have an effect on growth? Mills has made a case for the gradual change in the world temperature to be at least partly responsible for the secular trend. He suggests that difficulty in heat loss may retard human growth as it does in experimental animals. However, current studies on children in the tropics and in temperate and cold regions do not seem to bear out this hypothesis. Race and climate are difficult factors to disentangle from nutrition and socioeconomic level. West African children (Mackay, 1952) are a good deal retarded in relation to American children, but white and Negroes in New York City in similar economic circumstances showed no appreciable differences (Michelson, 1944), indicating that race was not a significant factor here. But how about climate? Using age of menarche (see below) as a criterion, Ellis gives 14.3 years as the mean age at menarche in Nigerian school girls of upper socioeconomic level and Levine 14.4 years as that of Eskimo girls. Wilson and Sutherland found the expected class difference in school girls in Colombo, Ceylon, to range from 12.8 years for the menarche in the upper group to 14.4 years in the lower, about the same class differential as found in the temperate zone.

Japanese children (Ito, 1942) born and reared in California were taller and heavier than children of similar parentage who remained in Japan. The California-reared Japanese children were also more advanced in skeletal development than the children who remained in Japan. This difference is usually attributed to better food and generally better living conditions, although the possible effect of climate cannot be ignored.

The effect of climate, if any, on growth is difficult to distinguish from the other variables affecting the children measured; however, it is clear that season has a definite influence on growth (Palmer, 1933; Reynolds and Sontag, 1944). In the Northern Hemisphere, October, November, and December are the months of greatest weight gain, and it may be five or six times as much as during the months of April, May, and June, when weight gain is at a minimum (Fig. 8-11). About two-thirds of the annual gain in weight is made in the fall (the 6 months from September to February) and only one-third in the remaining 6 months of the year. Height gains are maximum in April, May, and June, and minimal in September, October, and November. The reason for the seasonal variation is quite unknown. It appears in well-nourished children as well as in poorly nourished ones. Suggestions have been made that hormone secretions are involved or that environmental temperatures or length of day are factors.

The age at which the changes of puberty take place is basically a genetically determined phenomenon; nevertheless, malnutrition can delay the events of puberty. In the secular trend the age of puberty is most pronounced. Maturation occurs earlier now than it did a century ago. Kiil found the average age of menarche of Norwegian girls in 1850 to be 17.0 years and in 1950 13.5 years. In the United States the average age of menarche has dropped from 14.2 years in 1900 to 12.9 years in 1950 (Mills, 1950) (Fig. 8-12). The effect of the economic depression as measured in Hagerstown, Maryland, was not sufficient to affect the growth of children measured. Nevertheless there was a demonstrable retardation of the age at which both boys and girls matured. Similar data were obtained both in France and in Belgium during World War II.

It would appear that the human body has to grow a certain amount before puberty can take place. If growth takes place rapidly, puberty comes early; if growth is slow, puberty must wait until the body has reached the requisite size, or more likely, maturity level.

The speed with which the human body *can* grow is doubtless genetically determined, but the actual speed is the resultant of the genetic potential and the opportunity afforded by the environment.

CONCLUSIONS

The following conclusions on the nature of human growth seem reasonably substantiated:

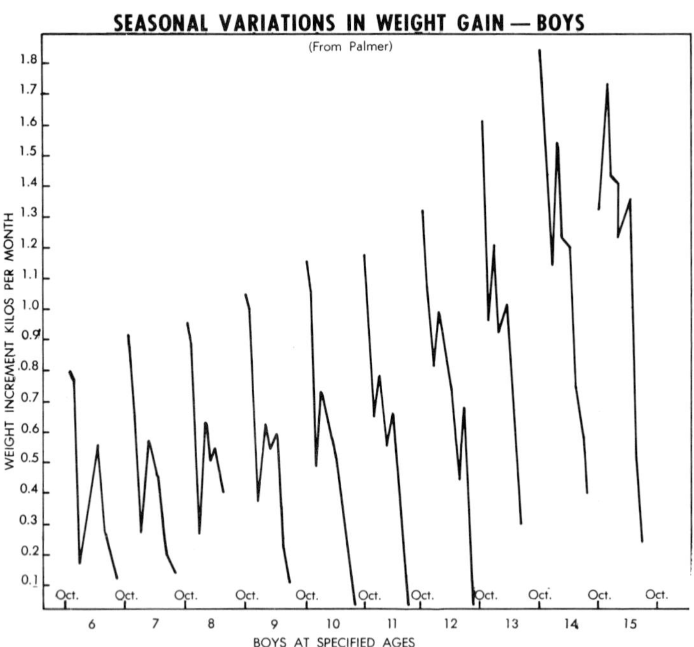

Fig. 8-11. Seasonal variations in weight gain in boys. (*From Palmer,* Seasonal variations in average growth in weight and height of elementary school children. (*Pub. Health Rep. Wash., 48:211, 1933.*)

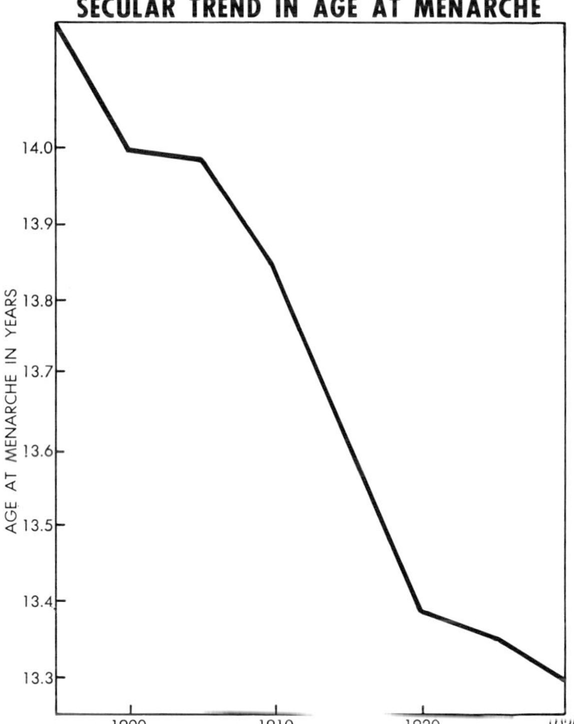

Fig. 8-12. Secular trend in age of menarche. *(From Mills, Temperature Influence on Human Growth and Development, Human Biol. 22:71, 1950, by permission of Wayne State Univ. Press.)*

1. All children possess the potential for a pattern of growth characteristically human; every child (barring those with gross defects) passes through the same stages as every other child. These stages are related to most of the measurable aspects of growth, such as physical measurements, development of organs, and maturation of function and behavior.

2. The differences among normal children, within the range of the human pattern, are large. These differences are reflected not only in the magnitude of the measurements but in the tempo of growth itself.

3. Correlations exist between various aspects of growth. A child who deviates from the mean with respect to one type of growth is apt to deviate proportionately in other aspects. While correlations between the various aspects of growth are frequent, they are by no means universal; in some children progression is less uniform than in others.

4. Genetic and endocrine factors are responsible for the basic patterns of growth and maturation. These patterns tend to persist through the life span, contributing to the uniformity of individual growth.

5. Genetic patterns can be modified by environmental factors, such as disease, nutrition, emotions. The effect of quantitatively similar environmental factors varies, depending both on the time in the life cycle when specific deprivations occur and, probably, on the genetic makeup of the individual on whom they are acting.

9

Assessment of Physical Growth

The use of physical size as a means of assessing health depends upon the assumption that each child has an inherent growth potential and that he will achieve his optimal size if the conditions of his life are satisfactory and, conversely, that he will fail in the attainment of his own optimum if he is subjected to stress. Size is a tricky criterion to use clinically, because the best estimates of an individual child's pattern are crude. Nevertheless, the physician, the parents, and the child himself all stand to profit from as much understanding as possible of what a child's inherited qualities with respect to size hold for him.

THE SEARCH FOR GROWTH STANDARDS

Over the years a good many different growth standards have been devised and used. In 1943 data from the Iowa Child Welfare Research Station were compiled by Meredith and published by Jackson and Kelly as charts. These charts give the median and the 16th and 84th percentile for weights of boys and girls. Charts for boys are shown in Figs. 9-1 and 9-2. The data for boys from the Harvard Growth Study, published by Stuart and Meredith are given in Figs. 9-3 and 9-4.

These charts are simple to use; it is not always so easy to interpret the results. If a child's height and weight are plotted on one of these standard charts, it is easy to see whether or not his growth is following a pattern similar to that of the standards. If the child's tempo of growth is within the range of the usual, it can be expected that his growth will be parallel to the standards, and deviations above and below the median can be attributed to his constitutional size. Big children can be expected to have growth curves approaching the upper percentile; little ones, the lower percentiles. However, these charts have only a limited usefulness in following the growth of children whose deviations from the norm are due to their tempo of growth, rather than to their constitutional size. A fast-maturing child will reach his full height earlier, but he may not attain a greater height than his more leisurely growing peers.

In 1956 Bayley introduced a set of standards based on longitudinally collected measurements of children which took into consideration not only body build but also the tempo of growth. These standards are reported

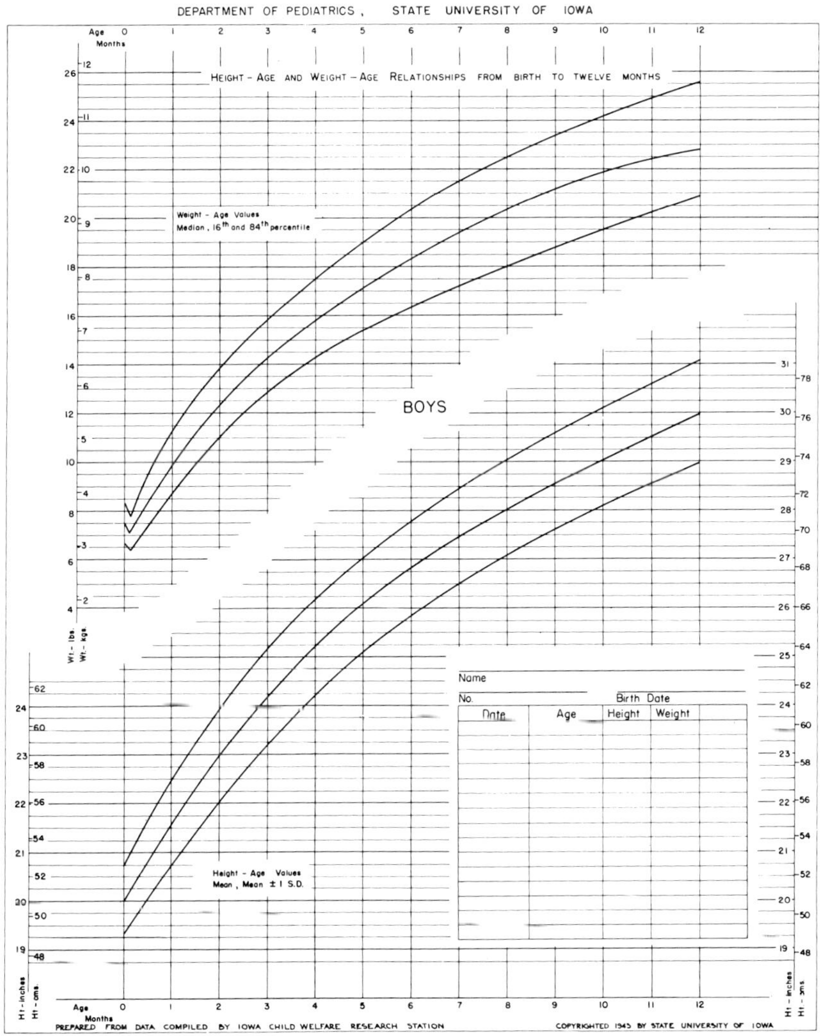

Fig. 9-1. University of Iowa chart of weight and height—boys age 0-1 year. (*From Jackson and Kelly Growth Charts for use in Pediatric Practice, J. Pediat., 27:215, 1945, and copyrighted by State University of Iowa.*)

together with other growth charts by Bayer and Bayley (1959) (Figs. 9-5 and 9-6). Three hundred healthy middle-class California children from European ancestry, an equal number from each sex, were followed from birth to maturity. Anthropometric measurements of these children were recorded periodically. After the children grew up, the data were sorted out, and various patterns of growth were identified.

In the study there were big children and little ones, fast maturers and slow maturers. It was found that the various identifiable patterns of growth were closely related to sex, weight at 1 year, and skeletal age.

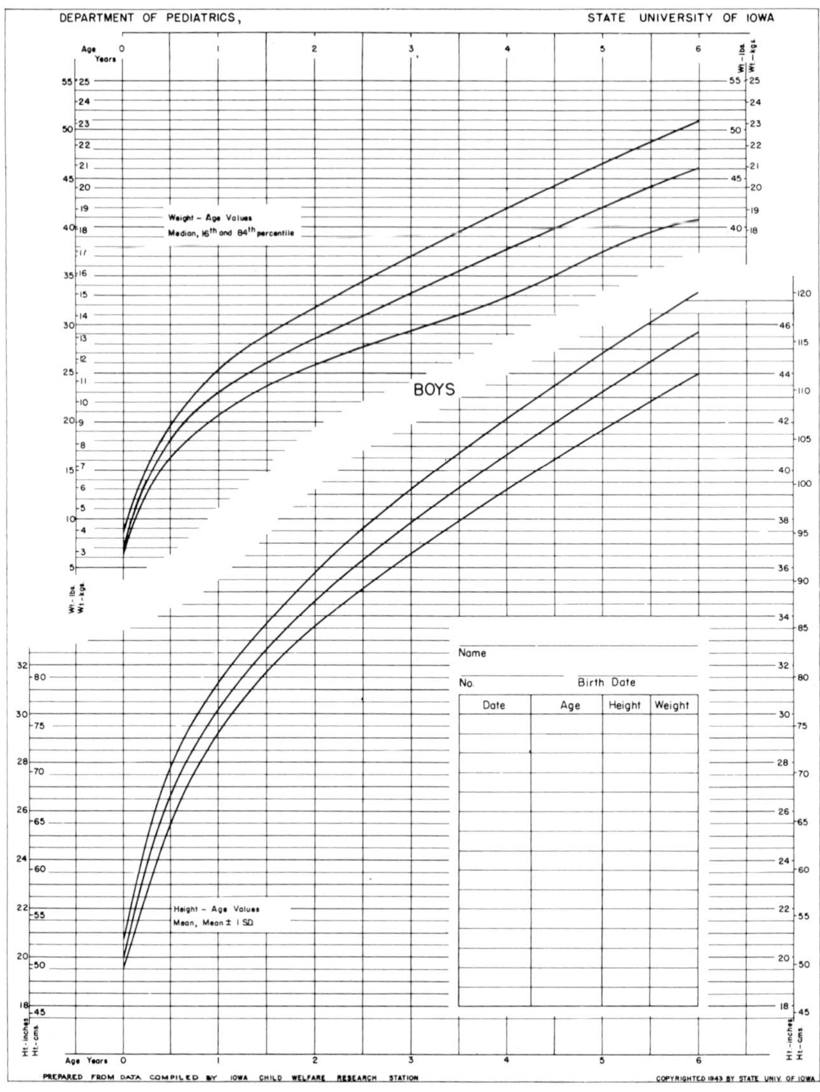

Fig. 9-2. University of Iowa chart of weight and height—boys 0-6 years.

These items seemed to represent criteria at an early age of inherent genetically determined growth potential. Data from children who fall within such genetic units were put together into groups and charts constructed of their growth performance. Against such standards, the performance of other children can be measured.

While most children maintained the same growth pattern throughout the growing years, there are exceptions in apparently healthy children. The time when a shift of pattern is most likely to take place is when the dominant influence on growth shifts from direct genetic control to endocrine control—to the hypophysis at about age 3 or 4 and to the gonads in early puberty. At these times slight endocrine shifts can slow down an accelerated youngster or speed up a retarded one. Such changes call for a clinical appraisal of the child to make sure there is no reason for his altered growth

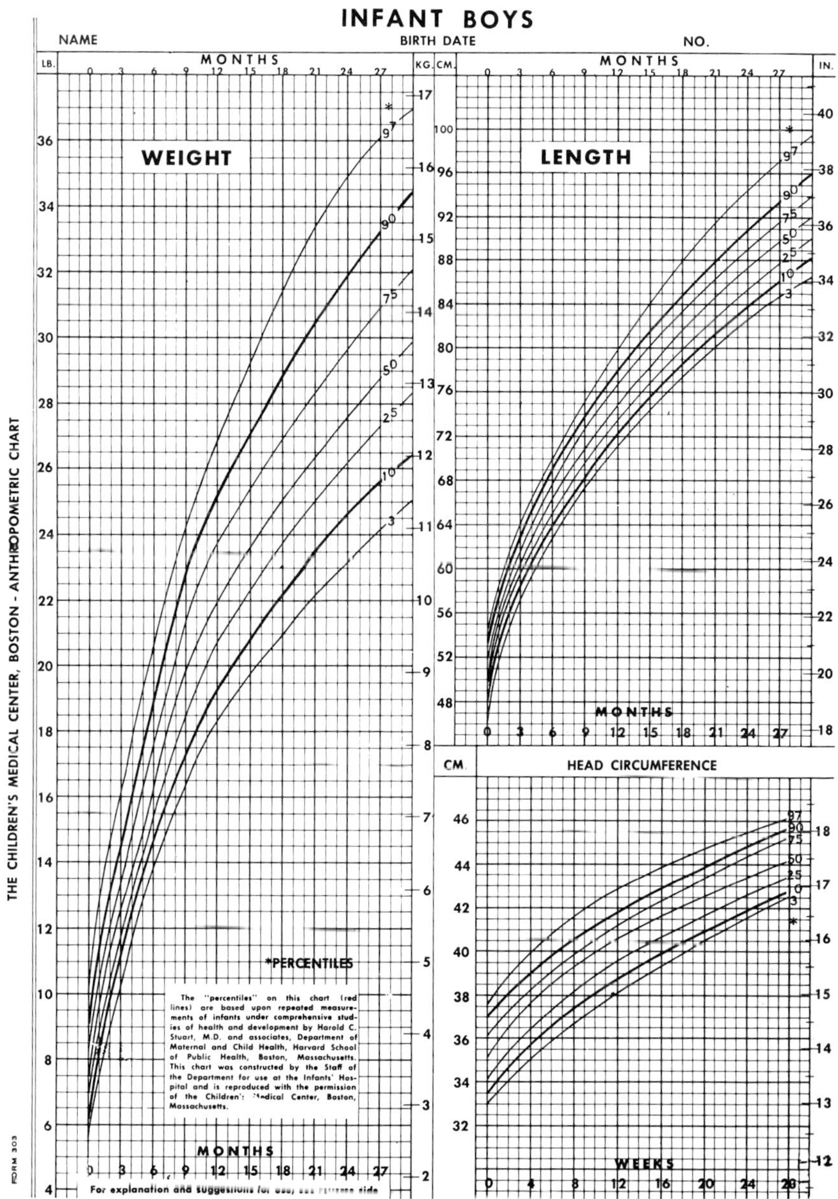

Fig. 9-3. Children's Medical Center, Boston, chart of weight and height—boys 0-1 year. (*From Reed and Stuart, Patterns of Growth in Height and Weight from Birth to Eighteen Years of Age, Pediatrics 24:supp., 904, 1959.*)

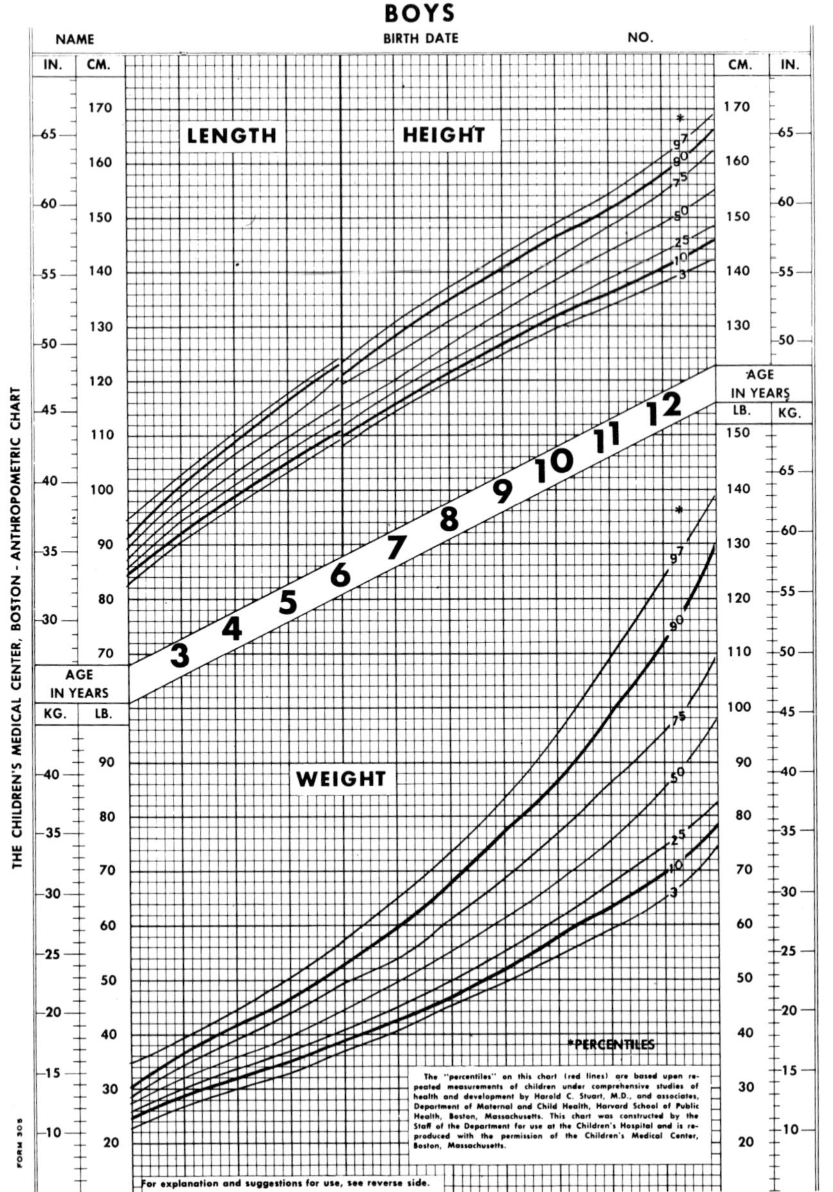

Fig. 9-4. Children's Medical Center, Boston, chart of weight and height—boys 2-12 years.

pattern other than the apparently normal growth shifts (Bayley, 1956).

For more extensive investigation of growth adequacy than can be achieved from weight, height, and skeletal age, Bayer and Bayley make use of additional measurements—shoulder breadth (biacromial), pelvic breadth (bicristal), and sitting height. From these measurements the following indices can be calculated: weight/height; sitting height/height; shoulder width/height; pelvic width/height and shoulder width.

Bayer and Bayley describe four types of profiles:

1. Normal—all measurements fall within one Standard Deviation of the norm.
2. Unusual in size but normal in proportion.
   Absolute measurements are consistently above or below 1 S.D. of the mean, but the indices fall within 1 S.D. These are the big children or the small children but average in tempo of growth.

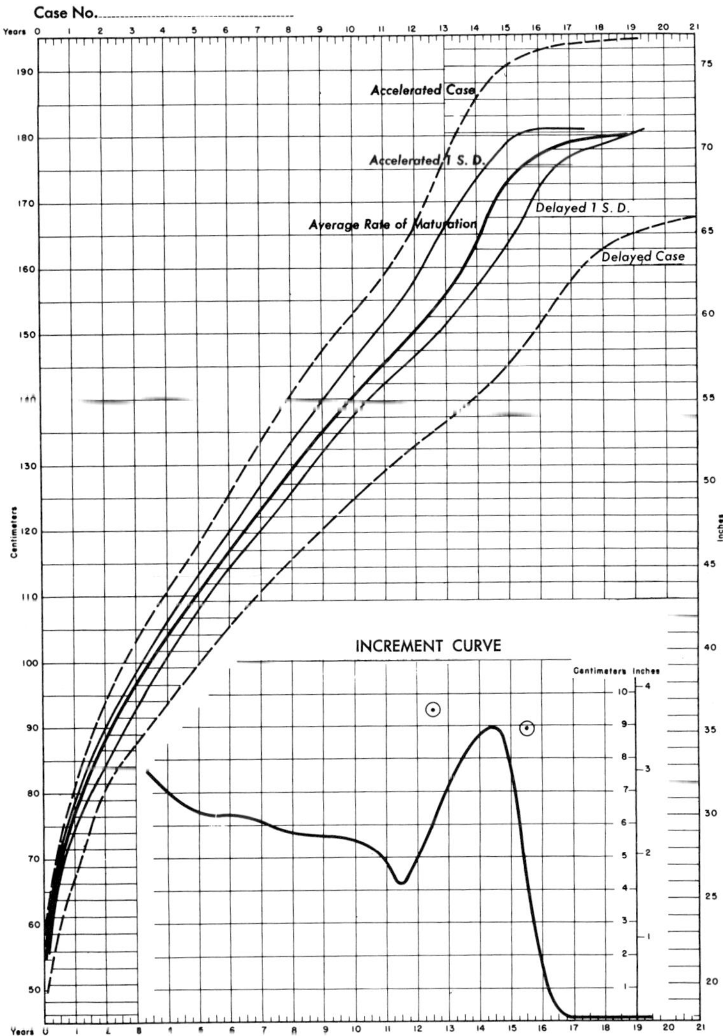

Fig. 9-5. Height chart by age for boys—average, accelerated, and retarded rates of maturation. (*From Bayley, J. Pediat., 48:187, 1956, with permission of C. V. Mosby Co., St. Louis.*)

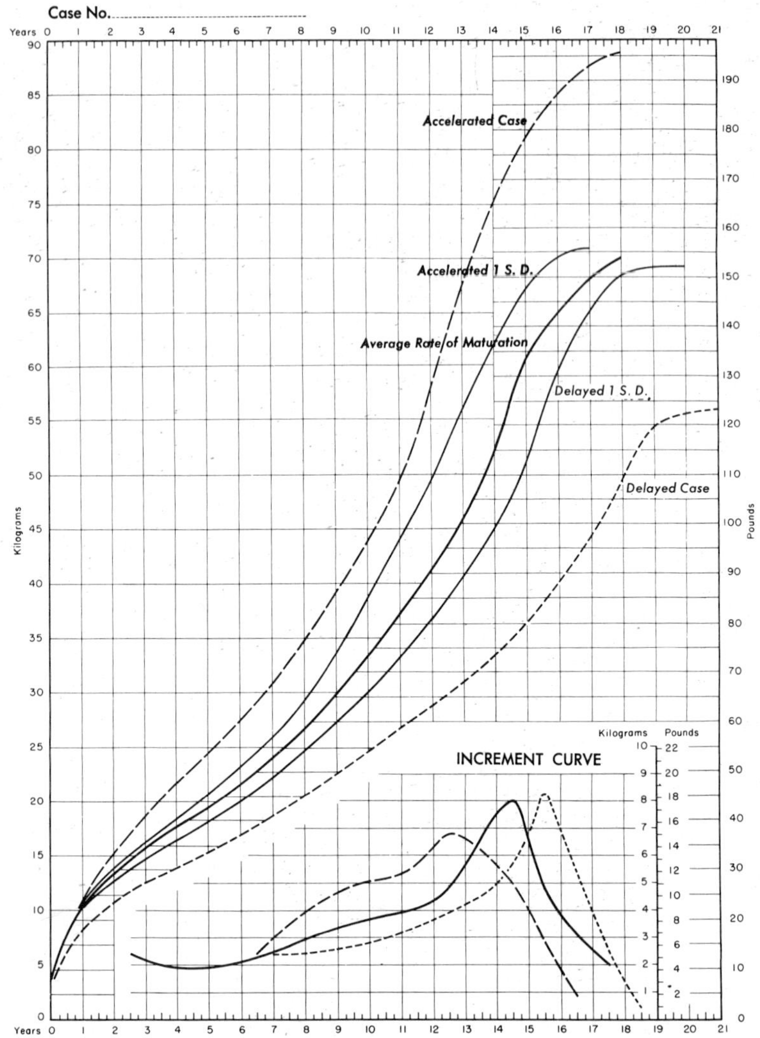

Fig. 9-6. Weight chart by age for boys—average, accelerated, and retarded rates of maturation. (*From Bayley, J. Pediat., 48:187, 1956, with permission of C. V. Mosby Co., St. Louis.*)

3. Unusual in both size and proportion.
   All measurements, both absolute and indices, fall outside plus or minus 1 S.D. of the mean. In such a record, if the child's measurements are replotted against the norms for his height peers, his whole profile moves toward the mean if the child's deviation is due to his tempo of growth. He is large or small because he is growing up faster or slower than the average.
4. Disharmonious—measurements fall erratically outside 1 S.D. of the mean and are not brought closer to the mean by adjustment to his height peers. Such a pattern calls for further investigation.

An individual child whose measurements fall in any one of the first three profiles can be considered to be growing satisfactorily. If he falls in group 4, his growth requires careful scrutiny.

PROCEDURES IN ASSESSING GROWTH

During the First Year

At birth, the child's weight, length, shoulder and pelvic breadth, and head and chest circumference are recorded. His measurements are of little immediate value in his general appraisal. They will be of greater value later on as reference points. The infant's health is determined from the general physical findings.

In the first few days after birth all infants lose some weight. The amount of this weight loss is variable and depends upon how soon after birth the infant is ready to eat. If the labor has been long and hard, the infant, as well as the mother, is tired out and needs rest before he is interested in sucking. Also if the mother has had a good deal of anesthesia during labor, the infant will be sleepy and uninterested in eating.

Once the infant begins to eat, he begins to gain weight. Usually by the end of the first week, the full-term infant has regained his birth weight and proceeds to add substance to his body. For the first few months gain in weight is rapid, and then it begins to slow down (Norval)

Just how rapid should this gain be for the particular infant under consideration? What is his inherent gene-determined potential? We do not know. It is necessary to use considerable caution in equating rate of growth with well-being during the first year. Criteria other than weight must always be considered.

At birth the child's sex is obvious, but this is not much help, since during infancy there is little difference between the growth of boys and girls. Birth weight is also known, but again this is not very helpful. The child may have greater potential for postnatal growth than his prenatal performance would indicate.

Among term infants the difference of a week or two before or after the calculated normal duration of pregnancy makes a difference in birth weight. The infant born slightly ahead of schedule is smaller than his "normal" birth weight, and probably his ability to grow is closer to that of the near-term fetus than to the slower rate of the slightly older-term infant. The converse, that the post-term infant has a greater birth weight, is not always true. Some infants appear to lose weight during an extra week or two in utero.

At birth there is no knowledge about an infant's tempo of growth, nor of his body constitution. About all that is known is that he is a human baby and will roughly follow the general human pattern. His growth increments will be progressively less each month during his first year. Average figures, compiled from large numbers of infants of all sorts of genetic backgrounds, are as follows:

Age, months	Increment, lb/month
0–3	2
3–6	1½
6–9	1
9–12	½

In very few individual infants will weight gain be exactly like these averages; nevertheless, the figures may be of some small use to the physician as he plots monthly increments on a graph and attempts to estimate a child's potential. If an infant's growth curve begins to flatten out appreciably more than that of children of his initial size, the physician is alerted to look for the cause of growth failure, although deviation in the curve of an individual infant from published standards may prove nothing more than that the infant is establishing his true growth potential. Figure 9-7 shows the growth data of two infants whose growth deviated appreciably from the expected figures. Infant K. P. gained both height and weight more rapidly than his initial size suggested. Careful scrutiny of his physical organism and his home climate revealed no cause for excessive growth. By the end of the first year he had established the pattern which he then maintained.

Infant B. C., on the other hand, gained both height and weight as expected for the first 2 months of life. His weight increment then became less than expected, although his height curve was as expected. Clinically the child looked well. He was neither apathetic nor irritable, nor was there any evidence of a pathologic condition. It was only the meager growth increments that suggested that he was not thriving as well as he might. He was a breast-fed infant. When supplements of cow's milk were given, his weight jumped up, an indication that the failure to gain was indeed due to malnutrition.

Growth of the Premature Infant

Weight curves for premature infants of varying gestational ages have been constructed by Lubchenco et al. (Fig. 9-8). With this chart it is possible to plot the weight of a premature infant of known gestational age and determine whether or not he is progressing after birth at about the rate that could have been expected from the weight he achieved during his abbreviated intrauterine stay. As with full-term infants, the weight gain of a premature must be interpreted with caution. Nevertheless marked deviations from expected growth constitute a danger signal that calls for investigation. In Fig. 9-9 is plotted the growth of I.O. against the Lubchenco chart. This child proved to have an atrial septic defect. It was the growth failure rather than a cardiac murmur that proved to be the earliest alerting sign of impending trouble.

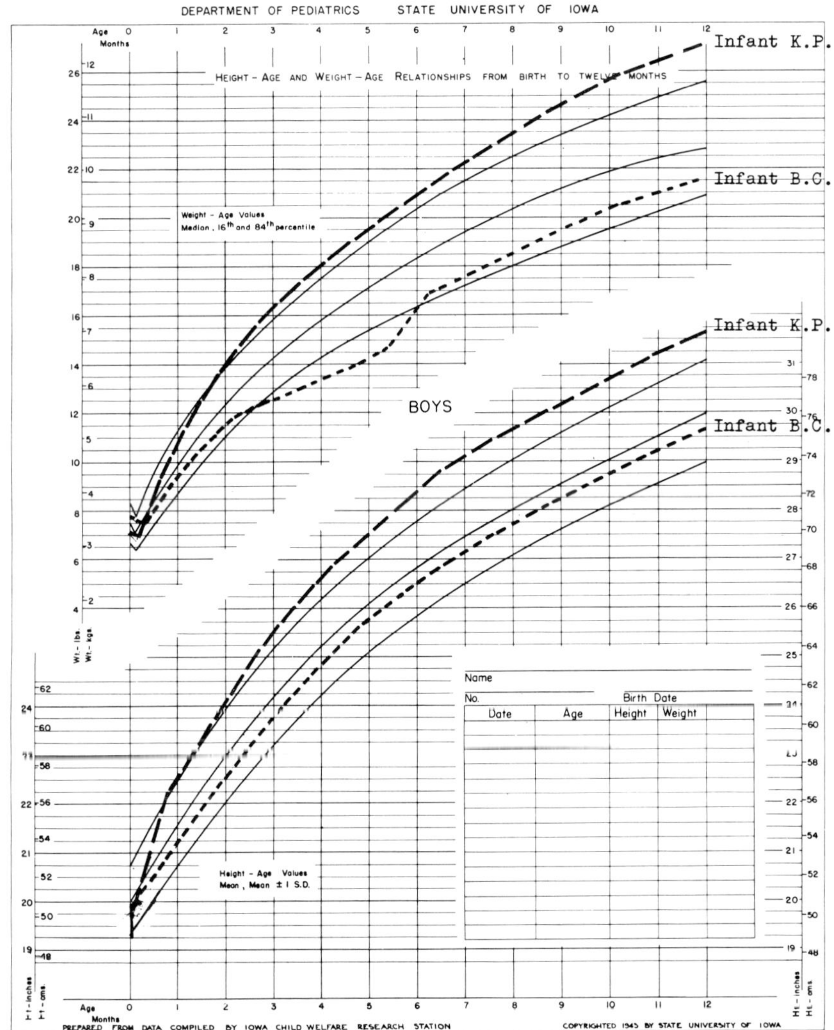

Fig. 9-7. Growth in weight and height of two infants whose measurements deviated appreciably from the standard.

Growth of Twins

It might be expected that monozygous twins would resemble each other in growth pattern both before and after birth, and in many cases they do; however, occasionally monozygous twins have markedly dissimilar weights at birth. Babson et al. studied a group of twins in whom one twin weighed 25 per cent less than the other at birth. He found not only that the runt seldom caught up to his twin but also that his IQ was appreciably lower. Babson postulates that this discrepancy in achievement of the pairs of twins is due to intrauterine environment and placental physiology. His work raises

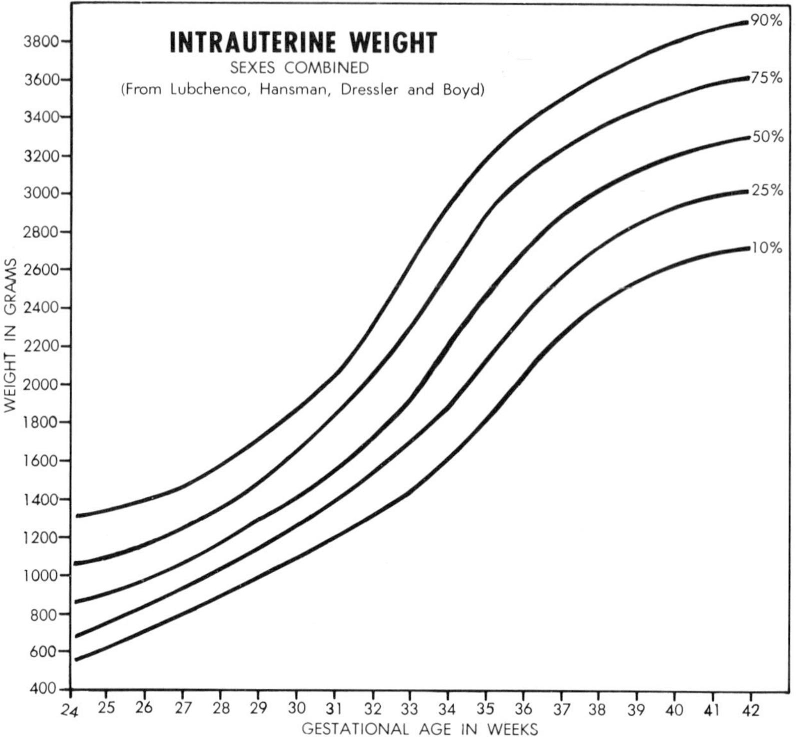

Fig. 9-8. Intrauterine weight. (*From Lubchenco, Hansman, Dressler, and Boyd, Intrauterine Growth as Estimated from Liveborn Birth Weight, Pediatrics 32:793, 1963.*)

the question of how often a single infant, smaller than expected at birth, may have suffered from similar intrauterine hazards.

After the First Year

After the first birthday, the Bayer and Bayley standards mentioned above can be used. In Figs. 9-5 and 9-6 the Bayley norms for boys from 1 to 21 years of age are given. The central curve represents the growth of average-sized children, maturing at an average rate. When plotted on the chart, most children's curves will be closely similar to these.

A child whose growth deviates considerably from the central curve needs to be further appraised. His tempo of growth can be roughly estimated clinically by his apparent maturity in muscular, emotional, and intellectual growth, but it can be much more accurately determined by an x-ray of his hand and wrist and estimation of his skeletal age (see Chap. 10). If his skeletal age and chronological age are less than 1 year apart, it can be assumed that he is either a large or a small person genetically and that his growth pattern will follow that of the large or small children in the graph. If the child's tempo of growth is accelerated or retarded by more than

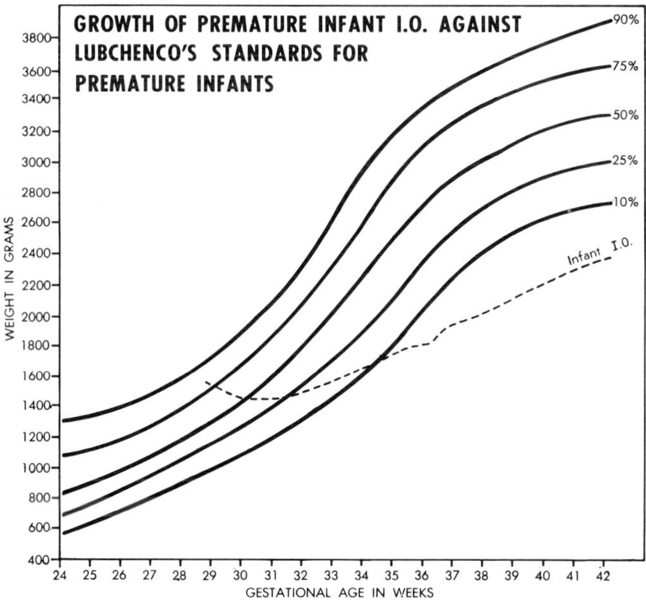

Fig. 9-9. Growth of premature infant "I.O." against Lubchenco's standards for premature infants.

1 year, his growth, when replotted according to his skeletal age, will approximate the standard more nearly like his own pattern. In Fig. 9-10 is plotted the growth of a boy who was large from an early age. This boy's skeletal age proved to be less than 6 months below his chronological age.

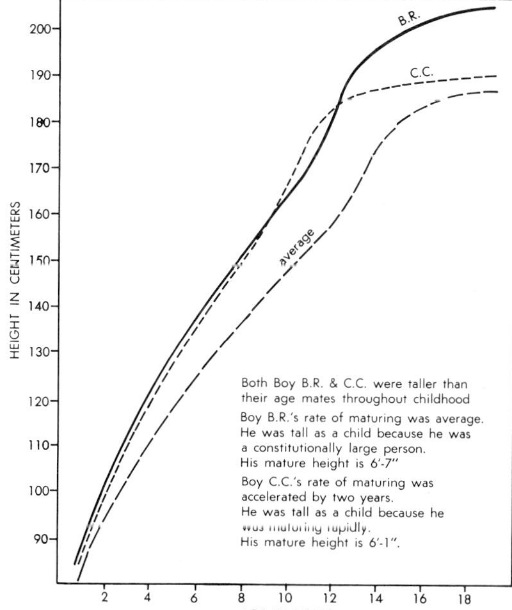

Fig. 9-10. Growth of two boys large for age in early childhood.

It could therefore be predicted before puberty that he would become an unusually large man. On the same chart is plotted the growth of another boy also larger than average in early childhood; however, this boy's skeletal age was 2 years advanced over his chronological age. When his height data was shifted to his skeletal rather than his chronological age, it became apparent that his ultimate height would fall far below that of the first boy.

More accurate predictions of adult height can be obtained by use of the Bayley and Pinneau height prediction tables reprinted in Table 9-1.

TABLE 9-1

Percent of Mature Height Achieved at Each Age

Age in years	BOYS			GIRLS		
	Average	Accelerated	Retarded	Average	Accelerated	Retarded
Birth	28.6			30.9		
1	42.2	44.5	40.4	44.7	48.0	42.2
2	49.5	51.3	47.0	52.8	54.7	50.0
3	53.8	55.6	51.6	57.0	60.0	55.0
4	58.0	60.0	58.0	61.8	64.9	59.8
5	61.8	64.0	59.7	66.2	69.3	63.8
6	65.2	67.8	63.8	79.3	73.4	67.8
7	69.0	70.5	66.8	74.0	76.0	71.5
8	72.0	73.5	69.8	77.5	79.5	74.5
9	75.0	76.5	73.2	80.7	83.5	77.7
10	78.0	79.7	76.4	84.4	87.9	81.0
11	81.1	83.4	79.5	88.4	92.9	84.9
12	84.2	87.2	82.2	92.9	96.6	88.2
13	87.3	91.3	84.6	96.5	98.2	91.1
14	91.5	95.8	87.6	98.3	99.1	95.2
15	96.1	98.3	91.6	99.1	99.5	97.8
16	98.3	99.4	95.7	99.6	99.5	98.9
16.5					100.0	
17	99.3	99.9	98.2	100.0		99.6
17.5		100.0				
18	99.8		99.2			100.0
18.5	100.0					
19.0			99.8			
20.0			100.0			

SOURCE: Bayley and Pinneau, Tables for Predicting Adult Height from Skeletal Age, revised for use with Greulich and Pyle, Hand Standards, *J. Pediat.*, 40:423, 1952. Permission of The C. V. Mosby Company, St. Louis and the University of California Institute of Human Development, Berkeley, Calif.

From data on sex, chronological age, height, and skeletal age, these tables give predicted adult stature. For children over the age of 9 years, the predictions are appreciably more accurate than for younger children.

While these standards are useful, they are far from absolute, and there is plenty of room for clinical judgment in the appraisal of any one child.

USE OF GROWTH DATA

Growth failure has many causes. Once a physician has determined that a child's growth pattern deviates more than can be accounted for on the basis of normal physiologic variations, it behooves him to ferret out the cause of the deviant growth. In Table 9-2 is given a list of possible causes

TABLE 9-2

Causes of Growth Deviations

Growth Failure
1. Malnutrition
   a. Inadequate ingestion
   b. Inadequate absorption
2. Metabolic disorders
   a. Congenital heart disease
   b. Renal disease (chronic)
   c. Pulmonary disease (chronic)
   d. Cystic fibrosis of pancreas
   e. Inborn errors of metabolism
   f. Endocrine diseases
3. Psychogenic causes
4. Primordial dwarfism

Excessive Growth
1. Endocrine gigantism
2. Primordial gigantism
3. Obesity
   a. Dietary
   b. Endocrine

of both retarded and excessive growth. Full discussion of the differential diagnoses of these various conditions is beyond the scope of this book.

Growth data, however, have another use. They are valuable in interpreting to parents the phenomenon of growth in general and their own child's particular pattern. A mother needs to know something about the overall human pattern of growth. She needs to know that growth normally slows down toward the end of the first year, that it is slow and steady through the years of childhood, and that it speeds up during puberty. A mother with this foreknowledge will not be tempted to try to force her child to eat more than he needs in early childhood, and she is alerted to the fact that in puberty refrigerator raiding is to be expected and had best be planned for.

A child whose size is larger or smaller than his peers is often a cause of anxiety to parents. Some parents go to extraordinary lengths to try to make a child conform to their idea of what he should be. They may pour tonics, vitamins, minerals, proteins into him, make him take extra naps and go to bed early. But if the child is plugging along according to the pattern in his genes, all the parents' efforts do is create tension and anxiety If the child's unusual size is due to his tempo of growth, this can be explained to his parents, and they can be assured that his ultimate size will be within the range of the usual.

A child whose potential appears to indicate that he will ultimately deviate considerably from the usual creates greater difficulty for the parents. The parents must be assured that no remediable pathologic condition is influencing the child's size (if this be the case). Then the child's pattern of growth *must* be accepted. It cannot be changed any more than can the color of his eyes be changed. Foreknowledge, explanation, sympathetic understanding of parental concern is of help in providing for the child an acceptance and appreciation of himself as he is. Satisfactions other than brawn must be found for the small boy if he is to grow up with a feeling of self-competency.

As the child reaches puberty, he himself is often concerned about his size, especially if he is different from his peers. This is an age when conformity is all-important to the youngster and when, if he is different, he will worry about his "abnormality." Such a child can be helped by explanations of the nature of growth, what his own pattern is, when he can be expected to mature, and how big he will probably become (see Chap. 12).

10

Tempo of Growth

Our usual orientation with respect to time is based on the clock and the calendar. The relativity of time, however, is recognized in common language. "Time flies" or "hangs heavy" according to inner feelings and quite regardless of the movement of the heavenly bodies.

The ticking of the clock is but one way of measuring time. It is the custom to measure life in terms of the calendar, but children do not grow by the calendar. Each child grows according to some mechanism deep within his genes which determines how much growing he will accomplish in each unit of conventionally measured time.

Look at the picture in Fig. 10-1. Each of these girls has spent 12 sun-measured years growing, but what different amounts of growing each has done. Girl A is still a child. Her body has been taking a leisurely pace. She shows no evidence of puberty; she has a lot of growing still to do. Girl D at the

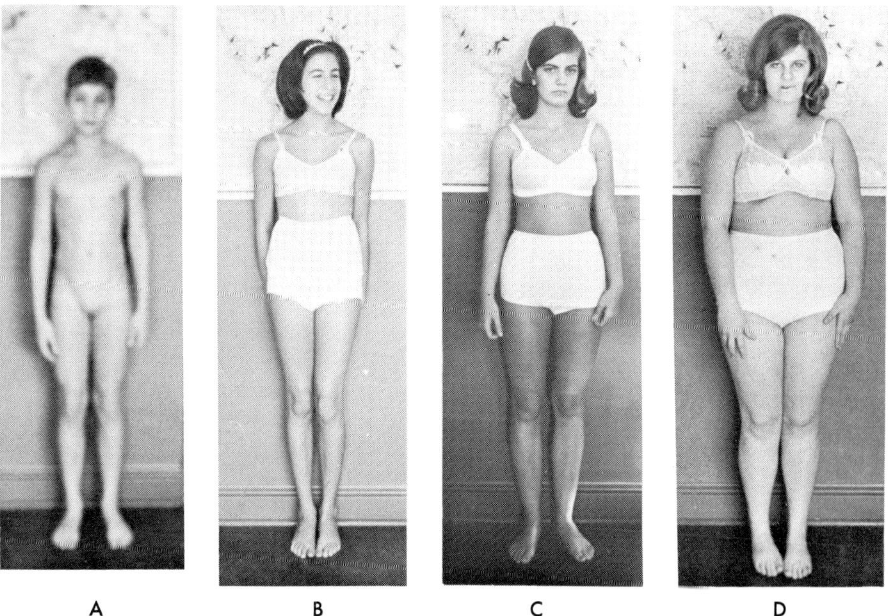

Fig. 10-1. Four girls who show different rates of maturing. *A.* Age 12 years 1 month, no menarche. *B.* Age 12 years 6 months, menarche age 12-6. C. Age 12 years 7 months, menarche age 11-6. *D.* Age 12 years 2 months, menarche age 9-6.

other extreme has an internal speedometer set at a higher speed. At 12 she has reached her adult height and is physically a woman. Girls B and C are neither as slow as A nor as speedy as D. To call all four of these girls "12" does not put them into a common group that has much significance.

This difference in speed is an inherent trait, probably present from the time of conception. Girl D's time mechanism has been crowding more than 60 seconds into each conventional minute all her life. At puberty it is easy to distinguish the A, B, C and D girls. At birth it is not so easy, though any observant person is aware that there is a difference in maturity of children of the same age. The early maturers are often larger than the slow maturers. Size, however, is an inadequate criterion of speed. There are genes for size which are not the same as the genes for speed; sometimes slow children are big and speedy ones small. To distinguish the speedy from the slow before puberty, some objective measure for development is needed other than chronological age.

While the speed of traveling through life varies from person to person, everyone does travel the same path. There is a fixed *order* in which development proceeds, even though there is variation in the age at which specific milestones are reached.

The regularity of the developmental pattern is obvious from conception. In the embryo, the heart always begins to beat before the organ is differentiated into its ultimate chambers, and spinal reflexes are established before nerve connections are made with the cerebrum. The order is genetically controlled and reflects the whole phylogenetic pattern that has led to man. It continues throughout the entire life span. The speed with which age brings about changes in one organ system reflects the speed of the organism as a whole.

The skeleton follows its genetically controlled developmental plan and can be used as an index of the speed of growth in the total organism. Maturation of bony tissue is relatively simple to follow by means of x-rays of the hand and wrist. Before birth, the bones of hand and wrist are laid down in cartilage, after which ossification begins. The process of ossification continues from midfetal life until maturity. At birth the shafts of the metacarpals and the phalanges are ossified and are visible in the x-ray. None of the carpal bones are ossified, and therefore they cannot be seen in the x-ray. Soon after birth, the carpal bones begin to ossify and can be seen as small opaque areas in the previously vacant space of the wrist, between metacarpals and radius and ulna. The capitate is always the first to be visible, soon followed by the hamate; the others follow in regular sequence (Table 10-1). In due course ossification centers appear in the epiphyses of radius, ulna, metacarpals, and phalanges, and ultimately these epiphyses fuse with the shaft of the bone. Epiphyseal fusion, like the appearance of ossification centers, appears first in one bone, later in another, in an orderly sequence (Fig. 10-2).

TABLE 10-1

Sequence of Ossification of the Bones of Hand and Wrist

Order of appearance	Ossification center	Mean average time of appearance in months	
		Girls	Boys
1.	Capitate	3.0	4.5
2.	Hamate	4.5	6.0
3.	Distal epiphysis of the radius	9.8	13.2
4.	Epiphysis of the proximal phalanx, digit 3	10.0	15.0
5.	Epiphysis of the proximal phalanx, digit 2	10.8	16.1
6.	Epiphysis of the proximal phalanx, digit 4	10.8	16.6
7.	Epiphysis of the second metacarpal	12.3	18.0
8.	Epiphysis of the distal phalanx, digit 1	12.1	18.3
9.	Epiphysis of the third metacarpal	13.8	20.5
10.	Epiphysis of the fourth metacarpal	15.6	23.3
11.	Epiphysis of the proximal phalanx, digit 5	14.3	21.5
12.	Epiphysis of the middle phalanx, digit 3	15.4	23.4
13.	Epiphysis of the middle phalanx, digit 4	15.6	23.8
14.	Epiphysis of the fifth metacarpal	17.1	26.0
15.	Epiphysis of the middle phalanx, digit 2	17.2	25.8
16.	Triquetral	22.7	29.3
17.	Epiphysis of the distal phalanx, digit 3	10.4	27.4
18.	Epiphysis of the distal phalanx, digit 4	18.7	27.7
19.	Epiphysis of the first metacarpal	19.1	31.8
20.	Epiphysis of the phalanx, digit 1	20.9	33.2
21.	Epiphysis of the distal phalanx, digit 5	23.7	37.3
22.	Epiphysis of the distal phalanx, digit 2	24.1	37.6
23.	Epiphysis of the middle phalanx, digit 5	23.6	39.2
24.	Lunate	36.0	44.4
25.	Trapezium	47.4	68.4
26.	Trapezoid	49.4	69.1
27.	Scaphoid	50.4	67.8
28.	Distal epiphysis of the ulna	68.3	82.4
29.	Pisiform	94.6	120.4
30.	Sesamoid of adductus pollicis	123.4	152.7

SOURCE: From "Radiograph Atlas of Skeletal Development of the Hand and Wrist," William Walter Greulich and S. Idell Pyle, with permission of the publishers, Stanford University Press, 1959, by the Board of Trustees of the Leland Stanford Junior University.

The amount of variation in the order is remarkably slight. The various investigators who have studied ossification of the bones of the hand and wrist in the United States have reported almost identical orders of ossification (Pyle and Sontag, 1943; Melman and Bakewin, 1950). In addition, studies of Dutch children (Mackay, 1952), of children from the Kenya coastal areas of East Africa, of children from Guam, of Japanese children in California (Sutow, 1953; Greulich, 1957) all indicate that the *order* of ossification is a universal phenomenon among human beings everywhere.

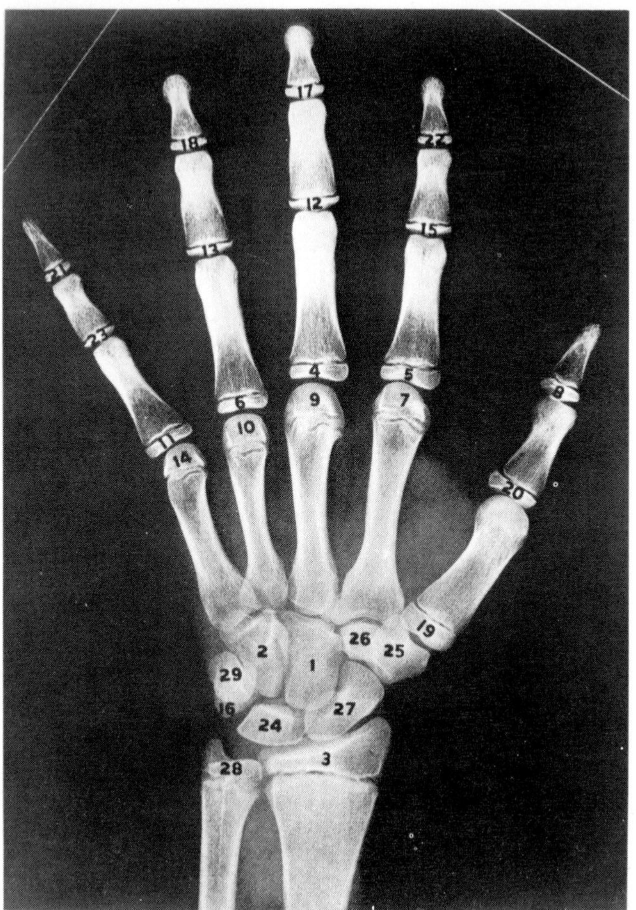

Fig. 10-2. X-ray film of hand and wrist showing sequence of appearance of ossification centers. (*From Radiograph Atlas of Skeletal Development of the Hand and Wrist by William Walter Greulich and S. Idell Pyle, with permission of the publishers, Stanford University Press, 1959, by the Board of Trustees of the Leland Stanford Junior University.*)

Though the order of ossification has been found quite constant in different groups of children, the amount of maturity found at specific ages has not been uniform. That is, the speed of growth has differed in different groups of children. It was thought that the more immature skeletal maturity of the Japanese children studied by Sutow was an indication of racial differences in the tempo of growth. However, a later study by Greulich of Japanese children reared in California but of very nearly the same genetic background showed maturity patterns very close to those of native American children. Since it is well known that malnutrition will retard development (Dreizen et al., 1954), the question is raised whether the slower growth tempo of the Japanese children in Japan was truly a racial difference or merely a nutritional one.

Greulich and Pyle were able to take an x-ray of the hand of a mummy of a young girl whom the archeologists estimated to have lived more than 3,000 years ago. The bones of this well-preserved specimen indicated that the order in which postnatal ossification occurs in the human body is the same today as it was thousands of years ago.

In 1937 Todd published a set of standards—x-rays of the hand and wrist of American children. These children were studied longitudinally from birth to maturity. The study of skeletal development was part of the Brush Foundation Study of Child Development. In 1959 Greulich and Pyle revised Todd's series and published a new atlas. The standards were selected by arranging 100 films of children of the same sex and chronological age in order of their relative skeletal maturity. The film selected as standard was, in the opinion of the investigators, the most representative of the central tendency. Since the 100 films of each array were of the same children, many of the standard films selected were of the same child. Skeletal age, therefore, as recorded in the atlas of Greulich and Pyle corresponds to the chronological age of the median child on whom the data were based.

In this atlas are published x-rays of the hand and wrist of boys and girls at specific ages from birth to maturity; there are 31 standards for the male and 27 for the female. The skeletal age of any child is determined by matching the x-ray of his hand and wrist with that of the standard most nearly like it.

Children from different genetic backgrounds may not be similar to the children in the series of Greulich and Pyle. That is, if a large number of children are assessed, it may be found that the median of the group is above or below that of those in the atlas. This does not invalidate the usefulness of these norms. A child whose tempo of growth may be called slow by these standards will grow as the slow children in this series grow, and it is possible to predict his future growth attainments.

Skeletal age is a useful measure of physiologic maturity. It is generally thought that growth hormone is concerned with increase in size and thyroid hormone with increase in differentiation (Becks et al., 1948). Malnutrition as well as endocrine disturbances can retard skeletal ossification (Dreizen et al., 1954).

Skeletal age is correlated with age of the menarche. The correlation is rather naturally more accurate in the later years than in the earlier ones, but even down to 2 years the correlation is significant. Girls whose menarche came between 10 and 12 years were found to have been consistently advanced in their skeletal development from the age of 2.

Skeletal age is, at the present time, a useful measure of the tempo of maturation. It appears to be reasonably well correlated with other measures of physiologic maturity, especially with the development of secondary sex signs, with full maturity, and with the mature height. Therefore, when combined with knowledge of chronological age and size, skeletal age is a means of predicting adult size and age of puberty (p. 112).

11

Differential Growth Rates

As a child grows, not only does his external shape change, but many of his internal organs change their relative proportions. Different parts of the body grow at different rates. Changes in external dimensions seem obvious today, nevertheless it has taken mankind centuries to realize this simple fact. Lack of awareness of the differences in shape between children and adults reflected a total attitude toward children prevalent in earlier centuries when it was generally believed that children were but miniature adults. Many of the beautiful madonnas of the Renaissance are shown with infants who have the shapes of full-grown men (Fig. 11-1).

EXTERNAL PROPORTIONS

Figure 11-2 shows the changing proportions from early fetal life to maturity. Total body growth prior to puberty follows the cephalocaudal law. Early growth in the fetus is greatest in the head. In infancy the trunk elongates. In childhood the legs are the most rapidly growing part. At puberty the trunk, once again, grows rapidly.

During the first year, when growth of the trunk dominates, the infant also broadens out by the accumulation of considerable masses of subcutaneous fat. He becomes round and chubby (see Adipose Tissue in Chap. 21). At about 1 year of age, when the child begins to walk, his big head, heavy trunk, and short, fat legs give him a top-heavy appearance. His legs are often bowed, his feet widely spaced, his abdomen protuberant.

After the first year the legs grow faster than any other part; subcutaneous fat is lost, the feet come together, the bowleggedness disappears, the abdomen is held in, and the slender, lithe build of the preschooler becomes evident. This long-legged, slender shape is characteristic of both boys and girls before the onset of puberty. Until puberty, differences in body shape and proportion have more to do with body constitution than with sex. The photographs in Fig. 11-3 demonstrate the neuter gender character of the body build of prepubescent children. When hairdos are eliminated, it is impossible to tell which of these children are boys and which are girls. After puberty (Fig. 11-4) their body shapes clearly identify their sex (Bayley, 1956).

The changes that take place at puberty involve almost every structure

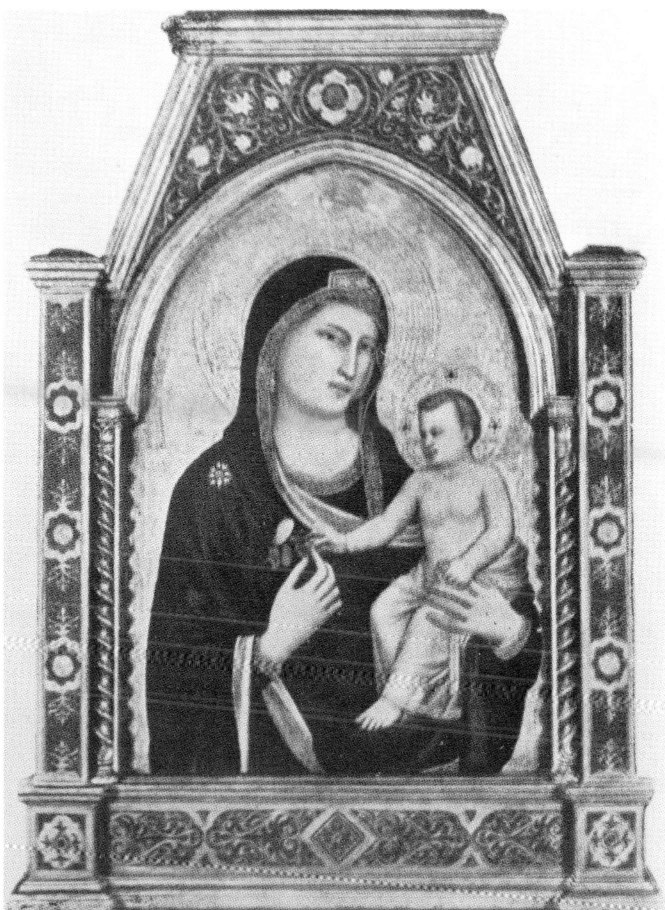

Fig. 11-1. Madonna and Child by Giotto painted before the proportions of the human figure were appreciated.

in the body. Puberty begins approximately 2½ years earlier in girls than in boys, so that for a few years girls are larger than boys of the same age. Growth of the skeleton and of the soft tissues is stimulated. Growth of the trunk is more rapid than that of the legs. The later puberty occurs, the longer the time that the legs grow rapidly. Those children who mature early end up with shorter legs than those who mature later. Boys, as a whole, maturing later than girls, have 2 to 2½ years more of rapid leg-growth time than do girls. Men are therefore longer-legged than women. This difference can be expressed quantitatively by the ratio of sitting height to total height (Fig. 11-5). Before puberty there is little difference between the sexes, but after puberty, women have a greater proportion of their total height above the waist than do men. As a result, when men and women are seated, their heads are much more nearly on the same level than when they are standing (Fig. 11-6).

The relation of shoulder breadth to pelvic breadth, similar in boys and girls in early childhood, changes markedly after puberty. Under the influence of androgens boys' shoulders grow rapidly during their growth spurt, much more rapidly than do those of girls, so that the mature man has shoulders considerably wider than those of the mature woman (Fig. 11-7). Pelvic diameter also increases in both sexes. The actual amount of widening at the hips (the bicristal diameter) is nearly the same in boys and girls (Fig. 11-7), but the shoulder growth is so much greater in boys that the ratio of pelvic breadth to shoulder breadth is considerably greater in women than in men.

Qualitatively the shoulder and hip growth is different in the two sexes. In boys, both shoulders and hips increase in size by growth of bone and muscle with little change in actual shape. In girls hip growth involves changes in the shape of the pelvis not found in boys; the female pelvis not only increases in total size under the influence of estrogen but it widens in the anterioposterior diameter, changing from an oval to a round shape (Greulich and Thoms, 1949). In addition to changes in bone and muscle, fat deposition is different in the two sexes (see Adipose Tissue in Chap. 21). Boys actually lose subcutaneous fat during the height of the growth spurt, while girls increase the amount of fat and lay it down in characteristically feminine patterns (p. 232, Fig. 21-3). It is the increased muscle mass in boys and the strategically placed adipose tissue in girls as well as skeletal differences that bring about the typically masculine and feminine figures.

The pelvic difference between men and women accounts for some differences in posture, most noticeable in the alignment of the legs. In feminine figures the broad pelvis and generous fat around hips and thighs result in

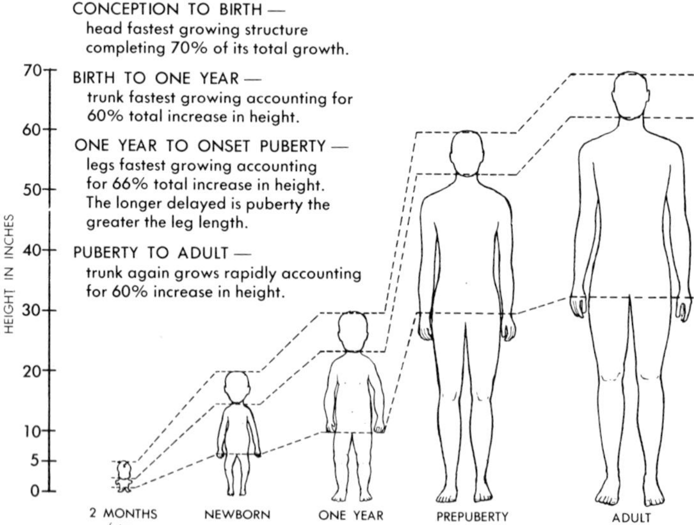

Fig. 11-2. Diagrammatic sketch of changing body proportions.

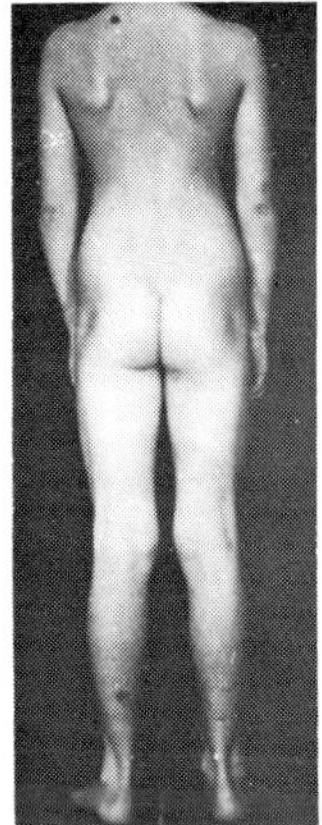
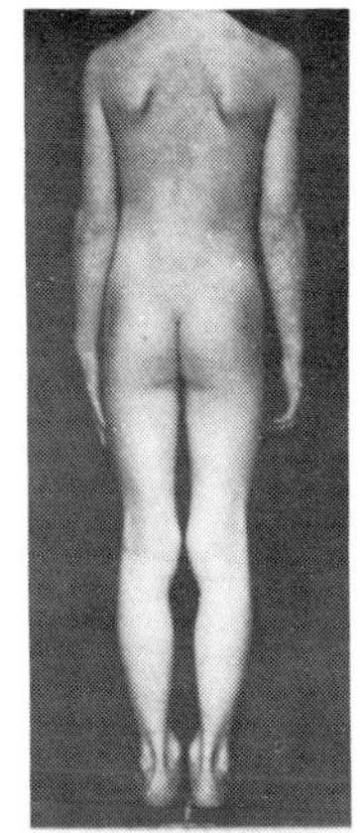
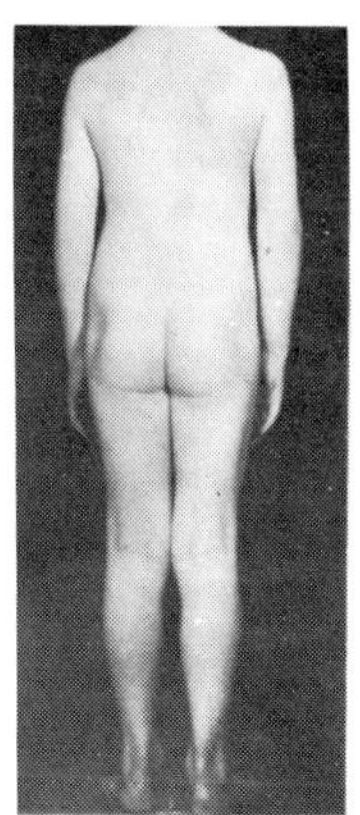
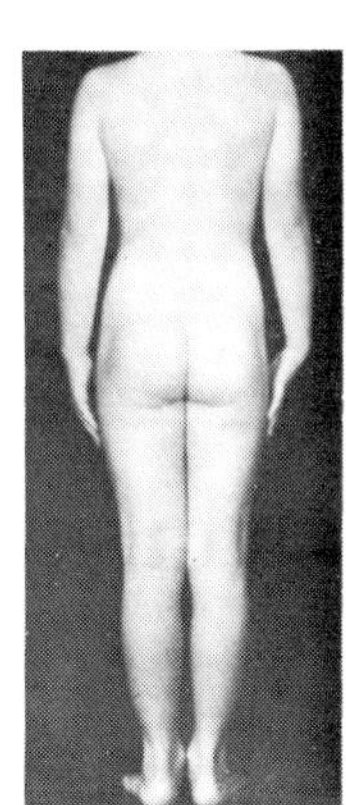

Fig. 11-3. Neuter gender character of body shape of prepubescent children. With hairdos eliminated it is impossible to tell which of these children are boys and which are girls.

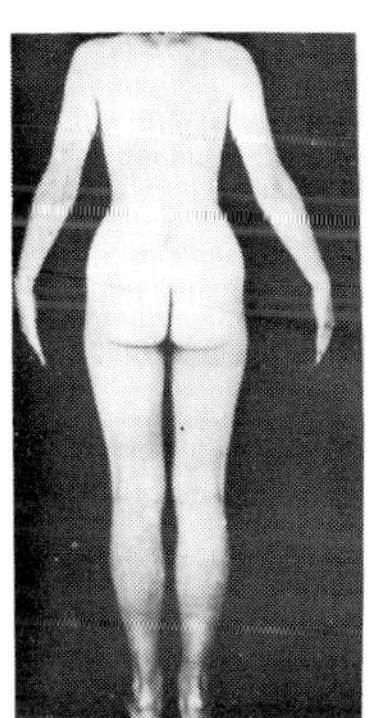
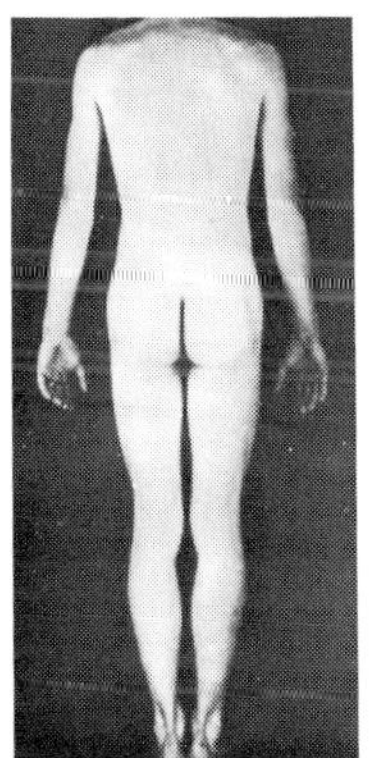
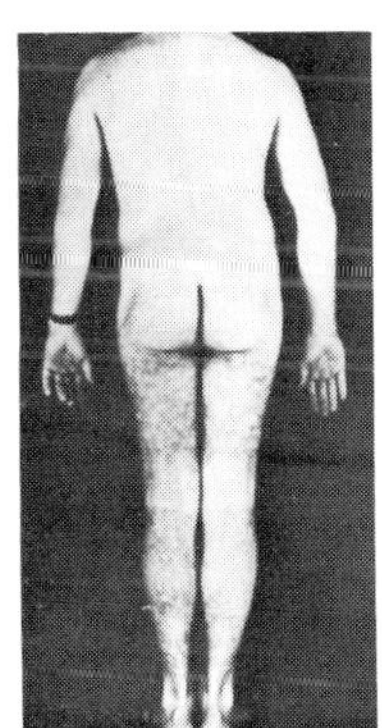
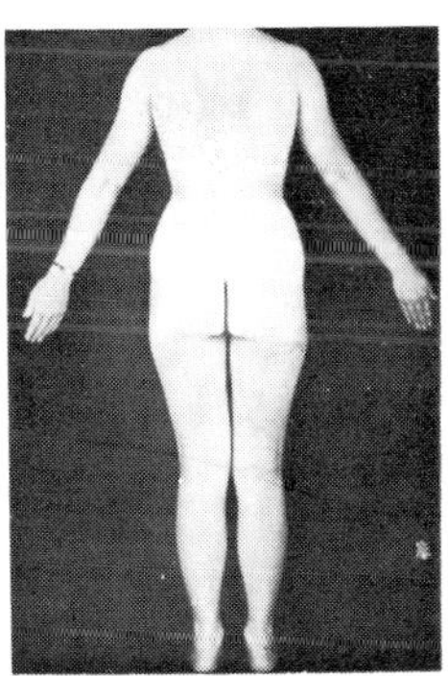

Fig. 11-4. Same children as in Fig. 11-3. After puberty sex can be identified by body shape. (*Photos in Figs. 11-3 and 11-4 supplied by Dr. Nancy Bayley from the files of one of the longitudinal studies of the Institute of Human Development, University of California, Berkeley.*)

closely approximated thighs and a tendency to knock-knees. In masculine figures the thighs are held further apart, and the knees are most apt to spread out and produce some bowleggedness.

In both sexes, the peak in weight comes after the peak in height; that is, the skeleton grows first, and the soft tissues expand later.

TISSUE AND ORGAN GROWTH

Changes in external shape and proportions come about concomitantly with changes in tissue and organ growth and reflect the changing functions brought about by maturation. Total body weight is of course the result of many different parts, each growing at its own rate (Figs. 11-8 and 11-9).

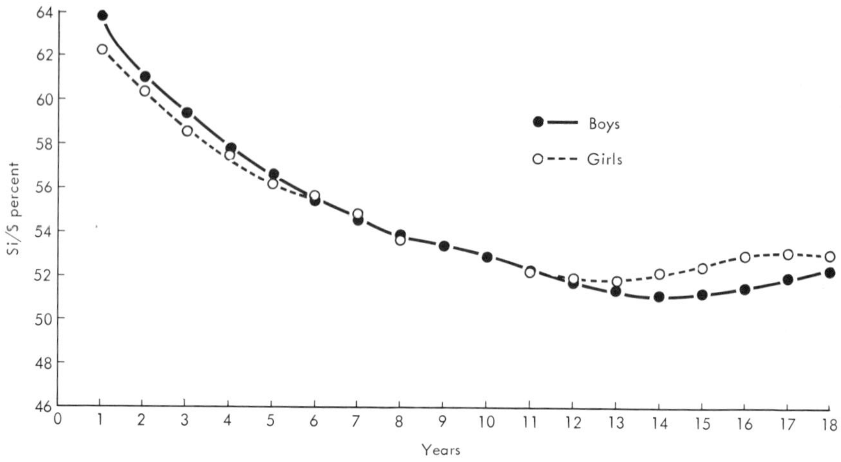

Fig. 11-5. Sitting height/stature ratio. *(Reprinted from Growth Diagnosis by Leona M. Bayer and Nancy Bayley, by permission of the University of Chicago Press.)*

The *muscle mass* constitutes the largest portion of the total body, hence its growth dominates the growth of the body as a whole. Muscle mass increases rapidly during infancy, grows slowly during childhood, spurts during puberty, and then increases slowly for a few years after sexual

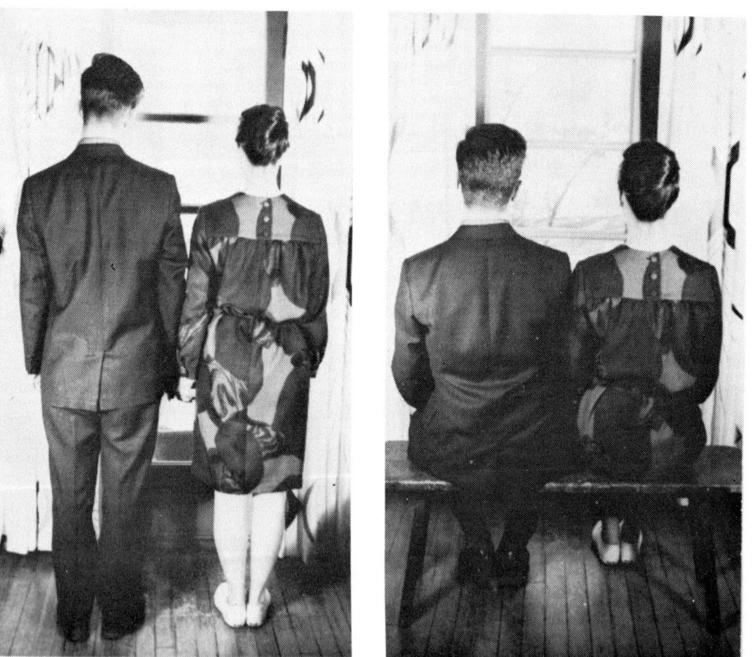

Fig. 11-6. When standing, the man is taller than the woman. When sitting, their shoulders and heads are at almost the same level.

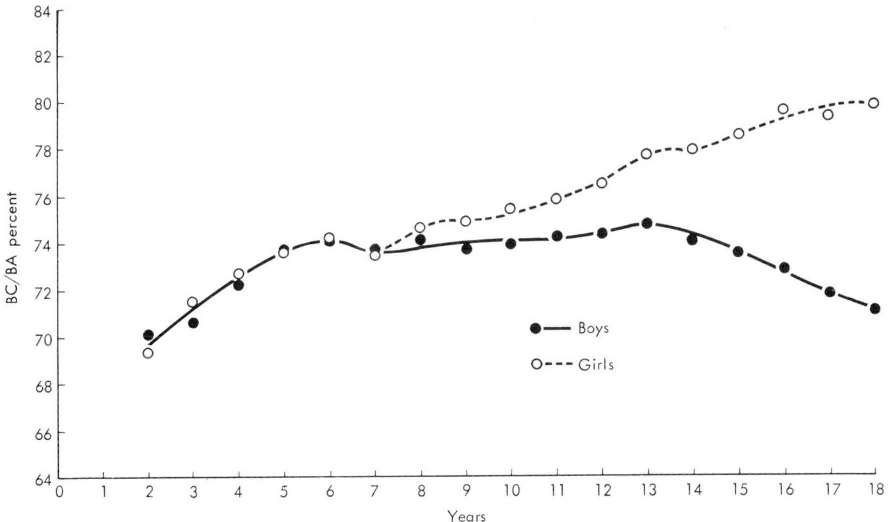

Fig. 11-7. Trunk-breadth index (bi-cristal/bi-acromial). As boys shoulders grow relatively wider, their ratio falls. As girls hips grow relatively broader, their ratio rises. (*Reprinted from Growth Diagnosis by Leona M. Bayer and Nancy Bayley, by permission of the University of Chicago Press.*)

maturation has been reached. Maximum muscle strength is not attained until a few years after muscle mass has reached maturity (p. 157). Muscular skills are dependent more upon the maturation of the nervous system than upon mere muscle size.

Like the muscle mass the *bones* follow a growth pattern similar to that of total body weight.

Although *adipose tissue* varies greatly from individual to individual, there is an overall lifetime pattern. Adipose tissue accumulates rapidly before birth and during early infancy, then decreases during childhood in both sexes. During puberty it reaccumulates in girls but not in boys (p. 230).

All the *neural tissues*—the brain, the cord, the peripheral nerves, and many of the sense organs—follow a growth pattern reflected by the changing size of the head. This growth is very rapid during intrauterine development and continues at a fast pace during infancy, reaching almost adult size by midchildhood. After that point there is a slow increase to full maturity. There is no spurt in neural growth at puberty.

Lymphoid tissue—lymph nodes, tonsils, thymus, and lymphocytes—constitutes a relatively small proportion of the total body weight. These tissues are widely scattered throughout the body; hence their unique growth is hardly reflected either in total body weight or in size of any easily measurable part of the body. Lymphoid tissue grows very rapidly during infancy and childhood, reaching its maximum size a few years before puberty; it then atrophies and is smaller in volume at full maturity than during child-

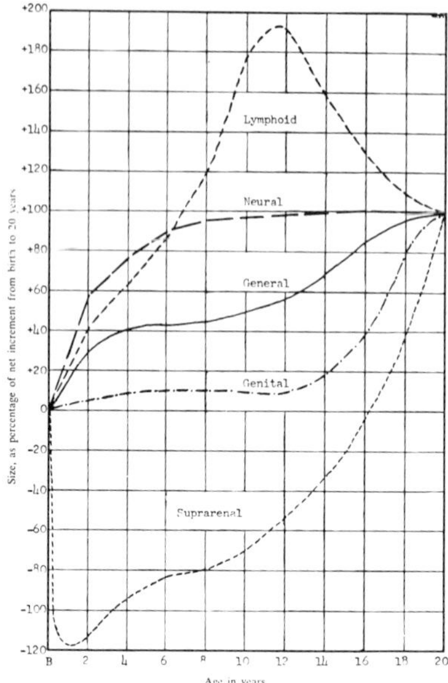

Fig. 11-8. Comparison of growth of five types of tissue. (*From The Measurement of the Body in Childhood by R. E. Scammon, in The Measurement of Man by J. A. Harris, C. M. Jackson, and R. E. Scammon, The University of Minnesota Press.*)

hood. The function of the lymphoid tissue is related to the development of immunity (p. 304).

The various *endocrine glands* do not have a common growth pattern. The *hypophysis* and *thyroid* glands grow at an almost constant rate from birth to maturity. The *adrenal cortex* undergoes a spurt in growth just prior to birth. After birth it decreases in size and reaches its smallest size several months postnatally. It hardly grows at all during the rest of infancy and childhood. At puberty it grows rapidly, reaching adult size within a few years.

The *genital organs* of both sexes, except the uterus, are small at birth. They remain at almost their birth size until puberty, at which time they grow very rapidly, achieving mature size and function during the years of puberty. The *uterus* has a growth pattern similar to that of the adrenal cortex.

During infancy the *heart* grows a little more slowly than the rest of the body. Its weight is doubled by 1 year of age, whereas total body weight is tripled. During childhood the heart grows steadily to about six times its birth size before puberty. The heart then takes part in the general rapid growth of puberty reaching its mature size concomitantly with that of the total body. The cardiothoracic index, the diameter of the heart divided by the internal diameter of the chest as determined by x-ray (Caffey, 1950) is often above 0.5 (0.6 to 0.4) before the age of 3. After this age the index in the normal child drops to below 0.5.

The *blood volume* increases roughly in proportion to body size. In the newborn, blood volume is between 100 and 130 ml per kg body weight depending upon the time after birth that the cord is clamped (p. 177). In the adult, blood volume is between 80 and 95 ml per kg.

Growth of the *respiratory system* parallels growth of the total body. Gaseous exchange, however, shows a sex difference which becomes apparent during the rapid spurt in growth at puberty (p. 157).

Growth of the *urinary system* as a whole parallels growth of the total body. The bladder doubles its capacity between 2 and 4 years of age (p. 415). While the kidneys function adequately at birth to maintain homeostasis when the body is not subjected to stress, their physiologic immaturity becomes obvious under adverse conditions (p. 214).

The proportion of body *water and solids* follows a pattern related to growth. The human organism dries out as life progresses. The young fetus is about 90 per cent water, the newborn infant about 70 per cent, the adult about 58 per cent. Sodium and chlorine, present in the extracellular fluids, accumulate as growth proceeds. Calcium increases as ossification of the skeleton takes place.

As a whole the *digestive system* grows as the total body grows, although certain parts of it have their individual spurts. The salivary glands grow rapidly in the early postnatal months. Saliva contributes relatively little to the digestion of sucked milk, but it is essential as soon as the infant is capable of consuming semisolid foods (p. 188). The stomach increases rapidly in the first months of postnatal life, then grows slowly and steadily throughout childhood. It shows a spurt of growth at puberty.

The ratio of size of the *liver* to that of total body weight is greatest in fetal life. By the time of birth the liver constitutes 4 per cent of the total body weight; in the adult, 2.5 to 3 per cent. The liver occupies a larger part of the abdominal cavity at birth than later in life. The liver edge can often be felt in the newborn. The liver decreases in size immediately after birth as the blood pouring in through the umbilical vessels is cut off. After the first postnatal months the liver increases steadily in weight until maturity. As growth progresses the anterior surface of the liver becomes covered by the diaphragm, and the liver edge is less often palpable. After the age of 2, growth of the liver, especially that of the right lobe, is sufficiently rapid to extend the organ below the costal margin. In middle childhood the liver edge of normal children can often be palpated. Beginning before puberty, the liver ascends slightly in the abdomen so that its edge can seldom be felt.

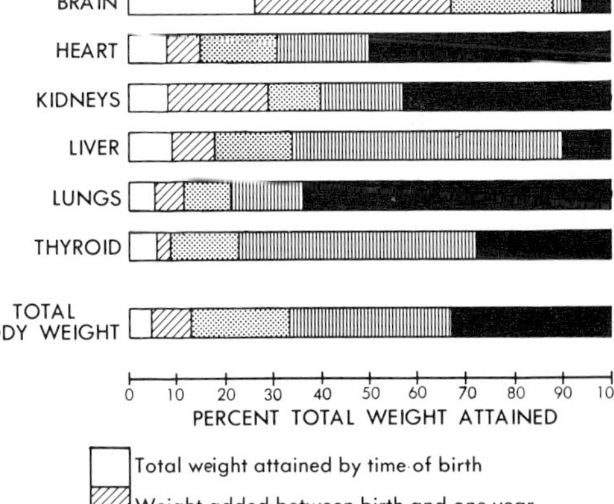

Fig. 11-9. Percent of mature weight attained by selected organs at specified ages.

12

Fringe Children

For most children growth poses no special problems when they and their parents understand the usual trends, but there are always some children whose growth deviates more than a little from the average. Many of these children are quite normal and healthy but are inherently larger or smaller than most of their peers.

THE LITTLE CHILD

Some children are genetically small individuals. Usually such children have small parents, but sometimes the genes for small size come from a more remote forebear. A complete physical appraisal is necessary to be very sure that the child's small size is due to his genes and not to some other factor interfering with his growth.

The parents need to accept the fact that the child is destined to be small. Considerable harm can be done a youngster by parents who try to force additional food into him to make him what it is impossible for him to be.

To the casual observer the small child does not look as old as he is, therefore there is a great tendency to baby him. He *looks* so tiny that parents, teachers, and casual friends are apt to treat him as a much younger child. He is not given a fair chance to grow up. It is of great importance to the child that he be treated according to his age and maturity, not according to his size. In ability to think, to reason, to assume responsibilities, the small child is the equal of his bigger age-mates. At the age of 8 he is not a cute little 6-year-old, he is an 8-year-old no matter how small he may be. He is perfectly capable of carrying on third grade work, walking to school alone, and crossing the intersections with the traffic light. He *is* an 8-year-old, and he needs the rights and privileges that go with this degree of maturity.

On the other hand, because of his small size he may not be able to compete successfully in games and playground activities. His agility, skills, and coordination are up to his age, but his muscles are not as big or as strong as those of bigger children. He needs a few skillful adults to steer him away from the activities he is apt to fail at and toward those things in which he can easily hold his own.

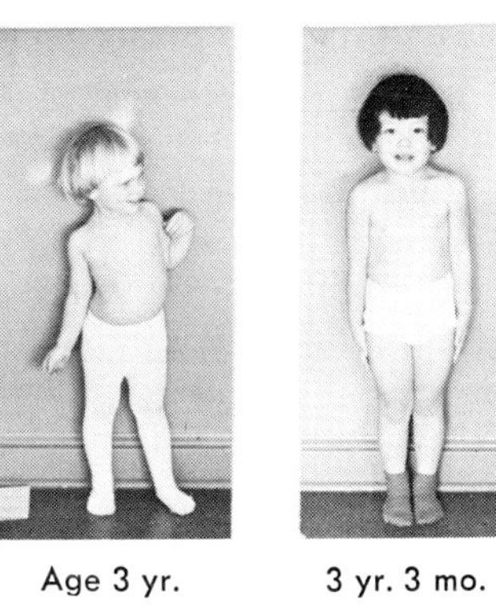

Age 3 yr. 3 yr. 3 mo.

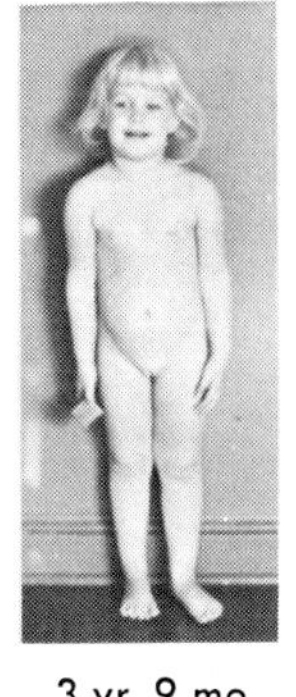

3 yr. 9 mo.

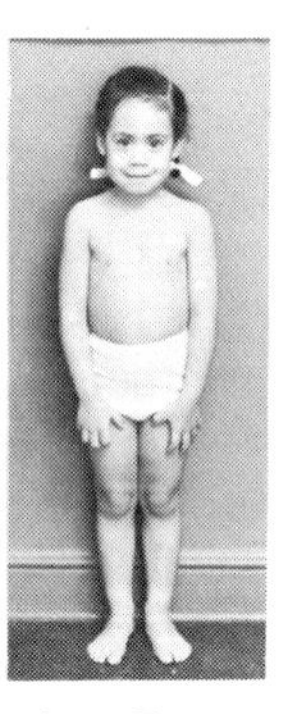

3 yr. 7 mo.

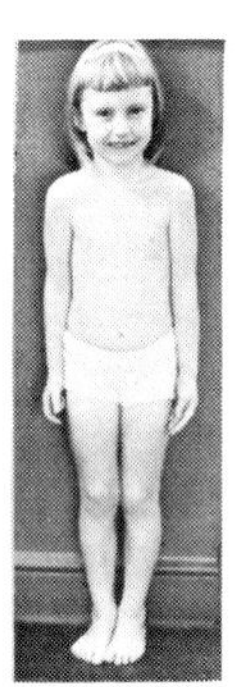

3 yr. 9 mo.

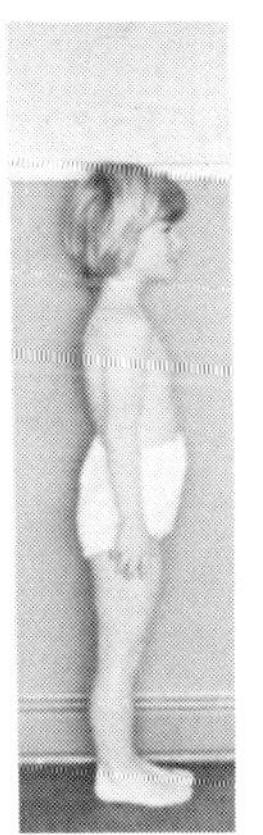

Age 9 yr. 3 mo.

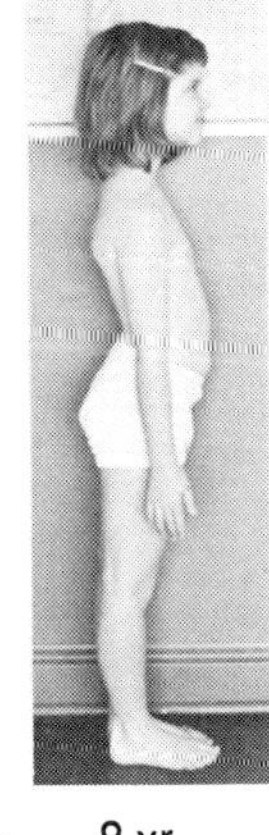

9 yr.

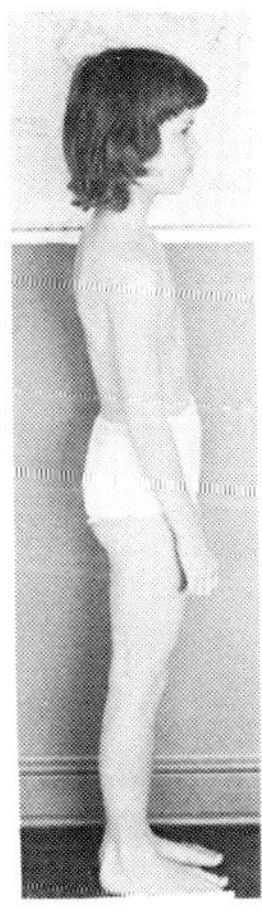

9 yr. 6 mo.

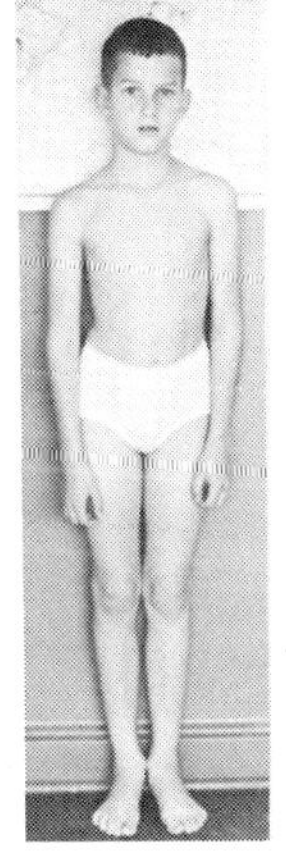

10 yr. 4 mo.

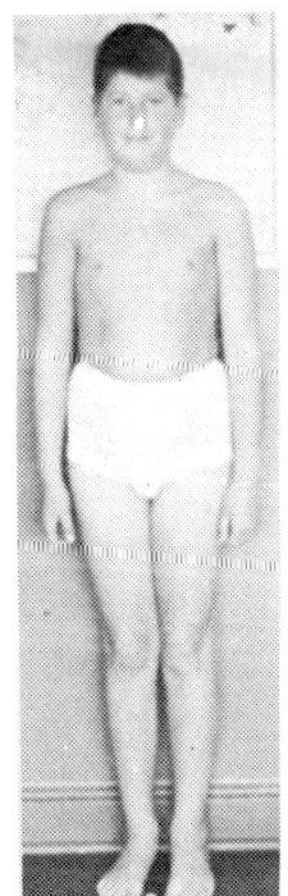

10 yr. 9 mo.

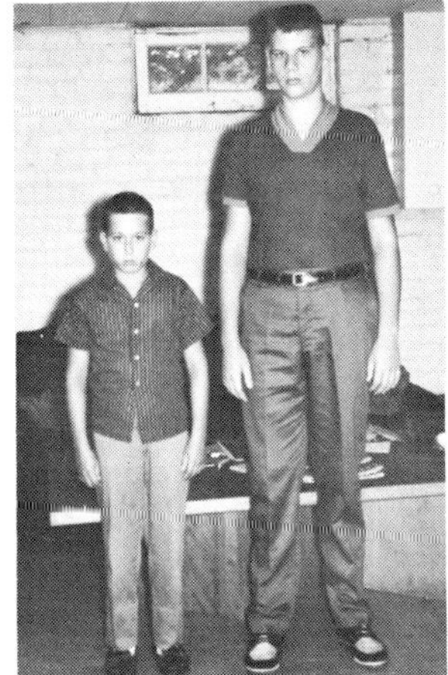

Age 13 yr. 1 mo. 13 yr.

Fig. 12-1. Children of approximately the same age and different sizes.

As he gets a little older, the child himself needs to understand that it is all right to be small, that there is nothing wrong with him. His acceptance of himself as he is will depend to a great extent upon his parents' attitude. If his parents are themselves small, as is so often the case, their own contentment with themselves in this regard and their acceptance of him will give him the knowledge that life is quite all right even if one is not a giant. But a parent who is determined that his son is going to make the college football team in spite of the fact that the youngster has a slim, small body build can do the child irremediable harm. Such a father is apt to call his small son a sissy, to urge him into attempts at physical feats that can only end in failure. When this happens, the boy grows up with an ever-present sense of his own inadequacy—his failure to measure up to his father's impossible demands.

THE BIG CHILD

The child who is oversized has no problems about food. Parents, by and large, are delighted with a good husky appetite. But the big child usually looks older than he is, again only to the casual observer who judges by size alone. The big child's round immature face tells the true story to anyone who really looks at him.

The big child is often pushed ahead faster than he can go. "A great big boy like you and you cannot tie your own shoe laces," or "What's the matter, only in third grade? You must have been left back a couple of times." It is next to impossible to protect the big child from the stupid remarks of some people.

The big child has trouble with children as well as with adults. He may

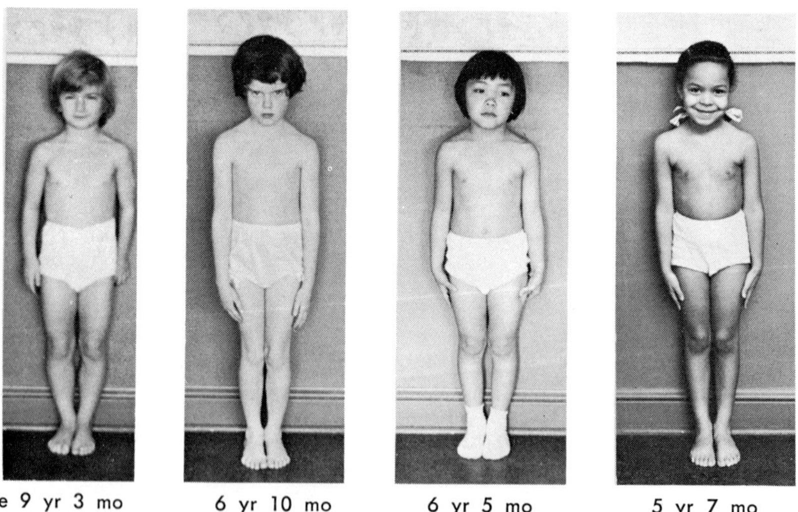

Age 9 yr 3 mo — 6 yr 10 mo — 6 yr 5 mo — 5 yr 7 mo

Fig. 12-2. Girls of approximately the same height and different ages.

look like a natural for a baseball team, but in spite of his big size he lacks the coordination of boys 2 or 3 years older than he is. So, with the cruelty of childhood, the older boys throw him off the team. He is too big and too strong to play with his age-mates and too immature and uncoordinated to compete with boys his own size.

If the important adults in a child's life—his parents, his teachers—can be helped to accept him for what he is, the child can be comfortable with himself. Like the small child, the big child needs to be treated according to his age and his degree of maturity.

RATE OF MATURING

Children vary in the speed with which they mature. This means that chronological age alone cannot be used as a measure of just how mature a child is (see Chap. 10).

There is a rough correlation between size and speed of maturing, some tendency for children who are bigger than their age-mates to be a little faster in maturing and for youngsters who are quite small to be a little slower. Insofar as this is true, it eases the problem of the child who is out of line in size. There are, however, so many exceptions to this correlation that caution needs to be used in judging a child's maturity from his size.

Maturing must be judged by what the child is capable of doing. Knowing how rapidly his skeleton is maturing is often a helpful, concrete guidepost. Bone age is more closely correlated with maturity than chronological age.

The age at which a child enters first grade is determined in many of our school systems on the basis of chronological age. Most children are ready to learn to read at 6 years of age, but a slow-maturing child may not have reached the developmental stage at which acquisition of this skill is possible. Pushing him into first grade before he is mature enough dooms him to failure. On the other hand, a rapidly maturing child may be quite ready and anxious to read at 5 years of age (p. 478).

The rate of maturation is important throughout the early years, but at puberty it assumes colossal importance. The "average" boy begins the changes of puberty at 13 years of age, but perfectly normal healthy boys may begin to mature as early as 12 or as late as 19. Girls mature earlier—the average is 12, but the normal fringe can be from 10 to 17. The slow maturers of both sexes often run into serious inner turmoil during the years when their age-mates are passing through puberty (Fig. 10-1).

The little girl is painfully aware of her flat chest and slim hips; she feels that this is the reason she is not let in on the giggles and boy talk of her erstwhile friends. She feels cheated because the other girls have experienced menstruation and she has not. She may well believe that she is doomed for a permanent position against the wall. Her fears and failures accentuate the normal doubts of this critical age period.

The slow-maturing boy is in a similar predicament. He is concerned because he remains so small and weak compared to his pals. He can no longer compete physically with them, and his high, childish voice compares very unfavorably with the deep tones of other boys. Some boys with these worries withdraw from all association with their peers; others turn to delinquent acts. Such a child feels he *must* somehow get back in with his crowd, and he will do anything to try to gain their acceptance.

A slow-maturing child may become so deeply worried that he (or she) is afraid to voice his fears. He *knows* that there is something terribly wrong with him. He does not ask because of fear that his doubts about himself will be confirmed. Many a child goes through years of needless turmoil and torment.

Slow-maturing youngsters need an understanding and sympathetic adult to explain to them that there is nothing wrong with them, that if they will but hold on and wait a few years, they too will grow and mature. The girl will get all the curves she craves; the boy will get size and strength and a deep voice. The waiting may be hard, but it need not be compounded by the awful fear that some permanent abnormality is preventing normal growing up.

Determination of skeletal age, a prediction of ultimate size and the time when puberty can be expected can do a great deal to bring inner peace to a frightened slow-maturing child.

Early-maturing as well as late-maturing children have their problems. Usually early-maturing children are large in comparison with their peers, and throughout early childhood they have the problems of the big child, softened a little by the fact that they really are a little more mature than their chronological age. Then they get their adolescent growth early. Already big, they soon tower over their age-mates. Size seldom creates a problem for the early-maturing boy—they enjoy being big, but the early-maturing girl does not enjoy being larger than her girl friends and larger than boys her own age. She often fears she will be uncomfortably tall when she is fully grown.

With puberty usually comes a change of interests. The adolescent is interested in more grownup thoughts and activities than the preadolescent. The early-maturing child is often pushed (or pushes himself) into the society of adolescents several years older. They may all be equal biologically, but the others, having lived at least a couple of years more, are more experienced. Thus the early-maturing child often struggles to keep up with a group somewhat beyond him. Again, the guidance of a perceptive adult can help the child accept the facts for what they are.

BIBLIOGRAPHY

Babson, S., John Kangas Gorham, Morton Young, and James L. Bramhall: Growth and Development of Twins of Dissimilar Size at Birth, *Pediatrics*, **33**:327, 1964.

Bayer, Leona M.: Weight and Menses in Adolescent Girls with Special Reference to Build, *J. Pediat.*, **17**:345, 1940.

———, and Nancy Bayley: "Growth Diagnosis," University of Chicago Press, Chicago, 1959.

———, and H. Grey: Plotting of a Graphic Record of Growth for Children Aged One to Nineteen Years, *Am. J. Dis. Child.*, **50**:1408, 1935.

Bayley, Nancy: Individual Patterns of Development, *Child Development*, **27**:45, 1956.

———: The Accurate Prediction of Growth and Adult Height, *Mod. Prob. Paediat.*, **7**:234, 1962.

———: Growth Curves for Height and Weight by Age for Boys and Girls Scaled According to Physical Maturity, *J. Pediat.*, **48**:187, 1956.

———, and Leona M. Bayer: The Assessment of Somatic Androgyny, *Am. J. Phys. Anthropol.*, N.S. **4**:433, 1946.

———, and Samuel R. Pinneau: Tables for Predicting Adult Height from Skeletal Age: Revised for Use with Greulich-Pyle Hand Standards, *J. Pediat.*, **40**:423, 1952.

Becks, H., and M. E. Simpson, R. O. Scow, C. W. Ashing, and H. M. Evans: Skeletal Changes in Rats, Thyroidectomized on the Day of Birth and the Effect of Growth Hormone in Such Animals, *Anat. Rec.*, **100**:561, 1948.

Boyd, E.: "An Introduction to Human Biology and Anatomy for First Year Medical Students," Child Research Council, Denver, Colo., 1952.

Broman, B., G. Dahlberg, and A. Lichtenstein: Heights and Weights During Growth, *Acta paediat.*, **30**:1, 1942.

Brozek, Joseph: "Body Measurement and Human Nutrition," Wayne State University Press, Detroit, Mich., 1956.

Caffey, J.: "Pediatric X-Ray Diagnosis," 2d ed., The Year Book Medical Publishers, Inc., Chicago, 1950.

Clements, E. M. B.: Changes in the Mean Stature and Weight of British Children over the Past 70 years, *Brit. M. J.*, **2**:897, 1953.

Cone, T. E. Symposium: A Survey of Growth Failure in Pediatrics, *Clin. Proc. Child. Hosp.*, **15**:75, 1959.

Dreizen, S., R. M. Snodgrasse, G. S. Parker, C. Currie, and T. D. Spies: Maturation of Bone Centers in Hand and Wrist of Children with Chronic Nutritive Failure, *Am. J. Dis. Child.*, **87**:429, 1954.

Dupertius, C. W., and N. B. Michael: Comparison of Growth in Height and Weight Between Ectomorphic and Mesomorphic Boys, *Child Development*, **24**:203, 1953.

Ellis, R. W. B.: Age of Puberty in the Tropics, *Brit. M. J.*, **1**:85, 1950.

Goldberg, Minnie B.: What Makes Us Grow As We Do, *J. Am. M. Women's A.*, **10**:110, 1955.

Greulich, William Walter, and Hubert Thoms: The Growth and Development of the Pelvis of Individual Girls, Before, During, and After, Puberty, *Yale J. Biol. & Med.*, **17**:91, 1944.

———: A Comparison of the Physical Growth and Development of the American Born and Native Japanese Children, *Am. J. Phys. Anthropol.*, N.S. **15**:489, 1957.

———, and S. Idell Pyle: "Radiograph Atlas of Skeletal Development of the Hand and Wrist," Stanford University Press, Stanford, Calif., 1959.

HATHAWAY, MILLICENT L.: Heights and Weights of Children and Youths in the U.S., Home Economics Research Report 2, U.S. Department of Agriculture, 1957.

ITO, P. K.: Comparative Biometrical Study of Physique of Japanese Women Born and Reared under Different Environments, *Human Biol.*, **14**:279, 1942.

JACKSON, R. L., and H. G. KELLY: Growth Charts for Use in Pediatric Practice, *J. Pediat.* **27**:215, 1945.

KIIL, V.: (Quoted by J. M. Tanner) in "Growth at Adolescence," Charles C Thomas, Publisher, Springfield, Ill., 1955.

KOGUT, MAURICE D., S. A. KAPLAN, and C. N. S. SHIMIZU: Growth Retardation, Use of Sulfation Factor as Bioassay for Growth Hormone, *Pediatrics,* **31**:538, 1963.

LEE, MARJORIE M. C., K. S. F. CHANG, and MARY M. C. CHAN: Sexual Maturation of Chinese Girls in Hong Kong, *Pediatrics,* **32**:389, 1963.

LEVINE, V. E.: Studies in Physiological Anthropology: III. The Age of Onset of Menstruation of the Alaska Eskimos, *Am. J. Phys. Anthropol.*, N.S. **2**:252, 1953.

LUBCHENCO, LULA O., CHARLOTTE HANSMAN, MARIAN DRESSLER, and EDITH BOYD: Intrauterine Growth as Estimated from Liveborn Birth Weight Data at 24–42 Weeks of Gestation, *Pediatrics,* **32**:793, 1963.

MACKAY, D. H.: Skeletal Maturation of the Hand. A Study of Development in East African Children, *Tr. Roy. Soc. Trop. Med. & Hyg.*, **46**:135, 1952.

MATTHEWS, C. A., and M. H. FOHRMAN: "Beltsville Standards for Growth of Jersey and Holstein Cattle," U.S. Department of Agriculture Technical Bulletin, Nos. 1098 and 1099, 1954.

MELMAN, D. H., and H. BAKEWIN: Ossification of the Metacarpal-Metatarsal Centers as a Measure of Maturation, *J. Pediat.*, **36**:617, 1950.

MEREDITH, H. V.: Stature and Weight of Children of the U.S. with Reference to Influence of Racial, Regional, Socio-Economic and Secular Trends, *Am. J. Dis. Child.*, **62**:909, 1941.

———: Stature and Weights of Private School Children in Two Successive Decades, *Am. J. Phys. Anthropol.*, **28**:1, 1941.

———: Birth Order and Body Size, *Am. J. Phys. Anthropol.*, **8**:195, 1950.

———, and E. M. MEREDITH: The Stature of Toronto Children Half a Century Ago and Today, *Human Biol.*, **16**:126, 1944.

MICHELSON, N.: Studies in Physical Development of Negroes: IV. Onset of Puberty, *Am. J. Phys. Anthropol.*, N.S. **2**:151, 1944.

MILLS, C. A.: Temperature Influence on Human Growth and Development, *Human Biol.*, **22**:71, 1950.

NICHOLSON, A. B., and C. HANLEY: Indices of Physiological Maturity Deviations and Interrelationships, *Child Development,* **24**:1, 1953.

NORVAL, M. A., R. L. J. KENNEDY, and J. BERKSON: Biometric Studies of the Growth of Children of Rochester, Minn., The First Year of Life, *Human Biol.*, **23**:273, 1951.

PALMER, C. E.: Seasonal Variations of Average Growth in Weight and Height of Elementary School Children, *Pub. Health Rep.*, **48**:211, 1933.

PYLE, S. IDELL, and L. W. SONTAG: Variability in Onset of Ossification in Epiphyses and Short Bones of the Extremities, *Am. J. Roentgenol.*, **49**:795, 1943.

———, ROBERT B. REED, HAROLD C. STUART: Patterns of Skeletal Development in the Hand, *J. Pediat.*, **24** (supp.): 886, 1959.

REED, R. B., and H. C. STUART: Patterns of Growth in Height and Weight from Birth to 18 Years of Age, *Pediatrics,* **24** (supp.): 904, 1959.

REYNOLDS, E. L., and L. W. SONTAG: Seasonal Variations in Weight, Height, and Appearance of Ossification Centers, *J. Pediat.,* **24**:524, 1944.

RICHEY, H. G.: The Relation of Accelerated, Normal, and Retarded Puberty to the Height and Weight of School Children, *Society for Research in Child Development Monograph,* vol. 2, no. 1, 1937.

ROBERT, C.: The Physical Requirements of Factory Children, *J. Statist. Soc.,* **39**: 681, 1876.

SCAMMON, RICHARD E.: The Measurement of the Body in Childhood, in J. A. Harris, C. M. Jackson, D. G. Patterson, and R. E. Scammon, "The Measurement of Man," The University of Minnesota Press, Minneapolis, 1930.

SHELDON, W. H.: "The Varieties of Human Physique," Harper & Row, Publishers, Incorporated, New York, 1940.

SHUTTLEWORTH, F. K.: Sexual Maturation and the Physical Growth of Girls 6–16, *Society for Research in Child Development Monograph,* vol. 2, no. 5, 253, 1937.

———: The Physical and Mental Growth of Boys and Girls Age 6–19 in Relation to Age at Maximum Growth, *Society for Research in Child Development Monograph,* vol. 4, no. 3, 1939.

SIMMONS, K.: The Brush Foundation Study of Child Growth and Development: II. Physical Growth and Development, *Society for Research in Child Development Monograph,* vol. 9, no. 1, 1944.

STUART, HAROLD C., and H. V. MEREDITH: Use of Body Measurements in the School Health Program, *Am. J. Pub. Health,* **36**:1365–1386, 1946.

STUART, HAROLD C., ROBERT B. REED, and ASSOCIATES: Longitudinal Studies of Child Health and Development. Series II. Reports Based on Completed Case Studies, *Pediatrics,* **24** (supp.): 875, 1959.

SUTOW, W. W.: Skeletal Maturation in Healthy Japanese Children 6–19 Years of Age: Comparison with Skeletal Maturation of American Children, *Hiroshima J. M. Sc.,* **2**:181, 1953.

SZALAY, GLENN C.: Intrauterine Growth Retardation versus Silver's Syndrome, *J. Pediat.,* **64**:234, 1964.

TANNER, J. M.: "Growth at Adolescence," Charles C Thomas, Publisher, Springfield, Ill., 1955.

———: Adult Body Measurements, *Arch. Dis. Childhood,* **31**:372, 1956.

TODD, T. W. "Atlas of Skeletal Maturation (Hand)," Kimpton, London, 1937.

WARKANY, JOSEF, B. B. MONROE, and B. S. SUTHERLAND: Intrauterine Growth Retardation, *Am. J. Dis. Child.,* **102**:249, 1961.

WETZEL, N. C.: Assessing the Physical Condition of Children, *J. Pediat.,* **22**:82, 208, 329, 1943.

WILSON, D. C., and I. SUTHERLAND: The Age of Menarche in the Tropics, *Brit. M. J.,* **2**:607, 1953.

Section IV

DEVELOPMENT OF ORGANIC STRUCTURE

13

The Nervous System

PHYLOGENETIC BACKGROUND

Some phylogenetic background is helpful in appreciating the ontogenic development of man's nervous system. Nervous tissue did not make its appearance phylogenetically until primitive forms became multicellular organisms. Squeezed in between the cells along the periphery of these early simple metazoa appeared a new kind of cell with two filaments, one projecting to the outside of the organism and the other extending backward into the body of the animal. The projecting filament was sensitive to physiochemical changes in the environment (Fig. 13-1). It connected directly with a nerve cell which sent its filament into some acting structure. The organism was thus able to act as a result of environmental changes. The earliest action system was a two-neuron chain, a sensory neuron and a motor neuron. As evolution advanced, several sensory neurons converged and made contact with a third and new kind of nerve cell—the association neuron (Fig. 13-2). This mechanism—a sensory neuron, an association neuron, and a motor neuron—is the basis of the nervous system of all animals from the simplest of the primitive metazoa to man. As the evo-

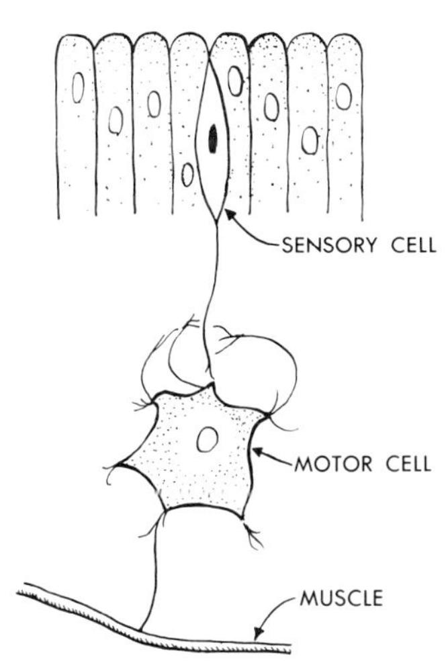

Fig. 13-1. Primative two-neuron chain.

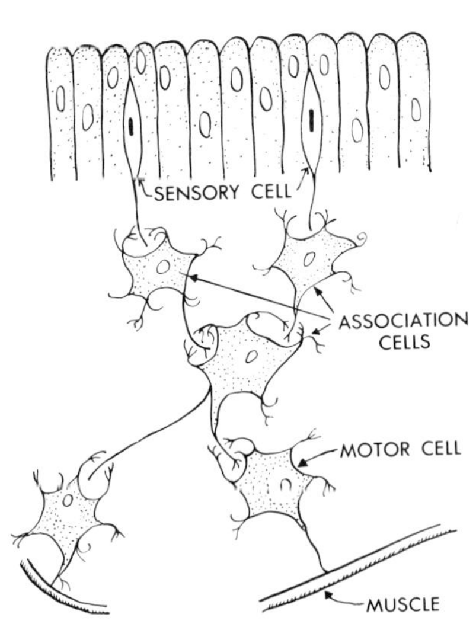

Fig. 13-2. Appearance of association neurons.

lutionary ladder is mounted, all three types of neurons have increased enormously in number and in the complexities of the pathways, but the fundamental structure has been maintained. Differences in nervous systems are quantitative; no essential qualitative difference has been found. Studies of neurons in the crayfish can shed much light on the function of the human brain (Russell, 1959).

The relative size of the central nervous system (CNS) in relation to body size gives animals their place in the evolutionary procession. This ratio provides an index of the controlling influence of the brain. The brain of the enormous dinosaurs which roamed the planet in the Age of Reptiles weighed only 2½ oz; the elephant of today, somewhere near the size of the dinosaurs, has a brain weighing 4 lb. The dinosaur had only about 1 oz of brain per ton of body weight, whereas the elephant has about 1 lb of brain per 500 lb body weight. Man has achieved about 1 lb per 50 lb body weight. Hence a man is 1,000 times more brilliant than an elephant and 100,000 times more brilliant than a dinosaur. As La Barre says, "the great dinosaurs had such enormous size that nothing could stop one of them when he was on his way; however, while it is all very well to be able to go where you are going, the reason for getting there and what is seen and understood on the way are even more important." [1]

A group of mammals who remained in, or returned to, the sea have evolved into the whales and dolphins of today. The dolphin's brain is almost as large as man's in proportion to his body size. According to W. N. Kellogg (1961) the dolphin has 1 lb of brain per 85 lb body weight and may well be man's closest intellectual rival (p. 456).

TABLE 13-1

Relative Sizes of Brain and Body

	Brain weight, lb	Body weight, lb	Ratio brain weight/body weight
Stegosaurs	0.0625	2,000	0.00003
Elephant	4.0	2,000	0.002
Primate (monkey)	0.77	110	0.70
Dolphin	3.5	300	1.17
Man	3.1	150	2.1

The primate evolved eyes that gave him a sense of depth, a hand with which to investigate, and, above all, a brain that allowed further development of association nerve fibers. Though the primate never achieved the relative brain size of the dolphin, it is through the primate that homo sapiens evolved.

[1] The correlation between brain weight and intelligence is a rough guide in comparing one species with another. It does not hold between individuals of the same species. The largest human brain on record was that of an imbecile.

Man began to emerge as a unique species when additional association fibers in his brain appeared, fibers that could block some of the hereditary paths of instinctive patterns. In the dim past of prehistory, an apelike creature, now back on the ground, walking erect on his hind legs, using his hands to feel, his eyes to explore, began to use his new-grown association nerve fibers to question his instinctive patterns. He could think up a better way to act than the inborn nervous pathways dictated. The ability to alter instinctive patterns by unique and individual thought diverted evolutionary progression in the direction that has led to man. This ability has its structural foundation in the cerebral cortex. Here there are masses of association nerve fibers which are, in a manner of speaking, free—free to direct the human into his own unique behavior. This freedom stands in contrast to the association fibers which are irrevocably tied by heredity into certain fixed patterns which the individual animal can never alter. Many animals have elaborate behavior patterns: the hive life of the bee, the migration of birds, the extraordinary journey of the eel to lay its eggs thousands of miles from the place where it spends most of its life. These and many others are rigid patterns built firmly into the neuron patterns and carried from generation to generation. With the advent of man, instincts began to lose their importance in determining behavior. Not only *can* man decide how to act; he *must* make decisions. With this equipment man has not only come to dominate the earth but is now beginning to chafe at the boundaries of a single planet.

Man is born with an immature brain which grows and develops as his body grows. His brain and his sense organs make it possible for him to gain an awareness of the world about him, of himself as a unique entity in the world. The full development of the power of the brain requires not only a structurally adequate mechanism but also a climate in which this mechanism can function to its full capacity.

DEVELOPMENT PRIOR TO BIRTH

The nervous system arises from the ectoderm, the outermost layer of the embryo. Phylogenetically it is the outer rim in the most primitive forms that makes contact with the environment, and this ancestral function of the periphery has been captured in the ontogenetic development of the nervous system of all animal species, including man.

No definite evidence of the nervous system is found in the embryo until the primitive streak is formed and the embryo has passed from a circular to a pear-shaped form. Then a thickened area of the ectoderm forms the neural plate, which soon folds inward, forming first the neural groove and later the neural tube. The tube extends the full length of the embryo. It is larger in the head area, where the brain will ultimately develop, and narrower in the parts destined to become the spinal cord (Patten, 1953, and Fig. 13-3).

The neuroblasts throughout the entire length of the neural tube arrange themselves into layers. This fundamental layered arrangement is quite remarkable in view of the very different functions that various parts of the central nervous system are to exercise. In the cortex the layered arrangement is recognizable throughout life; in the brain stem and cord, it is obvious in early development but becomes obscured in the mature organism.

The cord, the spinal nerves, the nerve sheaths, the autonomic system, and

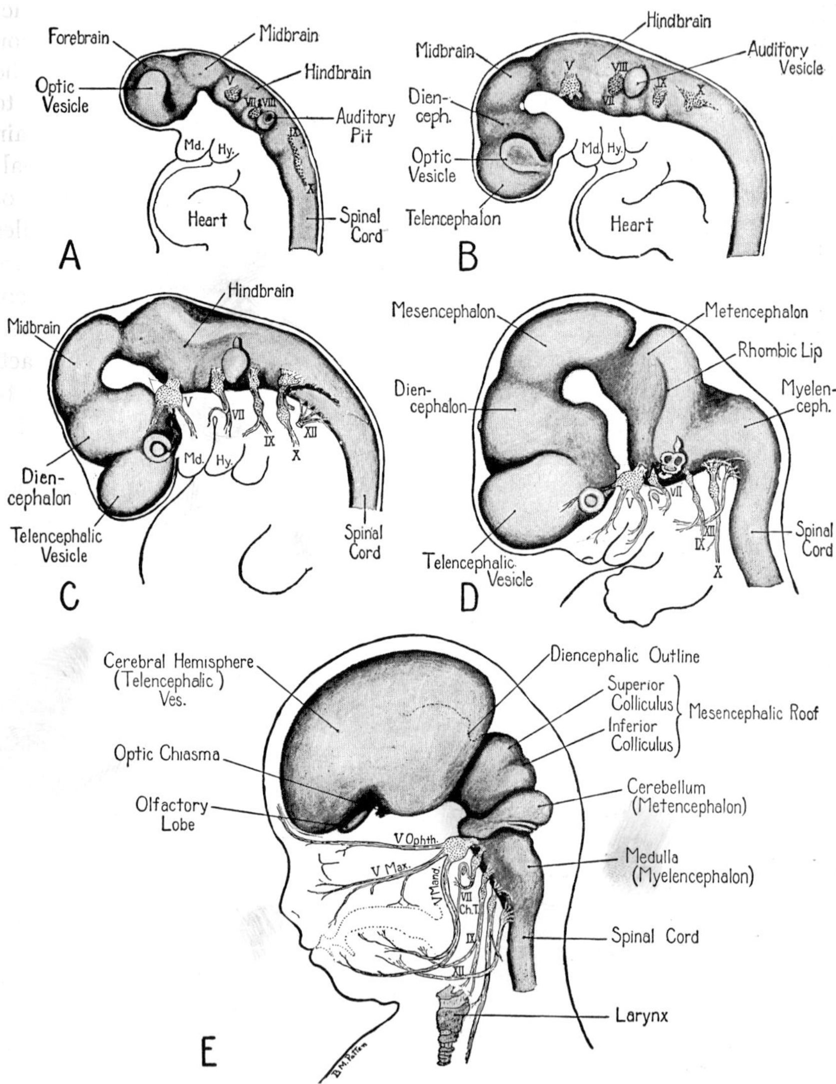

Fig. 13-3. Five stages in the early development of the brain and cranial nerves. *A*. 3½ weeks gestational age. *B*. 4 weeks. *C*. 5⅓ weeks. *D*. 7 Weeks. *E*. 11 weeks. (*From Human Embryology, 2d ed., by Bradley M. Patten, McGraw-Hill Book Company, Inc.*)

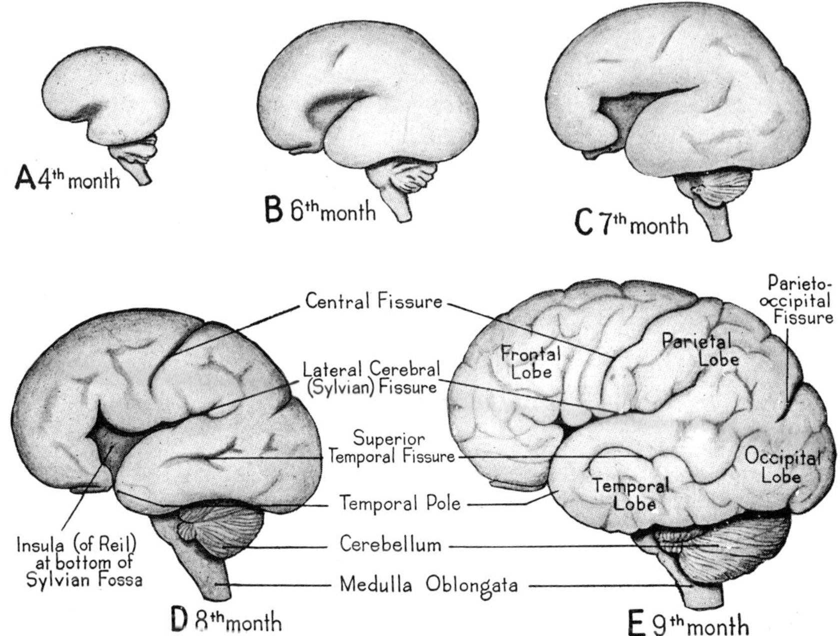

Fig. 13-4. Lateral views of the fetal brain at various stages in development. *(From Human Embryology, 2d ed., by Bradley M. Patten, McGraw-Hill Book Company, Inc.)*

the brain stem of man are quite similar to those of the higher mammals. It is in the most cephalad division of the neural tube, the telencephalon, that the greatest difference between the brain of man and that of other animals becomes apparent. This part of the neural tube starts off modestly as small paired outgrowths of the primitive tube, but by midfetal life these outgrowths have become the paired cerebral hemispheres and have so increased in size that they envelop the entire brain.

The outer surfaces of the hemispheres are smooth until about the sixth fetal month. As further increase in size takes place, the superficial areas begin to fold over, and fissures become evident. The first of these is the large sylvian fissure which divides the frontal and parietal lobes from the temporal lobe. By the seventh month, the Rolandic fissure appears dividing the frontal from the parietal lobes. The Rolandic fissure is not seen in brains below that of the primate. The large fissures and the smaller infoldings, the sulci, are evidence of the greatly increased brain surface of man. This infolding process goes on rapidly in the last months before birth and continues for the first few years of postnatal life.

THE NERVOUS SYSTEM AT BIRTH

From conception to birth the head increases in size at a much greater rate than the rest of the body. By the time of birth, the head has achieved almost three-fourths of the total mature size, while the rest of the body has attained but one-fourth of its adult size (p. 125).

In spite of this enormous growth in size of the head, only the phylogenetically older parts of the brain and nervous system have achieved sufficient maturity to carry on their predestined function.

The infant at birth must maintain physiologic independence. He must breathe, circulate his blood, eat, digest food, eliminate waste, and within limits maintain homeostasis. These functions are dependent upon the development of the viscera, the endocrine glands, the brain stem, and the autonomic and peripheral nerves. They are not dependent upon the cortex (Peiper, 1963).

The brain stem of the neonate shows varying degrees of maturity; those tracts going to the cortex are less mature than those leading to lower centers.

All the cranial nerves, with the exception of the optic and olfactory, appear myelinated and mature at birth.

The autonomic nervous system, including the hypothalamic supercontrols, are mature at birth and are capable of directing visceral function. Such visceral reflexes as sneezing, coughing, yawning are under control of the autonomic nervous system. A day-old baby can sneeze as effectively as a college graduate.

The segmented spinal nerves are mature, fully myelinated and functional at term birth. The neonate is capable of responding to sensory stimuli with characteristic and stereotyped motor behavior (p. 386) (Dekaban, 1959).

The cortex of the brain of the newborn shows all the major divisions of the adult brain as well as the primary fissures and sulci. The finer configurations, however, are missing. Many of the nerve tracts connecting the cortex with lower centers are immature at birth (Truex, 1964). The newborn functions primarily on a subcortical level, although his immature cortex is not entirely devoid of function.

POSTNATAL CHANGES IN THE NERVOUS SYSTEM

The brain grows rapidly after birth and by the age of 2 years has reached about 90 per cent of its total size. Most of the postnatal growth takes place within the cortex—that part of the brain most immature at birth.

In the first few postnatal months the sulci in all lobes of the cortex deepen, and by 3 months of age true tertiary sulci can be distinguished. By 1 year of age, the sulci are deep and prominent. They continue to increase through the years of childhood, though after 2 years of age the rate of increase is quite small (Conel, 1955).

The acquisition of myelin in the cortex, the brain stem, and also in the cord is closely correlated with the observed behavior of the infant (Langworthy, 1933). There is evidence that nerve fibers can conduct impulses before they have acquired a myelin sheath. The impulse goes down an uninsulated fiber at a slower pace than down a myelinated one. In addition there is some diffusion of the impulse carried by an unmyelinated pathway.

The corticospinal tract, which carries efferent fibers to the voluntary musculature, begins to acquire myelin soon after birth. Myelinization of this tract follows the cephalocaudal, proximodistal law. The infant becomes able to bring muscular structures under his will, first in the head, later in trunk, arms, hands, pelvic girdle, and finally, in the legs (p. 397). By the age of 2 years all structures of the spinal cord, brain stem, and cortex are myelinated. The sequence of development is similar in all human beings; the tempo, even within the limits of normal, can vary considerably. Gross failure of neuromuscular development suggests damage to the central nervous system.

As the brain matures, it begins to exercise some control, through association pathways, over much of reflex activity. Motor reflexes of the newborn, such as the Moro reflex, the grasping reflex, the tonic neck reflex, the rooting reflex, slowly fade out. Persistence of these reflexes after the age at which they should have disappeared suggests failure of normal cortical development (p. 388).

One of the simplest segmented reflexes present at all ages is the knee jerk. Afferent and efferent impulses are transmitted through a single segment of the cord; however, after the age of infancy, because of an association pathway to the cortex, the individual is aware that his knee jerks.

Not only does the brain exercise control over spinal reflexes, but also it may interfere with the smooth running of visceral function. For example, bowel evacuation can result from stimulation of autonomic nerves by a full rectum, or it can result from the response of a higher center to anxiety. In either case efferent impulses reach the rectum and cause it to discharge its contents. Likewise a cough can be stimulated by a drop of liquid on the uvula, or it can be stimulated by a desire to attract attention, in which case, though the cough mechanism is the same, the neural pathway is quite different. A yawn is a reflex produced when a sleepy person needs an increased supply of oxygen. Everyone has a tendency to yawn when he is sleepy, but sometime in childhood a cortical pathway begins to function so that the sight of someone else yawning will produce a yawn. Even reading about a yawn may produce the result!

At birth the cortex does not interfere with the functioning of the autonomic system, but during the first half year of life anxiety can interfere with the infant's visceral functions.

NEUROPHYSIOLOGY, MEMORY, EDUCATION, AND PERSONALITY

The ability to think, reason, remember, feel, and make decisions are man's highest achievements. That they have their reason for being within the nervous system seems highly probable (Brain, 1950). As more is learned about the physiology of this vastly complicated system, the justification for the dichotomy of mind and brain slips away; psychology is but physiology. This concept in no way detracts from the sense of awe inspired by the enormous complexity of the neural mechanisms; it does, however, increase the desire to know the knowable. Much is already understood about the functions of the nervous system, and this knowledge but whets the appetite for further insights into what makes man man and what makes each individual unique.

Some of this knowledge can be summarized. The basic structure of the entire nervous system consists of neuron chains, in which incoming sensations are received, shunted through channels of varying degrees of complexity, and finally discharged through an acting mechanism. Sensory stimulation is essential for both the development and maintenance of neural function (Hebb, 1958, p. 505).

In each cerebral hemisphere there are five major areas. Three have to do with sensation, one with motor control, and at least one area, possibly more, with psychic and emotional reactions. These cortical areas can be considered a kind of superstation in the whole network of control according to Penfield (1952). Impulses come into the organism by way of the basal ganglia; then by elaborate association pathways, some aspects, or maybe all, of the incoming data are sent to the cortex for analysis and coordination. From the higher cortical areas, again through the association pathways, impulses travel throughout the brain structure. Eventually an impulse reaches a basal structure in the brain stem from which an activating mechanism is set into operation. The cortex analyzes, modifies, and coordinates incoming sensory impulses in relation to previous experience, but it is neither the primary receiving station nor the primary acting station.

All activity of the CNS is referred to emotional mechanisms, which, according to Russell, are mediated through the hypothalamus and the frontal lobes of the cortex. In early childhood the feeling response is dominant in determining behavior; later, behavior becomes so complex that it is often difficult to see the connection between an overt act and the emotion that prompted it.

Motor memory consists of pathways facilitated by use (Russel). This may be as true of the relatively simple spinal cord reflexes as of the pathways in the higher centers. Memory is individual and, to a large extent, haphazard. Random activity of the infant becomes stylized; and once the stylized action is learned, it tends to persist because it is easier for the impulse to travel the remembered pathways. Most of our motor skills have individual characteristics. A person can often be recognized by his walk, by his voice, or by certain individual gestures. Handwriting is sufficiently individual to be useful in the legal identification of people.

Through pathways leading from the hypothalamus to the frontal lobe (or perhaps other pathways) each activity has a component of emotional gratification or frustration. The psychoanalyst, as well as the neurophysiologist, has explanations of why some past events are remembered and others forgotten. Freud and the early analysts felt that those things are forgotten (i.e., repressed) which, if remembered, would cause anxiety.

The hypothalamus is perhaps the area where, in lower forms, instinctive patterns are laid down. In man, the multiplicity of connections between hypothalamus and frontal lobes provides a mechanism of multiple choices, and hence breaks ancestral patterned behavior. Once patterns are established, it is possible for the individual to continue many routine activities on the basis of choices he made early in life. In a way he has established his own instincts (Hebb, 1949).

Much in the immediate environment goes unnoticed. We cannot possibly pay attention to every impression that constantly impinges upon our senses. We look, but we do not see unless alerted. Pavlov talked of a "What is it?" reaction.

A sudden change in sensory stimulation starts an impulse along a pathway to the reticular nucleus, and the individual is alerted, pays attention, and responds with the "What is it?" reaction. The impulse probably goes on to the hippocampus, where what Russel calls the "I have been there before" reaction comes into play.

In small children the alerting mechanism is powerful.

Schachtel has a good deal to say about what he calls *focal attention,* which he distinguishes from other kinds of attention. Focal attention, according to Schachtel, is man's ability "to center his attention on an object fully so that he can understand it from many sides as clearly as possible." Focal attention emerges slowly as the child matures. In early infancy the child's reaction is a total global response of ill- or well-being, in which there is no differentiation between the child and his environment; this slowly changes with time until discreet objects begin to emerge for the child and he can conceive of their existence even when he has no immediate contact with them; ultimately he can direct his focal attention to an idea or thought as well as to a concrete object. This faculty does not mature until the symbolism of language has developed, since an idea cannot be retained in memory without a symbol. Once the child has developed focal attention, he uses his ability to explore and assimilate the world about him—objects, people, ideas, relationships. This is the time when his curiosity is inexhaustible. Every stimulation gets the "What is it?" reaction, and since the child has not "been there before," his alert pushes him into giving the object focal attention. This is the age of discovery.

How much of this urge to explore the world of reality is retained as life goes on varies greatly, perhaps because of certain innate abilities but also because of environmental conditions. Focal attention is primarily time free from anxiety. The child does not dare concentrate on an object if he must constantly be on the alert to avoid dangerous aspects of reality. The anxious or fearful child glances at an object, recognizes some elements of familiarity, and lets it go at that. On the other hand, the relaxed child feels free to explore. He repeats and repeats what appears to the adult as the same experience, but each repetition is bringing to the exploring child ever-new aspects and new understanding. This urge to explore is the stuff out of which creativity is born. All little children (unless very seriously disturbed) show focal attention and inexhaustible curiosity. Some maintain for life a high measure of this ability. Such children grow up into imaginative, creative adults. Other children lose their early exploratory drive. Their curiosity becomes dampened, perhaps by anxiety, perhaps by other things. Their human potential to comprehend reality fully is suppressed. Such children grow into adults who accept a superficial acquaintance with reality as familiarity. They feel nothing is worthy of penetrating exploration.

ABERRATIONS OF DEVELOPMENT OF THE CNS

As pointed out above, normal development of the CNS depends not only upon adequate structure but also upon a suitable human climate. Structural damage is of infinite variety. It can be the result of faulty intrauterine development, of injuries at birth, or of injuries or disease in postnatal life (Truex, 1964; Dodgson, 1962).

Failure of adequate sensory stimulation after birth interferes with the normal development of the CNS (Kubzansky, 1961; Eccles, 1957; Edds, 1950; Granit, 1955). Emotional and neurotic disorders are considered primarily caused by environmental factors. Psychotic disorders are thought by some investigators (Krakowski) to have an organic base although this point of view is not universally accepted. Mental retardation is a syndrome with multiple causes and will be discussed here.

Mental Retardation

Incidence

At what point an individual is considered retarded depends upon cultural and environmental factors. A child with an IQ of 100 might be considered retarded in a family of Ph.D.s, whereas in a family of unskilled workers he might be thought of as very bright. Most children are expected to cope with life in about the same intellectual manner as the adults with whom they grow up. Any child whose intellectual endowment falls appreciably above or below this level may need help to make the best use of his potential. The "average" child born into a "superior" family is not usually classed as retarded, although his welfare is a challenge to those who care for him.

Children with IQs of 75 or below are the ones usually considered retarded. The degrees of retardation are classified as mild—IQ 50 to 75 (the educable), moderate—IQ 20 to 50 (the trainable), and severe—IQ below 20 (the untrainable).

The incidence of mental retardation varies according to the tests used and the population tested. Most surveys record the highest incidence in the 10 to 14 age group. Prior to age 10 many cases of mild retardation are missed. After school age, the apparent incidence of retardation declines, indicating that many who have been considered retarded on a basis of school performance are nonetheless capable of adjusting to society. There are no data to support the idea that actual retardation suddenly appears in the second decade and disappears in the late teens or early adult years.

TABLE 13-2

Recorded Incidence of Mental Retardation by Age

Age, years	Recorded incidence/1,000 pop.
0–4	0.7
5–9	12.0
10–14	44.0
15–19	30.0
20–29	8.0
30–39	8.0

SOURCE: From Paul A. Harper, "Preventive Pediatrics," Appleton-Century-Crofts, Inc., New York, 1962.

A conservative estimate of the number of children in the United States whose IQ, by reasonable standards, is below 75 is about 3 per cent; this means roughly 1,750,000 children under the age of 15. Each year approximately 126,000 mentally retarded infants are born. Because of decreased infant mortality and increased longevity, the total number of mentally retarded is increasing. In 1963 there were about 5½ million retarded persons in the total population of the United States. These people represent one of the nation's most serious health, education, and public welfare problems.

The mildly retarded far outnumber the more severely handicapped. Of the 3 per cent with IQs below 75, in 2.6 per cent retardation is classified as mild, in 0.3 per cent as moderate, and in only 0.1 per cent as severe.

Etiology

Mental retardation may follow structural alterations in neural or other tissue, or it can result from functional inadequacy of apparently adequate structures.

Structural alterations can be the result of infection, intoxication, or mechanical trauma taking place before birth, during birth, or after birth (Heber, 1961). Some metabolic, immunologic, and hormonal disorders, known to be genetic in origin, are associated with mental retardation (phenylketonuria, aminoaciduria, porphyria, galactosemia, idiopathic hypoglycemia, hyperglycemia). Chromosomal disorders have also been found associated with mental retardation—21 trisomy, or Down's disease; 18 trisomy; D-1 trisomy; and sex chromosome defects, Klinefelter's and Turner's syndromes.

A large group of the more mildly retarded appear to be the result of cultural and intellectual poverty in the home (Sarason and Gladwin, 1958). Children who live in a home where there are no books, where even pencil and paper are seldom to be found, where children's questions are brushed aside lack the motivation to pursue learning. It is to be noted that mild retardation is found to a much greater extent among the socially underprivileged than among the upper classes. Moderate and severe retardation on the other hand, is approximately equally distributed among all classes.

Another apparent cause of mental retardation is related to emotional disturbance or to psychotic personality disorders (Masland, 1958).

Doubtless there are other causes of mental retardation, and in many cases there are multiple factors (Sarasan, 1958).

Diagnosis

As in all diagnoses the first requirement is to be alert to the possibility of the disorder. Complete evaluation of the newborn with adequate history for possible suspicious genetic background and adequate urine and blood examinations will detect those inborn errors of metabolism with mechanisms that are understood. Early diagnosis of these diseases can, in some cases, lead to the institution of a regime that can reduce the amount of damage to the CNS. Other conditions suspected clinically in the neonatal period (chromosomal defects) are not amenable to present preventive techniques.

Many cases of mental retardation are suspected only as the child fails to develop as expected. Slow motor development, poor or inadequate speech in the preschool years are alerting signs (Penfield, 1959). Later, in the school years, inability to learn at a normal rate is suggestive. Mental retardation must be distinguished, however, from perceptual inadequacies, especially of hearing or vision, and emotional or psychotic disturbances. An evaluation of the intellectual, emotional, and cultural adequacy of the home can sometimes help one distinguish organic from cultural retardation.

Psychometric testing can aid in establishing a diagnosis of retardation and evaluating the degree of disability. To be valuable such tests must be performed by qualified psychologists and even then must be interpreted with caution, bearing in mind the many factors which can cause a poor showing on the tests.

An awareness on the part of the physician of a child's mental status is of value in helping him make maximum use of his endowments. It is also of use in pinpointing any possible remedial factors in a child's body or in his milieu (Krakowski, 1963).

BIBLIOGRAPHY

Brain, W. Russell: The Cerebral Basis of Consciousness, *Brain,* **73**:465, 1950.

Conel, J. Le Roy: "The Post-Natal Development of the Human Cerebral Cortex," vol. 1. The Cortex of the Newborn, 1939; vol. 2. The Cortex of the One-Month-Old, 1941; vol. 4. The Cortex of the Six-Month-Old, 1951; vol. 5. The Cortex of the Fifteen-Month-Old, 1955; Harvard University Press, Cambridge, Mass.

Dekaban, Anatole: "Neurology in Infancy," The Williams and Wilkins Company, Baltimore, 1959.

Dodgson, M. C. H.: "The Growing Brain, An Essay in Developmental Neurology," John Wright and Sons, Ltd., Bristol, England, 1962.

Eccles, John Carrew: "The Physiology of Nerve Cells," The Johns Hopkins Press, Baltimore, 1957.

Edds, Mac V., Jr.: Hypertrophy of Nerve Fibers due to Functionally Overloaded Muscles, *J. Comp. Neurol.,* **93**:259, 1950.

Granit, Ragnar: "Receptors and Sensory Perception," Yale University Press, New Haven, Conn., 1955.

Harper, Paul A.: "Preventive Pediatrics," Appleton-Century-Crofts, Inc., New York, 1962.

Hebb, D. O.: "The Organization of Behavior," John Wiley & Sons, Inc., New York, 1949.

———: The Motivating Effects of Extroceptive Stimulization, *Am. Psychol.,* **13**: 109, 1958.

Heber, Rick: Modifications in the Manual on Terminology and Classification in Mental Retardation, *Am. J. Ment. Deficiency,* **65**:499, 1961.

Kellogg, Winthrop N.: "Porpoises and Sonar," The University of Chicago Press, Chicago, 1961.

Krakowski, Adam J.: The Role of the Physician in the Management of the Emotionally Disturbed Child, *Psychosomatics,* **4**:215, 1963.

Kubzansky, Philip E., and P. Herbert Leiderman: "Sensory Deprivation," Harvard University Press, Cambridge, Mass., 1961.

La Barre, Weston: "The Human Animal," The University of Chicago Press, Chicago, 1954.

Langworthy, Orthello R.: Development of Behavior Patterns and Myelinization of the Nervous System in the Human Fetus and Infant, Contributions to Embryology XXIV, no. 139, 1933, and 163, 1941, Carnegie Institute of Washington, Washington, D.C.

Masland, Richard L., Seymour B. Sarason, and Thomas Gladwin: "Mental Subnormality," Basic Books, Inc., Publishers, New York, 1958.

Patten, Bradley M.: "Human Embryology," 2d ed., McGraw-Hill Book Company, New York, 1953.

Peiper, Albrecht: "Cerebral Function in Infancy and Childhood," translation of 3d revised German edition by Benedict Nagerand, Hilde Nagler, Consultants Bureau, New York, 1963.

Penfield, Wilder: Memory Mechanisms, *Arch. Neurol.,* **67**:178, 1952.

———, and Lamar Roberts: "Speech and Brain Mechanisms," Princeton University Press, Princeton, N.J., 1959.

14

The Respiratory System

Every living cell must have a continuous supply of oxygen and a usable organic carbon compound. It is the oxidation of the carbon that supplies the energy for staying alive.

Organic carbon compounds can be stored, small amounts in each individual cell, larger amounts in reservoirs throughout the body. There are no reservoirs for oxygen, however, neither in the individual cells nor in special storage facilities elsewhere in the organism. Oxygen must be supplied constantly. Any interference with its minute-by-minute supply threatens life.

Because of the imminent danger of death if oxygen supply is cut off, there is no terror so great as the fear that one cannot breathe. The fear that the supply of food may stop is insignificant compared with the terror caused by interference with oxygen supply.

Fortunately the supply of oxygen on the surface of this planet is abundant and ubiquitous. Neither animal nor man must seek for oxygen. If man ever establishes communities on the moon where imported oxygen will have to be rationed, profound changes in human values and personality may take place. On the surface of the earth, however, it is not the supply of oxygen but the organism's own apparatus for receiving and transmitting it to the tissues that is of concern.

The respiratory apparatus is a highly complicated system of organs which function, in coordination with the rest of the body, under nervous and hormonal regulation. Basically it consists of the entrance passageways – the nose, the sinuses, the larynx and trachea, and the deeper structures, the bronchi and lungs, with their surrounding thoracic cage. By means of these organs, oxygen enters the body, and gaseous waste products are eliminated. From the respiratory apparatus the vital gases are transported to the tissues of the body through the cardiovascular system.

Prior to birth, oxygen is supplied through the maternal circulation, but once the umbilical cord is cut, the individual must put his own breathing apparatus into operation.

RESPIRATION AT BIRTH

Before birth the air sacs do not contain air. There is evidence, however, that respiratory movements take place in utero and that the fetus "breathes in" amniotic fluid, which tends to stretch the alveoli (Patten).

Normally the infant takes his first breath as soon as his head is born, sometimes before the rest of his body has emerged from the birth canal. The onset of respiration is not completely understood. Doubtless there are several causes. One is certainly the sudden stimulation of the infant's tactile receptors as he emerges into air and also of his thermal receptors by the lowered temperature he meets as he leaves the uterus. These sensory stimuli cause an immediate increase in muscle tone, which, acting on the thoracic cage, causes the initial expiratory effort. This breathing out tends to clear the airways of accumulated amniotic fluid. As this is going on, the umbilical cord is compressed, oxygen level in the infant's circulation falls, and the resulting hypoxia stimulates the respiratory center. Under influence of the respiratory center, the thoracic muscles relax and inhalation takes place. If the airways are clear, the elasticity of the pulmonary tissues and the surface tension within the lungs is overcome, and inhalation rushes air into the lungs. After the initial respiratory effort the respiratory gases are diffused through the infant's body, the respiratory center continues to be stimulated, and regular in-and-out breathing is established. Normally this happens about 1 minute after delivery. Resuscitation in the newborn is discussed on p. 77. The mechanisms controlling initiation of respiration are similar in the term and premature infant. The immaturity of pulmonary tissue in the premature may interfere with the permanent establishment of regular respiration.

TABLE 14-1

Respiratory Rate

Age in years	Boys	Girls
0–1	31	30
1–2	23	27
2–3	25	25
3–4	24	24
4–5	23	22
5–6	22	21
6–7	21	21
7–8	20	20
8–9	20	20
9–10	19	19
10–11	19	19
11–12	19	19
12–13	19	19
13–14	19	19
14–15	18	18
15–16	17	18
16–17	17	17
17–18	16	17

SOURCE: Alberta Iliff and Virginia A. Lee, in *Child Development*, 23:237, 1952, by permission of the Society for Research in Child Development.

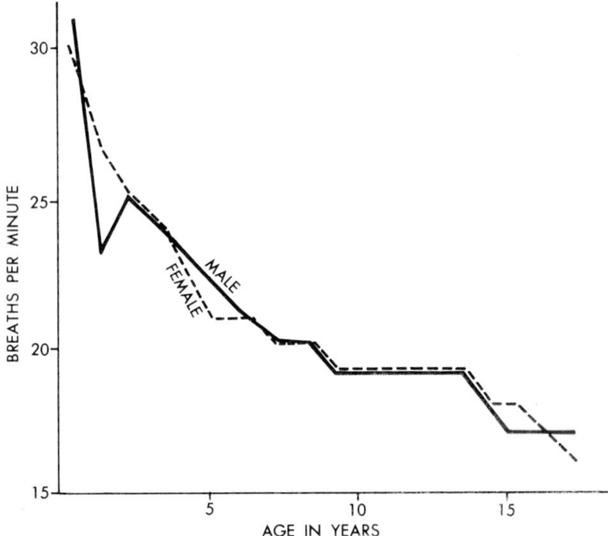

Fig. 14-1. Respiratory rate through the life span by sex. (*From Iliff and Lee, Pulse Rate and Body Temperature of Children between 2 Months and 18 Years of Age, in Child Development, 23:237, 1952, by permission from the Society for Research in Child Development, Inc.*)

RESPIRATORY CHANGES THROUGH THE LIFE SPAN

Respiratory rate, fast in infancy, gradually slows down through all the years of childhood (Iliff and Lee, 1952; Shock, 1946) (Table 14-1 and Fig. 14-1). The drop is faster in infancy and the preschool years than later. It continues to fall slowly until full maturity is reached. Puberty does not alter this downward trend. There is virtually no sex difference in respiratory rate at any time of life.

The respiratory exchange gradually becomes more efficient as life advances. From birth to puberty there is little difference between boys and girls in their acquisition of breathing efficiency, but after maturing men accomplish more with each breath than do women.

The actual volume of air inhaled with each breath increases, of course, as the size of the lungs increases with general body growth. Demuth found that lung volume increased approximately as the cube of the height. The vital capacity of the lungs (the number of liters of air in a maximum expiration following a maximum inspiration) and the maximum breathing capacity (the number of liters of air breathed during a 15-second test period) rise gradually with growth in both sexes. In boys these two measures of lung capacity increase during puberty to a greater extent than in girls (Fig. 14-2). The increase is more than can be accounted for by the greater size of boys after puberty. Morse et al. think that this represents an actual increase in lung tissue in boys concomitant with their increase in shoulder girth.

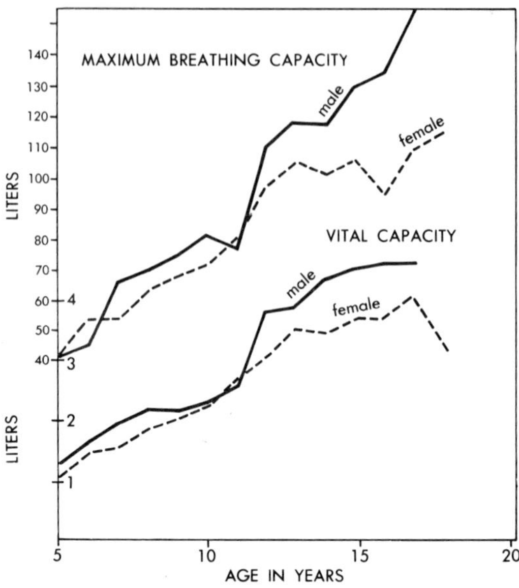

Fig. 14-2. Breathing capacity and vital capacity through the life span by sex. (*From Ferris, Whittenberger, and Gallagher, Maximum Breathing Capacity and Vital Capacity of Male Children and Adolescents, in Pediatrics, 9:659, 1952, and Ferris and Smith, Maximum Breathing Capacity and Vital Capacity of Female Children and Adolescents, in Pediatrics, 12:341, 1953.*)

There is also a qualitative difference in air expired at different ages. The amount of oxygen in the expired air decreases and the amount of CO_2 increases during all the years of childhood (Shock, 1941). Before puberty there is no sex difference in this qualitative change, but at puberty this trend in boys is accentuated to a greater extent than in girls, so that when maturity is reached, men lose less oxygen and get rid of more CO_2 with each breath than women do (Fig. 14-3). Since men expel more CO_2 with each breath, they have a bigger alkali reserve in their blood than women (Shock and Hastings, 1934). Therefore they absorb larger amounts of lactic acid and other muscle metabolites during exercise than women can without causing a change in blood pH or contracting an oxygen deficit. In other

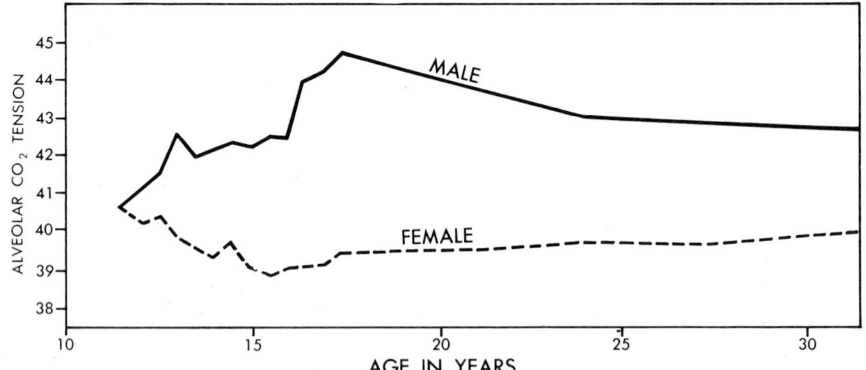

Fig. 14-3. Basal alveolar CO_2 tension through the life span by sex. (*From Shock, Age Changes and Sex Differences in Alveolar CO_2 Tension, in Am. J. Phy., 133:610, 1941.*)

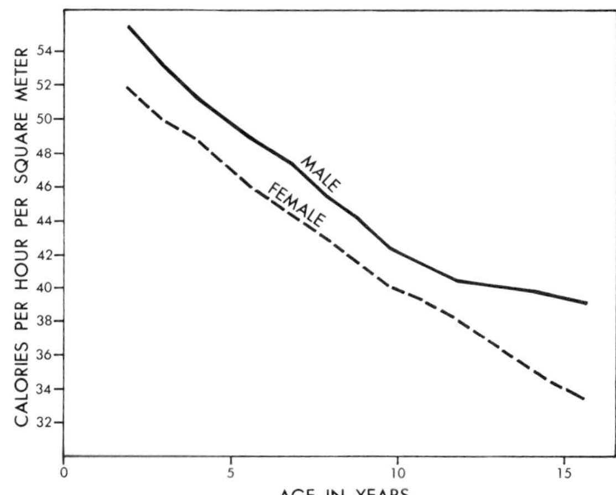

Fig. 14-4. Basal metabolism through the life span by sex. (*From Lewis, Kinsman, and Iliff, The Basal Metabolism of Normal Boys and Girls from Two to Twelve Inclusive, in Am. J. Dis. Child., 53:348, 1937, and Lewis, Duval, and Iliff, Effect of Adolescence on Basal Metabolism of Normal Children, in Am. J. Dis. Child., 66:396, 1943, and 65:834, 1943, by permission from the Society for Research in Child Development, Inc.*)

words the same amount of muscular exercise (muscle for muscle) is less fatiguing for a man than a woman.

In both sexes the basal metabolic rate falls continuously from birth onward (Talbot et al., 1937, and Lewis et al., 1937), not only to maturity, but on into old age (Fig. 14-4). The difference between the sexes is negligible until puberty. The decline in metabolic rate then flattens out in boys to a greater extent than in girls, so that adult men have a higher rate than adult women. This difference cannot be accounted for solely on the basis of the greater muscle mass in men than in women. Clark and Garn showed that boys have a higher oxygen consumption per kilogram of body weight than girls of the same muscular build from puberty on (Fig. 14-5). It is possible that the male acquires a specific metabolic stimulus, very likely from androgenic hormone (Tanner, 1955).

Because of these changes, as the child of either sex approaches puberty, he is capable of ever greater muscular exertion without exhaustion. The capacity for physical exertion increases markedly in boys after puberty. The preadolescent boy becomes exhausted appreciably more rapidly than the postadolescent boy. In adult life men are capable of greater feats of

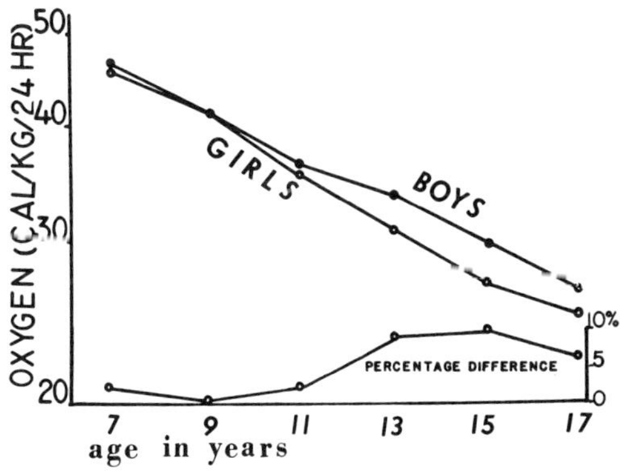

Fig. 14-5. Oxygen consumption in Calories per kilo by sex. (*From Garn, and Clark, The Sex Differences in Basal Metabolic Rate, in Child Development, 24:215, 1953, by permission of the Society for Research in Child Development, Inc.*)

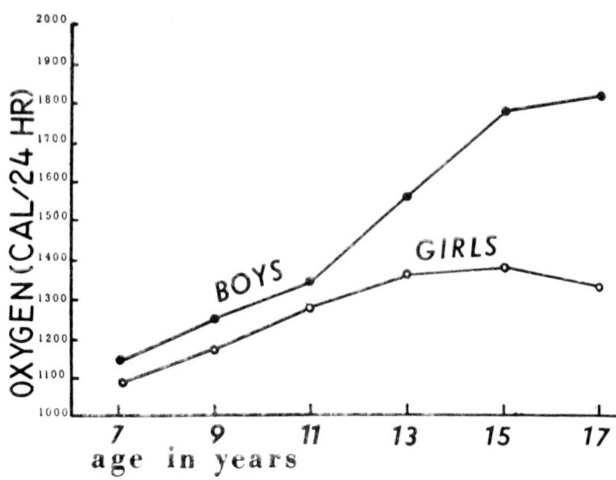

Fig. 14-6. Oxygen consumption in Calories per 24 hours by sex. *(From Garn, and Clark, The Sex Differences in Basal Metabolic Rate, in Child Development, 24:215, 1953, by permission of the Society for Research in Child Development, Inc.)*

muscular exertion than women, not only because they have bigger muscles, but also because their respiratory exchange is more efficient.

BIBLIOGRAPHY

CLARK, LELAND C., JR., and STANLEY M. GARN: Relationship between Ketosteroid Excretion and Basal Oxygen Consumption in Children, *J. Appl. Physiol.,* **6**:546, 1954.

DE MUTH, G. R., W. H. HOWATT, and B. M. HILL: The Growth of Lung Function, *Pediatrics,* **35** (supp.): 161, 1965.

FERRIS, B. G., and C. W. SMITH: Maximum Breathing Capacity and Vital Capacity of Female Children and Adolescents, *Pediatrics,* **12**:341, 1953.

———, J. L. WHITTENBERGER, and J. R. GALLAGHER: Maximum Breathing Capacity and Vital Capacity of Male Children and Adolescents, *Pediatrics,* **9**: 659, 1952.

GARN, STANLEY MARION, and LELAND C. CLARK: The Sex Difference in Basal Metabolic Rate, *Child Development,* **24**:215, 1953.

ILIFF, ALBERTA, and VIRGINIA A. LEE: Pulse Rate, Respiratory Rate, and Body Temperature of Children between 2 Months and 18 Years of Age, *Child Development,* **23**:237, 1952.

LEWIS, ROBERT C., GLADYS M. KINSMAN, and ALBERTA ILIFF: The Basal Metabolism of Normal Boys and Girls from Two to Twelve, Inclusive, *Am. J. Dis. Child.,* **53**:348, 1937.

———, ANNA MARIA DUVAL, and ALBERTA ILIFF: Basal Metabolism of Normal Children from Thirteen to Fifteen Years Old Inclusive, *Am. J. Dis. Child.,* **65**:805, 1943.

———, ANNA MARIA DUVAL, and ALBERTA ILIFF: Basal Metabolism of Normal Children, *Am. J. Dis. Child.,* **66**:396, 1943, and **65**:834, 1943.

MORSE, MINERVA, DONALD E. CASSELS, and MELBA HOLDER: The Position of the Oxygen Dissociation Curve of the Blood in Normal Children and Adults, *J. Clin. Invest.,* **29**:1091, 1952.

———, FREDERICK W. SCHULTZ, and DONALD E. CASSELS: Relation of Age to Physiological Response of the Older Boy (10–17) to Exercise, *J. Appl. Physiol.,* **1**:683, 1949.

PATTEN, BRADLEY M.: "Human Embryology," 2d ed., McGraw-Hill Book Company, New York, 1953.

SHOCK, NATHAN W., and A. BAIRD HASTINGS: Studies of the Acid-base Balance of the Blood, *J. Biol. Chem.*, **104**:585, 1934.

———: Age Changes and Sex Difference in Alveolar CO_2 Tension, *Am. J. Physiol.*, **133**:610, 1941.

———, and MAYO H. SOLEY: Average Values for Basal Respiratory Functions in Adolescents and Adults, *J. Nutrition*, **18**:143, 1939.

———: Some Physiological Aspects of Adolescence, *Texas Rep. Biol. & Med.* **4**:289, 1946, and **4**:368, 1946.

TALBOT, FRITZ B., EDWIN B. WILSON, and JANE WORCHESTER: Basal Metabolism in Girls, *Am. J. Dis. Child.*, **53**:273, 1937.

TANNER, J. M.: "Growth at Adolescence," Charles C Thomas, Publisher, Springfield, Ill., 1955.

15

The Cardiovascular System

Unicellular forms of life need oxygen and some organic carbon compound from which to liberate the energy necessary for their survival. Every cell of the metazoan body has these requirements, but the complexity of the many-celled animal makes it impossible for each cell to obtain its needs by diffusion from the surrounding environment. The simplest of the multicelled organisms had a system of open canals through which sea water flowed. By this device the nutrient fluid reached the inner cells which could not communicate directly through the periphery of the organism. As complexity of structure emerged, these open canals became a closed circuit, and a clump of muscle fibers developed which served the purpose of pumping the fluid through the closed system.

The cardiovascular system of man serves the same basic function as did the early primitive open canals. Blood shows its phylogenetic origin from sea water. It is essentially a saline solution modified by the presence of protein in colloidal suspension, emulsified fat, and other substances. Both the blood and the cardiovascular system of man have assumed many subsidiary functions.

Blood carries oxygen from the lungs to all the tissues and carries CO_2 back to the lungs. The blood also carries, from the gastrointestinal tract to the tissues, the digested nutrients of the food consumed. It takes away from the tissues nitrogenous waste products, carrying some to organs of excretion and others to areas of the body where these nitrogenous products are used for metabolic function. In addition blood transports hormones and antibodies.

The blood of warm-blooded animals is largely responsible for the maintenance of body temperature. It can spread out in thin layers in dilated superficial capillaries, dissipate the body heat to the surroundings, and thereby cool the body, or it can drain back into deep organs when the capillaries contract and thus conserve heat. The blood also aids in the control of the amount of fluid within the body tissues. The heart acts as a central pump which makes it possible for the blood to carry out its specific functions.

EMBRYOLOGY

In the heart, the vascular apparatus, and in the respiratory apparatus (Chap. 14) functioning units must develop that will serve the needs of the fetus before birth and yet be able to take over radically different functions at the moment of birth. That the cardiovascular system is apt to fail in its development is reflected in the fact that almost half of all congenital malformations that cause death within the first year are due to abnormalities of the circulatory system.

The fetus lives a parasitic existence. It depends upon the maternal organism to prepare its nutrients, supply its oxygen, and eliminate its waste. The source of supply for the fetus is the chorion. It is in this structure, outside its own body, that the fetus must build an elaborate series of blood vessels through which to receive its vital needs. At the moment of birth, when the umbilical cord is severed, these vascular plexuses are forced immediately to stop functioning. Not only must these channels be obliterated, but the fetus must have built up a sufficiently elaborate system of blood vessels in lungs, gut and kidneys to take over the now defunct umbilical circulation. It is not as though the blood vessels could slowly grow into these organs as they increase in size and need a larger flow of blood. The vascular network must grow into them without any immediate need. This is obviously a gene-directed phenomenon.

The heart is under the same kind of handicap. It begins to be formed about the third week of fetal life, and at about 2 months it has assumed essentially adult configuration (Fig. 15-1). The circulation at this age has two distinct parts—the intraembryonic and the extraembryonic. The intraembryonic circulation sends blood by way of the developing aorta to the emerging structures of the embryo where it is spread out in capillary beds. The blood is then collected into the venous channels and returned to the heart.

The extraembryonic circulation starts at the heart and passes through the aorta and out of the embryonic body to end in the capillary network of the chorion. In the beginning the extraembryonic circulation heads for the yolk sac. In the mammal the yolk sac is empty of nutrients; yet the embryo, retracing its phylogenetic origins, develops a circulation to this vestigial and useless structure. Rather quickly this circulation becomes obliterated, and the embryo directs its vascular structure toward the chorion, which takes over the nutritive function once inherent in the yolk sac. It is, however, in the yolk sac that the first blood islands appear; it is here that the first blood corpuscles are made.

The extraembryonic circulation is large during all of embryonic and fetal life. The return flow from the chorion passes through venous channels to the liver, where the veins break up into capillaries and traverse the tissues of the liver before again being collected into further venous channels and

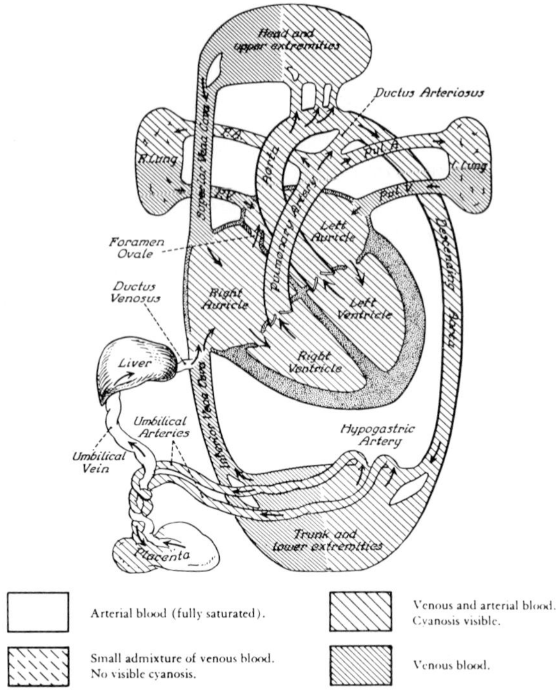

Fig. 15-1. Four stages in the fusion of paired primordia of the heart as seen in cross section. *(From Human Embryology, 2d ed., by Bradley M. Patten, McGraw-Hill Book Company, Inc.)*

returned to the heart. Because of the large volume of blood flowing through the liver during fetal life this organ reaches a relatively enormous size. After birth, when only the blood from the small intestine passes through the liver (the portal circulation), the liver gradually decreases in bulk.

From this early beginning the heart, the arteries, and the veins progress through complicated developmental stages until finally the fetus is ready to attempt existence on its own. At birth the circulatory pathways vital to fetal existence become rapidly obliterated, and the as-yet-untried channels get their opportunity to prove the adequacy of their preparation.

Radical as these changes are, the fetus has more or less prepared itself, and the transition is made with remarkable smoothness in the vast majority of newborn infants.

FETAL CIRCULATION JUST PRIOR TO BIRTH

Toward the end of intrauterine life the fetus has developed the potentiality of carrying on a self-sufficient circulation independent of supplies from the maternal circulation. Nevertheless, the fetus must maintain its aquatic, parasitic circulation up until the moment it is released from this phase of life.

Just prior to birth the circulation is as shown in Fig. 15-2. From the umbilical vein the blood flows through the liver to the right atrium. Before reaching the heart this blood is combined with that of the inferior vena cava, the chief venous return from the fetal body. Thus the blood entering the right atrium is oxygenated blood from the chorion plus deoxygenated blood from the vena cava. From the right atrium the blood has two possible passageways. Some of it passes to the right ventricle and heads toward the lungs. The lungs, prior to birth, are nonfunctional.

In the young fetus only a very small amount of blood goes through the lungs. As gestation advances and the lungs increase in size, the pulmonary flow becomes greater, though it remains small in comparison to what it will be after birth. Much of the blood in the fetal right atrium goes through the foramen ovale directly into the left atrium. The left atrium receives also blood which went through the fetal lungs. From the left atrium the blood passes to the left ventricle and then out the aorta to the fetal body. Since

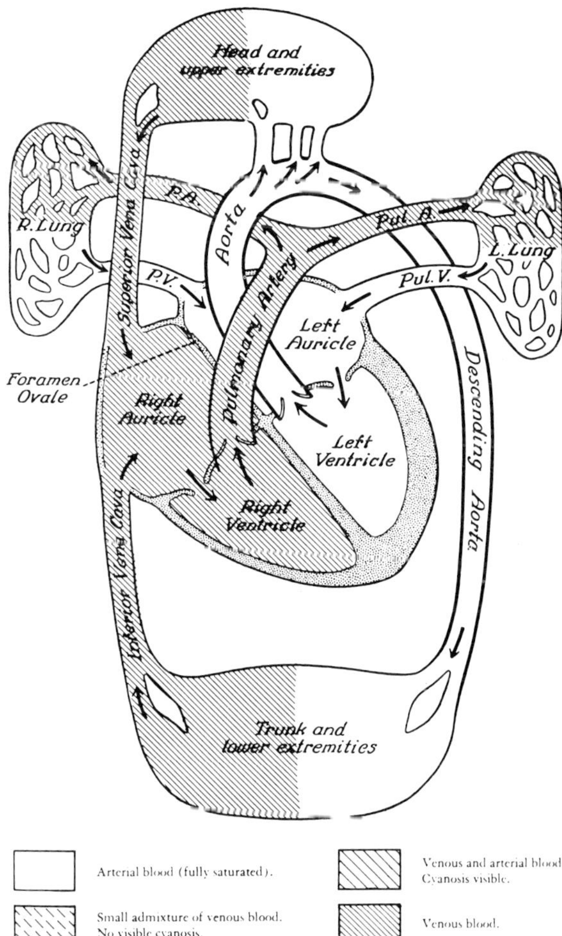

Fig. 15-2. Fetal circulation. (From *Congenital Malformation of the Heart,* by Helen B. Taussig, published by Harvard University Press for the Commonwealth Fund, Inc.)

more blood passes from right ventricle to the lungs than the lungs can take in their unexpanded condition, a shunt exists whereby some of the blood in the pulmonary artery bypasses the lungs and goes directly into the aorta. This is the ductus arteriosus. This shunt serves the purpose in the fetus of maintaining a larger flow through the right atrium and ventricle than would otherwise be possible. This volume of blood prepares the right side of the heart for its increased load as soon as breathing begins.

IMMEDIATE POSTNATAL CHANGES

As soon as the infant takes his first breath, the lungs demand more blood and the ductus arteriosus closes. This is soon followed by the shutting of the foramen ovale. All the blood entering the right side of the heart then proceeds through the lungs. The pressure in the pulmonary artery decreases as pulmonary resistance lessens and the blood bypasses the shunt, which becomes functionally closed almost at once. From the lungs the pulmonary vein deposits the blood in the left atrium, increasing the pressure in this organ. This increased pressure helps to keep the foramen ovale closed and prevents admixture of blood in the two atria. From the left atrium the blood flows to the left ventricle, then to the aorta. The ductus arteriosus is functionally closed by the changes in pressure relations, so that the aorta has only blood from the left ventricle.

Both the ductus arteriosus and the foramen ovale close functionally soon after birth. There is a contraction of the smooth muscle of the ductus which reduces the flow of blood through this channel. This is followed by anatomic closure and obliteration. The intima of the vessel slowly grows into the lumen and completely occludes it. The lumen is completely gone by the third or fourth month of postnatal life.

The foramen ovale likewise closes functionally as the pressure in the left antrum increases immediately after birth. This valve does not close anatomically until toward the end of the first year (Fig. 15-3).

In addition to the postnatal changes in circulation through the heart there are changes surrounding the umbilical vessels. Blood flow through these vessels stops abruptly when the umbilical cord is severed. Obliteration of the lumen of the vessel takes place slowly over the first few weeks of postnatal life.

CONGENITAL DEFECTS OF THE HEART

When the development of the circulatory system is appreciated, it is not surprising that there are occasions when the intricate coordinating mechanisms do not work out perfectly. Most congenital cardiac malformations are the result of failure of the system to time each move at exactly the right moment for everything to fall accurately into place. Three main types of failure are recognized:

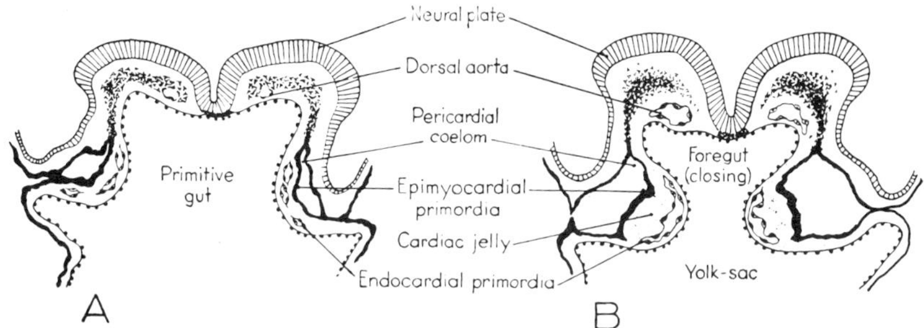

Fig. 15-3. Postnatal circulation. (*From Congenital Malformations of the Heart, by Helen B. Taussig, published by Harvard University Press for the Commonwealth Fund, Inc.*)

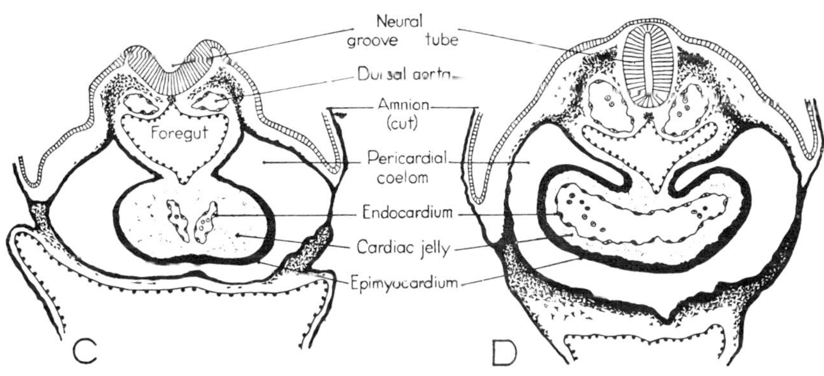

1. Failure of rotation of the heart. In the early weeks of fetal life the single-chambered tubular heart twists spirally; should this twisting fail to take place, a confusion between right and left sides of the heart comes into being. The blood in the aorta may flow into the lungs and that from the pulmonary artery into the body tissues.

2. Failures of development of the septums which separate the right and left chambers of the heart, and faulty development of the numerous valves that separate one compartment from another.

3. Persistence of structure, normal and essential in fetal life, but incompatible with existence independent of the placental circulation.

In addition to these main types of maldevelopment in the cardiac system other anomalies may occur in the intracardiac structure, such as aortic rings, coarctation of the aorta, anomalous coronary or pulmonary vessels.

Any one type of developmental failure may exist singly, or several forms of failure may be coexistent. Failures can be of all degrees of severity from minimal derangements with no clinical significance to such gross defects that independent life is impossible.

Any defect which alters the normal pressure relations within the heart is apt ultimately to cause serious trouble, even though clinical symptoms of cardiac embarrassment are not present in early life. If pressure in the right side of the heart is increased, as the result of increased blood flow because of septal defects or a persistent ductus arteriosus, pulmonary hypertension often results. It is generally agreed today that in some infants with or without associated cardiac defects, the fetal pattern of high pulmonary artery pressures and high resistance is maintained after birth. When there is no associated cardiac or vascular defect, this condition is known as *primary pulmonary hypertension.* In the wake of pulmonary hypertension and raised pulmonary resistance may come reversed flow into the right side of the heart and cyanosis. In addition there appears to be a relation between increased blood flow and pressure and the development of atherosclerosis (see below in the discussion of Cholesterol).

The last decade has seen enormous strides in cardiac surgical techniques. Most congenital cardiac defects are now repairable. The repair of a ductus arteriosus is a relatively simple operation hardly more serious than an appendectomy. Surgical operation on defective valves and septums is practical in most cases, though it is a more difficult procedure than that on extracardiac structures, such as a ductus. Repair of defects due to transposition of the great vessels is not possible with current techniques.

CARDIAC FUNCTION THROUGH THE LIFE SPAN

Pulse Rate and Its Controls

The action of the heart is under the control of the autonomic nervous system. The human cannot by an act of will retard or slow his own cardiac rate. Throughout life the cardiac rate is responsive to organ needs and also to the emotional state. Fear, anxiety, tension, increase the rate; depression slows it.

The heart rate falls steadily throughout childhood. It is very high in fetal life, about 150 beats per minute. It falls by the time of birth to about 130 beats per minute. From then on it falls through all of childhood, reaching the adult rate soon after puberty (Table 15-1).

In early life not only is the pulse rate rapid, but it is more variable than later in life. Sinus arrhythmia is considered a physiologic phenomenon during childhood. It appears to be related to respiration; the heart accelerates with inspiration and slows with expiration. It is more marked with slow respiration and usually disappears when breathing becomes rapid. Thus during sleep the pulse is often quite irregular, but with exercise the irregularities disappear. Absence of sinus arrhythmia in childhood is suggestive of cardiac abnormality—the normal young heart is irregular, whereas the

TABLE 15-1

Pulse Rate and Body Temperature

	Pulse		Body temperature	
Age, years	Boys	Girls	Boys	Girls
0–1	135	126	99.1	99.1
1–2	105	104	99.1	98.9
2–3	93	93	99.0	98.8
3–4	87	89	98.9	98.8
4–5	84	84	98.6	98.5
5–6	79	79	98.5	98.5
6–7	76	77	98.4	98.5
7–8	75	76	98.3	98.4
8–9	73	73	98.3	98.3
9–10	70	70	98.1	98.2
10–11	67	69	98.0	98.1
11–12	67	69	98.0	98.0
12–13	66	69	97.8	97.9
13–14	65	68	97.7	97.9
14–15	62	66	97.6	97.9
15–16	61	65	97.4	97.9
16–17	61	66	97.3	97.8
17–18	60	65	97.2	97.9

SOURCE: From Iliff and Lee, Pulse Rate, Respiratory Rate, and Body Temperature of Children between 2 months and 18 years, in Child Development, 23: 237, 1952, by permission of the Society for Research in Child Development, Inc.

abnormal heart is apt to be less responsive in the necessary reflex mechanism. Why this should be so is not clearly understood.

Adolescence marks the end of the downward trend in pulse rate and the cessation of the irregularities of the young heart (Fig. 15-4). Before puberty there is very little difference between the pulse rate in boys and girls, but after maturity has been reached, women have a slightly higher rate than men. Heart rate is related to the size of the organism. Children have a higher rate than men.[1]

In adult man the rate is about 60 beats per minute and in adult women about 65. This sex difference is established at adolescence. Why this difference exists between the sexes is not understood. It may be merely that men are a little bigger than women.

Increased body temperature increases the heart rate, and Tanner has suggested that the slightly higher heart rate of women may be related to their slightly higher body temperature. Body temperature falls a little during childhood, boys and girls showing no difference until about the age

[1] It is interesting to note that this relationship seems to exist throughout the animal world. The heart rate of a canary is 1,000 beats per minute, while that of an elephant is but 25 (Best and Taylor, 1955).

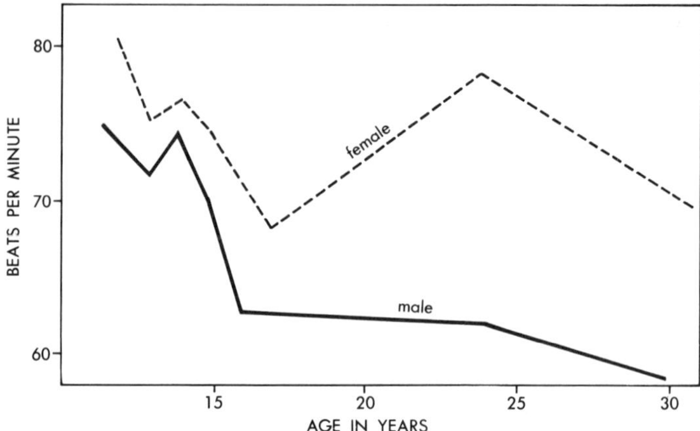

Fig. 15-4. Pulse rate at puberty by sex. (*From Iliff and Lee, Pulse Rate, Respiratory Rate, and Body Temperature of Children between 2 Months and 18 Years of Age, in Child Development, 23:237, 1952, by permission of the Society for Research in Child Development, Inc.*)

of 12. At this time the body temperature of girls remains stationary, but that of boys continues to fall for another few years before it flattens out into adult values. Tanner points out that a difference of 0.7°F in the body temperature of men and women would account for a difference of five beats per minute in heart rate.

The cause of the sex difference in body temperature is quite unknown. Whether or not the difference in body temperature is the sole cause of the difference in heart rate between the sexes is not known. It is possible that heart rate could reflect the higher systolic blood pressures in the male and be related to a greater stimulation of the vagus nerve (which serves the heart) because of the higher blood pressure.

Blood Pressure

Immediately after birth the systolic pressure is lower than at any other time during life. This reflects the fact that the left ventricle has not as yet had to pump a full quota of blood through the arterial system. In fact the pressure in the pulmonary system is about equal to that in the systemic system for the first weeks of life. Quite rapidly, however, the left ventricle builds up strength and power, and the systolic pressure rises from the low of about 40 mm Hg at birth to about 70 mm Hg at 2 weeks of age. After this the rise in systolic pressure is slower but reaches about 80 mm Hg toward the end of the first month of life. From then on the pressure increases very gradually during childhood, reaching roughly 100 mm Hg several years before puberty. At puberty the basal systolic pressure rises rapidly, and adult values are reached. The rise is related to the age of puberty, rather than to the chronological age, early-maturing children showing a s[illegible] in systolic pressure sooner than late-maturing ones. Boys, maturing as they do later than girls, show an increase in systolic pressure some years after the girls but always in relation to the age at which they mature. When the rise occurs, it is greater in boys than in girls, establishing a sex difference which persists through the mature years. The increase in blood pressure is almost entirely in the systolic pressure; the diastolic pressure shows little change during the adolescent years and is the same in boys and girls, which means that pulse pressure in men is somewhat higher than in women from the time of puberty on through the mature years.

CHOLESTEROL

Within the last few years there has been much discussion of the role of cholesterol in the production of atherosclerosis. Atheromatous plaques contain this sterol, and high levels of blood cholesterol have been found to be associated with atherosclerosis in older people. It has also been demonstrated that replacement of a significant proportion of dietary saturated fats with vegetable oils, high in linoleic acid (the polyunsaturated fats), reduces serum cholesterol in many individuals whose serum cholesterol level is higher than normal.

Cholesterol in the blood is low at birth; it rises during infancy and reaches approximately adult levels by about 7 months of age (Wohl and Goodhart, 1960). Whether or not blood cholesterol levels rise higher with age in the healthy person is a matter of dispute. Page et al. found blood cholesterol levels approximately constant in a large group of healthy men, from 19 to 101 years of age. Similar results were obtained by Sperry and Webb in a longitudinal study lasting 15 years. Keys, on the other hand, believes that even in health, blood cholesterol levels rise with age.

There is much still unknown about the metabolism of this essential sterol and its relation to vascular disease. While it is true that there appears to be an association of atherosclerosis and high serum cholesterol levels in older people, it is also true that extreme atherosclerosis has been demonstrated in infants whose cholesterol values were low. It is possible that increased intravascular pressure due to congenitally stenosed valves was related to the development of the sclerosed plaques in these infants. It is also possible that increased intravascular pressure is a factor in the development of atherosclerosis in later life.

At the present state of knowledge, one must keep an open mind concerning the metabolic significance of cholesterol and its relation to atherosclerosis.

Over the age of 40 the failure of the cardiovascular system is the major cause of death. It appears that the heart and its vessels wear out more rapidly than any other system in the human body. One aspect of this degenerative process is the development of atherosclerosis. It is possible that this may be a gene-directed phenomenon; it does appear to "run in families." One can speculate that if those individuals prone to develop atherosclerosis in middle life could be detected before the process began to develop, it might be feasible to institute measures that would prevent its development.

Bloomfield and Liebman recently reported on a means of detecting idiopathic cardiomyopathy in apparently healthy children. The ultimate cardiac fate of children so affected may provide insight into cardiac problems of middle age.

All investigators agree that preformed dietary cholesterol (such as exists in eggs and liver) has relatively little influence on the blood level of cholesterol. There seems to be no justification, therefore, at the present time, in limiting the intake of eggs, liver, and whole milk in the diet of children. Such limitations may cause more nutritional damage than the hypothetical advantage of cholesterol limitation.

BIBLIOGRAPHY

Best, Charles H., and Norman Burke Taylor: "The Physiological Basis of Medical Practice," The Williams and Wilkins Company, Baltimore, 1955.

Bloomfield, Daniel K., and Jerome Liebman: Idiopathic Cardiomyopathy in Children, *Circulation,* **27**:1071, 1963.

Eicharn, Dorothy H., and John P. McKee: Oral Temperatures and Subcutaneous Fat During Adolescence, *Child Development,* **24**:235, 1953.

Iliff, Alberta, and Virginia D. Lee: Pulse Rate, Respiratory Rate, and Body Temperature of Children between 2 Months and 18 Years of Age, *Child Development,* **23**:237, 1952.

Keys, Ancel, Flaminio Fidanza, Vicenzo Scardi, Gino Bergami, Margaret Keys, and Ferruccio DiLorenzo: Studies on Serum Cholesterol and Other Characteristics of Clinically Healthy Men in Naples, *Arch. Intern. Med.,* **93**: 328, 1954.

Page, Irvine H., Esben Kirk, William H. Lewis, Jr., William R. Thompson, and Donald D. Van Slyke: Plasma Lipids of Normal Men at Different Ages, *J. Biol. Chem.,* **111**:613, 1935.

Patten, Bradley M.: "Human Embryology," 2d ed., McGraw-Hill Book Company, New York, 1953.

Shock, Nathan W.: Physiological Responses of Adolescents to Exercise, *Texas Rep. Biol. & Med.,* **4**:369, 1946.

———: Basal Blood Pressure and Pulse Rate in Adolescents, *Am. J. Dis. Child.,* **68**:16, 1944.

———: Some Physiological Aspects of Adolescence, *Texas Rep. Biol. & Med.,* **4**:289, 1946.

Sperry, Warren M., and Merrill Webb: The Effect of Increasing Age on Serum Cholesterol Concentrates, *J. Biol. Chem.,* **187**:107, 1950.

Tanner, J. M.: "Growth at Adolescence," Charles C Thomas, Publisher, Springfield, Ill., 1955.

Taussig, Helen B.: "Congenital Malformations of the Heart: I. General Considerations, II. Specific Malformations," Harvard University Press, Cambridge, Mass., 1960, published for the Commonwealth Fund.

Wohl, Michael G., and Robert S. Goodhart: "Modern Nutrition in Health and Disease," Lea and Febiger, Philadelphia, 1960.

16

Formed Elements in the Blood

Blood consists of a liquid medium, plasma, in which are suspended a variety of formed elements. In this chapter the formed elements will be considered with special attention to their developmental pattern and to alterations in these structures which are signs of trouble.

CLASSIFICATION OF FORMED ELEMENTS

The formed elements are divided into the following categories:

1. Erythrocytes, the cells that negotiate, minute by minute, the gaseous exchange upon which life depends.
2. Leukocytes, of three kinds which have in common the property of protecting the body against stress, particularly against infection. These are:
   a. Granulocytes
   b. Lymphocytes
   c. Monocytes
3. Thrombocytes, or platelets, small particles the function of which has to do primarily with the bleeding and clotting mechanisms.
4. Other formed elements occasionally seen during health but more frequently seen in disorders of the hematopoietic system.

ORIGINS OF THE FORMED BLOOD ELEMENTS

The origin of the formed elements of the blood is in dispute. Some maintain that all blood corpuscles have a common origin from a single primitive cell; others, that several primitive cells arise, each of which differentiates into a specific series of blood elements. A discussion of the various theories is given by Wintrobe.

Blood begins to form very early in the embryo. By the third week of intrauterine life, blood islands make their appearance in the yolk sac. These islands are the beginnings both of the formed elements and of the blood channels. Blood islands are soon evident in many areas of the mesenchyme. From them the primitive blood cells spread to adjacent structures and colonize new blood-forming regions everywhere that structure is actively being formed. Reticuloendothelium appears around these areas, which grow rapidly while the structure is being formed and then, as metabolic activity in the area subsides, become less active and finally disappear (Patten, 1953). By the sixth to eighth week of fetal life the original primitive hemangioblasts have become concentrated in reticuloendothelium in various parts of the organism and begin to differentiate into the precursors of some of the mature blood elements: erythroblasts containing hemoglobin (the precursors of the erythrocytes), granuloblasts (the precursors of the granulocytes), and megakaryocytes (the precursors of the platelets).

The liver is the most active hematopoietic organ from the second month to midfetal life. The spleen begins to produce blood cells soon after the liver, and bone marrow comes into action at about the fourth month. By the time of birth, formation of erythrocytes, granulocytes, and thrombocytes has all but ceased everywhere except in the bone marrow (Wintrobe). The ribs, the sternum, and the bodies of the vertebrae remain for life the main site for formation of the erythrocytic and granulocytic series of blood corpuscles.

While these areas are the normal site for the formation of erythrocytes and granulocytes after birth, some of the fetal blood-forming areas, notably the liver and spleen, retain their potential for the manufacture of these blood elements in time of hematopoietic stress during the years of early childhood.

ERYTHROCYTES

The outstanding feature of the erythrocyte is the fact that it synthesizes hemoglobin in its cytoplasm. It is the only formed blood element that does acquire this substance. The immature cells of the series are quite large, but as they mature by successive cell divisions, each cell becomes progressively smaller—the nucleus becomes more compact and deeper-staining. As the last stage in maturation is reached, the nucleus of the cell is extruded, but a fine network of basophilic material is still retained. An erythrocyte with a basophilic network is called a *reticulocyte*. The mature erythrocyte, now devoid of nucleus, is expelled into the bloodstream, and soon afterward its basophilic network is lost.

In early fetal life many of the erythrocytes in the circulatory blood are nucleated; that is, they are expelled from the reticuloendothelial tissue in an immature form. Maturation, however, proceeds rapidly, and by about the tenth week of fetal life, approximately 90 per cent of the circulating erythrocytes are nonnucleated. By the time of birth, only occasional nucleated red cells are present.

The erythrocytes of the newborn, either full-term or premature, are reasonably mature and capable of carrying oxygen from lungs to tissue and CO_2 from tissue to lungs. The immaturity of the hematopoietic system is reflected by the presence of nucleated red cells and of reticulocytes in the circulation.

Hemoglobin is synthesized in the blood-forming areas and transported by the erythrocytes. There is a close but not absolute correlation between the amount of hemoglobin and the number of red cells. At times when the body lacks the material from which to make hemoglobin, each cell will mature with a less than optimal amount of this substance. Erythrogenesis is influenced also by hormones from the adrenal, the thyroid, and the hypophysis. Synthesis of hemoglobin and other proteins occurs in the immature nucleated cell. After the nucleus is extruded and the cell enters the circulation, enzymatic activity decreases. The mature erythrocyte circulates for 100 to 120 days and is then broken down in the cells of the reticuloendothelial system, primarily those of the bone marrow and secondarily those of the spleen, although under some circumstances the erythrocyte can be catabolized in other reticuloendothelial sites.

The iron is split off from the hemoglobin molecule, bound to plasma proteins, retained in the bone marrow or transported to bone marrow, and reused for further hemoglobin manufacture. The heme fraction yields biliverdin, which is rapidly reduced to bilirubin, released into the bloodstream, and transported to the liver, where the insoluble bilirubin is converted into soluble forms and excreted in the bile. The globin passes into the general body amino acid pool.

In health the number of erythrocytes in the circulating blood and the amount of hemoglobin vary with age, with sex, and with altitude (Table 16-1). Anemia results if erythrogenesis is interfered with or if red cells once formed are destroyed or lost more rapidly than the erythropoietic organs can manufacture them.

When blood is mixed with an anticoagulant and allowed to stand in a vertical column, the red cells fall to the bottom of the tube, leaving a clear supernatant liquid. The speed with which red cells settle, the *sedimentation rate,* rises in certain disease conditions. More than a minimal amount of tissue destruction or exudative reaction anywhere in the body alters blood plasma in such a way that the red cells clump together and settle rapidly. A rise in sedimentation rate is not diagnostic of any specific disease but may be an indication that some disorder associated with tissue destruction is present.

Normal values for the sedimentation rate depend upon the method used, but even with the same method the normal constitutes a range rather than a single figure. Children show a slightly higher sedimentation rate than adults, regardless of the method used. There is no significant difference between boys and girls prior to puberty. Wolman gives the following figures as representing the upper limits of normal in prepubescent children: by the Westergren method, 15 to 20 mm in 1 hr; with the Wintrobe method, 10 mm; with the Cutler method, 15 mm. After puberty women have a somewhat higher rate than men.

LEUKOCYTES

Leukocytes are widely distributed in the reticuloendothelial tissue side by side with erythrocytes. This series of white blood cells probably originates from the primitive hemangioblasts.

Granulocytes

Early in development the precursor of the granulocyte can be distinguished from the precursor of the erythrocyte by the fact that no hemoglobin appears in the cytoplasm of the former. Granuloblasts soon separate into three types: neutrophils, eosinophils, and basophils, distinguishable by their staining reactions. Each type of granulocyte goes through maturation divisions and is finally expelled into the circulating blood. The granulocytes are quite mature in the last weeks of gestation, the blood of the newborn therefore contains all types of granulocytes, although a slightly larger proportion of immature forms are found in the blood of the newborn than in that of slightly older infants.

The neutrophils are active phagocytic cells. They engulf and transport particulate material. Bacteria and viruses are carried by neutrophils to lymph nodes, where pathogenic organisms are further dealt with (p. 289), fractions of disintegrating erythrocytes are carried by neutrophils to the bone marrow, where hematin is conserved for further hemoglobin synthesis. The number of neutrophils in the circulating blood during health varies with age. Neutrophils increase when there is an increase in foreign matter to be transported—i.e., in infection; they decrease in conditions in which the bone marrow is impaired and unable to respond to normal or accelerated demand for this type of cell.

The eosinophils, like the neutrophils, are phagocytic cells, although they are more sluggish in their action than the neutrophils. Eosinophils have, however, a predilection only for certain kinds of particulate matter, especially that occurring in the hypersensitive state (p. 301), which they remove and detoxify. In health the number of eosinophils is small. They increase in number under particular kinds of stress. In addition to the presence in the body of substances to which the eosinophils react, the concentration of eosinophils is influenced by the pituitary-adrenal mechanisms.

The function of basophils is not well understood. Their concentration in peripheral blood is normally low.

Lymphocytes

Lymphocytes do not appear in the circulating blood of the fetus until well after erythrocytes and granulocytes have been circulating for some time. Whether lymphoblasts arise from the primitive hemangioblasts or whether they arise directly from the epithelial primordium of the mesenchyme, they are ultimately to be found in all lymphoid tissues of the body—thymus, spleen, tonsils, lymph glands, and Peyer's patches in the intestine, where they mature by passing through a series of cell divisions, after which they are expelled, either directly into the blood or indirectly by means of the thoracic duct.

Recently, Fichtelius has presented data that indicates that the thymus may be the primary site of origin of the lymphocytes and that from the thymus lymphocytes are seeded to the other lymphoid organs. If this is true, primary thymic lymphocytes may not be identical with those from the secondary lymphoid tissue. Extending this theory, Burnet suggests that the thymus may be the primary immunologic organ of the body (p. 294).

Lymphocytes, unlike the granulocytes, do not phagocytize foreign material. Their presence, however, in lymph glands appears to increase the rate of phagocytosis of the neutrophils. Lymphocytes manufacture γ-globulin, a substance essential in the synthesis of antibodies (p. 295).

Lymphocytes are more abundant in the blood of healthy children than in the blood of older people and are doubtless related to the development of acquired immunity (see Table 16-2). Lymphocytosis and lymphopenia occur in certain disease states.

Thrombocytes

Platelets are small colorless bodies which may be spherical, oval, or rod-shaped. There have been many theories of their origin, but it is now generally accepted that they arise from megakaryocytes in the bone marrow. These large cells mature, and as they are expelled into the bloodstream, they rupture, and the small particles circulate as platelets.

The function of the platelets has to do with the complicated clotting mechanisms. Platelets agglutinate and aid in sealing an injured blood vessel; they probably also aid in the actual clotting of blood, although the mechanism of their action is not well understood.

BLOOD OF THE NEONATE

The blood of the newborn has many more immature forms than that of older infants. Reticulocyte levels up to 5 per cent of all red blood cells occur frequently. These fall to less than 2 per cent within a few days and less than 1 per cent after the second week. In addition, nucleated red cells may be present in the newborn but disappear in the first few days of life. Immature leukocytes also appear in the blood of the newborn, but they too disappear within the first week of life (Wolman, 1957).

Immediately after birth the number of erythrocytes, the amount of hemoglobin, and the number of all types of leukocytes in the circulating blood are at an all-time high. The red cell count ranges from 4.8 to 6.6

million, the white cell count from 7,000 to 35,000 (Table 16-1). These values remain high or even rise during the first week and then begin to fall. It is possible that the values really begin to decline from the first day on, but the values are obscured by the general shrinkage in blood volume due to the initial loss of weight (Wolman, 1957). In the premature the number of erythrocytes depends upon the amount of the prematurity, but it is always lower than that of the full-term infant.

Both red cell count and hemoglobin values at birth are influenced by a number of factors, chief of which is the time after birth that the umbilical cord is clamped. Immediately after birth the placenta contains a large amount of blood. If the cord is clamped immediately, this blood fails to enter the infant's circulation. On the other hand if a delay of 2 or 3 minutes is allowed to take place, much of the blood in the placenta will pass through the umbilical veins into the infant's circulation. The amount of this blood ranges from 75 to 135 ml. Two factors facilitate this transfer: the first is the postbirth contraction of the uterus which mechanically propels the blood from placenta to infant; the second is the low systolic blood pressure in the infant immediately after birth due to the greatly increased pulmonary blood flow.

TABLE 16-1

Red Cells, Hemoglobin and Hematocrit: Approximate Optimal Mean Values for Healthy, Well-Nourished Full Term Infants and Children

Age	Hemoglobin, Gm per 100 ml	RBC, millions per cu mm	Hematocrit, %
6–48 hours	16–22	4.8–6.6	53–63
3–7 days	13–20	4.6–6.4	50–60
2 weeks	18	5.5	57
3 weeks	17	5.2	52
4 weeks	16	4.8	47
5 weeks	15	4.6	43
6 weeks	14	4.4	39
7 weeks	13	4.2	36
8 weeks	12	4.0	34
3 months	11.5	4.1	34
4 months	11.8	4.4	35
5 months	11.8	4.5	35
6 months	12	4.7	36
9–12 months	12	4.8	36
18 months	12.5	5.0	37
2–6 years	13	5.0	38
7–12 years	14	5.2	41
13–17 years (girls)	14	5.2	41
13–17 years (boys)	15	5.7	44

SOURCE: From Laboratory Applications in Clinical Pediatrics by Irving J. Wolman, McGraw-Hill Book Company, Inc., 1957.

TABLE 16-2

Normal Values of Leucocytes*

Age	Total all leucocytes		Neutrophils			Eosinophils			Lymphocytes			Monocytes		
			Absolute total		% Total WBC	Absolute total		% Total WBC	Absolute total		% Total WBC	Absolute total		% Total WBC
	Range	Average	Range	Average		Range	Average		Range	Average		Range	Average	
1 day	7,000–35,000	18,000	2,500–27,000	11,000	50–85	100–1,000	400	1–5	1,500–10,000	5,400	15–45	200–2,500	850	1–5
2 days	8,000–40,000	22,000	3,000–32,000	14,000	50–85	100–1,000	400	1–5	1,500–12,000	6,400	15–45	200–2,500	850	1–5
7–14 days	4,000–20,000	10,000	1,000–10,000	3,000	30–50	100–800	300	1–5	1,200–13,000	5,500	45–65	200–2,500	850	2–7
2 weeks–6 months	5,500–20,000	12,500	1,000–8,000	3,700	30–50	100–700	300	1–5	1,500–13,000	7,500	45–65	200–2,500	800	2–7
6 months–1 year	6,000–16,000	11,000	1,500–7,000	3,800	30–50	100–700	300	1–5	3,000–10,000	5,900	45–65	400–2,000	750	2–7
1–2 years	6,000–15,000	10,300	1,500–7,000	4,000	30–50	100–600	300	1–5	3,000–8,000	5,000	40–60	400–2,000	700	2–7
2–3 years	5,000–14,000	9,500	1,500–7,000	4,100	30–50	100–600	250	1–5	2,500–7,000	4,200	40–60	400–2,000	600	2–7
4–6 years	5,000–13,000	9,000	1,500–7,500	4,300	30–50	100–600	250	1–5	1,500–7,000	4,000	40–60	300–1,800	550	1–6
7–12 years	4,000–13,000	8,500	1,500–8,000	4,300	40–60	100–600	250	1–5	1,000–6,500	3,300	35–55	300–1,500	500	1–6
Adult	5,000–10,000	7,000	3,200–6,200	4,300	45–65	100–300	200	1–5	1,500–3,000	2,000	30–50	300–500	400	1–6

* Basophils range from 0–300 cells at all ages. Blast forms range from 0–1,000 cells during first few days of life, then drop to 0–600 cells.
SOURCE: From Laboratory Applications in Clinical Pediatrics, by Irving J. Wolman, McGraw-Hill Book Company, Inc., 1957.

De Marsh, Alt, and Windle compared two groups of infants with respect to time of clamping the cord. They found that in those infants in whom the cord was clamped immediately after birth the red cells and hemoglobin during the first week of life averaged 5.45 million red cells and 19.5 Gm hemoglobin, compared with 8.01 million red cells and 22.1 Gm hemoglobin in those infants who received the placental blood. They also found that the group in which the cord was immediately clamped maintained a high reticulocyte count (6 to 8 per cent) for the first days of life, whereas the group in which the tying of the cord was delayed had a peak reticulocyte count (5.8 per cent) at 24 hours which dropped to 4 per cent at 48 hours of life. Buckels and Usher found that infants with immediate cord clamping had anemia, hypotension, and acidosis compared with infants permitted to receive placental transfusion. Milking or stripping of the umbilical cord can provide the newborn with even more blood than mere delayed clamping of the cord (Born et al., 1954).

Since prematurely born infants have an appreciably lower hemoglobin than term infants, the delayed tying of the umbilical cord in premature infants may be of more significance than in term infants, since a larger supply of the blood of the premature lies within the umbilical veins than is the case in the term infant.

Whether or not the polycythemia induced by delayed clamping of the cord and/or milking of the umbilical veins is an unmitigated advantage to the newborn is not altogether clear. McKeon is of the opinion that it is possible that the added blood volume may be something of a hazard to the newborn struggling under the cardiopulmonary alteration that must take place as air breathing begins. It is true, however, that the added iron received by the newborn from placental transfusion may represent as much as 50 per cent of the iron requirement of a premature infant for his first 6 months of life.

Other factors influence *initial* hemoglobin in the blood but little. Woodruff and Bridgeforth found that the maternal hemoglobin level did not appear to affect the synthesis of fetal hemoglobin until very low levels were reached in the maternal blood. Infants born to mothers whose hemoglobin averaged 13 Gm showed no higher levels than those to mothers whose hemoglobin was only 10 Gm. However, when the maternal hemoglobin dropped to 5 Gm, the incidence of anemia during the neonatal period was considerably greater (Strauss). (For further discussion of the effect of maternal hemoglobin on anemia of infancy, see Chap. 26.)

DEVELOPMENTAL PATTERN

Erythrocytes and Hemoglobin

After the first week of life hemoglobin values fall. This is a physiologic phenomenon and occurs in all infants. The high hemoglobin levels at birth help tide the newborn over the initial period when respiration is being established. They probably reflect the polycythemia present in the prenatal state when low oxygen and high CO_2 tensions exist. After the neonatal period, hemoglobin continues to drop for the first 6 months of life (for factors influencing this drop, see Chap. 26); then there is a slow and steady increase up to the time of puberty (Fig. 16-1). During childhood there is no sex difference in either hemoglobin or red cells. Coincident with the pubertal growth spurt in boys there is a rapid rise in both hemoglobin and red cells, mature levels being reached in the postpubertal period. In girls there is no pubertal rise, so that in adult women hemoglobin and red cell values are appreciably below those of men. These are the trends; when it comes to reporting actual values for hemoglobin and red cells there is difficulty of distinguishing between "usual," "normal," and "optimal."

Iron is essential for the formation of the hemoglobin molecule, but so are amino acids and other dietary substances, among which can be named copper, cobalt, pyridoxine, niacin, vitamin B_{12}, and probably others. Malnutrition is reflected in the hemoglobin levels. Iron is by far the most frequently inadequate dietary ingredient (p. 333) (Wiehl, 1941).

People living in high altitudes have more circulating hemoglobin than those living at sea level (Wintrobe, 1961). Recent infections, amount of exercise, time of day, season of the year, emotional factors all play a role in the amount of hemoglobin present at any given time. Therefore random samples on a large population group are unsatisfactory data from which to draw conclusions concerning the optimal level of hemoglobin at any given age. Even longitudinal studies, unless carefully controlled with respect to the known factors influencing hemoglobin, are to be viewed with some skepticism. Table 16-1 gives data for healthy, well-nourished children and is as well-controlled as possible to ensure reasonably optimal health in the subjects and comparability of data. Similar data from Mugrage show the adolescent changes in hemoglobin and red cells for both boys and girls (Fig. 16-1).

The red cell count follows hemoglobin values fairly closely. It reaches its low point several months before the hemoglobin values are lowest. It rises more rapidly than hemoglobin and reaches a plateau about the end of the second year, where it remains until puberty, at which time, like the hemoglobin, there is a rapid spurt in boys but nothing comparable in girls.

Leukocytes

The total number of leukocytes is high at birth but rises even higher within the first few days of life (Table 16-2). Then it falls more or less continuously during the years of childhood, reaching adult values at puberty. There are no remarkable changes at adolescence and no appreciable sex difference in the total number of leukocytes.

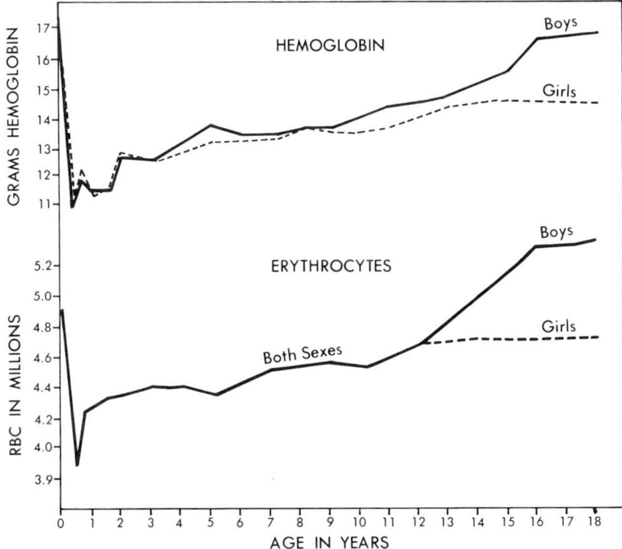

Fig. 16-1. Life patterns of hemoglobin and erythrocytes. (*From Mugrage and Andersen, Red Blood Cell Values in Adolescence, in Am. J. Dis. Child., 56:997, 1938.*)

Granulocytes

Throughout life the number of neutrophils is many times greater than that of the other types of granulocytes, and hence their developmental pattern is more readily detected. The total number of neutrophils is high at birth but rises even higher within the first few days of life; then it falls precipitously and by the age of 2 weeks reaches a lifetime low. It then rises slowly and more or less continuously during the years of childhood, reaching adult levels at puberty. There is no remarkable change at puberty, nor is there an appreciable sex difference in the number of neutrophils.

Eosinophil levels drop slowly and continuously throughout all of childhood, from the high levels at birth to their adult levels which are reached at puberty.

Basophils remain more or less at their birth levels until puberty, when they drop to adult levels.

Lymphocytes

The life pattern of the number of circulating lymphocytes is different from that of the other formed blood elements. Lymphocytes are high at birth, rise slightly a day or two after birth, and then fall by 2 weeks of age. Then, unlike other formed elements, lymphocyte levels rise, reaching a lifetime high within the first half year. After this peak, the number of lymphocytes decreases in the circulating blood and reaches adult levels at puberty.

Relative Proportion of Leukocytes

It has long been customary to report the total number of all types of leukocytes per cubic millimeter of blood and then the per cent of the total represented by each type of cell (the differential count). A newer procedure (Wolman, 1957) slowly coming into acceptance is to report the absolute number of the various types of leukocytes, a figure obtained by multiplying the percentages from the differential distribution by the total

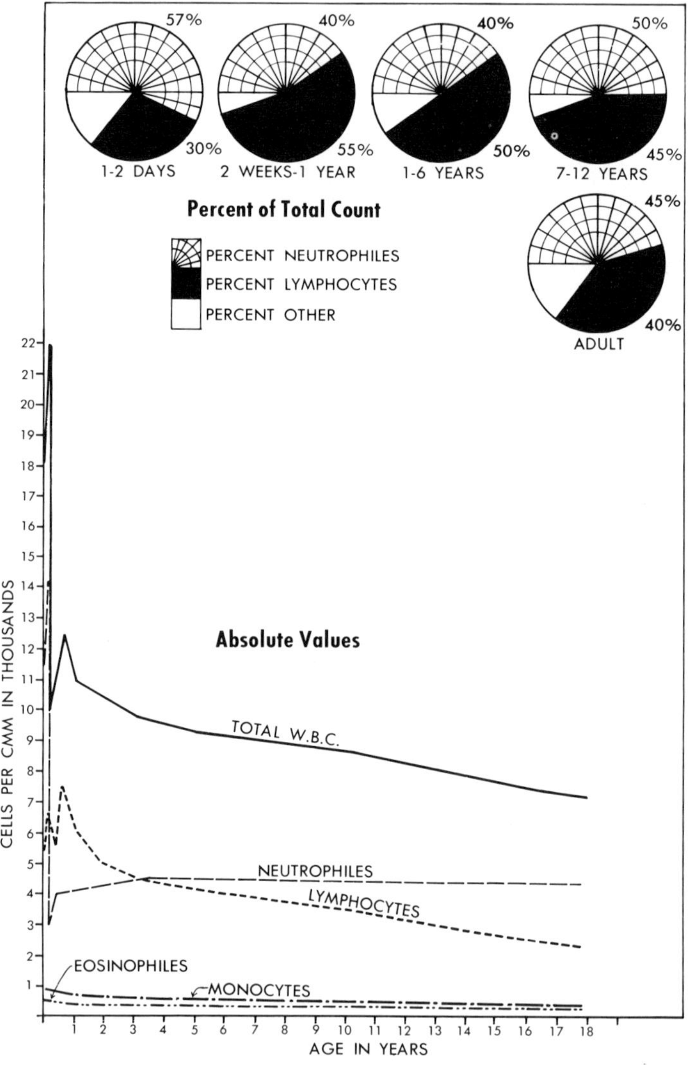

Fig. 16-2. Life patterns of leucocytes. (*Chart drawn from data in Laboratory Applications in Clinical Pediatrics, by Irving J. Wolman, McGraw-Hill Book Company, Inc.*)

leukocyte count. Since the various kinds of leukocytes vary independently of each other, more useful information is obtained by referring to absolute values.

INTERPRETING THE HEMOGRAM

Blood is a mobile organ which is in minute-by-minute contact with virtually every other tissue in the body. It therefore reflects metabolic changes not only in itself but also in the body as a whole. Blood is easily accessible, and its examination is a simple procedure; hence the hemogram is a useful addition to a physical appraisal.

As a screening test, a hemogram consisting of a determination of the hematocrit and the sedimentation rate can contribute much useful information. In the interpretation of the hemogram it is essential to bear in mind the normal developmental pattern of the blood elements. Changes which are alerting signs that development is not progressing in optimal fashion can then be noted.

Normal values (see Table 16-1) for the hematocrit indicate that erythrocyte function is adequate. High values suggest a polycythemia. High values may also be indicative of any condition in which the blood volume has been lowered. Such conditions as hemorrhage, shock, dehydration, and burns are accompanied by a rise in hematocrit.

Low values of the hematocrit are indicative of anemia, and such findings call for further studies. While pallor of the skin and mucous membranes may be a sign of anemia, it is a notoriously unreliable one. Rosy cheeks and pink gums may be associated with a lower hematocrit than that of a child of more sallow complexion.

In the screening hemogram, a sedimentation rate that falls within normal limits is presumptive evidence that the patient is free of certain diseases. An elevated sedimentation rate calls for further investigation. The sedimentation rate is a useful but by no means infallible guide. The rate is elevated in acute infections only after a few days elapse and then only if inflammation accompanies the infection. The rate is elevated in such subacute and chronic infections as rheumatic fever, atypical pneumonia, active tuberculosis, malaria, histoplasmosis, and nephritis. A count of the leukocytes and of each of the several varieties is called for when a patient's sedimentation rate has been found elevated. Developmental patterns must be kept in mind in deciding whether any of the leukocytes is present in abnormal numbers.

BIBLIOGRAPHY

Born, G. V. R., G. S. Dawes, J. C. Mott, and J. G. Widdicome: Changes in the Heart and Lungs at Birth, *Cold Spring Harbor Symp. Quant. Biol.*, **19**:102, 1954.

BUCKELS, L. J., and ROBERT USHER: Cardiopulmonary Effects of Placental Transfusion, *J. Pediat.*, **67**:239, 1965.

BURNET, MACFARLAND: The Immunological Significance of the Thymus, *Australasian Ann. Med.*, **11**:79, 1962.

DEMARSH, Q. B., H. L. ALT, and W. F. WINDLE: Factors Influencing the Blood Picture of the Newborn, *Am. J. Dis. Child.*, **75**:860, 1948.

———: Effects of Depriving an Infant of Its Placental Blood on Blood Picture in the First Week of Life, *J.A.M.A.*, **116**:2568, 1941.

———, W. F. WINDLE, and H. L. ALT: Blood Volume of the Newborn in Relation to Early and Late Clamping of the Umbilical Cord, *Am. J. Dis. Child.*, **63**:1123, 1942.

FICHTELIUS, KARL ERIK: A Difference between Lymph Nodal and Thymic Lymphocytes Shown by Transfusion of Labelled Cells, *Acta Anat.*, **32**:114, 1958.

———: Further Studies on the Difference between Lymphocytes of Lymph Nodes and Thymus, *Acta Haemat.*, **19**:187, 1958, and **22**:322, 1959.

MCKEON, CHARLES: The Value of the Placenta Transfusion in Full Term and Premature Infants, *Quart. Rev. Pediat.*, **11**:81, 1960.

MUGRAGE, EDWARD R., and MARJORY I. ANDERSON: Red Blood Cell Values in Adolescence, *Am. J. Dis. Child.*, **56**:997, 1938.

PATTEN, BRADLEY M.: "Human Embryology," 2d ed., McGraw-Hill Book Company, New York, 1953.

STRAUSS, MAURICE B.: Anemia of Infancy from Maternal Iron Deficiency in Pregnancy, *J. Clin. Invest.*, **12**:345, 1933.

TANNER, J. M.: "Growth at Adolescence," Charles C Thomas, Publisher, Springfield, Ill., 1955.

WIEHL, DOROTHY G.: Hemoglobin and Erythrocyte Values for Adolescents in High Income Families, *Milbank Mem. Fund Quart.*, **19**:45, 1941.

WINTROBE, MAXWELL M.: "Clinical Hematology," Lea and Febiger, Philadelphia, 1961.

WOLMAN, IRVING J.: "Laboratory Applications in Clinical Pediatrics," McGraw-Hill Book Company, New York, 1957.

WOODRUFF, CALVIN W., and EDWIN B. BRIDGEFORTH: Relationship between the Hemogram of the Infant and That of the Mother during Pregnancy, **12**:681, 1953.

17

The Gastrointestinal Tract

The gastrointestinal tract is a refining plant for the processing of raw fuel and the absorption of nutrients. The system acts also as an organ of excretion, not only for the undigested residue of the ingested material, but also for other waste products, some of which are poured into the large bowel from the blood while others are excreted into the intestine by way of the bile. The gastrointestinal tract participates in maintaining the water and electrolyte balance of the body.

Events in the mouth and in the anus (eating and defecating) come under control of the will, as the child matures, and play a role in the development of personality. All the actions of the gastrointestinal tract—food intake, digestion, absorption, and elimination—not only respond to physiologic needs but from birth to old age are sensitive to tensions and anxiety.

THE GASTROINTESTINAL TRACT AT BIRTH AND IN EARLY INFANCY

Prior to birth, nutrients are supplied to the fetus through the placental circulation, and the gastrointestinal tract is not called upon for digestion or absorption of food materials. The lumen of the gut, however, is not empty at the time of birth. It contains cast-off epithelial cells, "practice secretions" from the various digestive glands, and the residue of swallowed amniotic fluid. This material, the meconium, is eliminated through the rectum during the first few days of life. It is a thick, sticky, greenish black substance, quite unlike later feces. Its passage provides evidence of the patency of the intestinal tract. During the first few days the infant takes in no food, although he does swallow air, which aids in opening the tract and may contribute to the establishment of the intestinal flora.

By the second or third day of life the infant is ready to eat. The infant ingests his food by sucking. Milk is deposited in the back of the pharynx, and swallowing is an automatic reflex act. The newborn produces a small amount of saliva, which lubricates his mouth and throat. His saliva contains a measurable, though small, quantity of ptyalin, the starch-splitting enzyme. However, there is little opportunity for this enzyme to act upon the rapidly swallowed food.

Once swallowed, the food is pushed down the esophagus to the stomach by a peristaltic wave. Being a hollow muscular sac, the stomach can stretch

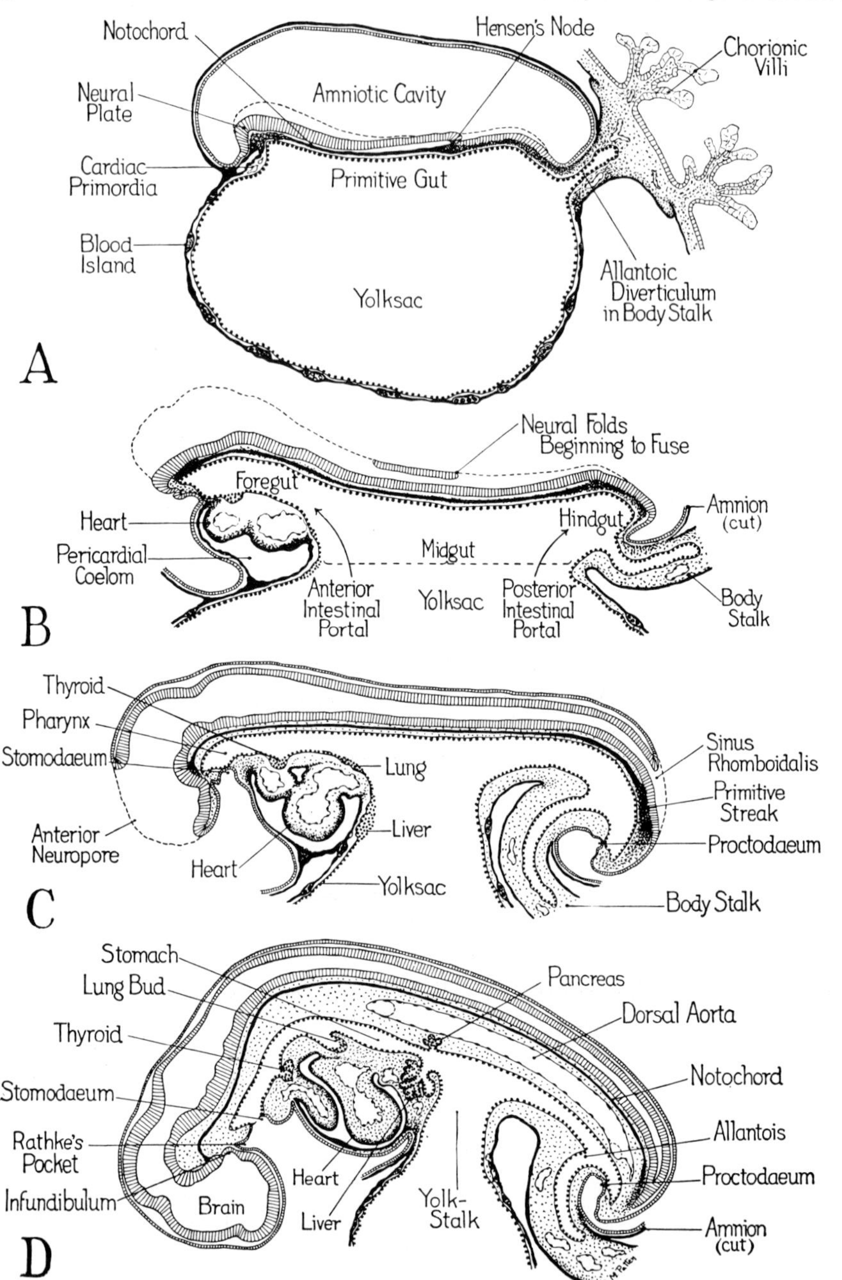

Fig. 17-1. Formation of the gastrointestinal tract. *A.* About 16 days gestational age. *B.* 18 days. *C.* 22 days. *D.* 1 month. (*From Human Embryology, 2d ed., by Bradley M. Patten, McGraw-Hill Book Company, Inc.*)

to accommodate the ingested food. At birth, most infants cannot take much more than 20 to 30 ml fluid into the stomach; in the course of the first 10 days, the stomach enlarges to accommodate 75 to 100 ml, and by 1 month of age most infants can take between 90 and 150 ml.

In the stomach the milk is curdled by the action of HCl and rennin. Food does not stay long in the infant's stomach. Within 5 to 10 minutes a considerable part of the food has been pushed on through the pylorus into the duodenum. After half an hour the greater part of the meal has left the stomach, and by 2½ to 3 hours the stomach is usually empty.

Because of the relatively short time that food remains in the stomach, gastric digestion consists primarily of the curdling of milk, with a minimal amount of digestion of the protein into shorter-chain molecules. Very little digestion of fat or carbohydrate takes place in the infant's stomach, and virtually no absorption of nutrients takes place there; however, in some infants, who have inherited the hypersensitive state, certain whole proteins are absorbed unchanged from the stomach in sufficient amounts to cause allergic response (p. 301).

Once the food is pushed through the pylorus into the duodenum, it meets pancreatic juice and bile. The pancreatic enzyme trypsin acts quickly on the partially digested protein but more slowly on the full protein molecule. Because of the rapid passage through the stomach in the infant, a larger proportion of undigested protein reaches the duodenum of the infant than that of the more mature individual. Trypsin is capable of digesting the full protein to polypeptides and also of breaking down some of the polypeptides to di- and tripeptides and then into amino acids.

The pancreatic juice in early infancy does not contain the starch-splitting enzyme amylase. Since starch digestion in the mouth is scanty and amylase is absent in pancreatic secretion, the infant has little ability to handle the long-chain polysaccharides.

Fat is emulsified in the duodenum by means of bile. Bile contains no enzymes in infancy or at any time of life. Its function is the breaking up of fat globules into such tiny morsels that the pancreatic lipase can penetrate and break the fat down into fatty acids and glycerol. As the chyme is pushed on down the intestinal tract, it meets the intestinal juices, which are essentially similar to those of the mature organism.

At birth the gastrointestinal tract is sterile. However, bacteria may enter by both mouth and rectum, and within a few days of life the characteristic flora becomes apparent. The colon-aerogenes group of organisms makes its appearance in the lower bowel. *Lactobacillus bifidus* is often the predominant organism in the bowel of the breast-fed infant and of infants in whose diet lactose is the principal carbohydrate. These organisms give way to members of the colon-aerogenes-proteus group when the diet becomes more varied. Various streptococci and staphylococci as well as the protolytic organisms are found in both the large and small intestines. Once the diet of the infant has become mixed, the intestinal flora is similar to that of the adult.

In the newborn, the digestive apparatus exhibits its immaturity by the rapid pace with which food passes through the tract. Not infrequently peristaltic waves go in the reverse direction for no apparent reason, producing spitting up of a mouthful or two of food, or at times more vigorous waves may result in the complete emptying of the stomach by vomiting. Some spitting up and some vomiting are almost universal in early infancy and are usually related to the lability of the muscular action and not to failure in digestion. There is apparently no sense of nausea associated with this infantile vomiting. Some quite healthy, normal infants spit up a good deal more than others. As maturity advances, the muscular action of the upper gut stabilizes, and reverse peristalsis ceases.

During early infancy reverse peristalsis in the small intestine may be sufficiently strong to push chyme back to an area where the conditions are unsuitable for digestion, and failure of digestion, combined with over-vigorous contractions, may thus contribute to colic (p. 193).

At the lowest end of the gastrointestinal tract the food residues are expelled as stool. Stools of the young infant are softer, more liquid and more frequent than they will be in a month or more. During the first month of life, and before the infant's diet has changed, the stools become firmer and less frequent. They remain soft and bright yellow as long as milk is the main dietary ingredient. As soon as a mixed diet is taken, the stools begin to take on adult consistency. The rectum is emptied as a reflex in early infancy (p. 409).

While the gastrointestinal tract of the infant is quite competent to handle the normal food of infancy, it is less able to cope with external adversity than is the more mature tract. Temperature changes which alter the body fluids interfere with digestion and absorption in the immature system. Infection, either in the tract or elsewhere in the body, which causes elevation of body temperature interferes with the ability of the gastrointestinal tract to maintain an adequate fluid and electrolyte balance. The immature tract, speedy under optimal conditions, further speeds up its processes in response to adversity, with the result that there is less opportunity for absorption, both of water and of nutrients, and the infant begins to suffer from dehydration. Actual digestion seldom fails; digestive juices are secreted in normal amounts, but the chyme is pushed through the tract so rapidly that absorption fails. The too vigorous muscular action of the insulted immature tract is not confined to pushing the chyme toward the rectum; the muscular action may go in the reverse direction and add vomiting to the diarrhea.

SUBSEQUENT DEVELOPMENTAL CHANGES

Swallowing becomes a voluntary act. By about the age of 6 weeks, the striated muscles in the pharynx begin to establish their cerebral connections, and by 6 months the infant can swallow if he wants to, or he can hold the food in his mouth, or if the fancy strikes him, he is quite capable of spitting it out.

Taste buds are present at birth, and there is evidence that infants are capable of experiencing taste soon after birth; however, they do not exhibit much taste discrimination until after the first few months, when mature connections between the taste buds and the cortex have been established. The infant then begins to express his likes and dislikes for the flavors of the foods offered him.

The teeth begin to erupt through the gums toward the middle of the first year of life. Prior to their eruption the gums swell and frequently cause irritation, which stimulates such an excessive flow of saliva from the rapidly growing salivary glands that the child is unable to swallow the secretion and it dribbles from his mouth. Not infrequently the irritated gums are painful, and the child may chew on his fingers and demonstrate other evidence of discomfort.

The time of appearance of the teeth varies considerably from infant to infant, but the order of their appearance is fairly regular (Table 17-1). The two lower central incisors are the first to appear. They may erupt as early as 4 months or as late as 1 year—in perfectly normal children. The average age is about 7 months. The appearance of the first teeth may precipitate trouble with a breast-fed baby, who may experiment with

TABLE 17-1

Chronology of Human Dentition

Tooth	First evidence of calcification	Crown completed	Average age of eruption	Root completed
Deciduous dentition				
Lower central incisors	4–5 months in utero	4–5 months	6–8 months	1½–2 years
Upper central and lateral incisors	4–5 months in utero	4–5 months	7–9 months	1½–2 years
Lower lateral incisors	4–5 months in utero	4–5 months	7½–10 months	1½–2 years
First molars	5 months in utero	6 months	12–16 months	2–2½ years
Cuspids	5–5½ months in utero	9 months	16–20 months	2½–3 years
Second molars	6 months in utero	10–12 months	20–30 months	3 years
Permanent dentition				
First molars	birth	2½–3 years	6–7 years	9–10 years
Lower central incisors	3–4 months	4–5 years	6–7 years	9 years
Lower lateral incisors	3–4 months	4–5 years	7–8 years	10 years
Upper central incisors	3–4 months	4–5 years	7–8 years	10 years
Upper lateral incisors	10 months	4–5 years	8–9 years	11 years
First bicuspids	1½–1¾ years	5–6 years	10–11 years	12–15 years
Second biscuspids	2–2¼ years	6–7 years	10–12 years	12–14 years
Second molars	2½–3 years	7–8 years	12–13 years	14–16 years
Third molars	7–9 years	12–16 years	17–21 years	18–25 years

SOURCE: From Harold J. Noyes (slightly modified), in Brenneman's Practice of Pediatrics, Vol. 3, W. F. Prior Company, Inc., 1957.

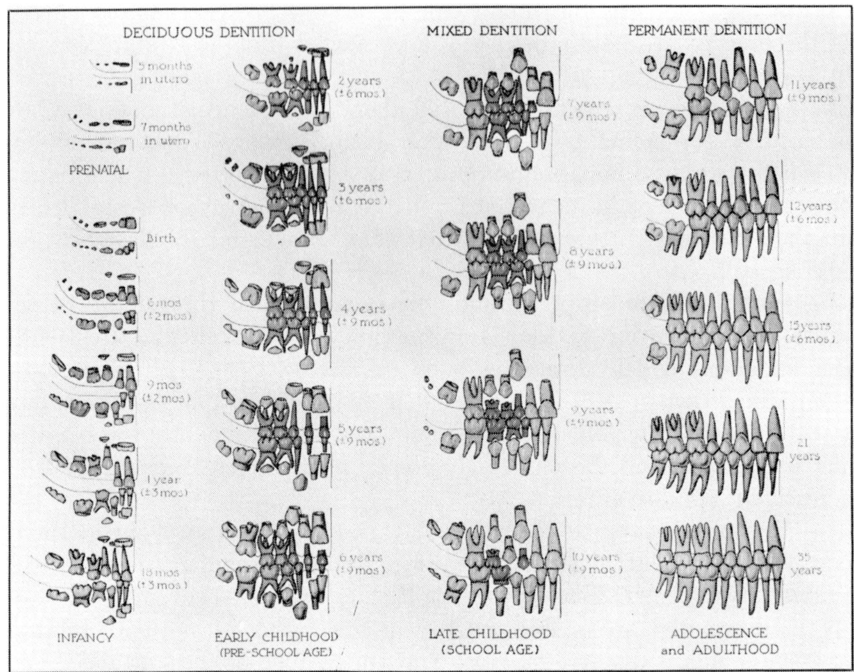

Fig. 17-2. Development of human dentition. *(Reprinted with permission of the American Dental Association.)*

biting his mother's nipple (p. 373). The eruption of the first teeth usually heralds the child's interest in chewing (p. 372).

After the lower incisors appear, there is usually a period of a month or more before the next teeth erupt, which are the four upper incisors. Usually the central ones come in before the lateral ones, but not infrequently the lateral incisors appear a week or two before the central ones. Again there is a waiting period before the lower lateral incisors erupt. On the average these eight teeth are present at about 1 year of age. A month or so later the four first molars erupt, soon followed by the four cuspids. The second molars seldom appear until after the second birthday. They complete the set of deciduous teeth.

The permanent teeth begin to erupt at about the age of 6. The first teeth of the permanent set are the 6-year molars, which come in behind the deciduous molars and therefore do not replace any teeth of the first set. In general the earlier a child gets his deciduous teeth, the earlier he will get his permanent teeth. After the eruption of the 6-year molars, other permanent teeth make their appearance in about the same order as the deciduous teeth. By the age of 10 years all the deciduous teeth usually have been lost. Two more sets of molars complete the permanent teeth. One set comes in at about the age of 12. The last set (the wisdom teeth) do not erupt until the early twenties.

The salivary glands, small at birth, increase rapidly in weight during the first 3 months of life, considerably faster than that of the body as a whole. After 3 months they continue to grow rapidly, although at a slower rate than during the very early period. By 2 years of age they have increased about five times their birth size and have reached about the relative proportion they will maintain until the senescent changes of old age make their appearance (Clement, 1922).

Secretion of saliva is under control of the autonomic nervous system. There are two types of reflex arcs which induce salivation, the inherent, or unconditioned, reflex and the acquired, or conditioned reflex. The unconditioned salivary response is inaugurated by substances placed in the mouth. Substances with a pleasant taste are strong stimuli, but any substance which impinges on the tactile nerve endings of tongue or cheeks will initiate the salivary reflex. Chewing or other movement of tongue and jaws are sufficient to induce salivation. As was noted above, the eruption of teeth in infancy, with its irritation of gingival surfaces, is a powerful stimulant to unconditioned salivation. Conditioned salivary secretion does not exist at birth. The infant must learn through experience what sensations mean a good eating experience is soon to come. Then his mouth "waters" in anticipation of gustatory delights.

Gastric juice is constantly secreted in the stomach. The amount is greatly increased under specific stimulation. There are three types of stimulus to the secretion of gastric juice: psychic stimulation, the actual presence of food in the mouth, and the presence of food in the stomach and duodenum.

The presence of food in the mouth sets up a reflex stimulation of the gastric glands, and the juice pours into the stomach. This is an unconditioned, inherent response and is present in the newborn. Conditioned responses, however, soon make their appearance. Gastric juice, like saliva, begins to flow in response to any sensation that means food is soon to come. Culture has an enormous impact on these learned responses. The look, smell, or thought of a fried caterpillar is not likely to make an American's mouth water. In the infant, the smell of breast milk, the sound of the mother's voice, the feel of arms picking up the infant—all these things become associated with food and stimulate the flow of digestive juices. As age advances, the list of sensations that can invoke gastric reaction becomes large indeed. One thing which all these excitatory mechanisms have in common is anticipatory pleasure. Unpleasant odors, sights, or sounds connected with the idea of eating inhibit the flow of gastric juice. Such stimuli are nauseating—they destroy the desire to eat, and they destroy it physiologically by inhibiting the flow of saliva and gastric juice. Not only does gastric juice fail to flow, but reverse peristalsis may take place and can result in vomiting.

Psychic states other than those directly concerned with food have an effect on gastric secretions and motility. Fear, depression, grief, anxiety, nervous tension all tend to decrease the flow of gastric juice and sometimes to induce vomiting as well. A child agitated over facing the world of school may be nauseated when he gets up in the morning. If forced to eat his breakfast, he may vomit it on the way to school. The psychic stimuli to gastric secretion account for about half of the total amount of juice secreted. They are an essential part of adequate digestion. In their absence gastric digestion does not proceed normally.

The acidity of gastric juice varies over the life span. It is low during infancy and rises during childhood, reaching a plateau at about the age of 10. Boys consistently show a slightly greater free acidity than do girls. At puberty there is a marked rise in the free gastric acidity in boys, paralleling the adolescent growth spurt (Vanzant et al., 1932). It is at this time that boys consume huge quantities of food. In girls there is an increase in free gastric acidity at puberty, but it is not as marked as in boys (Fig. 17-3).

Pancreatic juice, by 3 months of age, probably contains as much amylase as does the secretion of the adult. The other pancreatic and intestinal digestive juices are relatively mature by the middle of the first year of life.

Peristalsis remains vigorous throughout infancy. Occasionally a too vigorous wave of peristalsis will cause the intestine to fold in on itself, producing an intussusception. This leads to serious difficulties. The pinched-off intestine loses its blood supply if the intussusception is not quickly reduced; the flow of chyme through the intestine is stopped, and obstruction results. The gastrointestinal tract is overwhelmed and needs the immediate help of the surgeon.

The appendix not infrequently causes trouble during the years of childhood. At birth the appendix contains a relatively large amount of *lymphoid tissue,* which, like lymphoid tissue elsewhere in the body, increases rapidly during the early years and then begins to atrophy at the time of puberty. The appendix grows rapidly during the first year, and then its growth slows down. At birth the appendix has a lumen that extends to its tip, but this lumen is gradually obliterated as age advances. During childhood, when the lumen is patent, especially if the opening into the caecum is small, ejection of the intestinal contents pushed into the appendix is difficult. The stasis of this material may result in painful ulceration of the wall of the appendix. An ulcerated appendix must, of course, be removed surgically to prevent its rupture and the resulting peritonitis. Because of the anatomic arrangements, appendicitis is more common during the years of childhood than later in life. However, the lumen may

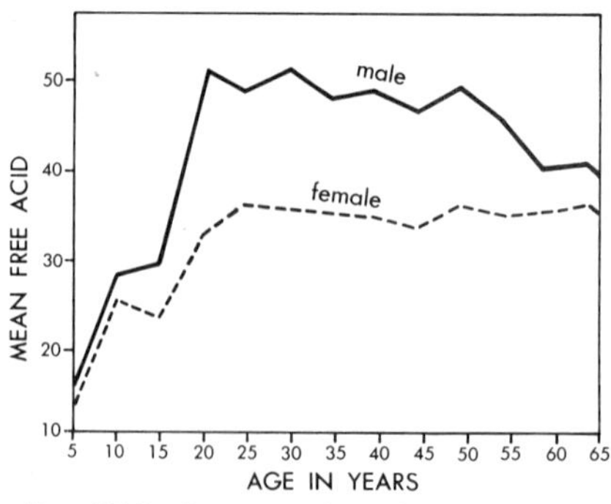

Fig. 17-3. Gastricacidity through life by sex. *(From Vanzant, Alvarez, and Eusterman, Dunn, and Berkson, in Arch. Int. Med., 49:345, 1932.)*

remain patent after puberty. If appendicitis occurs in middle life and the appendix ruptures, the infection spreads rapidly because the protective lymphoid tissue has decreased at this age (p. 304).

The large amount of lymphoid tissue in the intestinal wall and in the mesentery surrounding the small intestine during the years of childhood may also cause trouble. It occasionally becomes inflamed and produces symptoms difficult to distinguish from those of inflammation of the appendix. This condition, known as mesenteric adenitis, is a frequent cause of "stomach ache" during childhood.

A Meckel's diverticulum, if present, may become ulcerated during childhood. This aberrant structure occasionally contains gastric secretory glands. Gastric juice secreted in this area of the intestinal tract is almost sure to cause ulceration. Unlike ulceration of the appendix, an ulcerated Meckel's diverticulum frequently bleeds, and often the first sign of its presence is blood in the stool.

Fecal matter stays longer in the rectum by the end of the first year, so that stools are drier and less frequent. Defecation, however, remains under reflex control, long after mastication and swallowing have become completely voluntary. In accordance with the cephalocaudal law of growth, nerve pathways to the caudal end of the body are the last to mature. A year-old infant can control the events in his mouth quite adequately, but he may be close to 2 before he can bring his will to bear on the events in his rectum (p. 409).

There is evidence that the various parts of the gastrointestinal system undergo periods of growth, maturity, and senescence. There is much that is not known about this process; but the suggestion is ever present in the available data that a generalized atrophy of the entire gastrointestinal tract is one of the concomitants of advancing age. However, the process is slow, and failure of the functions of alimentation is seldom a cause of death (Ivy, 1939, and Meyer, 1937).

PSYCHOSOMATIC DISORDERS OF THE GASTROINTESTINAL SYSTEM

Whatever may be the relation between organic competency and emotional stress, psychosomatic disorders of the gastrointestinal tract are among the most common complaints of mankind. They may appear at any time of life. In addition to "stomach aches" and vomiting due to school phobias, mentioned above, the following are common in childhood:

Peptic ulcer, once thought to be a disorder of middle age, has been found with increasing frequency in children.

Ulcerative colitis, thought by some investigators to be primarily psychosomatic, becomes manifest during the pediatric years in approximately 10 per cent of all cases (Hijman, 1962).

Colic remains a baffling disease. By many it is thought to be primarily psychosomatic and related to maternal anxiety. Colic occurs in 15 to 20 per cent of babies, in boys more frequently than girls, and in most cases disappears dramatically at about 3 months of age. Innumerable mechanical or digestive factors have been suggested as causative—overfeeding, underfeeding, too much sugar, too much fat, nipples too big or too small. Alterations in these and other mechanical items and changes in formulas have had remarkably little effect upon the course of this distressing syndrome. Once in a great while a colicky infant recovers miraculously when taken off cow's milk.

Clark et al. have recently made a unique suggestion. They found in colicky babies a deficiency of circulatory progesterone hormone. They devised a urine test for a metabolite of this hormone and found that after ingestion of the hormone, colicky infants who previously had excreted none of the metabolite began to excrete it and simultaneously had a remission of symptoms. Progesterone exerts a relaxing effect on smooth muscle.

The gastrointestinal tract in early infancy is characterized by hypermotility. It is possible that colicky infants have a more than usual motility and that some of the contractions are sufficiently powerful to cause pain. Lack of progesterone may be a factor in that such infants are deprived of the relaxing effect of this substance. Maternal anxiety may have similar effects in these infants or in others.

In an overall view, the gastrointestinal system is a functional unit remarkably adapted to the needs of the organism. It is an extraordinarily complicated system with a highly intricate system of controls and balances. It must take on its complicated tasks in infancy, while it is still immature. As the infant matures into childhood, his gastrointestinal tract gains considerable stability and becomes more and more able to withstand minor vicissitudes. The general slowing down of the passage of food through his gastrointestinal tract permits the child to have an infection with fever without developing diarrhea or vomiting. By about the age of 2, he has teeth and can chew his food. Food stays in the mouth long enough to benefit from salivary digestion. The digestive juices are quite mature and effective. His gastric acidity is not as high as it will be a few years later, but it can function adequately. Other digestive juices are about at their adult level. A child of 2 can digest and assimilate almost everything normally present in a mixed diet.

Throughout life the organic competency of the gastrointestinal tract is maintained in most people. While organic failures of the tract are relatively infrequent, functional disorders are many. It is almost as though nature needed some way of alerting man to the problems of his emotional state and picked out the strongest system in the organism to bear the brunt of his wayward emotions.

THE LIVER

The liver takes part in a great many life-sustaining functions in addition to its role as a gland secreting bile into the gastrointestinal tract. The liver stands guard, as it were, at the entrance to the physiologic interior of the body. Food elements and fluids are absorbed from the gut into the splanchnic capillaries. These vessels drain into the portal vein which leads to the liver. The liver permits immediately needed substances to pass without delay into the general circulation and holds back nutrients and fluids in excess of immediate demands. This rapid action aids in maintaining homeostasis. The liver has temporary storage facilities for some substances (glycogen, fat, protein, iron) and is able to release them as needed for metabolism.

The liver detoxifies potentially harmful substances, plays a role in the blood coagulation mechanisms, contributes to body heat, aids in regulation of blood volume. It synthesizes glucose from amino acids and fat; it builds up glucose into glycogen, it deaminates some amino acids, synthesizes others, and manufactures urea; it synthesizes enzymes, some of which are used in the liver, some of which are released into the circulation. Thus the liver participates in the utilization and metabolism of incoming protein, carbohydrates, fat, inorganic substance, and vitamins. The controls of these multitudinous functions are mediated through chemical, hormonal, and nervous mechanisms. In addition to its role in metabolism, the liver acts as an organ of excretion by means of the secretion of bile (Rouiller, 1964).

The unit of structure of the liver is a system of two interdigitating lobules. In the secretory lobule a central duct receives bile formed in the liver cells and passes it on for storage in the gallbladder. In the center of the vascular lobe is a vein from the portal circulation—one of two afferent blood supplies. Blood is distributed from this vein to the interspaces between the glandular cells. This is the portal blood which, after birth, has passed through a capillary bed surrounding gut, spleen, and pancreas, and is laden with food elements to be processed by the liver cells before being released into the general circulation. A second and smaller afferent supply to the liver comes from the hepatic artery. This blood flows directly from the aorta and carries the oxygen needed for liver metabolism. Thus the trinity of channels in the liver lobules consists of a bile duct, a branch of the portal vein, and a branch of the hepatic artery. The efferent return of blood from both the portal vein and the hepatic artery is drained into the hepatic veins which ultimately reach the vena cava (Fig. 17-4).

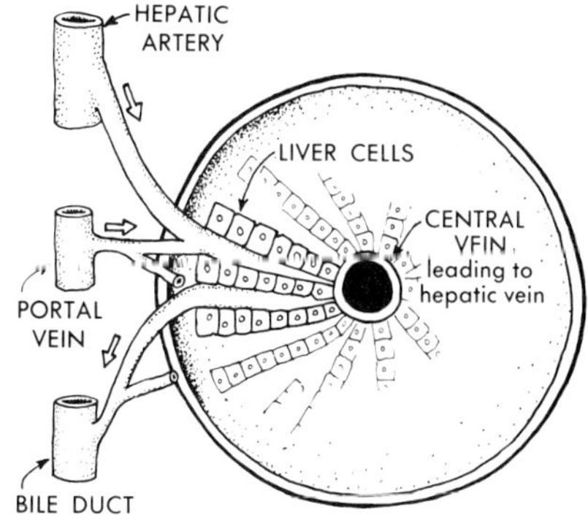

Fig. 17-4. Schematic representation of circulation within the liver lobule.

In spite of their multitudinous functions the glandular cells of the liver appear histologically alike. Crowded in between these glandular cells and lying within the blood sinuses are a group of large flattened stellate cells—the Kupffer cells. These cells are part of the reticuloendothelial system.

The liver appears in the embryo toward the end of the third week of gestation as a diverticulum on the ventral side of the primitive gut. At this early age the embryo has not yet established its own circulation. Blood islands appear in the developing liver as well as in the yolk sac. Soon blood channels are formed which connect the liver with the umbilical vessels. In the later part of gestation the liver ceases to make blood cells. This function is taken over by bone marrow and lymphatic tissue (p. 173).

Before birth the interdigitating system of liver lobules is formed. There is, however, considerable immaturity of function in the liver of the neonate. This may in part be accounted for by the different conditions under which the liver operates pre- and postnatally. The source of nutrients and also the source of oxygen for the fetus is from the umbilical vessels. The portal circulation is formed in utero, but because of the nonfunctional character of the intestine before birth the blood from the splanchnic area is much smaller in volume than it will be once alimentation takes place.

In the fetus the umbilical vessels join the portal veins and pour placental blood into the liver. Immediately after birth the umbilical vessels are obliterated, and the portal circulation must take over the task of bringing to the liver blood from the infant's splanchnic area, rich in food substances processed in the infant's gastrointestinal tract. The hepatic artery is formed also in utero, although the fetal liver depends upon placental blood for its oxygen supply.

The glandular cells of the liver do secrete bile in the later months of gestation, as is evident from its presence in the meconium. Since the intestinal tract does not digest food prior to birth, it is not dependent upon the presence of bile. The bile of the fetus contains bile pigment, but this function too is immature in the liver of the neonate. The immaturity of bile secretion may be a factor in the hyperbilirubinemia observed in the full-term infant and more markedly in the premature infant.

Other functions of the liver cells are also probably immature at birth. There is evidence that the liver of the neonate is not as efficient as that of an older person in glucogenesis, in ketone body formation, in deaminization of amino acids. It is probably less able to act as temporary storage reservoir for nutritional substances. In addition, the various hormones that participate in liver function are immature in the young infant.

The liver matures rapidly after birth, and by 1 year of age it functions almost as efficiently as in the adult. It is somewhat less able to store temporarily supplies of vitamins than is the fully mature liver; hence the child is more dependent upon a day-to-day supply of these accessory food substances than is the adult.

In the last month of gestation the liver becomes a large vascular organ. Immediately after birth the liver shrinks in size and does not begin to grow until the second to the third month of postnatal life. It then grows steadily through all of childhood, reaching about 90 per cent of its mature size by the onset of puberty.

BIBLIOGRAPHY

BEST, CHARLES H., and NORMAN BURKE TAYLOR: "The Physiological Basis of Medical Practice," The Williams and Wilkins Company, Baltimore, 1955.

CLARK, ROBERT L., A. B. FRANK GANIS, and WILLIAM I. BRADFORD: A Study of the Possible Relationship of Progesterone to Colic, *Pediatrics,* **31**:64, 1963.

CLEMENT, NICORY: Salivary Secretions in Infants, *Biochem J.,* **16**:387, 1922.

HIJMAN, J. C., and N. B. ENZER: Ulcerative Colitis in Childhood. A Study of 43 Cases, *Pediatrics,* **29**:389, 1962.

IVY, C. A.: The Digestive System, in E. V. Cowdry (ed.), "Problems of Aging," The Williams and Wilkins Company, Baltimore, 1939.

LATTIMER, JOHN K. AURELIO, C. USON, and MEYER M. MELICOW: Urological Emergencies in Newborn Infants, *Pediatrics,* **29**:310, 1962.

MANN, FRANK C., JESSE L. BOLLMAN, THOMAS MAGATH: Studies on the Physiology of the Liver: IX. The Formation of Bile Pigment after Total Removal of the Liver, The Site of Formation of Bilirubin, *Am. J. Physiol.,* **69**:393, 1924.

MEYER, JACOB, J. S. GOLDEN, N. STEINER, and H. NECHELES: Ptylin Content of Human Saliva in Old Age, *Am. J. Physiol.,* **119**:600, 1937.

NOYES, HAROLD J.: The Teeth, Jaws, and Oral Structures, in "Brenneman's Practice of Pediatrics," vol. 3, W. F. Prior Company, Inc., Hagerstown, Md., 1957.

PATTEN, BRADLEY M.: "Human Embryology," 2d ed., McGraw-Hill Book Company, New York, 1953.

ROUILLER, C. E.: "The Liver, Morphology, Bio-Chemistry, Physiology," vol. 1, 1963, vol. 2, 1964, Academic Press, Inc., New York.

TANNER, J. M.: "Growth at Adolescence," Charles C Thomas, Publisher, Springfield, Ill., 1955.

VANZANT, FRANCIS R., WALTER C. ALVAREZ, GEORGE B. EUSTERMAN, H. L. DUNN, and J. BERKSON: The Normal Range of Gastric Acidity from Youth to Old Age, *Arch. Intern. Med.,* **49**:345, 1932.

18

The Reproductive System

THE GERM PLASM

The primary organs of the reproductive system are the testes of the male and the ovaries of the female, collectively called the *gonads*. In the gonads is segregated the germ plasm, the tissue which carries all the ancestral potentialities of life in an unbroken line since organisms first appeared on the planet. The rest of the body, the heart, lungs, brain, muscles —the myriad of somatic cells which make up an individual, cease to exist after the individual dies, but the germ cells live from generation to generation in descendents carrying imprints of all that has gone before.

DEVELOPMENT PRIOR TO BIRTH

The segregation of the germ plasm occurs very early in embryonic life. Soon after the formation of the germinal layers, cells are seen in the endoderm of the yolk sac which are believed to be primordial sex cells. These cells migrate, probably through the primitive blood channels, and come to lie in the gonads (Patten, 1953). Once in the gonads, they seem not to be subject to the hazards of existence, the brunt of which is borne by the somatic cells. Why they should be safe in the gonads is not at all clear.[1]

Whether an embryo is to become a male or a female is a fact determined by his chromosomes at the time of conception. In spite of this initial biologic decision about its sex, the embryo is quite slow in differentiating itself into male or female. It gives the impression of keeping one foot in either camp of maleness and femaleness. The earliest gonad in both sexes is an undifferentiated structure, consisting of a central medulla and a surrounding cortex. Two sets of ducts form adjacent to the gonads. If the embryo is destined to become a male, the Wolffian ducts develop epididymis, vas deferens, seminal vesicles, and ejaculatory duct, and the Müllerian ducts remain rudimentary. On the other hand in an embryo with female potential the Müllerian ducts develop fallopian tubes, uterus, and vagina, and the Wolffian ducts remain rudimentary (Fig. 18-1).

There has been much controversy concerning the stimulus that pushes

[1] For discussion of those aspects of the environment that *do* penetrate to the germ cells, see p. 64.

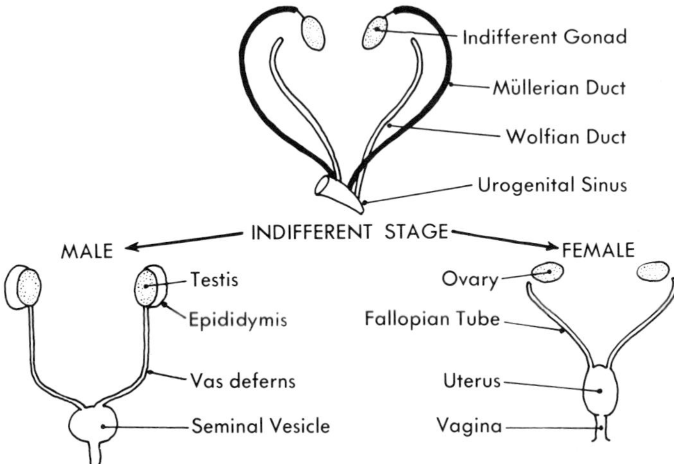

Fig. 18-1. Development of the sex ducts.

the sexually indifferent embryo into either maleness or femaleness. The consensus at the present time (Wilkins, 1964) is that in the embryo with XY chromosome, the medulla of the gonad forms cells of Leydig, which soon begin to secrete androgen. The presence of this hormone is responsible for the further development of the medulla, the suppression of the cortex, and the formation of male structures. In the absence of hormone the cortex of the gonad develops, the medulla is suppressed, and female development takes place. It is this hormone rather than the chromosome configuration per se which apparently is the deciding factor in pushing the embryo toward maleness. In castrated embryos with either XX or XY chromosomes female structures develop (Jost, 1959). Injections of androgens into the mother during early pregnancy masculinize a female embryo (Wilkins, 1960).

Once formed, the gonads of either sex migrate from their original position. The testes move caudally, and at about the seventh month they slip into the scrotal sac. Failure of the last part of this migration results in cryptorchism. The ovaries migrate slightly caudally, but the greatest extent of their migration is to the side, so that ultimately they come to lie quite widely spaced, one on either side of the lower abdominal cavity, behind the peritoneum and embedded in the broad ligament.

The external sex organs of both male and female begin their development from the genital tubercle, which lies in close proximity to the cloaca, the common exit of primitive urinary and gastrointestinal systems. As with the differentiation of the ducts, the differentiation of the external genitalia into the male organs is dependent upon the presence of androgens. In the absence of androgens, female external genitalia develop. Two folds of tissue appear at the sides of the tubercle which become the scrotum in the male or the labia majora in the female. The genital tubercle itself becomes the

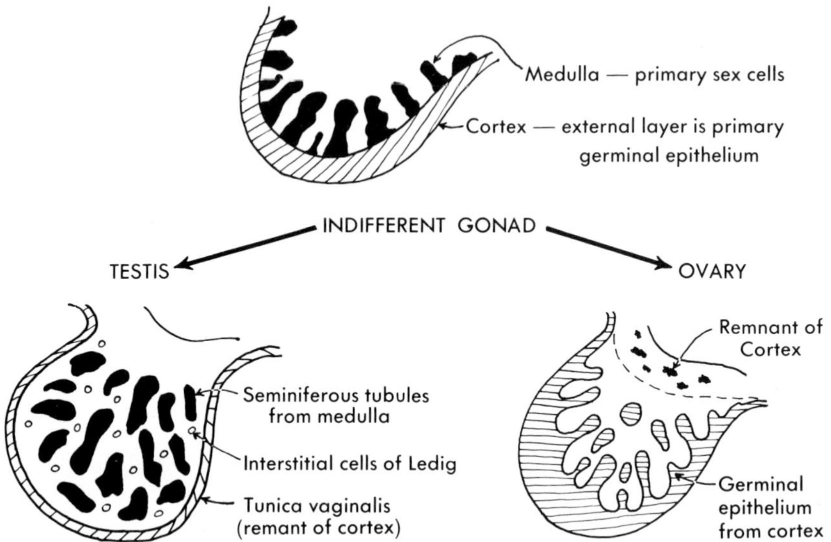

Fig. 18-2. Development of testis and ovary from indifferent gonad.

penis in the male, the clitoris in the female. In the female, the clitoris remains small, and the urethral opening stays in its original position at the base. In the male, the structure grows considerably larger than in the female, and on the underside a groove forms which ultimately connects with the bladder. Finally the groove closes over and extends the urethra the length of the penis, moving the urogenital outlet from the base to the tip of the penis. A scarlike vestige of the closure remains on the underside of the penis. Various degrees of failure of the growth and closure of this groove lead to hypospadias. As the urethra is being formed, an ingrowth around the tip of the penis forms the prepuce. The prepuce is usually adherent to the glans penis at the time of birth.

In the male the accessory sex glands are the seminal vesicles, the prostate gland, and the bulbourethral glands. The seminal vesicles are small outpouchings from the proximal part of the urethra. The prostate comes from multiple outgrowths along the base of the urethra and forms a ring around the urethra. These glands in the adult male secrete a mucoid substance in which the spermatozoa are suspended. The bulbourethral glands lie along the length of the urethra. They produce a mucoid secretion in the adult male. At the time of birth all these glands are well differentiated and show evidence of the production of mucin.

In the female the accessory glands are not as well developed as in the male, since the female has no need for a fluid in which to suspend her germ cells. There are, however, glands in the female vestibule, the glands of Skene (probably the homologue of the prostate in the male) and the bulbourethral glands, the glands of Bartholin. In the adult female these glands secrete a lubricating mucoid substance. At birth the glands are present and may secrete a small amount of mucin.

THE SEX ORGANS AT BIRTH AND DURING CHILDHOOD

In normal newborn infants the sex organs are well differentiated into male and female. Unlike such structures as the respiratory tract, the cardiovascular system, and the kidney system, the sex organs do not have a vital function to play in the immediate postnatal adjustment of the infant. However, the full quota of sensory nerves to the reproductive apparatus is present in the infant. In the glans penis in the male and in the clitoris in the female are large venous channels and smooth muscle fibers which, when stimulated, cause erection. Throughout childhood the penis and the clitoris respond to local stimulation and exercise their power of erection. At no time in life is erectile tissue under voluntary control. Erections are probably accomplished through reflex arcs in the sacral segment of the spinal cord. As the nervous system matures, pathways develop from the cord to the cerebral cortex. When this degree of maturity is reached, long before puberty, the child becomes aware of sensations in his genital area. This awareness plays a significant role in the child's emerging understanding of his body, of his gender, and of himself (p. 423).

THE FEMALE ORGANS THROUGH THE LIFE SPAN

The basic sex organ in the female is the ovary. Without an ovary femininity does not develop; nevertheless the ovary itself is under the supercontrol of the hypothalamic-hypophysis mechanism. Accessory organs are the uterus, the vagina, the fallopian tubes, the clitoris, the labia majora and labia minora, and the associated glands of Skene and Bartholin. The breast and the mammary tissues take part in reproductive function and, like the rest of the accessory apparatus, are under the control of the ovary.

Most of the secondary sex characteristics, the body shape and form, much of the psychic and emotional attributes, the things that make an individual feminine rather than neuter, get their immediate cues from the ovary.

The Ovaries

In the embryo when the indifferent gonad begins to take on the characteristic structure of an ovary, it becomes an oval-shaped structure and is surrounded by a layer of germinal epithelium. This epithelium penetrates into the stroma of the ovary in cords and then becomes broken up into islands of germ tissue. In each of these islands one cell develops into a primitive ovum around which the other cells of the group become arranged in a circular layer. This body is the primitive follicle, and such follicles begin to form in midembryonic life. It has been estimated that at the time of birth each human ovary contains some 400,000 follicles.

The primitive follicles formed in the embryo go through a rapid development in the last weeks of gestation in response to maternal gonad-stimulating hormone which has seeped from the mother's body to that of the fetus. This early development, however, ceases soon after birth; the ovary shrinks a little in size and remains in an immature form throughout the period of childhood, not even increasing in size sufficiently to keep pace with the general somatic growth.

With the beginning of puberty, which takes place any time between the ninth and seventeenth year, great changes take place in the ovary. At the onset of puberty, the anterior lobe of the hypophysis begins to secrete two hormones—ACTH, which stimulates the adrenal to produce androgens, and gonadotropin, which stimulates the ovary. The maturation of the ovary is concomitant with the development of the primitive follicles and the production of the female sex hormone, estrogen. Androgens stimulate the growth of pubic and axillary hair. Androgens and estrogens have an effect on many structures in the body: the long bones grow, muscles increase in size, fat accumulates and becomes so redistributed that the body curves of femininity make their appearance, and the breasts enlarge. The emotions and the psyche further mature. The little girl becomes a woman. The primitive follicles in the ovaries, lying dormant since fetal life, are now ready to form mature ova capable of carrying on the race. The maturation of ova leads to menstruation, the overt evidence of sexual maturity.

Deep within the stroma a single follicle begins to enlarge, and soon it becomes surrounded with two additional layers of cells. The outermost layer is a fibrous coat. The next layer, now the middle layer of the follicle, is highly vascular and the place where estrogen probably is produced. The innermost layer of the follicle, the one surrounding the primitive follicle and immediately adjacent to the ovum, grows, and soon a cavity around the ovum is formed which becomes filled with fluid. The whole follicle, now called the graafian follicle, continues to enlarge. When finally mature, the follicle migrates toward the surface of the ovary, ruptures, and expels the ovum into the peritoneal cavity where it is almost immediately picked up by the waving end of the fallopian tube. After rupture the graafian follicle becomes filled with a clot of blood; soon a yellow lipid material, the corpus luteum, is secreted into this space. At this time a second hormone from the hypophysis, the luteinizing hormone, is secreted and acts upon the corpus luteum, making possible its development. Surrounding the corpus luteum is a mass of blood vessels, many of which penetrate into the yellow cell mass. A hormone, progesterone, is secreted from the corpus luteum and absorbed by these vessels into the bloodstream. The corpus luteum is active for about 10 days, then degenerates; the blood vessels disappear, and nothing is left but a small scar.

As soon as the ovum is picked up by the fallopian tube, it begins its journey to the uterus. During the journey the ovum completes its own maturation (p. 44).

During the formation of the graafian follicle, estrogen secreted by the follicle acts upon the mucosa of the uterus, which responds by building up a thick layer of blood-filled tissue. The hypertrophy of the endometrium of the uterus begins before the rupture of the follicle and continues after the formation of the corpus luteum, under the influence of the progesterone excreted by the graafian follicle, now empty of ovum, from which the traveling ovum came.

The ovum finally reaches the well-prepared uterus. If it has not been fertilized, the ovum has already begun to degenerate, since the life of the ovum is measured in hours and that of the journey to the uterus in days. A degenerating ovum has no attraction for the endometrium; it passes through the uterus and is expelled from the body by way of the vagina. Once the ovum has begun to degenerate, the corpus luteum atrophies, and progesterone ceases to be made. In the absence of progesterone the uterus has no incentive to retain its hypertrophied endometrium. This excess tissue pulls away from the uterine wall, and the uterus contracts and expels it. The passage of this blood-filled tissue through the vagina is menstruation.

To recapitulate, the menstrual cycle is divided into three stages: the proliferative stage (about 12 days), the secretory stage, also about 12 days, and the menstrual stage (about 3 to 4 days).

If the ovum becomes fertilized on its journey down the fallopian tube, pregnancy ensues. A powerful attraction exists between the fertilized ovum and the endometrium. Instead of passing quickly through the uterus, the developing embryo buries itself in the endometrium, and the fetal membranes soon begin to form under the stimulation of progesterone from the corpus luteum. As soon as the placenta forms, it secretes additional progesterone, which maintains the corpus luteum in the ovary until the last trimester of pregnancy.

Four major hormones are directly involved in female sexual function; in addition, hormones from thyroid and adrenal play a part (Tepperman):

1. Follicle-stimulating hormone from the hypophysis which initiates maturation of the follicle.
2. Estrogen, which is produced in the graafian follicles and also in the stroma of the mature ovary and in large quantities in the placenta. It is widely distributed throughout the body. It is found in the blood, in urine, and in muscles and adrenal cortex of adult women. Estrogen, the basic female sex hormone, has a host of actions:
   a. It stimulates the hypertrophy of the endometrium of the uterus.
   b. It stimulates growth of mammary tissue, first in puberty, later after childbirth.
   c. It is responsible for many of the secondary sex characteristics.
   d. It stimulates the adrenal glands.

3. Luteinizing hormone from the hypophysis. The luteinizing hormone has several actions:
   a. It depresses the first part of the ovarian cycle—the maturation of the graafian follicle.
   b. It stimulates the second part of the cycle—the maturation of the corpus luteum.
   c. It stimulates the production of progesterone in the corpus luteum.
4. Progesterone from several sources. Progesterone also has several actions:
   a. It stimulates the changes in the uterine mucosa preparatory to implantation of the ovum.
   b. It is necessary for the development of the placenta.
   c. It is necessary for maintaining the fetus in utero.
   d. It has an influence on growth of mammary glands and, especially, of the alveoli of the glands.
   e. It suppresses ovulation.

Progesterone is produced in the corpus luteum. It is also produced in large quantities in the placenta. While the corpus luteum is present and progesterone is in the circulation, the hormone inhibits the action of the follicle-stimulating hormone from the hypophysis. As a result no new graafian follicles come to maturity as long as the corpus luteum is intact. Once it degenerates, either after menstruation or after the termination of pregnancy, this influence over the hypophysis ceases, and the cycle starts again. The end product of progesterone is an inert substance secreted in the urine. This fact has been utilized in the so-called "rabbit test" for pregnancy.

Progesterone has also been used as an oral contraceptive. When this hormone is given in the late menstrual phase and continued in the preovulatory and ovulatory phases of the cycle, it inhibits ovulation by suppressing the follicle-stimulating hormone from the hypophysis. When the drug is discontinued in the late phase of the menstrual cycle, withdrawal bleeding occurs.

Throughout the reproductive life of a woman graafian follicles come to maturity periodically. The germinal epithelium covering the ovary maintains its embryonic ability to penetrate the stroma of the ovary and create new ova, which go through their maturation cycles as described above.

However, there comes a time when the germinal epithelium ceases to have the ability to create new ova. Under the microscope such epithelium fails to show the mitotic figures of cell division so characteristic of the young tissue. When there are no longer primitive follicles in the ovary there is nothing more for the hypophyseal hormone to stimulate. Ovarian function slowly comes to an end, and the gland shows atrophic changes; the stimulation to the uterus ceases, and menstruation does not take place. Atrophic changes take place in all the sexual organs. The cessation of menstruation, the outward manifestation of the termination of ovarian function, is the menopause. Like puberty, it is quite variable in its times of appearance. The average age is about 45 but it may occur as early as 40 or as late as 55.

It is of interest to note that this cessation of ovarian function occurs in most women well before the age of general senescence. Many organs in the human body appear, develop, make their contribution to the total organism, then cease to function and atrophy. Among organs of this class may be mentioned the cartilaginous skeleton (p. 234), the tonsil (p. 304), and the placenta. Cessation of function of an organ often heralds a new stage of development.

The menopause does not usher in old age, as many people have been wont to believe. Women in American society, and especially now with our increased longevity, have several decades of productive life ahead of them after the menopause.

The Mammary Glands

Even though the mammary glands can function only in the female, they are developed by both sexes during fetal life, a further reflection of the neuter gender character of the early embryo. As early as the sixth week of fetal life bandlike thickenings of ectoderm appear along the ventrolateral body walls extending all the way from the axilla to the groin. These are the so-called "milk lines" which echo their phylogenetic history in mammals. In the human the actual breasts develop only in the pectoral region, although accessory glands appear at various levels of the milk line in a few people, oddly enough about twice as frequently in the male as in the female (Patten, 1953). By a process of invagination of epithelium into the underlying mesenchyme the glands take form. By the time of birth cords of cells have pushed out and formed the main ducts of the gland. No secretory acini form before birth. Development of the mammary glands is identical in the two sexes up to the time of birth.

Soon after birth in both sexes there is frequently an enlargement of the breasts. Presumably this takes place under the influence of estrogen, spilled over from the mother into the infant's circulation. This hormone activates the infant's hypophysis to manufacture lactogenic hormone, which in turn stimulates the growth of the mammary tissue. The infant's duct system increases, some secretory acini are formed, and milk is actually produced. This is the so-called "witches' milk," a substance rich in the tradition of folklore. As the estrogen from the mother is dissipated in the infant's body in a few days and as he has no further supply of the hormone, the enlargement of the infant's breasts subsides. No treatment of the infant is needed except what Williams called "skillful neglect."

After the initial burst of activity the mammary glands return to their nonsecretory status and so remain in both sexes through the years of childhood. At the time of puberty the glands are once again awakened by hormonal activity, but this time the estrogen is manufactured in the child's own body.

There is sometimes a slight mammary development in boys at puberty, usually due to upsets in hormonal balance. As the boy becomes a little older, his androgens and estrogens achieve a better relation, and his breasts retreat to acceptably masculine contours (Karsner, 1946). While seldom an organic problem gynecomastia (enlarged breasts in the male) is often a cause of considerable emotional disturbance to the body-conscious young adolescent trying to achieve ideal masculinity.

In girls puberty brings real mammary development. The maturing ovary manufactures estrogen, which stimulates the production of lactogenic hormone in the hypophysis, which in turn acts upon the breast. In spite of the distinctly hormonal nature of the immediate stimulus, the early enlargement of the breasts at puberty is quite largely adipose tissue, though there is some increase in mammary ducts and also of the nipple. The budding of the breasts is usually the first outward sign of puberty in girls and predates the menarche by a year or a little more.

Pubertal breast development is divided into four stages as follows:

1. Prepubertal breast—elevated papella only
2. Elevated areola, or minimal breast swelling
3. First swelling of the breast to a small mound formation
4. Final stage, after which no further development of the breasts occurs until pregnancy and lactation brings them into functional activity (Fig. 18-3).

While the breasts of all girls undergo pubescent changes, the actual size of the mature breast is largely dependent upon the amount of fat in the organ, which, in turn, is related to the general body constitution. The nipple and the areolar area mature in direct response to the estrogen secreted by the maturing organism and are therefore more accurately correlated with emerging puberty than mere breast size. Once the breasts have reached their adult size and contours, the rest of the sexual development has also attained maturity, and the girl soon has her first menstrual period.

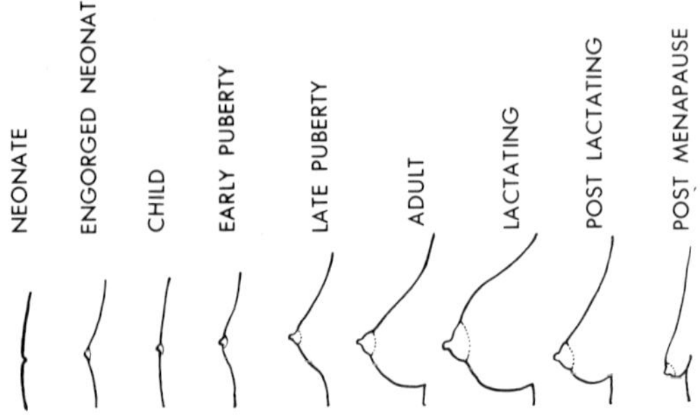

Fig. 18-3. Mammary development.

With each menstrual cycle there is often a slight temporary mammary enlargement. It occurs during the premenstrual period and is thought to be a progesterone effect.

During pregnancy the breasts increase in size considerably more than they do during each menstrual cycle; not only do the breasts become larger, but there is development of the alveoli as well as of the ducts. It is thought that this is due to a hormone from the placenta, possibly progesterone. At the termination of pregnancy, spectacular development of the breasts takes place. For the first few days after delivery the breasts remain quiescent; then rather suddenly the "milk comes in." The alveoli fill up with secretion and the entire breast swells and becomes firm. The hormonal control of the event is probably quite complicated. There is a lactogenic hormone secreted by the anterior lobe—prolactin—which is released when the amount of estrogen and progesterone is reduced soon after parturition. In addition, both the thyroid and the adrenal cortex secrete hormones which are essential for the secretion of milk.

In lower animals prolactin seems to have some bearing on maternal instincts. Animals deprived of the hormone experimentally refuse to suckle or care for their young. It has been suggested that prolactin may have some influence on the human being in the care given by the mother to her infant; however, comparison of the "instincts" of the human being with those of other species is a hazardous speculation.

Milk secretion doubtless is also under nervous as well as hormonal control. The nipple area is richly supplied with nerve plexuses from both the sympathetic and parasympathetic systems, as well as general sensory nerves. Stimulation of the nipple by sucking activates these nerves and increases the flow of milk. Whether the mechanism of this stimulation is through the nervous system or whether these nerves in turn stimulate hormonal mechanism is not known. However, it is certainly true that milk secretions can be inhibited by anxiety, fear, and nervous tensions, emotions quite often present in the postpartum period of women in our culture.

The nipple contains smooth muscle fibers which are arranged vertically as well as circularly. The vertical fibers cause the erection of the nipple under stimulation. The sensations aroused in the nipple are a diffuse, whole-body reaction. They have been compared to those arising in the erectile tissue of the glans penis or clitoris. Such sensations are aroused during the sucking of the infant, as well as during the precoital period of sexual excitation. It is certainly true that for many women the experience of suckling a baby is one of profound emotional satisfaction.

Lactation is maintained by the stimulation of sucking. If the milk-filled breast is not emptied by periodic sucking, the secretion dries up.

Irritated, cracked nipples are an extraordinarily common complaint of nursing mothers in our society. Such nipples are not only excruciatingly painful, but they can be dangerous, since breaks in the mucous membrane predispose them to infection. This condition can, in the main, be attributed to our modern mania for cleanliness and asepsis, increased in the last few years by new gadgets in nursing brassieres.

The largest sweat and sebaceous glands in the body are found around the nipple (MacKenna, 1948). Secretions of these glands are bactericidal. Washing with soap and water removes these secretions and deprives the nipple of their benefits. Alcohol does the same and in addition is irritating. Boric acid solution not only removes the natural secretions and irritates the nipple but, in one well-documented case in a lying-in hospital, was found responsible for an epidemic of diarrhea in newborn infants (Wegman, 1951).

Plain tap water is the most desirable prenursing treatment for the nipple (Newton, 1955). After nursing, exposure to the air is desirable. Exposure to an electric light is an additional aid in toughening the nipples.

Many modern nursing brassieres have a waterproof protection over the nipple area, which creates a warm moist atmosphere and prevents the nipples from toughening. The ideal type of nursing brassiere is one that supports the heavy breasts but has a flap that can be left open, thus exposing the nipple to the air.

A most satisfactory adjunct for the mother whose nipples have become a little tender is to drink a glass of wine or a bottle of beer 15 minutes before nursing time.

FEMALE SEX FUNCTION

The biologic function of the sexual apparatus is the procreation of the race. In the strictly biologic sense this in the female includes coitus, pregnancy, and lactation. Menstruation, in a very loose analogy, may be compared with the phenomenon of muscle tonus: it keeps the organism ready to function during periods of quiescence.

As has been said, ova mature one at a time; there is a mechanism for the expulsion of an unused ovum, and no pressure and tension build up because of an accumulated mass of ova. In addition, ova are matured at a regular pace, quite regardless of any sexual stimulation. The process is continuous from menarche to menopause, plodding along regardless of the life the woman leads. In the pubescent girl with a physiologically mature reproductive apparatus, mild sexual stimulation produces, primarily, a pleasing allover sensation and relatively little local genital feeling. More strenuous stimulation, kissing, necking, may produce "butterflies in the stomach," but in the young girl such stimulation does not build up pressures due to the rapid production of trapped ova and does not necessarily lead to a desire for coitus. The difference between postadolescent girls and boys with respect to the response to sexual stimulation has profound cultural ramifications.

In the human female the initiation of desire for coitus is not solely (perhaps not at all) under hormonal control, as evidenced by the fact that it can be brought about at any time during the menstrual cycle and has no relation to readiness of the genital tract for fecundation. Sex desire in the human female is largely under the domination of the cortex, not of the genital tract (Ford and Beach, 1951).

In mature women precoital stimulation activates neural pathways to the cortex. From the brain, not from the genital tract, further neural pathways activate the autonomic nervous system and the hormones, and organic preparations for the sex act are brought about. There is engorgement of the vulva, erection of the clitoris, relaxation of the adductor muscles of thigh and vaginal orifice, and secretions of mucus from the glands of Skene and Bartholin; concomitantly there is an acceleration of pulse and respiration, and a rise in blood pressure. When these processes are at their peak, the cortex has relinquished its control to the genital apparatus. When intromission takes place, rhythmic contractions of the uterus constitute the female orgasm, after which the above physiologic processes are reversed and the woman's body returns to its nonstimulated state (Wright, 1952).

The development of sexuality in the human female has a greater significance than the execution of the sex act; the genital apparatus is the tool through which many aspects of the personality emerge (p. 439). The milestones in the developmental history of the woman's genital organs are their formation during uterine life, quiescence during childhood, maturation at puberty, fulfillment of reproductive function in maturity, and final involution at the menopause. Throughout life these organs have human dimensions of function.

THE MALE SEX ORGANS THROUGH THE LIFE SPAN

The male sex organs are far less complicated than the female. The mature function of the male organs is the single act of coitus. The basic essential sex organ in the male is the testis. The accessory organs are the penis, the duct system and its associated glands, by means of which the germ cells are expelled to the outside, suspended in a fluid.

The secondary sex characteristics, the body shape and form, the hair on face, the deep voice, and much of the psychic and emotional attitudes of the man are due to the growth and maturation of the testes. Pubic and axillary hair are dependent upon androgens from the adrenal cortex in the male, as in the female.

The Testes

In the embryo the indifferent gonads begin to take on the characteristic structure of the testes at about the ninth week of gestation. They become oval in shape and are surrounded by a layer of germinal epithelium. It is this epithelium that contains the germ plasm from which the actual sex cells will develop. Cords of this substance penetrate the gland and break up into an elaborate series of tubules. During embryonic life these tubules contain a solid cord of potential germ cells but nothing comparable to the primitive follicle of the female. In the female the cell which will ultimately develop into a mature gamete can be identified, but in the male no such differentiation can be detected. Once the tubular structure of the testes is established and connections are made with their ducts, the epididymis and vas deferens, no further development of the germinal tissue takes place during fetal life.

In the developing testes, as was noted above, very early in embryonic life, lying between the seminiferous tubules, the cells of Leydig can be seen. After birth the only significant change in the testes is the disappearance of these cells. Once the organism has taken on its maleness under the influence of the hormone from these cells, evident by the development of the male and suppression of the female organs, the hormone seems unnecessary. During all of childhood the testes, like the ovary, remain dormant and small, not even growing in proportion to the rest of the body.

At the onset of puberty the testes awaken. The stimulus comes from the anterior lobes of the hypophysis and is the same hormone that maintains the corpus luteum in the female—the luteinizing hormone. The testes increase in size, and simultaneously the interstitial cells of Leydig reappear. These cells begin to secrete testosterone, the male sex hormone, and under its influence and that of adrenal androgens, the testes and penis continue to increase in size, and pubic hair makes its appearance. Testosterone (like estrogen in the female) influences the whole body. Not only do the genitalia grow, but long bones increase in length, muscles increase, the larynx enlarges and the voice deepens, hair appears on the face, the emotions change, the psyche matures—the boy becomes a man.

Growth of the external genitalia is the first evidence of puberty in the boy. The stages of sexual maturing are described as follows:

Stage 1: Penis, testes, and scrotum are essentially the same as in early childhood.

Stage 2: Testis and penis have noticeably enlarged; lightly pigmented downy hair has appeared.

Stage 3: The penis has appreciably lengthened; downy hair is interspersed with stronger, coarse, pigmented hair.

Stage 4: Larger testes and penis of increased diameter; pubic hair looks adult, but its area is smaller.

Stage 5: Genitalia are adult in size and shape; pubic hair is adult.

The growth of the testes is due largely to actual increase in the seminiferous tubules, the actual sex elements of the gland. In these tubules are the germinal cells which pass through several stages until the mature spermatozoa are formed. Spermatozoa mature within the testis (the ovum does not reach final maturation until it has been expelled from the ovary and is on its way down the tube). The mature spermatozoa, detached from the wall of the tubules, are pushed through the lumen to the epididymis—a transient storage reservoir for the mature germ cells. Toward the end of puberty the epididymis probably has a goodly supply of mature spermatozoa.

When maturity is reached, there is a sufficient accumulation of spermatozoa in the epididymis to initiate an ejaculation. For an ejaculation the spermatozoa must be suspended in a fluid medium. The fluid comes from the various accessory glands. When an ejaculation takes place, the smooth muscles of the testes contract, completely emptying the glands of accumulated germ cells, which are pushed through, first to the epididymis and then on into the duct of the vas deferens; here they meet the secretions of this gland and the secretions of prostate and seminal vessels. These glands, like the tubules of the testes, contract and empty under the impetus of the ejaculatory reflex. Finally the suspended spermatozoa are pushed through the ejaculatory duct and out through the erect penis. A single ejaculation of semen (the germ cells and the fluid) has been estimated to contain 300 million sperm cells.

The early ejaculations of the adolescent boy usually occur during sleep and are termed *nocturnal seminal emissions.* For some years these physiologic ejaculations take place at periodic intervals of roughly 2 weeks. They occur independently of sexual stimulation.

MALE SEX FUNCTION

Once a boy has reached full sexual maturity, his reproductive organs become very responsive to sexual stimulation. It is then that the look or even the thought of an attractive girl sends a tingle through his genitals. Greater stimulation, kissing, physical contact, precoital play stimulate the production of spermatozoa and the abundant flow of secretions from the accessory glands, all of which build up pressures and tension that excite the ejaculatory reflex, which physiologically terminates in ejaculation. In the boy, unlike in the girl, sexual stimulation is felt as a localized genital experience and is directed toward relief of tension by ejaculation. Culturally determined mores offer little opportunity for coitus for the young postadolescent. His constantly stimulated sex drives frequently lead him into masturbation—a device whereby his body is relieved of the inevitable biologic tensions (p. 437).

Sexual drives are probably at their height during the late teens and early twenties; however, they remain a powerful drive all through the years of a man's maturity. Gradually, as old age is reached, sexual drives become less powerful and in many men subside as the last decades are reached. Concomitant with lessening of the ability for sexual arousal there is a slow atrophy of testicular tissue. Many men, though certainly not all, do pass through a climacteric, after which there is no more production of spermatozoa and no more sexual power. However, the male climacteric is nowhere near as definite and as sure of fulfillment as the female climacteric. In addition, the termination of sexual activity in the male takes place later in life than in the female. When it does occur, it may bring with it hormonal imbalances capable of producing somatic and psychic symptoms similar to those of the menopause in women.

Sexual function in the male, as in the female, has a developmental cycle, and throughout life it has human dimensions of functions (p. 439).

BIBLIOGRAPHY

Best, Charles Herbert, and Norman Burke Taylor: "The Physiological Basis of Medical Practice," The Williams and Wilkins Company, Baltimore, 1955.

Ford, Clellan, and Frank A. Beach: "Patterns of Sexual Behavior," Harper & Row, Publishers, New York, 1951.

Gross, Robert E., and Robert L. Replogle: Treatment of the Undescended Testes, *Postgrad. Med.*, **34**:266, 1963.

Grumbach, Melvin M., and Murray L. Barr: Cytologic Tests of Chromosomal Sex in Relation to Sexual Anomalies in Man, *Recent Prog. Hormone Res.*, **14**:255, 1958.

Jost, A.: Hormonal Influences in Sex Development of Bird and Mammalian Embryos, in C. R. Austin (ed.), "Sex Differentiation and Development," Cambridge University Press, London, 1959.

Karsner, Howard T.: Gynecomastia, *Am. J. Path.*, **22**:235, 1946.

Keele, Curil, and Eric Neil: "Samson Wright's Applied Physiology," 10th ed., Oxford University Press, New York, 1961.

MacKenna, R. M. B.: "Modern Trends in Dermatology," Paul B. Hoeber, Inc., New York, 1954.

Newton, Niles: "Maternal Emotions," Paul B. Hoeber, Inc., New York, 1955.

———: Nipple Pain and Nipple Damage, *J. Pediat.*, **41**:411, 1952.

Patten, Bradley M.: "Human Embryology," 2d ed., McGraw-Hill Book Company, New York, 1953.

Pronove, Pacita: Sex Chromatin Pattern and Ultimate Sex Determination, *Clin. Proc. Child. Hosp.*, **16**:252, 1960.

Randolph, Judson: Surgical Aspects of Intersex, *Clin. Proc. Child. Hosp.*, **20**:33, 1964.

Tepperman, Jay: "Metabolic and Endocrine Physiology," The Year Book Medical Publishers, Inc., Chicago, 1962.

Wegman, Myron E.: An Epidemic of Diarrhea Among Breast-fed Newborn Infants, *J.A.M.A.*, **145**:962, 1951.

Wilkins, Lawson: Embryonic Sex Differentiation Controlling Factors and Abnormalities, Diagnosis, and Treatment, *Clin. Proc. Child. Hosp.*, **20**:1, 1964.

———: Masculinization of Female Fetus Due to the Use of Orally Given Progestine, *J.A.M.A.*, **172**:1028, 1960.

Wright, Samson: "Applied Physiology," Oxford University Press, London, 1952.

19

The Urinary System

DEVELOPMENT OF THE KIDNEY

The urinary system begins to develop in the embryo within the first few weeks of existence but does not complete its full development until about the end of the first year of extrauterine life. The earliest urinary structure, the pronephros, makes its appearance at about 3 weeks, continues to develop for a few weeks, then degenerates without ever assuming any function. It leaves as a legacy the Wolffian ducts, which become the vas deferens in the adult male. The pronephros is replaced by the mesonephros, another abortive urinary structure, which, however, may function in a rudimentary fashion before it too degenerates and is replaced by the metanephros, which is the beginning of the permanent kidney (Patten, 1953).

The ureters develop as buds from the Wolffian duct. These buds elongate and become ureters, renal pelvis, and collecting tubules. Failure or incomplete development of these buds or duplication of a bud accounts for many of the anomalies found in the ureters, renal pelvis, and collecting tubules. The glomeruli and their capsules and all the tubular system proximal to the collecting tubules develop from the metanephros. The two sets of tubules unite to form a continuous channel from Bowman's capsule to the bladder. Failure of adequate union of the two sets of tubules results in obstruction to the flow of urine and is thought to be a cause of polycystic kidneys.

While all this minute development of glomerular capsules and tubules is taking place, the organ shifts its position in the abdomen. The kidney begins to develop near the caudal end of the organism but migrates upward and rotates until it comes to rest at about the level of the fourth lumbar vertebra (Fig. 19-1).

Once the permanent kidney makes its appearance in the embryo, development consists mainly in the rapid formation of more and more of the individual renal units—the nephrons. The normal kidney at birth has probably its full quota of nephrons, although the kidney of the prematurely born infant may still be developing new nephrons (McCance, 1948, Campbell, 1963, Fig. 19-2.)

It is probable that the kidney of the normal fetus functions before birth and that fetal urine contributes to the amniotic fluid. However, the job the fetal kidney must accomplish is simple compared with that which the

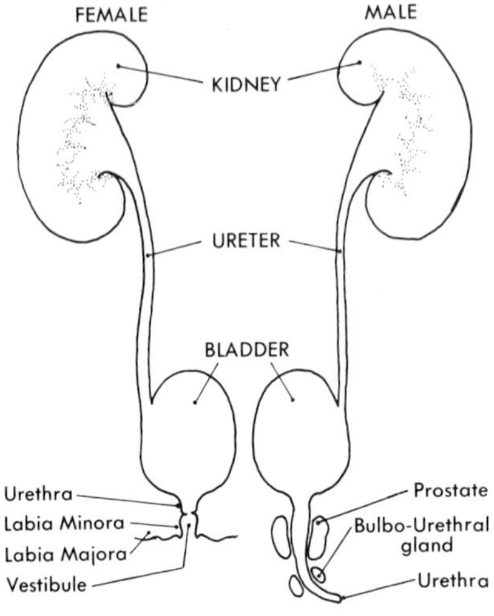

Fig. 19-1. Schematic representation of the urinary tract in the male and female.

kidney is called upon to perform after the maternal circulation is cut off. During fetal life, if the mother is in normal health, she supplies the fetus with the constituents of her plasma which are in equilibrium; the fetus can accept them as they are. His urine therefore bears a constant relation to his plasma. The fetal kidney is not called upon to adjust his electrolyte balance. While the fetal kidney does produce urine, this is not a survival function during intrauterine life; infants have been born with such rudimentary kidneys that little or no function was possible. Such infants survived, during fetal life, without any renal functions of their own (McCance, 1941).

Though all the renal units are probably formed by the end of fetal life, they are still immature. Anatomically, the glomeruli are more developed at birth than the tubules which are both short in length and narrow in diameter (Fetterman et al.). The tubules "grow up" rapidly and by approximately five months of age, the relative size of glomeruli and tubules approaches an adult ratio. Functionally, Calcagno and Rubin demonstrated slow tubular clearance in the early months of life which increased to almost adult levels after the first half year. The epithelium of both the glomeruli and the tubules in the newborn infant is composed of tall, columnar cells (McCory, 1959). In the older child and adult it has changed to a very thin pavement epithelium. It seems probable that filtration and absorption are more readily accomplished through the thin adult type of epithelium than through the relatively thick membrane of the newborn. At roughly 1 year to 18 months after birth, the histologic structure of the kidney resembles that of the adult (Colby, 1961).

Not only is the kidney structure itself immature but the endocrine mechanisms of the newborn also are immature (p. 221). His kidney is able to cope with solute loads if they do not vary too widely from physiologic norms, but he is under a distinct disadvantage if he loses excess water and electrolytes through vomiting or diarrhea or sweating. He may also get into trouble if his food contains an electrolyte balance very different from that of breast milk (p. 226).

CONGENITAL ABNORMALITIES OF THE URINARY TRACT

Abnormalities of the genitourinary tract account for about one-third of all congenital abnormalities (Potter, 1952; Ashley and Mostofi, 1960).

Some developmental mistakes have to do with agenesis, hypoplasia, or dysplasia of renal tissue and are often found in conjunction with abnormalities in other organ systems and suggests a fetal insult at a critical time in development (Rubenstein et al., 1961). Other abnormalities have to do primarily with obstruction to the flow of urine at some point in the tract from Bowman's capsule to the urethra. Adequate drainage is essential for normal function. Any obstruction builds up abnormal pressures which in time cause degeneration of kidney parenchyma (Rallner, 1963).

Many urinary tract anomalies appear to cause a predisposition to infection. Even what appears to be a minor abnormality such as a slight narrowing of the urethra appears to invite bacteria. The resulting inflammation and edema augments the preexisting interference with the free flow of urine.

Plastic procedures perfected within the last few years are making it possible to repair many urinary tract abnormalities, especially those of the lower tract. If such abnormalities can be detected before permanent damage to kidney parenchyma has taken place, many a potentially inadequate urinary tract can be salvaged for a normal life span (Leadbetter, 1963).

Obstruction of the vesical neck, due to narrowing of the lumen or to urethral valves, sometimes causes symptoms which readily alert the physician to possible pathologic condition; unfortunately, many of the anomalies are relatively silent until permanent damage has been done (McDonald et al., 1961).

Bender, Rice, and Guin point out that any child with even a minor

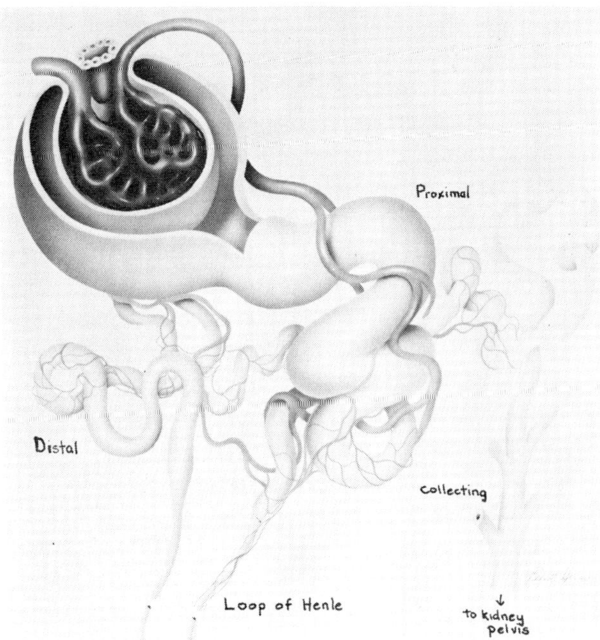

Fig. 19-2. The nephron. (*Courtesy of Eaton Laboratories, Norwich, New York.*)

abnormality in his external genitalia should be suspect. A boy with hypospadias or cryptorchism, a girl with a clitoris adherent to the urinary meatus, or a tiny meatus in either sex are signs often associated with other abnormalities of the urinary tract.

A small and narrow stream of urine or a prolonged time of urination are signs of trouble. Since a child makes no complaint of these signs, the mother should be quizzed routinely concerning her child's urinary performance. As a child with partial obstruction sits on the toilet, he may bend forward and press both hands over his bladder. This apparently helps him to urinate. McDonald makes a plea for cystourethroscopic examination of all children with signs or symptoms that point toward urinary obstruction.

Obvious symptoms such as dysuria and frequency point to urinary abnormalities. Pyuria is almost always associated sooner or later with obstruction to the flow of urine; however, pyuria can exist for prolonged periods without causing overt symptoms and will be detected only if urine examinations on uncomplaining children are routine. Urinary infections are frequently the cause of "fevers of unknown origin" in small children. They exist without causing localized symptoms and are detected only by urine examination (Ross et al., 1957).

THE URINE OF THE NEONATE

The bladder of the newborn usually contains urine which is passed within 24 hours after delivery. This first act of urination gives evidence that there is no gross obstruction in the urinary tract. Failure to urinate within 48 hours calls for investigation of the patency of the tract. The first urine represents that formed under fetal conditions; it shows a specific gravity of about 1.015; in other respects it is more or less similar to that of the maternal urine (Thomson, 1964).

Subsequent urine is formed by the infant's own machinery unaided by the placental circulation. Since the breast-fed infant receives little food during his first few days, his urine during this time is the result of catabolism of his own tissues; as soon as he begins to eat, his urine reflects his dietary intake. During the first weeks urine is scanty, but it is also quite dilute, with a specific gravity approaching that of a patient with diabetes insipidus—1.001 to 1.003. Heller has found that the amount of antidiuretic hormone recoverable from the newborn infant's posterior hypophysis is relatively small compared with that recoverable from the glands of older people. Lack of this hormone is one factor in the infant's inability to concentrate his urine. However, even if antidiuretic hormone is administered to a newborn, he is still unable to concentrate his urine, a fact which McCance attributes to immaturity of the tubules.

The urine of the neonate reflects the immaturity of his renal mechanism. Glomerular filtration rates are low, which results in lower concentration in the urine of those substances such as urea which are fractionally reabsorbed. Tubular reabsorption is less efficient than it will be later; this causes failure to reabsorb completely threshold substances such as albumin and sugar which may appear in small amounts in the urine of healthy infants.

While the urine of the healthy neonate may show small amounts of glucose or of albumin because of immaturity of his renal mechanism, there are a few substances which, if present, indicate not renal immaturity but basic errors in metabolism. Among these substances are galactose, fructose, cystine, phenylpyruvic acid.

URINE AFTER THE NEONATAL PERIOD

Not only does the composition of urine reflect the adequacy of kidney function, but since glomerular filtrate bears a constant relation to blood plasma, urine reflects many aspects of total metabolism. It is therefore desirable to include a urinalysis, at least once a year, in routine examinations of healthy children. Such a urinalysis should include, as a minimum, color, specific gravity, pH, sugar, protein, and microscopic sediment. Other tests can be done if and when indicated. The composition of urine in the healthy child after the age of 2 years changes but little as the child matures.

The most significant urine to examine is a "clean catch"[1] specimen collected first thing in the morning (after an overnight fast). This urine is formed under relatively basal conditions and gives the truest picture of what the kidney can do with minimum interference from activity, diet, or emotions. If such a urine shows values which fall within normal limits (see below) and the child shows no signs or symptoms suggesting pathology, further tests are seldom needed.

TABLE 19-1

Average Daily Secretion of Urine

Age	Milliliters/24 hr
0–2 days	15–50
3–10 days	50–300
10 days–2 mos.	250–400
2 mos.–1 yr.	400–500
1–3 yrs.	500–600
3–5 yrs.	600–750
5–8 yrs.	700–1,000
8–14 yrs.	700–1,500

In health, urine volume rises after the first month of life, as body size increases. It varies with the amount of fluid ingested, the environmental temperature, and the activity.

[1] Technique of obtaining a "clean catch": wash the genitals with soap and water; discard the first part of the urinary stream; collect the mid-stream urine in a sterile container.

TABLE 19-2

Renal Function and Urinalysis as a Monitor of Well-being

Small, thin stream of urine, prolonged duration of act of micturation, gesture of clutching abdomen are signs of possible urinary obstruction.

Frequency, pain on micturation, straining to void suggest infection in lower part of urinary tract.

Fever may be the only sign of urinary infection in young children.

Infection and/or signs of obstruction call for investigation of urinary tract.

Frequency without other symptoms suggests emotional stress.

Edema, especially around the eyes, suggests nephritis.

Volume of urine:
- Increase (to be distinguished from frequency)
  - With decreased specific gravity suggests:
    - Advanced nephritis.
    - Diabetes insipidus.
  - With increased specific gravity suggests.
    - Diabetes mellitus.
- Decrease suggests:
  - Dehydration.
  - Kidney damage.

Specific gravity:
- Decrease suggests:
  - Kidney damage.
  - Diabetes insipidus.
- Increase suggests:
  - Diabetes mellitus.
  - Any condition with proteinuria.

Color:
- Normal urine is yellow.
- Pink urine suggests excessive bilirubin from liver disease or hemolysis.
- Brown urine suggests excessive bilirubin from bile obstruction or hemolysis; rarely, from alkaptan bodies.
- Red urine suggests hemoglobin due to hemolysis or RBC due to bleeding anywhere in urinary tract; rarely, due to ingestion of beets.
- Black urine suggests reduced hemoglobin.

Protein:
- Normal urine is protein-free.
- Protein may be present transiently because of:
  - Intense physical exercise.
  - Exposure to extreme cold.
  - Emotional stress.
  - Orthostatic albuminuria.
- Protein constantly present suggests:
  - Renal damage, especially of the glomeruli.
  - Cystitis or pyletitis

Acetone:
- Normal urine is free of acetone.
- Its presence suggests ketosis due to starvation or diabetes mellitus.

Glucose:
- Normal urine is glucose free.
- Glucose may be present transiently because of:
  - Intense physical activity.
  - Emotional stress.
- Glucose usually present suggests:
  - Diabetes mellitus.

TABLE 19-2 (cont.)

Renal Function and Urinalysis as a Monitor of Well-being

Other reducing substances:
- Normal urine is free of all reducing substances.
- Reducing substances other than glucose need identification—all are signs of metabolic error.

Formed elements in urinary sediment:
- RBC:
  - Normal urine contains no RBC.
  - RBC may be present transiently after vigorous physical exercise.
  - Persistent presence of RBC even in small numbers suggests bleeding anywhere in the urinary tract.
- WBC:
  - Normal urine is free from WBC. Care must be exercised to distinguish WBC actually present in urine from contamination from vagina or meatus.
  - Large numbers of WBC, especially if clumped, suggest infection in lower urinary tract.
  - Occasional WBC suggest infection in kidney.
- Casts:
  - Normal urine is free from casts.
  - Presence suggests renal damage.
- Bacteria:
  - Normal urine is sterile. Bacteria present in urine and not due to contamination indicates infection.

BIBLIOGRAPHY

ASHLEY, DAVID J. B., and F. K. MOSTOFI: Renal Agenesis and Dysgenesis, *J. Urol.*, **83**:211, 1960.

BENDER, PAUL B., E. CLARENCE RICE, and GRACE H. GUIN: Genito-urinary Anomalies, *Clin. Proc. Child. Hosp.*, **13**:17, 1957.

BEST, CHARLES H., and NORMAN B. TAYLOR: "Physiologic Basis of Medical Practice," The Williams and Wilkins Company, Baltimore, 1955.

CALCAGNO, P. L., and M. I. RUBIN: Renal Extraction of Para-aminohippurate in Infants and Children, *J. Clin. Invest.*, **42**:1632, 1963.

CAMPBELL, MEREDITH F.: Urology in Infancy and Childhood, in "Urology," vol. III, 2d ed., W. B. Saunders Company, Philadelphia, 1963.

COLBY, FLETCHER H.: "Essential Urology," The Williams and Wilkins Company, Baltimore, 1961.

FETTERMAN, G. H., N. A. SHUPLACK, F. G. PHILIPP, and H. S. GREGG: The Growth and Maturation of Human Glomeruli and Proximal Convolutions from Term to Adulthood, *Pediatrics*, **35**:601, 1965.

HELLER, H.: Renal Function in Newborn Infants, *J. Physiol.*, **102**:429, 1944.

LEADBETTER, GUY L.: The Etiology, Symptoms, and Treatment of Urethral Strictures in Male Children, *Pediatrics*, **31**:80, 1963.

MCCANCE, R. A., and W. F. YOUNG: Secretion of Urine by Newborn Infants, *J. Physiol.*, **99**:265, 1941.

———: Renal Function in Early Life, *Physiol. Rev.*, **28**:331, 1948.

MCCORY, WALLACE W.: Maturation of Processes for Renal Tubular Transport, in J. J. Foman (ed.), "Disturbances of Cellular Metabolism in Infancy," Report of 33rd Ross Conference on Pediatric Research, Ross Laboratories, Columbus, Ohio, 1959.

MCDONALD, HAROLD P., WILBORN E. UPCHURCH, and CARLOS L. CELAYA: Vesical Neck Obstructions in Children, *Am. Surgeon*, **27**:603, 1961.

Ostow, Mortimer, and Seymour Philo: Chief Urinary Pigment: Relationship between Rate of Excretion of the Yellow Urinary Pigment and Metabolism Rate, *Am. J. M. Sc.*, **207**:507, 1944.

Patten, Bradley M.: "Human Embryology," 2d ed., McGraw-Hill Book Company, New York, 1953.

Potter, Edith L.: "Pathology of the Fetus and Newborn," 2d ed., The Yearbook Medical Publishers, Inc., Chicago, 1952.

Rattner, William H., Ruben Meyer, and Jay Bernstein: Congenital Abnormalities of the Urinary System: IV. Valvular Obstruction of the Posterior Urethra, *J. Pediat.*, **63**:84, 1963.

Ross, Sidney, Leonard B. Berman, Allan B. Coleman, Hamilton P. Dorman: Pyuria in Children, *Clin. Proc. Child. Hosp.*, **13**:181, 1957.

Rubenstein, Marc, Ruben Meyer, and Jay Bernstein: Congenital Abnormalities In the Urinary System, A Post-mortem Survey of Development Anomalies and Acquired Congenital Lesions in a Children's Hospital, *J. Pediat.*, **58**:356, 1961.

Smith, Homer W.: "The Kidney: Structure and Function in Health and Disease," Oxford University Press, New York, 1951.

Thomson, John: Observations on the Urine of the Newborn Infant, *Arch. Dis. Childhood,* **19**:169, 1944.

Vorzimer, Jefferson, Ira B. Cohen, and J. Jaskow: The Use of Urinary Pigment Excretion for the Measurement of Basal Metabolic Rate, *J. Lab. & Clin. Med.,* **34**:482, 1949.

Wolman, Irving J.: "Laboratory Applications in Clinical Pediatrics," McGraw-Hill Book Company, New York, 1957.

20

The Endocrine System

The endocrine system consists of a number of glandular structures scattered throughout the body. Although the mass of these glands is small in comparison with that of the total body mass, the hormones produced in them influence the whole conduct of the organism. These hormones are intimately related one to the other and are sensitive to the total metabolism. The hypothalamus exercises a subtle control over endocrine function. The relationships are so involved that, as Tepperman says, endocrinology has become one long and complicated exercise in correlation. Some hormones are essential for growth and differentiation of structure; others serve their greatest usefulness in metabolic adjustments, and still others maintain homeostasis under conditions of stress.

The fetus is seldom under physiologic or biochemical stress. He receives his nourishment from the maternal blood plasma; if the mother is healthy, her plasma is in biochemical equilibrium. She transmits to her child nourishment, electrolytes, and fluids in almost exactly the concentration that is optimum for use in fetal tissue. The fetal endocrine glands develop in utero; some are essential for normal intrauterine development, but many function little, if at all, prior to birth (Williams, 1962).

The neonate is able to cope quite well if his internal functioning does not deviate appreciably from a physiologic equilibrium, but he is at a severe disadvantage if he must adjust to wide fluctuations in concentration of water, of electrolytes, of glucose, or of amino acids. Hormones, which later in life will bring about homeostasis easily, are not available to the young infant in adequate amounts. The immaturity of his endocrine system adds to his difficulty in coping with adversity.

The endocrine glands to be considered are (1) the thyroid, (2) the adrenals, (3) the gonads, (4) the hypophysis, (5) the parathyroids, and (6) the islets of Langerhans.

The thyroid, the adrenals, and the gonads take their cues from the hypophysis. The parathyroids, while anatomically closely related to the thyroid, are functionally dependent only slightly on the hypophysis. The islets of Langerhans are more or less independent of other glands although in times of stress their function becomes intertwined with that of the rest of the neurohormonal mechanisms.

THE THYROID GLAND

Toward the end of the fourth month of gestation the thyroid gland has developed sufficient maturity to be responsive to thyroid-stimulating hormone from the hypophysis. From this age on through life thyroxin is poured into the blood in accordance with a feedback mechanism operating between the hypophysis and the thyroid gland. The thyroid gland increases in size from midfetal life to maturity; the gland in boys is always a little larger in proportion to body size than is that of girls. At adolescence the thyroid gland takes part in the general growth spurt (Tanner, 1955). In the normal adult male it weighs about 25 Gm.

Thyroid deficiency can occur at any age after midfetal life and may be due to primary defects in the gland or in the hypophysis. Such defects are usually genetic. Thyroid deficiency can develop because of deficiency in the raw material out of which thyroxin is made, iodine and the amino acid tyrosine. Iodine is the most likely to be lacking since tyrosine is an amino acid that can be synthesized in the body from other amino acids. Iodine is deficient in certain parts of the world, and in these areas thyroid deficiency is more common than in areas with larger amounts of iodine. In the United States the addition of iodine to table salt has almost eliminated hypoiodinism as a cause of thyroid deficiency.

Thyroid deficiency during fetal life can result from treatment of the pregnant mother with thiouracil or similar preparations. Thyroid deficiency from any cause occurring before birth may result in the birth of a child with cretinism. The stigmata of this disease in the newborn are enlarged tongue, potbelly, umbilical hernia, and characteristic fat pads in the neck. The clinical suspicion of this disease can be verified by several tests (see below). Treatment consists of administration of the hormone. However, if the deficiency has existed for some time during fetal life, prognosis for normal development is poor; irreparable damage to the nervous system may have already taken place.

Thyroid deficiency beginning after birth is suspected by a general slowing down of metabolic processes. Cardiac rate is slow, appetite is poor and gain in weight skimpy, the extremities are short and inadequate. Motor development is slow, the teeth appear late, and the child is slow-moving and easily fatigued. He is mentally as well as physically sluggish; he is usually constipated, has a low hemoglobin, and suffers from cold extremities. Sexual maturation is considerably delayed. In fact, every major organ system in the body is affected when thyroid secretion is inadequate.

Obesity in children is almost never due to thyroid deficiency, although in the adult excess weight, water retention, and excess adipose tissue may be related to inadequate amounts of thyroid secretion.

A child small for his chronological age, especially if he is a little sluggish, may be suspected of hypothyroidism. It then becomes necessary to distinguish short stature due to a constitutionally slow rate of maturing (p. 115) from that due to a true thyroid deficiency. Diagnosis of thyroid deficiency can be arrived at by determination of protein-bound iodine, by iodine uptake tests, and by clinical conditions other than stature (Wolman, 1957).

The administration of thyroid to a child with a thyroid deficiency will increase his growth and general well-being. However, the administration of thyroid to a normally slow-maturing child will not only do him no good but may serve to inhibit his normal thyroid secretion. Now that accurate tests are available for diagnosis of a thyroid deficiency, there is no excuse for the indiscriminate administration of the hormone to any child who seems a little short or slow or dull.

THE ADRENAL GLANDS

The adrenal glands are small bilaterally placed structures lying on the top of each kidney. Each adrenal gland consists of two parts, (1) a central area or medulla, and (2) the peripheral area or cortex. The two parts lie in such close proximity that they constitute a single gland morphologically; nevertheless they maintain their embryonic identity, an identity which is reflected not only by the production of different hormones but by the fact that they respond to different stimuli.

The adrenal gland goes through definite morphologic changes during the life cycle. Immediately after birth, it decreases in size, and this decrease continues throughout the first year of life. The gland then begins to increase in size (Fig. 11-8). During childhood the adrenal is smaller than it was at birth. In puberty the gland spurts in growth as the somatic tissues grow, reaching its adult size at about the same time as the rest of the body. Throughout life, from the age of about 1 year when adrenal size begins to increase, males have slightly larger adrenals than females, a difference accentuated at adolescence when the male spurt is greater than the female.

The medulla of the adrenal secretes epinephrine and norepinephrine. The cortex of the adrenal secretes many hormones. They are of three types, and each type is produced in a different area of the cortex, as follows:

From the outer layer, hormones that influence metabolism of water, sodium, and potassium: aldosterone and deoxycorticosterone. The function of these hormones is to restore homeostasis in times of physiologic stress. The immaturity of this mechanism in the young infant renders him prone to derangements of his electrolyte balance under stress.

From the middle layer, a hormone that influences metabolism of proteins, fat, and carbohydrates: cortisol. Cortisol is needed under stress. The types of stress that call it forth are excessive muscular exercise, profound infection, extremes of heat and cold, trauma, and emotional states of fear and anger. The stress mechanism is immature during infancy.

Androgens are not produced normally by the adrenal cortex until puberty.

While the hormone produced in males and females appears to be the same, it stimulates male pubic hair in boys and female pubic hair in girls. Axillary hair is similar in the two sexes. Androgens also act upon sebaceous glands of the face and shoulders predisposing them to the development of acne (p. 251).

THE GONADS

The ovary in the female and the testis in the male can be considered endocrine glands as well as reproductive organs, since both secrete hormones. Their secretions are discussed on p. 203.

THE HYPOPHYSIS, OR PITUITARY BODY

The hypophysis is a small structure weighing, in the adult, only about 0.5 Gm. It lies in a special bony encasement at the base of the skull, the sella turcica. The hypophysis is the smallest of all the endocrine glands, yet it influences profoundly almost every organ in the body either by direct action or through the intermediary of other endocrine glands (Table 20-1).

TABLE 20-1

Hormones from the Anterior Lobe of the Hypophysis

Hormone	Action
Thyroid stimulating (TSH)	Release of thyroid hormone into blood by means of action on thyroglobin in thyroid gland
Adrenocorticotrophins (ACTH)	Synthesis in adrenal cortex and release into blood of: Cortisol Androgens
Gonadotropins	
Follicle stimulating (FSH)	Development of Graafian follicles and production of estrogen
Luteotrophins in female	Development of corpus luteum and production of progesterone Mammary development
Luteotrophins in male	Development of cells of Leydig and production of testosterone
Pituitary growth (PGH)	Protoplasmic growth

The hypophysis consists of two parts, one neural, the posterior lobe, and the other glandular, the anterior lobe.

The Anterior Lobe

The anterior lobe has often been referred to as the master gland of the body. This is a misnomer because the anterior lobe initiates very little. It is directed by impulses (neural or hormonal) from the hypothalamus. It is the hypothalamus which probably exercises supreme control.

At a lower level of function the anterior lobe and the glands (thyroid, adrenal cortex, gonads) on which its secretions act relation. A feedback mechanism controls the secretion lobe and its target gland. When the amount of a spec. lating in the blood drops, the anterior lobe pours out i mone; when the hormone level becomes adequate, the an secreting.

In addition to hormones which act upon a target gland produces PGH, pituitary growth hormone, which acts dire tissue. The effect of PGH is to stimulate protein synthesis (...aben, 1962). It exerts marked effect upon the growth of bone, muscle, liver, kidney, and adipose tissue. Its effect on bone is the stimulation of growth of cartilage, especially at the epiphysis, although it acts also on bone matrix. Excess PGH prior to closure of the epiphysis results in gigantism; after closure, excess PGH produces a general thickening of bone and increased disposition of calcium, a condition called acromegaly. Decreased PGH prior to closure of the epiphysis results in dwarfism.

It is difficult to disentangle the effects of nutrition, other hormones, and PGH on the growth of a child. Doubtless there are genetic influences also which play a role in growth potential. PGH does not cease to be produced when the animal stops growing. It seems probable that PGH aids in some mechanism that permits adaptation to periods of food deprivation (Tepperman, 1962).

The Posterior Lobe

Two hormones are produced in the posterior lobe of the hypophysis: (1) antidiuretic hormone (ADH), or vasopressin, which inhibits water diuresis in the renal tubule and (2) oxytocin, which is concerned with the process of lactation and also the contraction of the smooth muscle of the uterus (Sawyer, 1961).

The posterior lobe of the newborn infant's hypophysis shows its immaturity by its inability to secrete more than minimal amounts of diuretic hormone. As with some of the other hormones, the fetus has little or no need for them, and the glands are immature prior to birth. The deficiency of the diuretic hormone in the neonate is another aspect of his inability to cope with stress. Lack of ability to conserve water predisposes him to dehydration under minor conditions of stress. Fluid for correction of dehydration in young infants should be hypotonic in view of the infant's inability to retain his fluids.

THE PARATHYROIDS

The parathyroids are four small symmetrically placed glands lying in close proximity to the thyroid. The hormone produced by these glands maintains homeostasis of calcium and phosphorus (Rasmussen, 1961).

g fetal life the mother (if her parathyroids are normal) maintains rmal balance between calcium and phosphorus for the fetus. After irth the newborn begins ingesting milk, and he must then cope with the calcium and phosphorus in it. If the infant is fed breast milk, the demand on his parathyroids is not great. Cow's milk presents the newborn with a slightly greater problem since the actual amounts of calcium and phosphorus are greater in cow's milk than in breast milk, and in addition the ratio between them is quite different. The calcium-phosphorus ratio in breast milk is 2.25:1 and in cow's milk 1.35:1 (Talbot et al., 1952). Since most infants do tolerate cow's milk quite satisfactorily, it is evident that the parathyroids rise to the occasion in normal infants.

While relatively rare, tetany in the newborn does occur, due to imbalance between calcium and phosphorus as a result of immaturity in the parathyroids. It occurs with greater frequency in infants fed cow's milk than in breast-fed infants. Why an occasional infant is born with parathyroids unable to come into function is unknown.

THE ISLETS OF LANGERHANS

Unlike the other endocrine glands the islets of Langerhans do not constitute a discrete gland. This tissue consists of masses of specialized cells dispersed more or less at random through the structure of the pancreas.

In the embryo the islets of Langerhans arise as buds from the same cords of epithelium that give rise to the secretory cells of the pancreas. They separate at an early age and mature independently of the pancreatic tissue. It has been estimated (Patten, 1953) that about a million of these clusters of cells develop, each with a series of dilated capillaries in their interstices.

Two hormones are produced by the islets of Langerhans, insulin and glucagon, both of which facilitate the utilization of glucose. Immediately after birth and for approximately the first week of life blood sugar levels are low in the normal infant. Levels range from 20 to 60 mg per 100 ml (Talbot et al., 1952). Since this degree of hypoglycemia is not accompanied by clinical manifestations of blood glucose deficiency, it can be considered physiologic for this age group. By the end of the first week of life, blood sugar rises to the levels found throughout life, 80 to 120 mg per 100 ml.

Throughout childhood blood sugar is apt to be somewhat more labile than later in life. It is not unusual to find a faint trace of sugar in the urine an hour after the ingestion of excessively large amounts of sweets, and hypoglycemia may occur in little children several hours after a meal, especially if they have been extremely active (which they usually are). This is not to be considered pathologic; such a condition merely reflects the immaturity of the endocrine system. Small carbohydrate snacks midmorning and midafternoon raise blood sugar and relieve the fatigue and irritability of slight hypoglycemia.

BIBLIOGRAPHY

Best, Charles N., and Norman B. Taylor: "The Physiological Basis of Medical Practice," The Williams and Wilkins Company, Baltimore, 1955.

Patten, Bradley M.: "Human Embryology," 2d ed., McGraw-Hill Book Company, New York, 1955.

Raben, M. S.: Growth Hormone, Physiologic Aspects, *New England J. Med.*, **266**:31, 1962.

Rasmussen, Howard: Parathyroid Hormone, *Am. J. Med.*, **30**:112, 1961.

Sawyer, Wilbur H.: Neurohypophysical Hormones, *Pharmacol. Rev.*, **13**:225, 1961.

Talbot, Nathan B., Edna H. Sobel, Janet W. McArthur, and John D. Crawford: "Functional Endocrinology from Birth Through Adolescence," Harvard University Press, Cambridge, Mass., published for the Commonwealth Fund, 1952.

Tanner, J. M.: "Growth at Adolescence," Charles C Thomas, Publisher, Springfield, Ill., 1955.

Tepperman, Jay: "Metabolic and Endocrine Physiology," The Year Book Medical Publishers, Inc., Chicago, 1962.

Wolman, Irving J.: "Laboratory Applications in Clinical Pediatrics," McGraw-Hill Book Company, New York, 1957.

Williams, Robert H.: "Endocrinology," 3d ed., W. B. Saunders Company, Philadelphia, 1962.

21

Connective, Adipose, Supportive, and Muscular Tissue

Posture, locomotion, and body shape are dependent, in large measure, on the skeleton, the muscles, and the connective and adipose tissues.

PHYLOGENETIC BACKGROUND

The phylogenetic history of posture and locomotion is a story of adaptation. The earliest vertebrates were fish whose bodies were buoyed up by the sea and whose locomotion was achieved by means of inundatory movements aided by paddlelike fins. Their skeletons were composed almost entirely of pliable and relatively soft cartilage adequate for their marine environment. When the early amphibians crawled out of the sea, their soft skeletons and short limbs permitted but a lumbering close-to-the-ground locomotion in the muddy flats near the shore. The higher vertebrates, who became true quadrupeds, had to have more skeletal support, and ultimately rigid bone evolved.

The appearance of primates who took to the trees introduced a new postural accomplishment. Primates achieved a part-time erect posture, albeit that posture came about by suspension of weight from the forward extremities. Ultimately the final descent from the trees took place, and man established a permanent erect posture based on weight bearing instead of weight suspension. The muscles which hold the skeleton in an erect position with a center of gravity not too far from the spine were evolved with the dual purpose of maintaining posture and of providing strength for survival in a rugged environment.

Discussion of body mechanics begins with consideration of the tissues involved. Connective and supportive tissues have a different life history from that of muscle and will be considered first.

CONNECTIVE AND SUPPORTIVE TISSUE

The connective and supportive tissue consists of fibroelastic tissue, adipose tissue, cartilage, and bone. In the mature organism, these tissues have very different functions, and yet all have a common origin in the embryo and maintain for life some fundamental common attributes. In all these tissues the secreted substance within the cell, rather than the cell body itself, performs the functions of the tissue. The cell extracts what is needed from the surrounding medium, then manufactures fibers or fat or bone and builds the various organ systems. The cell bodies continue to be of importance as a means of maintaining the nourishment of the tissue and replenishing the tissue itself, but the cells do not themselves perform the function of the organ. This state of affairs stands in marked contrast to that in muscle, where it is the actual cell body that does the work of the tissue. A corollary of the fact that secreted substances perform the functions of the connective and supportive tissues is the phenomenon of repair after injury. A muscle cell that is destroyed is gone forever; there is no possibility of regeneration of it or its function. On the other hand, while a fibroblast that is destroyed is gone, adjacent fibroblasts continue to manufacture fibers and heal a wound with tissue exactly like the destroyed tissue. Bones heal with new bone formation, whereas muscles heal only by proliferation of scar tissue.

Fibroblasts, adipose cells, chondroblasts all originate from what appears to be the same kind of mesenchymal cells; once differentiated, each maintains its own individuality. Fibroblasts never accumulate fat, adipose cells never grow fibers, and neither ever deposit cartilage (Patten, 1953).

FIBROELASTIC TISSUE

The fibroelastic tissue is widespread throughout the entire organism. It is composed, as its name implies, of interlacing bundles of collagenous and elastic fibers which hold the various structures together and give them resilience and the ability to adapt to changes in position. Where toughness is required, the collagenous fibers predominate, as in the periosteum; where greater mobility is needed, the elastic fibers are most abundant, as in the sheaths around muscle fibers, nerves, and blood vessels. Fibroelastic tissue penetrates into the innermost parts of almost every structure binding the functional units together. It is found in between the follicles in the ovary, between the glomeruli and the tubules of the kidney, in the interspaces between the alveoli of the lung. It is also in the spaces between the organs, in the peritoneum, in the thorax, in fact, almost everywhere.

Much recent interest has been directed toward a group of diseases collectively known as *collagen diseases*. Some of these diseases are acquired, others are genetic in origin (McKusick, 1960), but all have in common alterations in connective tissue.

ADIPOSE TISSUE

Adipose tissue is an active participant in the body economy and is now considered an organ formed by specific cells (Wells, 1940). This is a relatively recent concept. For many generations fat was thought to be inert storage material, laid down in connective tissue, whenever the energy intake exceeded the energy output. It is now accepted that fat is only deposited by adipose cells, not by connective tissue in general, and can only accumulate where adipose cells are present; the more adipose cells, the greater the potential fat stores. Even in extreme obesity, there is no accumulation of fat in the eyelids, the nose, or the cerebral membranes; the hands and feet never store fat to the same extent as the abdominal wall, the buttocks, or the subcutaneous areas. Adipose cells exist in certain areas of the body, not in others (Wertheimer, 1948).

The Overall Life Pattern of Fat Accumulation

While there are enormous differences in the degree of fatness or leanness of human being at all ages, nevertheless, there is a lifetime cycle of fat accumulation against which it is convenient to discuss the many variations (Fig. 21-1). This pattern can be divided into several epochs (Reynolds, 1950).

1. Rapid accumulation of fat occurs in both sexes from the seventh prenatal month to about the sixth postnatal month. Fat droplets can be detected in adipose tissue by the fourth month of gestation, but fat storage is scanty until the seventh month, when fat begins to accumulate rapidly. Infants born prematurely have an old and wizened appearance because they were born before much, if any, subcutaneous fat had been accumulated. After birth, fat stores continue to increase for the first half year. It is during this time that the infant becomes round and chubby (Fig. 21-2).

There are large individual differences between infants in the amount of subcutaneous fat. Obese infants may have more than twice as much subcutaneous fat as lean infants. At birth there is a correlation between the

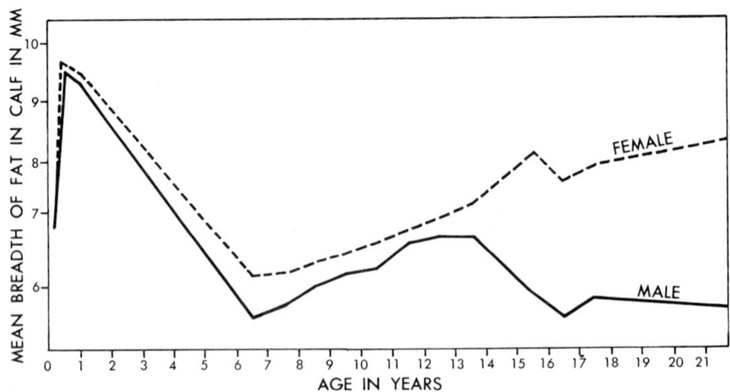

Fig. 21-1. Life patterns of adipose tissue. (*From Reynolds, The Distribution of Subcutaneous Fat in Childhood and Adolescence, Monograph of the Society for Research in Child Development, Inc., 15 Serial 50, 1950, with permission of the Society for Research in Child Development, Inc.*)

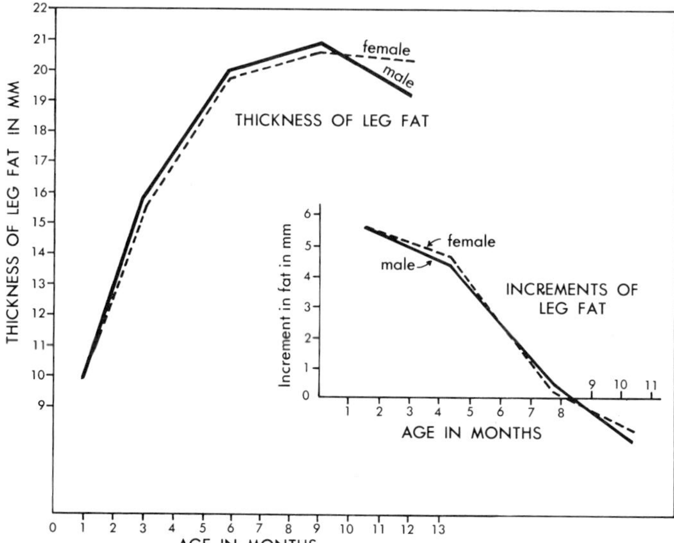

Fig. 21-2. Fat deposition in the first year of life. *(From Garn, Fat Thickness and Growth Process during Infancy, Table on p. 235, Human Biology, 28:232, 1956, by permission of Wayne State University Press.)*

amount of fat and the weight of the infant, but this correlation is not maintained; the leaner infants have a tendency to catch up with the fatter ones. When length and muscle mass are compared toward the end of the first year, it is found that the initially leaner infants are approximately the same length and may have even more muscle mass than the initially fatter infants. Since muscle mass is a better guide to nutritional adequacy than adipose tissue, it is evident that depth of subcutaneous fat is no guide to nutritional well-being in infancy (Garn and Young, 1956).

2. Deceleration of fat accumulation and even fat loss takes place in both sexes from the middle of the first year to 6 or 7 years of age (Fig. 21-1). Soon after the first birthday all children begin to slim down. The chubby appearance of the toddler merges into the lithe build of the preschooler. There are wide individual differences, but even the fat child becomes less fat during the years between 1 and about 6 or 7. Girls have a tendency to maintain slightly more fat than boys, but the differences, due to sex, are slight in early childhood.

3. In both sexes from the age of 6 or 7 to early puberty, fat begins to accumulate slowly; girls become slightly fatter than boys, but the difference between boys and girls is small in the years before puberty. These are the years when true obesity begins to make its appearance in some children.

4. Beginning in early puberty the pattern of the deposition of fat is different in the two sexes. At the time of the maximum growth spurt in boys, the amount of fat decreases sharply (the increase in weight in boys

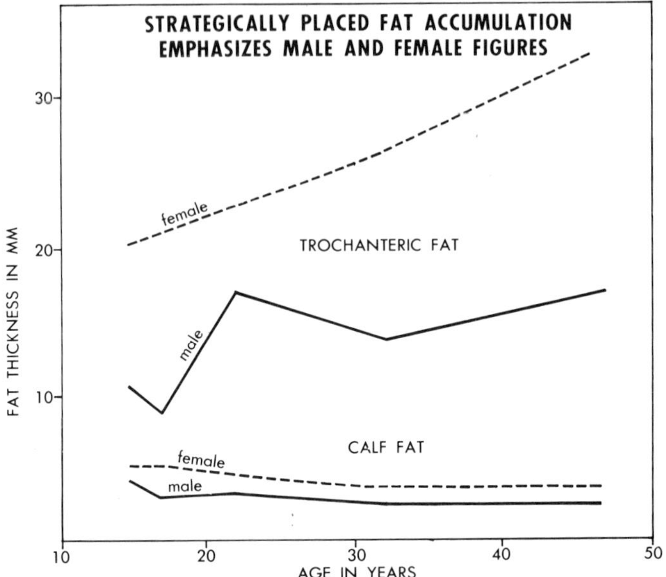

Fig. 21-3. Strategically placed fat accumulation emphasizes masculine and feminine figures. (*Drawn from data in Table 1, p. 499, Garn and Young, Concurrent Fat Loss and Fat Gain, Am. J. Phys. Anthropology, 14:497, 1956. Courtesy of the Wistar Institute of Anatomy and Biology, Philadelphia.*)

is due largely to increase in muscle mass and bone). The pubescent boy becomes tall and thin (Fig. 21-3).

In the female, accumulation of fat stores begins in prepuberty and is uninterrupted by sexual maturation. It is the accumulation of strategically placed subcutaneous fat that produces the feminine curves in girls, and adipose tissue accounts for an appreciable amount of the pubertal spurt in weight in girls (Fig. 21-4).

5. In the male, after full maturation fat loss comes to an end and fat accumulation begins. It continues slowly through the mature years. In the female after full maturation some girls slim down somewhat; others maintain about the same amount of adipose tissue they had before puberty. In the mature years women have a tendency to add slowly to their subcutaneous fat stores.

6. In both sexes fat stores are lost in those individuals who live beyond the seventh decade.

Individual Variations

While the above epochs describe the overall human life pattern of fat accumulation, there are enormous individual variations. Some people are thin, others fat, throughout life; some lose or gain fat at different ages.

Body constitution is the most significant factor correlated with fat deposition. During childhood the tempo of growth influences the amount of fat accumulated, although this is not independent of body constitution. Health, both physical and emotional, influences the consumption of food and its utilization. In addition, such things as culturally determined diets have a bearing on calorie consumption, and, finally, the amount of exercise determines what proportion of ingested food is used and what is stored as fat.

Fat accumulation varies greatly with body build. Reynolds compared the fat deposition of three boys who roughly fit into Sheldon's three classifications of ectomorphy, endomorphy, and mesomorphy. These boys were studied longitudinally, from 6 to 18 years of age. The ectomorph had considerably less fat than the endomorph, and the stocky mesomorph had fat stores between these two extremes. These differences were maintained throughout the period of the study. All three boys gained fat before puberty, lost fat during puberty, and began to add fat after full maturation, although the absolute amounts varied considerably.

Caloric intake has something to do with fat deposition, but it is certainly not the whole answer. On isocaloric diets the endomorph deposits more fat than the ectomorph. Doubtless there are hormonal or neural mechanisms involved about which little is known at the present time. Exercise is also a factor; in general endomorphs move more conservatively than ectomorphs and do not use as many calories for what appears to be the same amount of exertion. In addition endomorphs are inclined not to engage in as much physical activity as either mesomorphs or ectomorphs. It is also possible (though certainly not proved) that during embryonic life, when the original undifferentiated mesenchyme was developing into specific types of cells, more adipose cells were formed in the endomorph than the ectomorph.

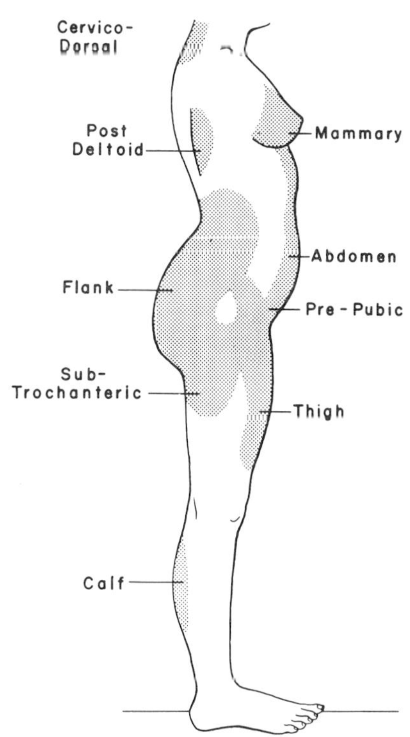

Fig. 21-4. Distribution of subcutaneous fat in girls. (*From Bayer, Weights and Menses in Adolescent Girls with Special Reference to Build, J. Pediat., 17:345, 1940, and The C. V. Mosby Company, St. Louis.*)

While experimental work has shown that ectomorphs and endomorphs utilize isocaloric diets differently, it is only under experimental conditions that the diets of individuals of these two body types are isocaloric. The endomorph, left to his own devices, eats more than the ectomorph. His appetite is bigger, he wants more food, he loves to eat. The endomorph is more viscerally oriented than the ectomorph. His gastrointestinal system occupies a larger part of his total body; his intestinal tract may be 20 ft longer than that of an ectomorph of the same height. His body is geared to alimentation. But why does he crave so much food that he has an excess to store as fatty tissue? This question at present is unanswered.

In both sexes early-maturing children are advanced in the rate at which they accumulate fat. Tempo of growth, however, is highly correlated with body build, so that the plumper appearance of the fast-maturing child is doubtless related to the nature of his physical constitution as well as the fact that he is getting where he is going at a faster rate.

Both physical and emotional health have an effect on fat deposition and are discussed elsewhere (p. 383).

BONE AND CARTILAGE

Bone is a special kind of connective tissue which ultimately becomes rigid by the deposition of mineral salts instead of elastic fibers. Most of the skeleton is outlined first in densely packed connective tissue; cartilage is then deposited in this connective tissue; finally the cartilage is destroyed and replaced by mineral salts, thus transforming the pliable cartilage into rigid bone. This is the phylogenetic pattern of bone formation, and it is repeated in the ontogenic development of the entire skeleton of man, with the exception of the bones of the face and the cranial vault.

Kinds of Bone

Phylogenetically bone evolved in the early amphibians whose small skulls were inadequate for the much bigger brains of higher forms. Though the organism had "learned" how to make bone via cartilage, when the larger cranium was needed, it was laid out in a tough membrane and directly ossified. Membranous bone formation seems a more efficient device for forming a bony structure, but only a small part of the skeleton is formed in this way. All the rest goes through the cumbersome process of being laid out in cartilage, then having the cartilage destroyed and replaced with bone (Stein, 1955).

Cartilage to Bone

When mature, cartilage and membranous bone are similar structures; they do, however, have different developmental patterns. Ossification of cartilage starts in embryonic life and continues until the end of puberty when the last epiphysis becomes rigidly attached to the shaft of its bone. At this time growth in height comes to an end. Unlike most other structures in the body, bone continues to form *new* material throughout the entire growing period. This is in marked contrast to such structures as the muscles, where the individual fibers are almost all formed before birth and growth is due to increase in size of the individual fibers, not increase in their number.

The timetable of ossification is discussed in Chap. 10.

MUSCLE MASS THROUGH THE LIFE SPAN

The number of striated muscle fibers is roughly the same in all human beings (Walls, 1960). The tremendous difference in size, not only from fetus to adult but between adults, is due to the ability of individual muscle fibers to increase in size. There is a growth potential inherent in the genes, influenced by hormones, by nutrition, by exercise, and possibly by other factors as well.

From about the fourth or fifth month of fetal life up to the beginning of puberty, the hormones that influence growth in size of the individual muscle fibers are the growth hormone from the anterior lobe of the pituitary, thyroxin, and insulin (Russell and Wilhelm, 1960). During this period of childhood the sex hormones play little part in the growth of muscle. As a result no appreciable difference in muscle mass is directly attributable to sex. Differences in muscle mass between children are more closely related to general body constitution than to sex. The lean, slender child has a smaller muscle mass than has the stocky, rounder child. These constitutional differences are carried through life.

At the onset of puberty in both sexes there is increase in growth hormone and in androgen from the adrenal. It is these hormones that are thought to stimulate the pubertal growth in size of muscle fibers in both sexes. In boys, muscle growth is further stimulated by testosterone. Since this hormone does not appear in the female, growth of muscle fiber (and other growth as well) proceeds further in boys than in girls (Tanner, 1955; Russell and Wilhelm, 1960) (Karpovich, 1959).

The increased size of muscle fibers in both sexes means that children increase in strength during these years. However, the increase in strength is greater in boys than in girls. Muscle size in boys precedes muscle strength (p. 157).

Muscle fibers achieve their maximum size and strength in early adult life, after which they decline slightly, but in general they remain in about the same state until the process of senescence begins to manifest itself (Rubinstein, 1960). Secondary changes in skeletal muscles occur as a result of wasting illness, nutritional deficiency, or disuse, but these are not primary evidence of muscle senility. Throughout life muscles are remarkably responsive to training. Muscle fibers increase in bulk, and therefore in strength, as they are used; conversely, they shrink when allowed to remain relatively unused (Hettinger, 1961) (Hines, 1961).

MECHANICS OF HUMAN POSTURE

Bones, joints, tendons, muscles are all involved in enabling the body to assume and maintain its many possible positions and in facilitating locomotion. The spinal column is the upright support. The load of the body which must be supported can be divided into several body regions: (1) the head, (2) the shoulders and arms, (3) the thorax, and (4) the pelvis.

All these body regions exert their pull forward of the spinal column. The large and heavy head is balanced on the cervical spine, but it pulls in a forward direction. The shoulders exert their pull vertically. The thorax is rigidly supported and attached to the spine; nevertheless, its pull is forward. The loosely attached viscera constitute a heavy load pulling forward from their nonrigid attachments. The spine, the pelvis, the legs, and feet must counteract the forward pull of the rest of the body and bring the center of gravity as near the supporting spine as possible. This is accomplished largely by muscles (Jones, 1955).

Optimal posture in the adult as usually described consists of the following:

1. A plumb line from the vertex falls through the ear, the acromial joint, the hip, the knee, to a point just forward of the ankle.
2. The feet and legs are straight, and the line of the heel cord perpendicular. The Achilles tendon is long enough to permit a 15° dorsiflexion of the foot.
3. The knees are straight, with no tendency to hyperextension.
4. The pelvis is tilted, about 30° from the horizontal.
5. The lumbar spine is slightly concave.
6. The thoracic spine is slightly convex backward.
7. The neck is inclined forward slightly beyond the perpendicular.
8. The spine has no lateral curvature.
9. The legs are of the same length.
10. The chest is moderately elevated.
11. The abdomen is flat.

With this posture the human body uses a minimum of muscular exertion. Deviations from optimal posture bring about related anatomic distortion, increased muscle tensions, and inequality in weight bearing. These structural strains lead to fatigue and pain (Lockhart, 1964).

The human prepares for the adult posture through all his period of growth (Sweet, 1938).

Fetal Posture

Flexion characterizes posture in utero. The fetus lies curled up in the narrow confines of the uterus, pushed on all sides by the elastic resistance of the uterus. Not only is his vertebral column flexed, but his large head is pulled forward on his chest, his extremities bent at shoulder and hip,

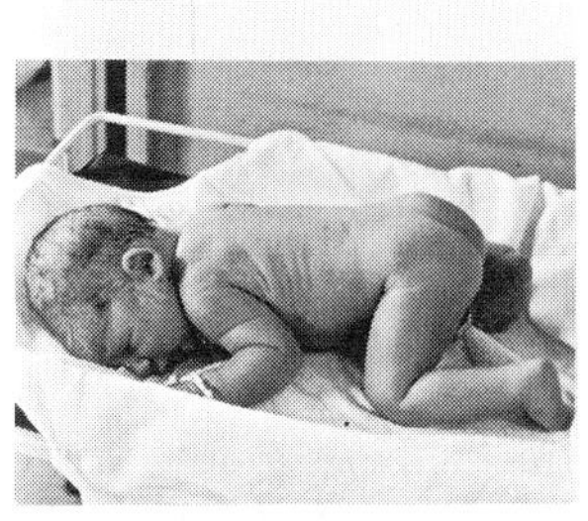
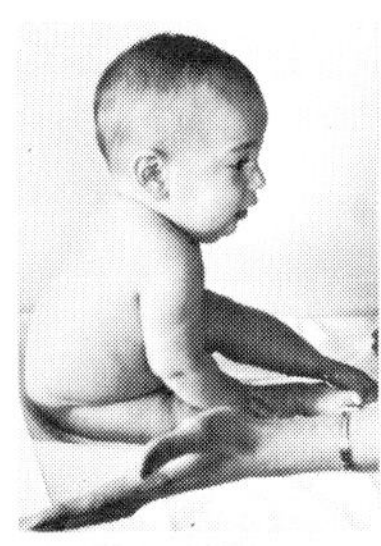
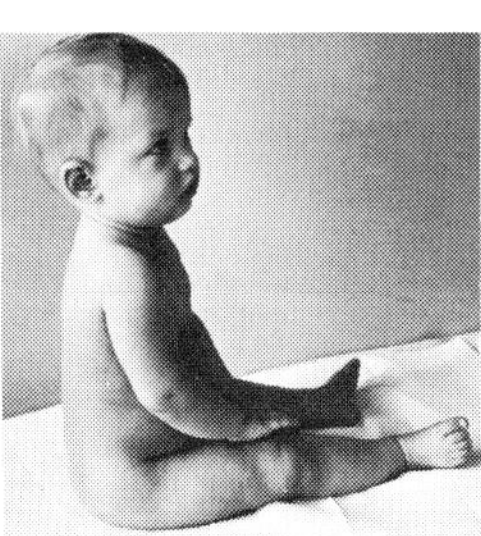
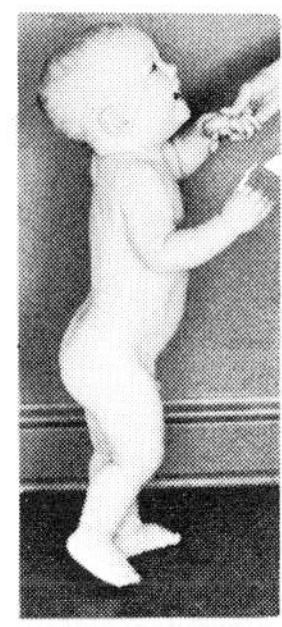

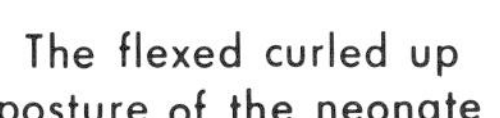

The flexed curled up posture of the neonate

A single curve from neck to buttocks

Straight back

Early erect posture

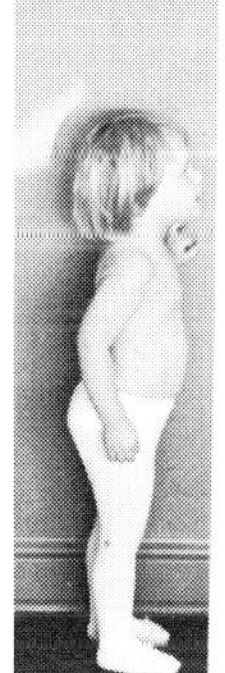
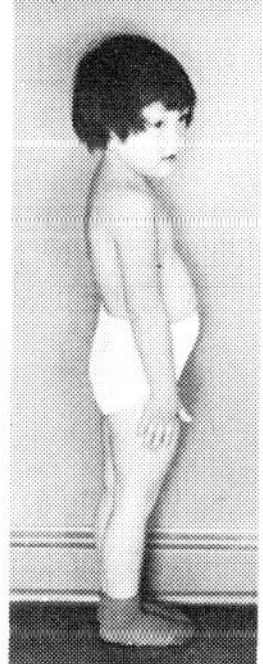
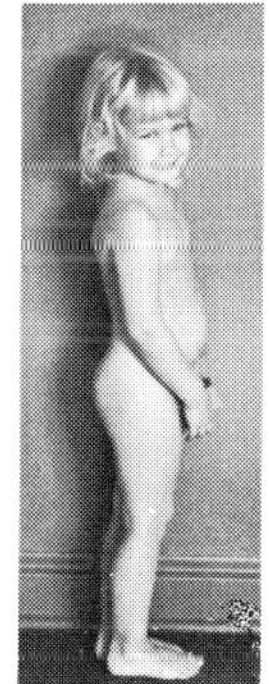
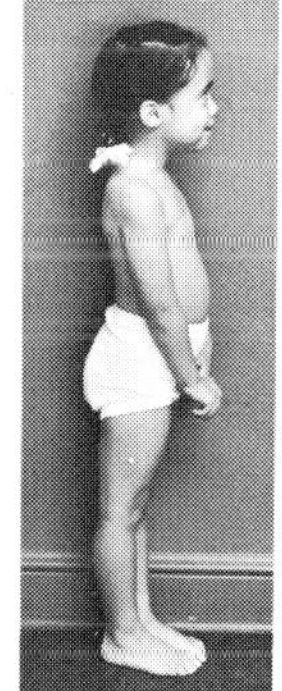
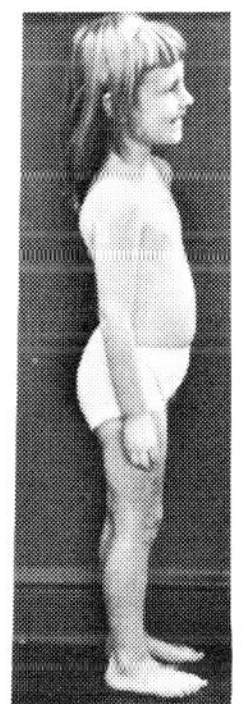

Toddler and preschool posture

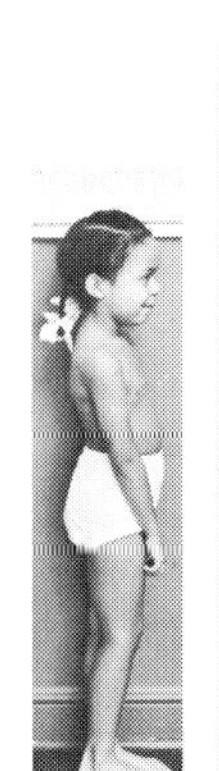
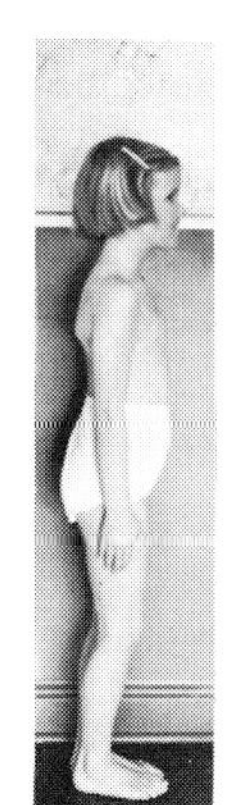
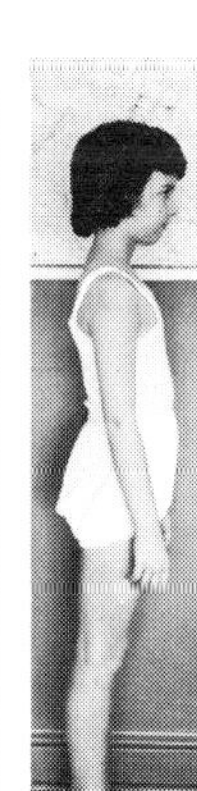
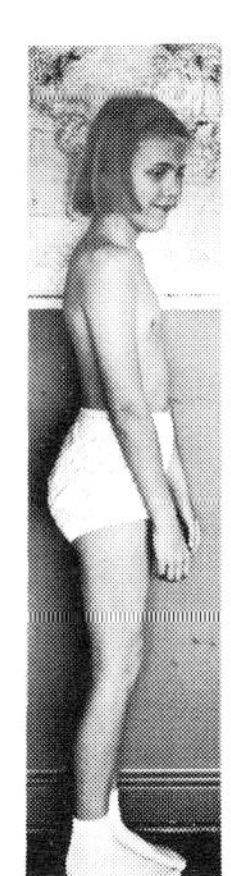
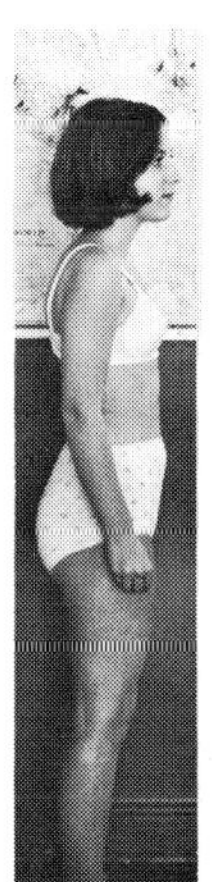
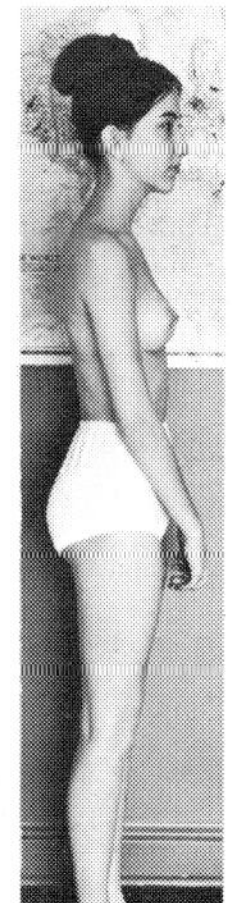
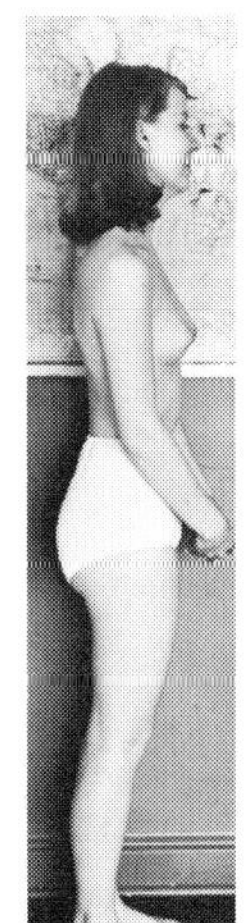
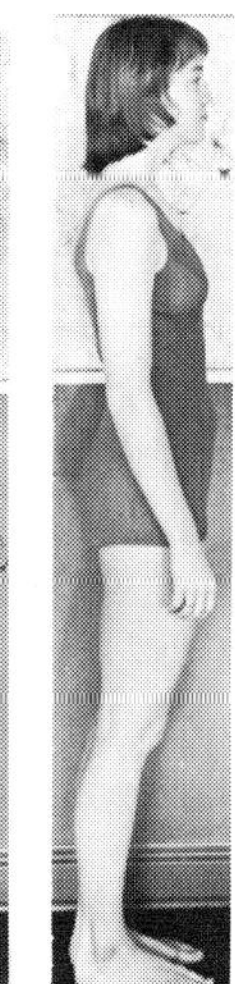

Posture from school age through puberty

Fig. 21-5. Posture changes with growth.

so that his whole body is in the shape of an ellipse. The pliability of his cartilagenous skeleton, the elastic quality of his tendons and connective tissue all contribute to the ease with which this posture is maintained in the aquatic environment of the uterus.

Neonatal Posture

Once released from the constant pressure of the uterus which pushed him into a ball-like shape, the newborn infant assumes a horizontal posture. Air is less buoyant than amniotic fluid; therefore the pull of gravity helps to straighten out the curled-up fetal position. The head and the back lie flat on the mattress of the crib; extremities remain flexed for some months, but they too become more extended as the months pass.

Much of the skeleton of the infant is still pliable and will take on the shape of constantly held positions. In early infancy the baby's position needs to be changed for him, so that undue molding of bone does not take place. This is especially true of the feet. An infant who lies always on his abdomen everts his feet and stretches the ligaments, holding the feet at right angles to the leg. This has a tendency to produce pronation when weight bearing is accomplished.

Infant Posture

As the infant is able to bring his striated muscles under control, he begins to compete with the pull of gravity. He pulls up his head, then his back, and soon achieves a sitting position. At first the back is held in a convex curve from head to hips with part of the weight supported on the arms. The arm support is soon abandoned, and the infant sits erect with a relatively straight spine. Soon he manages to pull himself to his feet and achieves his human heritage of erect posture.

Toddler Posture

As he first stands, the baby has a protuberant abdomen, a lumbar lordosis, and a relatively straight or slightly convex upper spine. He rotates his pelvis forward with the aid of his gluteus maximus and stands with feet apart and flat on the floor. Often the feet are mildly pronated.

The toddler will walk, run, jump, climb, pull, and push. He will use and develop every muscle fiber in his body. He needs a safe place and freedom. A few toys such as big blocks, a swing, a tricycle, boards, a jungle gym, are helpful, but little children will make use of any handy articles.

Preschool Posture

Loss of adipose tissue and development of a lithe body characterize the posture of the early years. The abdomen is somewhat flattened as abdominal muscles strengthen, although the little child has a more protuberant abdomen than he will have a few years hence. Lumbar lordosis is still marked, the upper spine is straight, and the head shows a slight lordotic curve but is not inclined forward. The chest is flat, the shoulders held well back of the chest. The feet often show a slight pronation; knees are fully extended, but hips show less extension than they will later.

The constant activity of little children is their best assurance of good posture. Like toddlers, their need is for space, freedom, and some equipment.

Posture in Early School Years

The adult posture is being approximated; slight lumbar curvature has become apparent, and the thoracic spine is convex backward. Looked at from the rear, the spine should be straight from neck to buttocks, with no lateral curvature. The chest is elevated, the abdomen still protrudes slightly. The knees are straight and held in full extension. The Achilles tendon should be perpendicular, the early tendency to pronation outgrown.

Posture in Puberty

The rapid growth of puberty brings increased muscular strength, and the full adult posture is assumed.

EXERCISE AND PHYSICAL FITNESS

If the little child is given ample opportunity for physical activity, good posture usually develops. Beginning in the school years and continuing on through adult life many children in the United States do not engage in enough vigorous activity to permit optimal development of their muscles. The child's muscles increase in length to take care of his growing height, but if they are not exercised, they remain slender and do not develop the power needed to hold the body in an efficient posture: the head sags, the shoulders fall forward, the abdomen protrudes.

Our culture does not demand much physical exertion; there is no wood to cut and bring in, no ashes to carry out; vacuum cleaners take the place of brooms; automobiles and buses make walking unnecessary. School takes up most of the child's day, and television all too frequently fills in the gaps.

Beginning during the school years and continuing through life, a conscious effort has to be made to ensure adequate physical exercise. During the growing years, muscles need exercise to develop; after growth has ceased, some exercise is still needed for maintenance of adequate muscular strength (Phelps, 1956).

Adequate exercise can be achieved in several ways. The least time-consuming is a regular daily period of calisthenics. The Kraus-Weber tests and exercises are adequate (Kraus and Hurschland, 1954). While this takes relatively little time, calisthenics are not much fun, and it is difficult to maintain a regular program. In some areas schools have instituted such programs as part of the day's activities.

A program more likely to be maintained is some active sport that is enjoyed. In cities this creates problems of space and equipment and often of money. Community programs for playgrounds, gymnasiums, swimming pools, tennis courts, ball fields, and the like are needed in greater abundance than now exists. During the school years most children enjoy sports and will learn skills if they have the opportunity. Athletic skills learned during childhood will serve the individual well throughout his life.

Every person—child and adult—needs a minimum muscular strength to maintain good posture easily. The amount of exercise needed over and above this depends upon the individual. Active sports are enjoyed by many people. Such people need sufficient strength to participate in this form of relaxation without fatigue.

But some people, again both child and adult, get more pleasure from quiet activities—they may enjoy a game of chess more than a game of tennis. Such people can maintain good health and have a good life with a much smaller muscle mass than the people who wish to hike 50 miles. There is no need to try to force everyone into the same mold.

BIBLIOGRAPHY

Bayer, Leona: Weights and Menses in Adolescent Girls with Special Reference to Build, *J. Pediat.*, **17**:345, 1940.

Garn, Stanley M.: Fat Patterning and Fat Intercorrelations in the Adult Male, *Human Biol.*, **26**:59, 1954.

———: Fat Thickness and Growth Progress During Infancy, *Human Biol.*, **28**: 232, 1956.

———, and Richard W. Young: Concurrent Fat Loss and Fat Gain, *Am. J. Phys. Anthropol.*, **14**:497, 1956.

Hettinger, Theodor: "Physiology of Strength," Charles C Thomas, Publisher, Springfield, Ill., 1961.

Hines, Marion: The Control of Muscular Activity by the Central Nervous System, in G. H. Bourne (ed.), "The Structure and Function of Muscle," vol. 2, Academic Press, Inc., New York, 1960, p. 467.

Jones, Laurence: "The Postural Complex," Charles C Thomas, Publisher, Springfield, Ill., 1955.

Karpovich, Peter V.: "Physiology of Muscular Activity," 5th ed., W. B. Saunders Company, Philadelphia, 1959.

Kraus, Hans, and Ruth P. Hurschland: Minimum Muscular Fitness Tests in School Children, *Res. Quart.*, **25**:178, 1954.

Lockhart, R. D.: The Anatomy of Muscles and Their Relation to Movement and Posture, in G. H. Bourne (ed.), "The Structure and the Function of Muscle," vol. 1, Academic Press, Inc., New York, 1960.

McKusick, Victor A.: "Heritable Diseases of Connective Tissue," 2d ed., C. V. Mosby Company, St. Louis, 1960.

Patten, Bradley M.: "Human Embryology," 2d ed., McGraw-Hill Book Company, New York, 1953.

Phelps, Winthrop M., Robert J. H. Kiphuth, and Charles W. Goff: "The Diagnosis and Treatment of Postural Defects," 2d ed., Charles C Thomas, Publisher, Springfield, Ill., 1956.

Reynolds, Earle L.: Sexual Maturation and the Growth of Fat, Muscle and Bone in Girls, *Child Development,* **17**:121, 1946.

———: The Distribution of Subcutaneous Fat in Childhood and Adolescence, Society for Research in Child Development Monograph, vol. 15, no. 50, 1950.

Rubinstein, J. L.: Aging Changes in Muscle, in G. H. Bourne (ed.), "The Structure and Function of Muscle," vol. 3, Academic Press, Inc., New York, 1960, p. 209.

Russell, Jane A., and Alfred E. Wilhelm: Endocrines and Muscle, in G. H. Bourne (ed.), "The Structure and Function of Muscle," vol. 2, Academic Press, Inc., New York, 1960, p. 142.

Stein, Irvin, Raymond O. Stein, and Martin L. Beller: "Living Bone in Health and Disease," J. B. Lippincott Company, Philadelphia, 1955.

Sweet, Clifford: The Teaching of Body Mechanics in Pediatric Practice, *J.A.M.A.*, **110**:419, 1938.

Tanner, J. M.: "Growth at Adolescence," Charles C Thomas, Publisher, Springfield, Ill., 1955.

Walls, E. W.: The Micro-anatomy of Muscles, in G. H. Bourne (ed.), "The Structure and Function of Muscles," vol. 1, Academic Press, Inc., New York, 1960, p. 21.

Wells, H. Gideon: Adipose Tissue, A Neglected Subject, *J.A.M.A.*, **114**:2177, 1940.

Wertheimer, E., and B. Shapiro: The Physiology of Adipose Tissue, *Physiol. Rev.*, **28**:451, 1948.

22

The Integumentary System

GENERAL STATEMENT

The skin and its appendages and adnexa (nails, hair, sebaceous glands, eccrine and apocrine sweat glands) constitute the integumentary system. In addition to the strictly integumentary elements of this organ, the skin contains vascular networks, sensory nerve endings, autonomic nerve fibers, muscles, and connective and adipose tissue.

Skin is a remarkably thin structure. In the infant, over most of the body it is only about 1 mm thick and only about 2 mm in the thickest spots—the palms and soles. In the adult the skin is only about twice as thick as in the infant. At birth, Leider has estimated, the entire skin of the body weighs roughly ½ lb; at maturity it increases to about 10 lb.

This thin, stretched-out organ is composed of three layers. The outermost layer, the epidermis, consists of stratified epithelium, and even though it is extremely narrow, it is divided into five distinct strata, though not all the layers can be detected in all parts of the body. The middle layer of the skin—the corium, or dermis—constitutes the bulk of the organ, being about twenty times greater in width than the epidermis. In the dermis are crowded masses of organized structures, blood vessels, nerves, hair follicles, glands, and muscles. The innermost layer, the subcutaneous fatty layer, is a band of fatty tissue of varying thickness which separates the skin from the underlying subcutaneous tissues.

While there is a similarity to all skin, this organ shows considerable variability. It varies in different parts of the body of the same individual; it varies from individual to individual; and it varies during the life span. Skin may be thick, thin, horny, taut, pliable, hairy, glabrous, moist, dry, rough, smooth, or light- or dark-colored. These variations account for some of the clinical manifestations of disorders of the skin. Many skin diseases have distinct regional distributions, others are related to specific age periods, and still others are more prevalent in some individuals (and some races) than others.

The integumentary system has many diverse functions. Physiologically its functions are (1) protection, (2) maintenance of homeostasis, (3) contact with the environment. Psychologically and emotionally its functions are (1) cosmetic, (2) expressive.

The epidermis is relatively impenetrable, from within and from without. It prevents the leaking out of body contents, and it protects internal structures, mechanically and immunologically, from environmental hazards. The pigment in the lower layers of the epidermis and the keratin in the superficial layers, protect against ultraviolet light. The texture of the epidermis is of cosmetic importance.

Sebaceous glands keep the skin moist by virtue of the ability of sebum to prevent evaporation of water from keratin. Their secretions may aid in bactericidal protection. Apocrine sweat glands contribute to body odors. In spite of the fear of "B.O." induced by mass media even civilized man is neither insensitive to, nor unresponsive to, body odors. The main function of the eccrine sweat glands is that of temperature regulation; in addition, these glands aid in maintaining electrolyte balance and are of some value in protection against infection. The vascular networks in the dermis aid in temperature regulation. The adipose tissue cushions and protects against

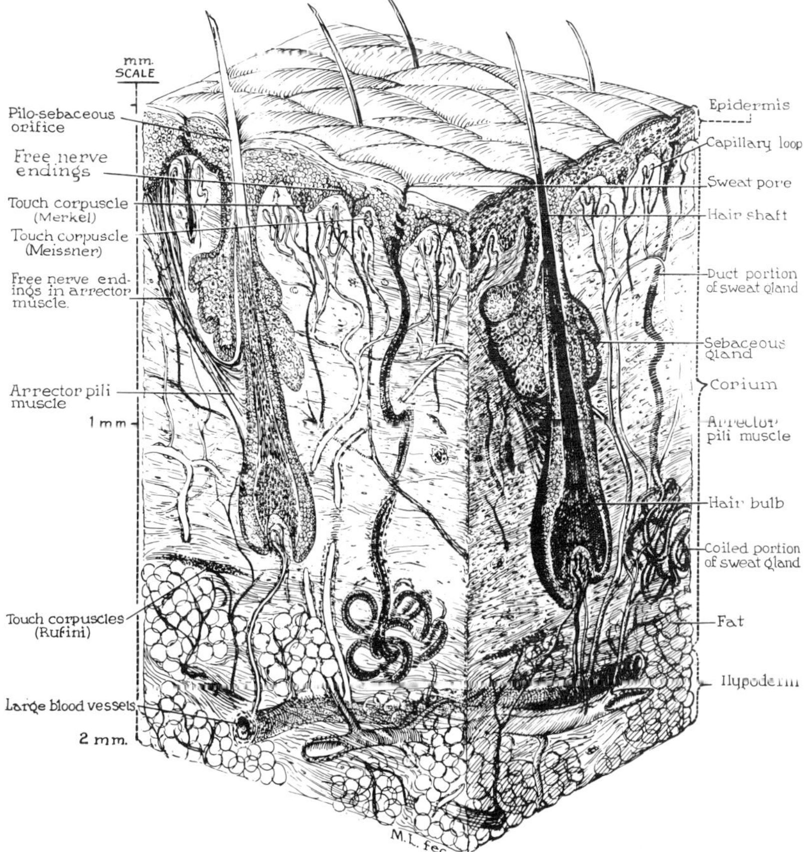

Fig. 22-1. Diagram of the skin. (*From Practical Pediatric Dermatology, 2d ed., by Morris Leider, The C. V. Mosby Company, St. Louis.*)

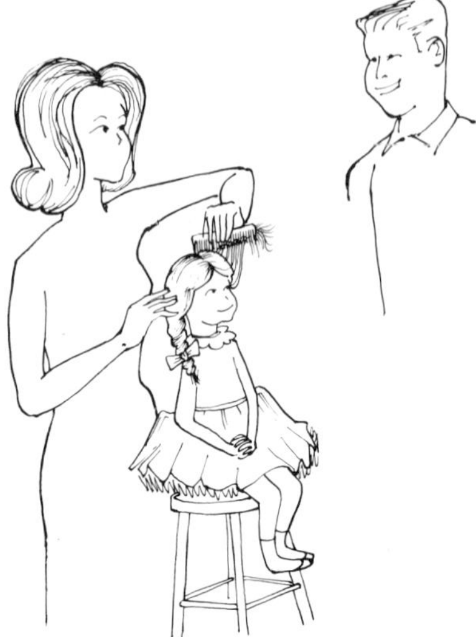

Fig. 22-2. The function of hair on the scalp is to beautify.

cold. Sensory nerve endings in the skin maintain the individual's contact with his environment.

In modern society the most important function of nails and hair in the human being is to beautify. Fingernails do aid in some fine movements of the fingers, especially in picking up small objects. They are also useful to scratch. Toenails, however, have no utilitarian function. Hair in eyelashes and eyebrows helps keep foreign matter from the eyes, but body hair is so sparse that it has almost no ability to protect as does fur in lower species. Hair is, however, very important cosmetically and contributes to, or detracts from, the individual's concept of his own adequacy. Hair on face and chest adds to an adolescent boy's feeling of manliness; hair on the face may destroy a girl's feeling of femininity.

The skin, as a whole, is the organ with which man faces the world. His self-confidence is tied up with how he looks. The enormous amount of money spent in beauty parlors and the time spent acquiring a suntan give evidence of the importance of the appearance of the skin to women. The huge number of cures for baldness is testimony that men are not unconcerned about their external appearance.

Many of the structures of the skin are under the control of the autonomic nervous system and the endocrines. The biologic purpose of these systems is to maintain homeostasis. But the skin, like other parts of the body, is responsive to emotional states. Involuntary mechanisms, mediated through the autonomic nervous system, make use of the skin as a target area for betraying emotions. Embarrassment causes blushing; anger, redness; anxiety, sweating; and fear, blanching or "goose bumps."

Striated muscle fibers in the dermis, especially of the face, as well as larger muscle bundles in and below the subcutaneous tissue, give rise to the variety of facial expressions.

The skin is an integral part of the entire body and, as such, is responsive to changes throughout the organism. At times the skin is a barometer of events taking place below its surface (e.g., the rashes of the exanthemas, jaundice, edema).

The skin is thus seen to be an organ that participates in, and contributes to, physical health and well-being. It is also an organ that plays a role in ego development, through sensory perception, emotional expression, and outward appearance.

DEVELOPMENT OF THE SKIN BEFORE BIRTH

The two main areas of the skin, the epidermis and the dermis, have different embryologic origins. The epidermis comes from the ectoderm; the connective tissue of the dermis, from the mesoderm. However, the skin appendages and adnexa, the nails, the hair follicles, the sebaceous and sweat glands, which lie deep within the dermis, all originate from the ectoderm by invaginations of the superficial epidermis (Montagna, 1962).

In the early differentiation of the embryo, the superficial ectoderm covers the entire body surface with a single layer of cuboidal epithelial cells. As the months pass, this epithelium thickens and arranges itself, first into two, then three, and finally five layers of the epidermis. The outer layer in the fetus is the periderm, a moderately hard covering which protects the fetus during embryonic life. This layer is shed just before birth (Patten, 1953). The innermost layer of the primitive skin remains soft and pliable and develops into the germinative layer, from which the epidermis continues to proliferate throughout life. By the end of gestation the five layers of the epidermis are recognizable.

Simultaneously with the development of the epidermis, a mass of fibroelastic connective tissue from the mesenchyme accumulates immediately below the stratified layers of the epidermis and comes to form the dermis. In the beginning the line between these two parts of the skin is a flat plane, but as development proceeds, the stratum germinatum of the epidermis develops a wavelike contour, and the dermis responds by pushing up into the hills and valleys of this layer, forming the dermal papillae. These irregularities make themselves obvious on the surface of the skin. It is to them that the intricate pattern of lines on fingers and toes is due. Fingerprint patterns are individualized by the sixth month of fetal life (Cummins and Middo, 1961).

Hair shafts arise from down growth of the epidermis during fetal life. Along the shaft of the hair further invaginations of ectodermal tissues form sebaceous glands. The combined hair and gland constitute the pilosebaceous apparatus. By the last month of fetal life, hair and sebaceous glands are widespread over the entire body except on the palms and soles. While the pilosebaceous apparatus continues to mature after birth, no new units are formed once the fetus has left the uterus. The early fetal hair is a thick, downy coat almost like a fine fur. This is the lanugo. It reaches its maximum development between the seventh and eighth fetal months. At this time the sebaceous glands are active. Their secretion contributes to the vernix caseosa.

In certain areas of the body, notably the axilla and around the genitals, the apocrine sweat glands differentiate from other buds on the hair sheath during the latter part of fetal life. The apocrine glands, once formed, lie dormant until puberty, when their development is completed.

A fourth type of invagination of the epidermis penetrates the dermis in the latter part of fetal life and forms the eccrine sweat glands. Unlike the sebaceous glands and apocrine sweat glands, the eccrine sweat glands are not anatomically connected with hair shafts.

The eccrine sweat glands are structurally mature by the seventh month of fetal life. After birth no additional glands are formed. Eccrine sweat glands are distributed over the entire body surface except the lips, glans clitoris, and inner surface of the prepuce; they are especially abundant in the palms of the hands and the soles of the feet.

Blood vessels from the developing vascular tree pass through the subcutaneous tissues and penetrate the dermis from below. An arteriole and a venule anastomose in a dermal loop, at which point a group of special cells within the capillaries forms the glomus body. This structure is capable of dilating or contracting in response to changes in environmental temperature or to emotional states.

Sensory nerves from the nuclei of the dorsal roots of the spinal cord wend their way from their central origin to the skin and terminate in a variety of sensory nerve end organs, which are located at all levels, in the epidermis, in the dermis, and in the subcutaneous tissues. Sensory nerves are especially abundant about the hair follicles (see The Tactile Senses, Chap. 23).

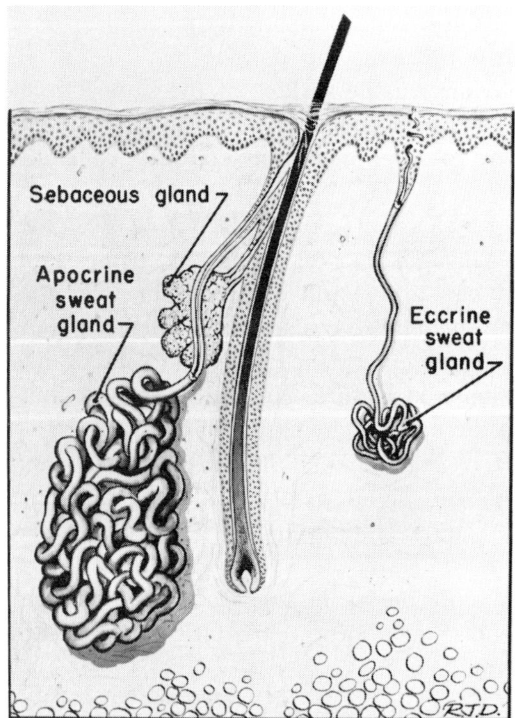

Fig. 22-3. Glandular appendages of the skin. (*From Manual of Cutaneous Medicine, by Donald M. Pillsbury, Walter A. Shelley, and Albert M. Kligman, W. B. Saunders Company, Philadelphia.*)

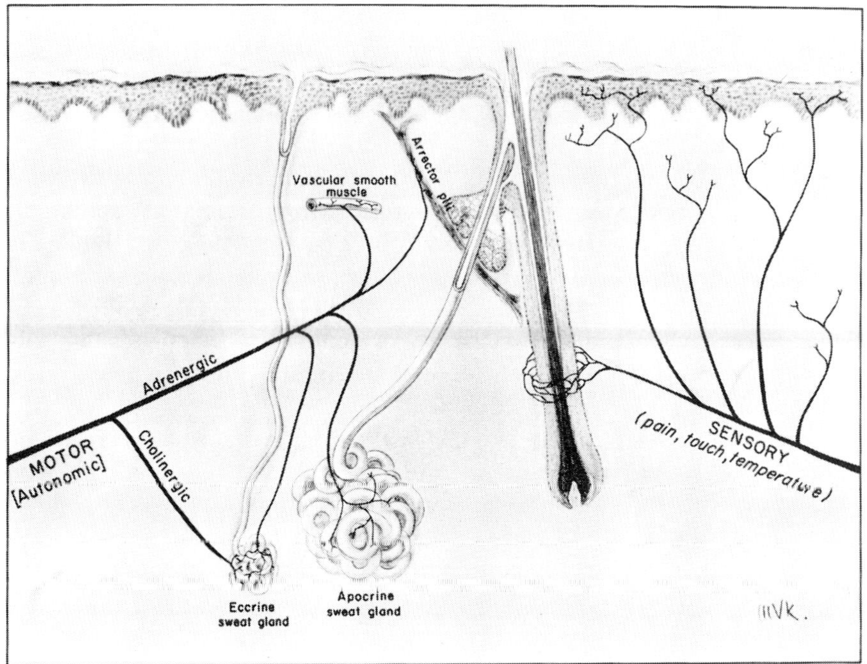

Fig. 22-4. Cutaneous innervation. (*From Manual of Cutaneous Medicine, by Donald M. Pillsbury, Walter A. Shelley, and Albert M. Kligman, W. B. Saunders Company, Philadelphia.*)

Motor nerves to the skin arise from the efferent sympathetic system. They contain both cholinergic and adrenergic fibers. Cholinergic fibers innervate the eccrine sweat glands; adrenergic fibers innervate the tiny muscles on the hair sheaths, the apocrine sweat glands, and the glomus bodies of the vascular system. The hair follicles and the sebaceous glands have no neural supply. All the efferent nerves to the skin carry stimulatory impulses (Pillsbury et al., 1961).

DEVELOPMENTAL CHANGES IN THE SKIN AFTER BIRTH

By the time of birth the skin contains all the various structures known to exist in adult skin; nevertheless the skin of the child, and especially that of the infant, is far from mature.

Immediately after birth the vernix caseosa covers the entire surface of the skin. This substance, composed of sebum and epidermal debris, possesses bactericidal properties. It wears off in a day or two, leaving the skin soft and velvety. The sebaceous glands, active in utero, gradually decrease their activity after birth. The lanugo begins to decrease before birth and continues its regression during the early weeks of life, to be replaced by body hair of a less extensive distribution.

At birth the skin is about 1 mm thick over most of the body surfaces. During all of childhood it increases in depth by not more than ¼ mm. The stratum corneum, the outmost layer of the epidermis, responsible for the major protective role of the skin, is no more than 0.01 mm in depth at birth (Montagna, 1962).

The epidermis is loosely bound to the dermis in early life. For this reason it will separate and form blisters as a result of inflammatory conditions, which in later life would produce only a localized edema or swelling. The epidermis contains relatively little pigment at birth. In dark-skinned races, pigment forms, under genetic influences, during early infancy. In light-skinned races, while pigment cells are present, they function sluggishly, if at all, even under ultraviolet stimulation. Infants sunburn much more readily than older children or adults.

Eccrine sweat secretion is skimpy in early life and has a relatively high pH. Apocrine sweat is absent in infancy.

The immaturity of the skin in early life makes infants and young children more prone than adults to rashes from physical, chemical, thermal, and bacterial agents. It also augments cutaneous manifestations of systemic conditions.

The skin matures slowly from infancy to puberty; at puberty there is a rapid spurt in maturation of the skin and all its many structures. Later in life senescent changes in the skin are among the most obvious signs of old age.

During puberty the growth and increased activity of the sebaceous glands makes this period of life one of vulnerability to acne.

The maturation of the skin will be discussed with reference to each of the various structures which participate in the developmental changes.

THE EPIDERMIS

The classic five layers of the epidermis can be thought of as essentially two functionally different units: (1) the outside horny cells, the stratum corneum, and (2) the living cells of the rest of the epidermis, the function of which is to build the stratum corneum.

The stratum corneum can be considered the excretion product of the living cells (Pillsbury et al., 1956). It consists of flat, dead, cornified cells devoid of nuclei, which have been pushed up from below by the living cells. The stratum corneum contains keratin and other by-products cast off by the living cells as these cells die and migrate outward. Lying between the dead and living cells is a transitional zone which is thought to contribute significantly to the impermeability of the skin.

In addition to cells which form keratin, the lower layers of the epidermis contain cells whose function it is to form pigment—melanin. Melanin is made exclusively by melanocytes. Pillsbury states that it is the activity of these cells, rather than their anatomic presence, that determines the degree of pigmentation. In albinism melanocytes are present, but they do not function. In dark-skinned races there are no more of these cells than in fair-skinned races; the cells are simply more active. The first step in melanin formation is the action of an enzyme, tyrosinase, on the amino acid tyrosine. Subsequent steps in the synthesis of melanin involve complicated mechanisms influenced by local and systemic conditions, by hormones, and also by the genetic makeup of the individual.

The primary function of the epidermis is that of being a barrier, a function it owes to its impermeability. It is this function which both prevents the body contents from leaking out and prevents noxious agents from the environment from entering the physiologic interior of the body.

This impermeability is not absolute at any time of life. It is, however, much greater in mature skin than in the thin immature skin of the infant and young child. The stratum corneum, with its high concentration of keratin and its coating of sebum and sweat, is the first defense against substances trying to enter the body from the outside. The transitional zone is the first defense against substances trying to leave the body. Each barrier reinforces the other.

In order to maintain homeostasis, fluid must be kept within the body. Small amounts of water do leave the body constantly by seeping directly through the skin (this is in addition to sweat). The lower layers of the epidermis in the adult are about 70 per cent water. The transitional zone prevents most of this water from entering the stratum corneum, which is only about 15 per cent water. Water in the stratum corneum evaporates, the amount depending upon environmental temperature and humidity. If the amount of water in the layer drops below 10 per cent, symptoms of chapping occur. In the young child the transitional zone is not as effective a barrier as it is in the adult, and more water seeps into the horny layer from the wet layers of the epidermis; hence more is available for evaporation. The loss of water by the transepidermal route is most marked in the premature infant. This is one reason the premature infant does best in an atmosphere of high humidity. In the full-term infant the mechanism is more mature; nevertheless, throughout infancy more water is lost by the transepidermal route than later in life. To some extent this water loss is compensated for by inactivity of the eccrine sweat glands during infancy.

The stratum corneum is the first line of defense against the penetration of agents from the outside. Neither water nor electrolytes enter the body through the skin in appreciable amounts. Some lipids and steroids can penetrate the skin. Vitamin D is synthesized on the surface of the skin by the action of sunlight on its precursor and absorbed directly into the body. Estrogen and testosterone can be absorbed from the surface of intact skin. It is thought that these substances penetrate the skin by gaining entrance through the follicular orifice to the sebaceous gland and thus bypass the barrier of the horny layer and the transitional zone. Many gases can penetrate the intact skin readily, and much remains to be learned about how small amounts of other materials penetrate. If the epidermis is sufficiently damaged, its vital resistance to the passage of noxious materials into the body may be seriously impaired.

Bacterial protection comes about through the action of the keratin, the sebum, and the eccrine sweat (Rothman, 1954). The outer surface of normal skin is acid; it has a pH between 4.5 and 6.5. The inner surface of the skin lying against the subcutaneous tissue has a pH between 7.25 and 7.35, like that of all the rest of the internal structure. The acidity of the skin may confer on it some of its bactericidal properties, since most pathogenic bacteria require a higher pH for their growth. However, the dryness of the skin surface and its physical intactness are much more important factors in fending off the bacteria growing on its surface. It is of interest to note that both stomach and vagina, which, like the skin, are part of the physiologic exterior of the body, are endowed with a low pH, which aids these organs in withstanding bacterial invasion.

The acidity of skin is brought about by the evaporation of sebum and eccrine sweat, both of which are in contact with keratin. Evaporation is essential for optimum lowering of skin pH. In those areas of the body where skin folds prevent ready access of air, sweat does not evaporate as readily as in the more exposed areas; hence such areas are more prone to infection—behind the ears, in the axilla, in the groin, between the toes. The diaper area in infants is under the increased stress of moisture from urine as well as the inhibition of evaporation by waterproof pants.

In early life, the secretion of sebum and eccrine sweat is skimpy; hence there is less to evaporate than later in life. As a result the pH of the skin drops as age advances (Rothman, 1954). These facts contribute to the greater susceptibility of the young child to skin infections.

The thinness of the stratum corneum, the meager secretion of sebum and eccrine sweat, the relatively high pH make the skin of the infant vulnerable to injury from chemical and thermal insults. Infants react with dermatitis to many substances that the more mature skin can withstand.

SEBACEOUS GLANDS

The sebaceous glands produce sebum. This is a complex mixture of free fatty acids, lipids, and sterols. Sebum contains the precursor of vitamin D, which, when exposed to sunlight, is transformed into vitamin D and then absorbed into the body.

Sebum is formed constantly, not intermittently as is the secretion of the sweat glands. It is not under control of the autonomic nervous system but is responsive to secretions from the endocrine glands. Androgens maintain a small constant supply of sebum; increased androgen secretion causes an increase in sebaceous gland activity. Estrogens diminish sebaceous gland activity, but only when extremely large doses are given.

Sebaceous glands are formed in connection with hair follicles as stated above. However, there is often an inverse ratio between the size of the gland and that of the hair. The distribution of the actively functioning sebaceous glands is independent of the conspicuous hair. Sebaceous glands are most abundant on the scalp, the face, and the genitals. They occur in fewer numbers on the trunk and sparsely on the extremities. They do not occur at all on the palms and soles. Sebum formation, therefore, has a regional distribution.

Sebum formation is influenced by environmental conditions. It is greater in hot, humid climates than in dry, cold ones. There is also a sex factor: men produce more sebum than women. This sex difference is more striking after puberty. There is relatively little difference attributable to sex in young children. There is also a genetic factor that influences sebum formation; some people produce appreciably more sebum than others under identical conditions.

In addition to these variants in sebum formation, there is a developmental cycle. Sebaceous glands are active in the last month of fetal life. After birth they slowly subside. The "cradle cap" of some infants is an indication of active sebum formation in these infants. In early infancy it is not infrequent for a few sebaceous glands on the face to become clogged, resulting in the appearance of tiny whitish raised areas, which usually disappear without treatment. As infancy advances, sebum formation continues to decrease. The skin of young children tends to be dry.

With the advent of the hormonal changes of puberty, the sebaceous glands increase in size and secrete additional amounts of sebum. This predisposes to the development of acne (see below). After puberty, sebum formation decreases, and skin maintains a "normal" degree of oiliness throughout the mature years. In the last decades of life sebaceous glands undergo some atrophy, the secretion diminishes, and the skin becomes drier than in the earlier years.

Acne

Some disturbance of the sebum is extraordinarily common during the years of puberty. About 75 per cent of all pubescent children have some acne. In the majority of those affected, the disturbance is mild and disappears without physical sequelae as puberty comes to an end. In a few the disease is severe and is accompanied by secondary infection and permanent scarring.

While never a life-threatening disease acne can cause serious personality disturbance, since it comes at a most vulnerable time of life, when the youngster is absorbed with his inward and outward characteristics (p. 577). The emotional sequelae of acne are not always in proportion to the severity of the physical condition.

The pathogenesis of acne is far from being completely understood. The local lesion of acne (the comedo) consists of an abnormal amount of sebum and keratin within the dilated sebaceous gland. This mass blocks and dilates the orifice of the gland. The peripheral part of the comedo becomes blackened by oxidative changes (not by dirt) and forms the blackhead. The comedo enlarges by pressure from sebum in the lower part of the gland which cannot escape through the clogged orifice. Pressure on the walls of the follicle may cause rupture of the follicle. The mass of the sebum and keratin then pours into the dermis, where it sets up an inflammatory reaction. Secondary infection may occur in the comedo, and subsequently the infection may spread to the dermis.

Acne appears simultaneously with puberty, and it is generally believed that androgen is instrumental in ushering in the disease. Early-maturing children show evidence of acne at a younger chronological age than do late-maturing children.

Pillsbury et al. (1956) list the following facts known about hormonal excitation in acne:

1. ACTH injection in susceptible individuals of any age may produce acne.
2. Administration of large doses of testosterone either to men or to women may produce acne.
3. Androgen-producing tumors of the adrenal gland or ovary may produce acne.
4. Eunuchs do not develop acne.

In general the disease begins at puberty. While acne develops in response to hormonal stimulation, it develops only in those individuals with sensitive target areas. The sensitivity of the sebaceous glands to the development of acne is probably a gene-directed phenomenon.

Individuals with acne do not produce greater amounts of testosterone than those without acne, nor, says Pillsbury, is there solid evidence of an imbalance in estrogen/androgen ratio.

Treatment of acne at the present time is, on the whole, unsatisfactory. Hormones play a role in its development, but since excessive amounts of, or an imbalance in, hormones cannot be implicated, the injection of large enough doses of hormones to affect the disease is likely to cause derangements in other endocrine functions.

The principal primary infection in acne is by *Corynebacterium*, which is found abundantly beneath the surface, around the base follicles and sebaceous glands. Any technique which reduces the likelihood of such infection is beneficial. Thorough washing twice daily with an antibacterial soap and water is logical. It must be pointed out that while cleanliness may reduce secondary infection in the comedo, there is no evidence that it has any effect upon the initial formation of the comedo or of the cysts beneath the surface.

It has long been believed that diet influences the course of acne. There are few controlled studies on this point. Custom states that chocolate, nuts (including peanut butter), and soft drinks have a bad effect. The elimination of these substances can do no harm. Attention to the requirements of good nutrition during the rapid growth of puberty is desirable for general health.

Local treatment of acne has some value in removing superficial comedos but has no effect on deep inflammatory nodules. Systemic treatment with antibiotics is at times effective in deep-seated acne. X-ray treatment for acne is no longer considered a safe procedure. Doses of x-ray sufficient to diminish the size of the sebaceous gland are also likely to cause permanent damage to other structures in the skin. Altogether the treatment of severe acne leaves much to be desired.

Since the emotional aspects of facial disfigurement may be profound in adolescent boys and girls, the psychiatric aspects of this disease must be ever-present in the mind of anyone treating acne and puberty. Superstitions about the cause of acne persist even in sophisticated society. One of the most pernicious of these old wives' tales is that acne is the result of masturbation. It is understandable that an adolescent might hesitate to mention this fear. Tactful questioning to ferret out and eliminate this unnecessary guilt may not alter the course of the physical disease, but it will certainly improve the youngster's emotional outlook.

HAIR

As the lanugo hair is shed soon after birth, new hair is formed from the existing hair follicles. Throughout life hair is shed and regenerated. Hair has different characteristics in different parts of the body. In the eyebrow and eyelashes, the hair which replaces the lanugo is heavy and gradually becomes heavier until adult thickness is reached (Savill and Warren, 1962).

Some infants are born with a heavy growth of hair on their heads; others have only a fine fuzz. Scalp hair is lost during the first half year, only to be replaced slowly by more permanent hair. Those infants whose initial hair is but a fine fuzz may appear almost bald for some months before the new hair grows. Scalp hair gradually thickens and often darkens in color as childhood advances. At puberty the thickening and darkening process is accentuated.

Body hair, though of less extensive distribution than the lanugo, remains fine throughout infancy in both sexes. It coarsens slightly during childhood.

At the time of puberty in both sexes, under the influence of the sex hormones, there is a spurt in hair growth. Hormones, however, act in curious ways on the growth of hair. Androgenic hormones stimulate hair growth in the axilla and in the public region of both sexes. They also stimulate hair growth on the face of boys in early puberty, but not in girls. Body hair does not increase at the beginning of the pubertal spurt as does axillary, pubic, and male facial hair. It is not until the late teens or early twenties that boys do acquire hair on the chest. In the female body hair does not participate in this late spurt. For the most part it remains the same downy coat that has existed throughout childhood (Montagna, 1958).

Two syndromes relative to hair growth deserve special consideration. One is hirsutism in the female; the other, baldness in the male. Both may begin to make their appearance in affected individuals in the early post-pubertal years. The younger the individual when the first symptoms appear, the greater is the probability that the condition will be severe. Either condition can cause great emotional distress.

Hirsutism is seldom a true pathologic condition; rather, it is a physiologic variation of a normal process, doubtless with a genetic basis. In the vast majority of cases, hirsutism is due to normal androgens acting on sensitive target areas. Hirsutism, without evidence of other hormonal imbalances, is almost never due to disorders of endocrine function. For this reason, treatment of hirsutism with hormones is usually contraindicated.

Local treatment of the hair follicles is also unsatisfactory. In times past x-ray therapy has been used, but doses of x-ray sufficient to destroy hair follicles is no longer considered a safe procedure. Electrolysis destroys hair follicles. This procedure is practicable if the hairs are sparse, but it is not always successful if the growth is moderately heavy.

Depilatories or shaving are the only remaining methods. There are many good depilatories on the market, although their long-continued use results in skin irritation in some individuals. Shaving is probably the safest method, but most young girls will need considerable emotional support to accept this method without damage to their feminine image of themselves. They also need to be disabused of the old superstition that shaving stimulates growth and coarseness of hair.

Like hirsutism in the female, baldness in the male is a gene-determined condition. It develops only under the influence of androgenic hormones. The hormone which stimulates the growth of hair at puberty is the same hormone that stimulates the falling out of scalp hair after puberty in those individuals with a gene-determined sensitive target area.

In males carrying this gene, hair is normal during childhood, but scalp hair begins to thin in the early adult years. Castrated males with this gene do not become bald, but neither do they develop "manly" hair. Administration of testosterone to eunuchs stimulates male hair growth, but it also produces baldness if the gene for this condition is present. There is no known treatment for familial baldness. The bald young man may wear a wig, but he may need emotional support to accept himself as an adequate person.

ECCRINE SWEAT GLANDS

Montagna estimates that there are about 2 million sweat glands in the human body, averaging about 130 per sq cm. They are most numerous on the palms of the hands and soles of the feet, where they may reach a density of over 400 per sq cm.

These glands are present by the time of birth, but they function sparingly during infancy. Gradually, as childhood advances, more sweat is produced, but it is not until puberty that eccrine sweat glands exercise their full potential. Sulzberger and Hermann mapped the sweating areas and found that there was considerable uniformity in the areas of sweating from individual to individual, although the amount of sweat produced by the same stimulus was variable. Before puberty the individual differences in amount of sweat were not related to sex; after puberty men sweat more than women, although again individual differences are great.

Structurally, the sweat glands appear similar in all areas of the body, and the sweat produced has a similar composition in all areas. However, sweat glands in various parts of the body respond differently to different stimuli. In some areas, sweat is most responsive to heat; in other areas, sensory and psychic factors are the major cause of stimulation.

In response to heat, sweating is under control of the temperature center in the hypothalamus. Sweat appears within moments of an appropriate environmental temperature, first on the forehead, neck, dorsal, and ventral aspects of the trunk; later, if the heat stimulus continues, sweat appears on the back of the hands, the cheeks, the sides of the trunk, the extremities, and the axilla. Only under extreme thermal stimulation does sweat appear on the palms and soles. Sweat glands do not store sweat, but they come into activity rapidly when stimulated.

Sweating in response to psychic stimulation occurs first on the palms and soles and then in the axilla. Sulzberger suggests an atavistic explanation for the dampening of the hands and feet in response to emotion. He suggests that the mechanism facilitates the adherence of the animal to any grasped object in times of terror. Emotional sweating in the human serves

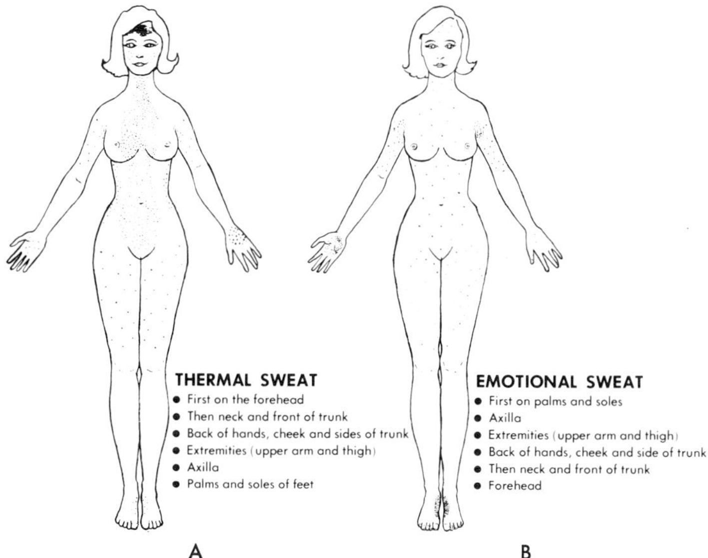

Fig. 22-5. Distribution of eccrine sweat (*A*) from thermal stimulation and (*B*) from emotional stimulation.

no useful purpose. It is of interest to note that it may have a phylogenetic background, unlike many other emotional autonomic reactions, which seem only to plague man. Under extreme conditions sweat may be poured out in enormous quantities.

Eccrine sweat is an aqueous solution 0.5 to 1.0 per cent of which is solids, half of which are inorganic salts and half organic substances (Montagna). Most of the inorganic material is sodium chloride, and about half of the organic material is urea. Sweat does not contain amino acids, glucose, or fat.

The composition of sweat depends to some extent on the composition of blood plasma. Sweat is not, however, a simple filtrate from plasma; it is the result of active secretion of the sweat glands. Lactate, urea, and ammonia are secreted in higher concentration than that which exists in blood plasma. Chloride in sweat shows considerable variation. Some people, when going to a hot climate, may lose significant amounts of sodium chloride in their suddenly increased volume of sweat. Within a few days the sweat glands adjust, possibly by the aid of NaK hormone from the adrenal cortex (p. 223), and reduce the amount of chloride in the sweat. This is doubtless a factor in acclimatization to a hot climate.

In cystic fibrosis of the pancreas the eccrine sweat glands are involved in the basic disorder and secrete large amounts of chloride. High chloride level in sweat is considered diagnostic of the disease.

APOCRINE SWEAT GLANDS

These glands have a limited distribution in man. They occur in the axilla, around the genitalia and anal areas, in the external auditory canal, around the umbilicus, and, in the female, around the aureola of the nipple. A few develop on the face. The mammary gland is morphologically an apocrine gland (Hurley and Shelley, 1960).

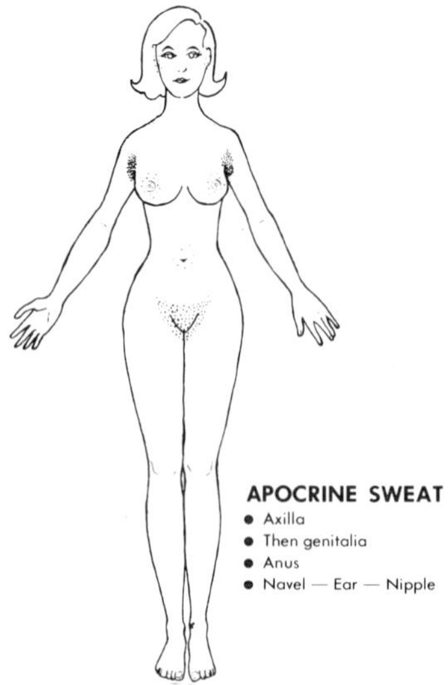

Fig. 22-6. Distribution of apocrine sweat.

These glands are formed in embryonic life in connection with hair follicles, but they do not mature until the pubertal growth spurt, at which time they increase in size and begin to secrete.

Unlike eccrine glands, once the apocrine glands mature, they form their secretion continuously and store it in the gland lumen. It is poured onto the skin in response to emotional stress (fear and anger, especially). Apocrine sweat is not responsive to temperature changes.

Apocrine sweat is a milkish white fluid, sterile and odorless as it comes from the gland. It contains fats which, when acted upon by bacteria, produce characteristic odors.

THE DERMIS

The dermis is considered part of the skin and anatomically composes by far the greater bulk of the organ; nevertheless the dermis is really part of the connective tissue matrix of the body. It protects and supports the many structures of the skin. It supplies the matrix through which blood vessels, nerves, and lymphocytes reach the skin structures. In the infant the dermis is thin and delicate and contains an abundance of elastin. As maturation takes place, the dermis thickens, and the proportion of collagen fibers increases. In old age the dermis becomes thinner than in the mature years and its elasticity decreases. These changes contribute to the development of wrinkles.

The primary unit of the epidermis is keratin; that of the sebaceous glands, lipid; that of the eccrine glands, water. Together they protect and maintain homeostasis. The primary unit of the dermis is the fibrocyte which supports and protects other units. The primary unit of the subcutaneous tissue is the adipose cell, which cushions and protects the entire body. Hair and nails have their primary function cosmetically—a function participated in by the entire epidermis.

BIBLIOGRAPHY

CUMMINS, HAROLD, and CHARLES MIDDO: "Finger Prints, Palms, and Soles," Dover Publications, Inc., New York, 1961.

HURLEY, HARRY J., and WALTER B. SHELLEY: "The Human Apocrine Sweat Glands in Health and Disease," Charles C Thomas, Publisher, Springfield, Ill., 1960.

LEIDER, MORRIS: "Practical Pediatric Dermatology," 2d ed., The C. V. Mosby Company, St. Louis, 1961.

MONTAGNA, WILLIAM: Cutaneous Innervation, in "Advances in the Biology of the Skin," vol. I, Pergamon Press, New York, 1960.

———: "The Structure and Function of the Skin," 2d ed., Academic Press, Inc., New York, 1962

———, and RICHARD A. ELLIS: "The Biology of Hair Growth," Academic Press, Inc., New York, 1958.

PILLSBURY, DONALD M., WALTER A. SHELLEY, and ALBERT M. KLIGMAN: "A Manual of Cutaneous Medicine," W. B. Saunders Company, Philadelphia, 1961.

———, ———, and ———: "Dermatology," W. B. Saunders Company, Philadelphia, 1956.

ROTHMAN, STEPHEN: "Physiology and Biochemistry of the Skin," The University of Chicago Press, Chicago, 1954.

Savill, Agnes, and Clara Warren: "The Hair and Scalp," 5th ed., Edward Arnold (Publishers), Ltd., London, 1962.

Sulzberger, Marion B., and Franz Hermann: "The Clinical Significance of Disturbances in the Delivery of Sweat," Charles C Thomas, Publisher, Springfield, Ill., 1954.

23

Organs of Special Sense

MAN'S SENSORY EQUIPMENT

It is generally stated that man possesses five senses: three proximity senses—touch, taste, and smell—and two distance senses—sight and hearing. All except the tactile senses are located in circumscribed areas of the body. Man tastes with the taste buds in his mouth, smells with the olfactory epithelium in his nose, sees with the retina of his eyes, hears with the auditory apparatus in his ears. But man *feels* over his entire body. The experience man obtains by feeling with his hands, however, is markedly different from the experience of feeling with the rest of his body. It is perhaps possible to say that the hand is the organ of feeling in the characteristically human way.

Taste, smell, sight, hearing, and tactation in the hand provide knowledge of the external world. All sensation coming from the outside is classed as exteroceptive.

The tactile senses, however, provide in addition information about internal as well as external events. There are sense receptors in muscles, joints, tendons, on the periosteum, and on the fascia around muscles. These receptors keep the organism alert to changes in position. They are classed as proprioceptive. In addition to the proprioceptive tactile receptors, the semicircular canals in the nonauditory labyrinth of the inner ear provide information about the body's movement in space and, together with the receptors in muscles and joints, are the means of maintaining body equilibrium.

In addition to tactile sensation classified as exteroceptive and proprioceptive, there are pain receptors in the viscera which alert the organism to undesirable events taking place in internal structure.

Man has sensations other than those mediated through sense receptors. He experiences hunger, satiety, thirst, sex desire, the urge to urinate or to defecate. These sensations—the interoceptive ones—are produced directly through the metabolic machinery of the viscera involved.

Unlike other parts of the nervous system, man's sensory equipment does not represent the pinnacle of evolutionary achievement. Dogs can smell more acutely than man, hawks have more acute vision than man, and bats and dolphins can detect sounds inaudible to the human ear (Smythe, 1961). However, with man's cerebral cortex, his ego, and his sense organs, his ability to perceive his world has transcended that of lower species. In this chapter the sense organs will be discussed. The nature of sensation is discussed in Chap. 34.

THE TACTILE SENSES

The Exteroceptive Tactile Senses

The feeling senses are of many kinds. In the skin, three systems of sensitivity are generally recognized: one for pressure reception, one for pain, and one which responds to temperature changes. Whether or not all kinds of cutaneous sensitivity can be squeezed into these three categories is debatable.

Nerve Endings

The nerve endings in the skin and mucous membranes which transmit sensation vary from the simplest of free nerve terminations to highly complicated tactile corpuscles. Some histologists believe that a continuum exists between the simplest and most complicated of these nerve endings; considerable anatomic evidence has been found to support this view. Some nerve endings, with tiny knoblike terminations, seem to represent the first degree of elaboration; others with flattened plates at the end of the nerve fibers are slightly more elaborate; then come the endings sufficiently complicated to be termed *corpuscles.* These vary, too, from the simplest encapsulated endings to elaborate structures. A catalogue of all the variety of tactile nerve endings in the skin has not as yet been completed, nor has it as yet been possible to correlate the infinite variety of sensation with the anatomic nature of the nerve termination. The distribution of the various kinds of sensory receptors gives some clue concerning their specific function.

It is believed that the simplest free nerve terminations transmit pain sensation, that the more complicated encapsulated endings are specific for various sensations. The Pacinian corpuscles are believed to transmit deep pressure sense; Meissner's corpuscles, which are abundant in the fingertips, are thought to transmit touch; Krause's end bulbs, cold; and the deeper-lying Ruffini's cylinders, warmth. A specific sensory receptor, the genital corpuscle, found only in the external genitalia, is thought to transmit the special sensations emanating from these organs. However, with a few exceptions, all types of sensory receptors are found in all areas, although the concentration of certain receptors is greater in some areas than in others.

Nerve Tracts of Sensory Stimulation

Impulses originating in sensory receptors are transmitted along primary sensory neurons to the central nervous system. Ropes of many of these neurons constitute the sensory nerves which carry neurons transmitting all the modalities of sensory impulses. The sensory nerves terminate in the primary cell bodies located in the dorsal root ganglia where each neuron synapses with the secondary sensory neurons, the axon of which enters the cord through the dorsal root. Once in the central nervous system, a regrouping of nerve tracks takes place whereby sensations of a particular kind are sorted out, regardless of the point of origin in the periphery. The axons of the secondary sensory neurons, after entering the cord, ascend for three or four segments, then cross the anterior commissure of the cord to find their places in one of the spinothalamic tracts, which one depending upon the nature of the sensory impulse being carried. Pain impulses are carried in the lateral, pressure in the posterior, and temperature in the anterior spinothalamic tracts. All these tracts ascend the cord and end in the thalamus, from whence the third sensory neuron conveys the impulses to the postcentral gyrus in the parietal lobe of the cortex. In this area of the cortex (the sensory cortex) sensory impulses are again sorted out into a neat geography of the periphery. This arrangement makes accurate localization of specific sensations possible.

Pressure

Felt sensation varies with the intensity of the stimulus and the extent of the area stimulated. It varies, too, with the duration of the stimulus, whether it is brief, long-continuing, or intermittent. It is possible that these variations in stimuli are responsible for all the variations in felt sensation; it is also possible, as indicated above, that different nerve endings pick up different stimuli (Nafe, 1941).

Tickle, itch and prick, are classified as pressure sensation (Geldard 1953). From the "feel" of an object (sensations transmitted through variations in pressure) it is possible to tell whether the object is soft, hard, rough, smooth, wet, dry, oily. While it is possible to obtain some recognition of the qualities of external objects from contact with them at any place on the body, it is man's hand which is the organ, par excellence, for appreciating the tactile attributes of the world about him. Man "handles" to understand (world-centered sensation). Pressure reception on the rest of the body primarily carries feeling tones of pleasure or displeasure (egocentric sensation—p. 505). Pressure reception is responsible for such divergent sensations as recognition of the shape of an object transmitted by handling it (world-centered sensation), and the sensation of pleasure from a back-rub (egocentric sensation).

Pain

Whether cutaneous pain is an independent sense transmitted by specific nerve endings, or whether it is an overstimulation of other cutaneous nerve endings, has long been in doubt (Goldschleder). Weddell's experimental evidence points toward the existence of independent cutaneous pain receptors.

Cutaneous pain is felt all over the skin, on the tongue, and in the mucous membranes of the mouth and nose. The stimulus for cutaneous pain can be mechanical, chemical, thermal, or electrical. It is only when the stimulus is sufficiently strong to produce tissue destruction that pain is felt. Pain from the skin is readily localized, due probably to the many overlapping sensory neurons in the skin as well as the sorting out of these impulses in the sensory cortex. Pain from cutaneous areas is sharp and results in reflex withdrawal. If the stimulus is brief, the sensation is reported as pricking pain; if it is long continued, it is reported as burning pain.

While pain can emanate from the viscera, these organs are amazingly free from pain. It has been learned through surgical procedures that abdominal viscera may be handled, cut, torn, cauterized, without any sensation of pain. Pain in the viscera is produced by inflammation of the mucosa (ulcers) by stretching or distention of a hollow viscus (passage of a gallstone or a kidney stone, accumulation of gas in the gastrointestinal tract), by spasms of smooth muscle, or by traction on the mesentery attached to the organ. The pain from the viscera is recognized as a "deep pain." It is experienced as dull or aching. It is poorly localized, due at least in part to the paucity of pain receptors in the deep structures compared with the abundance of these receptors on the skin. If deep pain is extreme, it is accompanied by slowing of the pulse, fall in blood pressure, sweating, nausea and finally, shock. Visceral accompaniments of pain can occur also with severe superficial cutaneous pain.

Muscles (smooth, striated or cardiac) are sensitive to eschemia. This local anemia is the cause of the pain of angina pectoris, and myocardial infarction and probably of much of the pain of parturition. It may be the cause of the pain of colic in the early months of life.

The Development of the Tactile Sense Organs Prior to Birth

The cells destined to form sensory tactile receptors develop from neuroblasts in the dorsal root ganglia.

From these ganglia, neurons grow out their delicate axons which slowly and unerringly wend their way out to the periphery of the organism where they terminate in one of the many varieties of sensory nerve end organs.

The free nerves are the first to make their appearance in the embryo and can be found toward the end of the third month of fetal life. These endings push in between the cells of the surface epithelium and in the nearby connective tissues. At first they are single nerve strands but by the 5th month of fetal life, these endings have become richly branched terminations, histologically mature.

The more complicated sensory receptors develop a little later in the embryo than the free nerve terminations.

TACTILE SENSATION AFTER BIRTH

At birth the neonate's *peripheral* sensory receptors are mature, and he is capable of receiving sensations of pressure, pain, and temperature from his entire body surface, from his mouth, and from his external genitalia. He is also equipped with mature pain receptors in his viscera as well as proprioceptive receptors in muscles, joints, tendons.

The cerebral components of tactile sensation are immature at birth. The neonate can receive sensation. Some sensations are the stimulus for the characteristic neuromuscular reflexes of the newborn, such as the rooting reflex (p. 306). The newborn is unable to localize sensation accurately, nor is he able to respond to it specifically (except in reflex action). He responds globally to tactile sensation.

TASTE

Taste is a chemical sense mediated by certain soluble substances which come in contact with the special sense receptors, the taste buds, located on the epithelium of the tongue and the posterior pharynx. Four kinds of taste buds are recognized both anatomically and functionally, one for each of the basic tastes: sweet, bitter, sour, and salt. When smell is eliminated, all gustatory sensations are combinations of these basic tastes (Fig. 23-1).

The taste apparatus makes its appearance in the human in the second month of fetal life. In the epithelium of the tongue small specialized masses of cells congregate along the papillae and make connection with the sensory neurons growing out from the sensory ganglia situated near the brain (Fox, 1932).

Neurons carrying the sensation of taste lie in 5th, 7th, 9th and 10th cranial nerves. From the primary sensory ganglia secondary sensory neurons converge to a nucleus in the thalamus and from there the tertiary neurons pass to the gustatory center of the cortex located in the postcentral gyrus of the parietal lobes (at considerable distance from the olfactory center—see below).

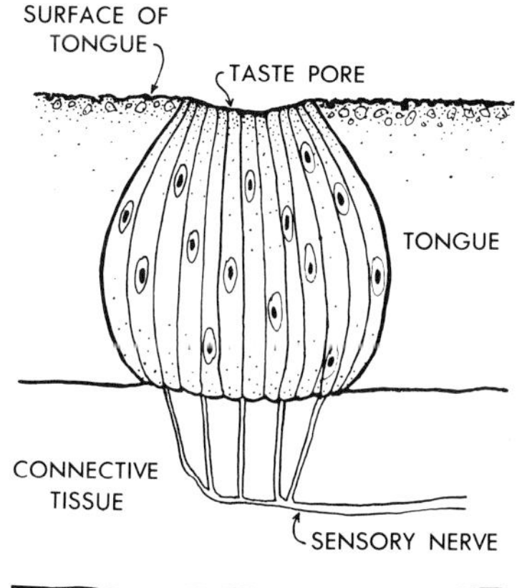

Fig. 23-1. Taste bud.

At birth the peripheral gustatory apparatus is mature; cortical pathways are incompletely myelinized. The neonate comes into the world fully equipped to taste what gets into his mouth. He lacks association

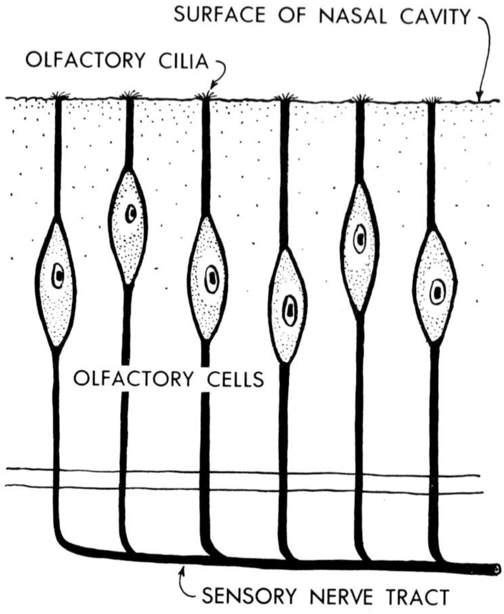

Fig. 23-2. Organ of smell.

pathways and is unable to bring motor activity into operation in response to his taste sensations. However, the neonate is quite capable of distinguishing the four basic tastes (Stirnimann, 1940)—and of reacting to them with pleasure or nonpleasure. Most infants will accept substance having a sweet taste, suck on such objects, and exhibit pleasure through general relaxation; infants refuse to suck on bitter substances (quinine solution) and respond with a global reaction of nonpleasure—crying and thrashing of extremities.

The infant and young child may be better equipped to taste than adults. There is some evidence that from birth onward there is a gradual diminution in the number of functionally adequate taste buds. The taste buds for the sweet taste are more abundant in early life and slowly decrease in number as adulthood is reached. This physiologic fact may have some bearing on the universal fondness of the young for sweets (Arey, 1935; Börnstein, 1940).

As maturity advances, the child sharpens his ability to react to gustatory sensation. It is not that he tastes any more acutely, but he is more able to do something specific about his feelings. When presented with an unpleasant taste, the neonate cries and thrashes his extremities. The 9-month-old child spits out food that has a taste he doesn't like. The toddler refuses to taste something which he does not like the look of—but this has to do with a different series of sensory reactions. Since taste is related to the pleasant and the unpleasant, taste preferences are apt to be related to taste experiences in early life associated with pleasant events (Cohen, 1949).

SMELL

Like taste, smell is a chemical sense mediated by certain soluble substances that impinge upon a tiny area in the nose in which lie the specific sensory receptors capable of reacting in such a way that an odor is perceived (Fig. 23-2).

Smell is called a proximity sense because the exciting stimulus must physically reach the receptor organ; however, since odoriferous substances are airborne, the sense of smell does transmit knowledge about objects at some distance from the individual.

Smell and taste are often confused subjectively. The confusion is due only to the close proximity, in the periphery, of the receiving organs, and to the fact that soluble substances capable of stimulating one set of receptors are often capable of stimulating the other. Food is often smelled before it is tasted and then smelled simultaneously with tasting. The actual receptors for these two sensations are completely separate, as are also the sensory nerve pathways and the cerebral areas of the brain which record the felt sensations.

Smelling apparatus appeared in evolution when animals first emerged from aquatic life and began to live on the land. Smell is highly developed in those animal forms which live close to the ground and depend upon odors to find food and detect danger. The receptors which pick up the tiny particles given off by odorous substances are large in animals like the dog. In addition, the part of the brain that records and remembers smells is likewise large and highly developed in such animals.

In primates, who took to the trees, smell became less needed for survival —there was less to smell high up in the trees than down on the ground. The olfactory receptors shrank in the primates, and the brain area occupied in lower forms by the smelling apparatus was displaced by the developing forebrain.

Development of Organs of Smell

The phylogenetic development of smell is repeated in the human fetus. In early embryonic life, scroll-like conchae develop along the walls of the nasal cavity. Five conchae appear during the early months, but only three remain in the mature nose: the inferior, median, and superior. Olfactory receptors appear only in a small area on the roof of the superior concha. They extend 8 to 10 mm and come to lie on the nasal septum and on the walls of the superior concha. The olfactory receptors are simple structures with cell bodies that lie within the nasal mucosa. Tiny bristle-like filaments from these cells project to the outside of the mucosa. At the proximal end of the cell body, filaments extend through the cribriform plate to synapse in the olfactory bulb; from this bulb the olfactory tract leads to the olfactory area in the brain.

The human infant is born with fully mature receptors for smelling. There is some evidence that the acuity of the sense of smell continues its fetal regression and that infants smell more odors and smell them more strongly than older children and adults do (Turk, 1954).

Later in life when association pathways from the smelling brain to the motor cortex mature, the child seeks the pleasant odors and tries to avoid unpleasant ones. However, what is pleasant or unpleasant is, to a very large extent, determined by what the child associates with odors. Hardly any infant in any culture reacts adversely to the odor of fecal material, but he learns that his adults find the odor disagreeable, and sometime in late toddlerhood most children have accepted the almost universal cultural belief that stool has an unpleasant smell.

Farmers who since childhood have associated barnyard smells with the normal activities of life accept them without aversion, while the city dweller is repelled by the odor of manure and yet accepts placidly the smell of automobile exhaust, which creates disgust in his country cousin.

HEARING

Sound waves enter the external ear and are conducted through the middle ear to the inner ear, where they impinge on the organ of Corti (the actual receptor organ). Here the sound waves are transformed into nerve impulses and conveyed along neural pathways to the auditory cortex of the brain. The ability to hear and interpret sound is dependent upon an intact mechanism from external ear to cortex (Fig. 23-3).

Development of the Auditory Apparatus

The ear develops in the embryo in three distinct parts, representing the divisions of the mature ear. The parts develop separately, and all fall into place in the last trimester of pregnancy. The middle ear is originally full

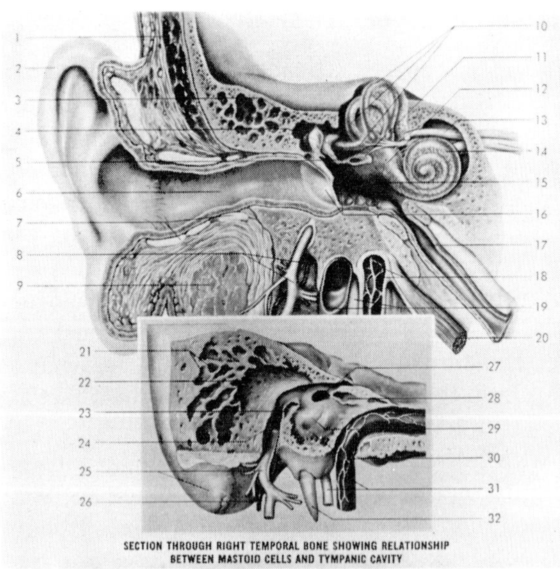

Fig. 23-3. The ear. (*Courtesy of Lederle Laboratories, A Division of American Cyanamid Company.*)

Temporal muscle
Helix
Epitympanic recess
Malleus
Incus
External acoustic meatus
Cartilaginous part of external acoustic meatus
Facial nerve and stylomastoid artery
Parotid gland
Semicircular canals
Stapes
Vestibule and vestibular nerve

13 Facial nerve
14 Cochlea and cochlear nerve
15 Cochlear (round) window
16 Tympanic membrane and tympanic cavity
17 Auditory (Eustachian) tube
18 Internal carotid artery and sympathetic nerve plexus
19 Glossopharyngeal nerve and internal jugular vein
20 Levator veli palatini muscle
21 Mastoid cells
22 Tympanic antrum

23 Cavity of the pyramidal eminence for the stapedius
24 Facial canal
25 Facial nerve and mastoid process
26 Stylomastoid artery
27 Vestibular (oval) window
28 Cochleariform process
29 Promontory
30 Cochlear fenestra
31 Internal carotid artery and glossopharyngeal nerve
32 Styloid process

of embryonal connective tissue in which the ossicles form in cartilage. These tiny bones ossify, and the connective tissue resorbs, leaving the ossicles suspended in the free air of the middle ear. This resorption is not quite complete until a month or so after birth; nevertheless, the ossicles are capable of transmitting sound waves before the middle ear is entirely free of connective tissue. The cortical auditory pathways, while all laid out at the end of gestation, are not myelinated beyond the midbrain by the time of birth.

Hearing After Birth

Normal infants hear almost immediately after birth. They respond to sounds at a subcortical level. A loud noise induces crying; soft sounds, relaxation. The neonate's reaction to sound, as to other sensory stimuli, is global.

By 2 months of age, an infant begins to bring voluntary muscular action into control and will turn his head toward a sound. As total maturity advances, the child learns to make finer auditory discrimination. He learns to bounce to a rhythm, develops auditory memory, and will stop crying as he hears his mother's footsteps. He listens to sounds, brings his vocal apparatus under control, and imitates what he hears. Ultimately he comprehends the symbolic meaning of speech and learns to talk (Chapter 32).

The hearing mechanism in the ear needs no further maturation after birth (except for the final resorption of the connective tissue in the middle ear). However, "hearing behavior," the ability to listen, to respond with discrimination to sound, to imitate what is heard, and to integrate sounds into symbolic meaning, matures only as total personality proceeds. Myklebust believes that full maturity of total auditory function does not take place until approximately 7 years of age.

Auditory Impairment

Normal auditory function depends upon a chain of structures from the outer ear to the auditory cortex. Deafness, partial or complete, results when there is malfunction in the cochlea or distal to it. *Aphasia* is the term used for malfunction of the cerebral components. *Autism* refers to failure to talk even though the auditory mechanism (as far as can be determined) is intact.

In the following discussion, the anatomy and physiology of interference with auditory mechanisms will be considered. The relation between deafness and ego development is discussed on p. 517.

The External Ear

Very occasionally the auditory canal is a site of congenital maldevelopment. The auditory canal may be missing or severely restricted in diameter.

If the middle and inner ear are normal, adequate hearing can be obtained if the surgeon can open up the occluded canal or even construct a new canal. However, congenital abnormality of the auditory canal is often accompanied by anomaly of the middle ear and sometimes of the inner ear as well, in which case, opening the auditory canal has little or no effect on ability to hear.

After birth, the auditory canal may become so impacted with cerumen that transmission of sound waves to the tympanic membrane is impaired. Removal of the plug of wax is the only treatment needed.

The Middle Ear

Faulty formation of the ossicles in the embryo may result in inadequate conduction of sound waves through this chamber.

After birth infections in the middle ear are a frequent sequela of upper respiratory infection. Such infections may erode the delicate ossicles, and when the acute condition subsides, scar tissue replaces active bone.

Normal conduction through the middle ear is dependent upon an equal pressure in this chamber and in the external auditory canal. Blockage of the pharyngeal end of the eustachian tube by an overgrowth of lymphoid tissue interferes with equalization of pressure. Adenoidectomy may open the proximal end of the eustachian tube and restore normal hearing. Adenoidectomy, however, does not always remove all the lymphoid tissue blocking the tube, since this tissue occasionally grows into the lumen of the eustachian tube, where it cannot be reached surgically. Nevertheless, adenoidectomy does benefit a sizable proportion of children whose hearing loss is associated with overgrowth of lymphoid tissue in the pharynx.

The ossicles are subject to otosclerosis, which may interfere with the free movement of these tiny bones and thus with conduction through the middle ear. Impairment of hearing due to otosclerosis appears to be a gene-directed phenomenon. It seldom becomes manifest in childhood; its usual time of appearance is early adult life, and it is frequently a progressive disease. Occasionally the bony changes may extend to the inner ear and cause destruction in the organ of Corti.

Malfunction of the middle ear, regardless of its cause, prevents airborne sound waves from reaching the sensory receptor organ. If the neural mechanisms are in working order, conduction deafness may be compensated for by the use of hearing aids, the function of which is to bypass the defective conduction apparatus.

The Inner Ear

The cochlea and its connections with the eighth nerve are subject to developmental aberrations prior to birth. Such failure may be due to faulty genes or to untoward events during the first trimester of pregnancy when these structures are forming (notably viral infections in the mother, especially German measles). Failure of development may be so extensive that total deafness results, or it may be less severe, so that the child's hearing is impaired rather than completely absent. Deafness due to defective genes may be present at birth, or it may make its appearance in childhood or later in life.

In the later decades of life, loss of hearing due to inner ear degeneration is common. There is some presumptive evidence that this failure may be at least partly genetic, since it seems more frequent in some families than in others.

The cochlea is well protected anatomically, lying deep in the temporal bone. Injury by trauma is rare. Injury from infections occurs occasionally. It is thought that damage to the cochlea from disease is brought about more by the toxic effect of the pathogenic organisms than the scarring resulting from tissue destruction, such as takes place within the middle ear. Meningitis and encephalitis are especially prone to affect the inner ear. Measles, mumps, whooping cough, diphtheria, and possibly other diseases occasionally cause cochlea damage. These diseases or their sequelae can also cause middle ear damage.

Regardless of its cause, malfunction of the inner ear impairs the ability to receive auditory sensations. If the organ of Corti is completely destroyed, hearing aids are of no value. This is seldom the case; if some cells remain functional, hearing aids may have a limited usefulness.

The Cerebral Components of Hearing

Damage or defect in the central nervous system components of hearing produce aphasia, which is essentially a disorder of language, not of hearing. Aphasia is of two major types: (1) receptive, or sensory, aphasia and (2) expressive, or motor, aphasia. The pathologic features of the two conditions are doubtless distinct, but present techniques have been unable to distinguish them anatomically. In sensory aphasia, the individual is unable to interpret sound and therefore unable to understand speech or to learn to talk. He may have a normal end organ for hearing, but his behavior is such that he is often considered deaf. In motor aphasia the individual hears and understands the speech of others but is unable to speak (Myklebust, 1960; Monsees, 1959).

Tests for Auditory Impairment

The objective in testing a patient suspected of hearing loss is to determine (1) the amount of loss, especially the amount of loss in the speech range, and (2) the location of the disorder in the auditory mechanism.

In a child too young to have developed speech, failure of normal progression in prespeech behavior is suggestive, though by no means diagnostic, of hearing loss (p. 470). A child with a moderate hearing loss may confine his prespeech sounds to those in the low pitch range. The area of the cochlea responsive to low-pitched sounds is less likely to be damaged than the areas responsive to high-pitched sounds. He may learn a few simple words as soon as the child with normal hearing; however, as soon as speech requires a significant number of high-pitched tones, the partially deaf child begins to show his inadequacy by distorted speech.

In a child who has developed normal speech, the first obvious sign of hearing loss is his failure to respond to ordinary verbal remarks. A young child who has become hard of hearing may demonstrate his handicap not so much by obvious signs of a hearing loss as by behavior problems of many kinds. Watch tick tests, conversation tests, and tests with a tuning fork are qualitative guides to hearing impairment. They may be used to screen individuals whose hearing should be further tested (Newby, 1958). Pure tone audiometer testing is the method used most frequently for testing individuals old enough to cooperate. In addition, instruments have been devised within recent years in which speech, rather than tones of known frequency, are used. These instruments have the advantage of testing directly the functionally useful hearing (Hirsh, 1952).

Occasionally it is necessary to test the hearing acuity of a child too young to cooperate in an audiometer test. It is also necessary from time to time to determine whether or not a child who has never learned to talk can actually hear. Bordley and Hardy devised a test using skin resistance. Essentially their test, known as PGSR (photogalvanic skin resistance), consists in introducing a reasonably loud tone of high frequency into the subject's ear by means of an earphone; 4 or 5 sec later an electric shock is administered, and the amount of sweating produced is measured on a galvanometer. Repetition of this series of events conditions the subject so that he responds to the tone by sweating without the administration of the electric shock. After he is conditioned, the loudness of the tone is reduced until the threshold is reached. Subsequently the frequency of the tone can be changed and the ability to hear in the entire speech range determined. The sound stimulus can be administered so as to test air conduction or bone conduction.

In addition to PGSR, tests using ectodermal (EDR) or electroencephalic responses (EER) have been introduced in recent years (Guilford and Haug, 1952). These tests indicate the subject's ability to respond to auditory stimuli, but they cannot be equated with ability to *hear.* In EDR, PGSR, and EER tests active participation of the subject is not required, and he is not asked to give any overt voluntary response to the test tones, as he is in audiometer testing. These objective tests measure the sensitivity of the individual to the test tone, that is, the adequacy of the end organ of hearing, but not his ability to recognize or respond meaningfully to sounds. It is not surprising, therefore, that results of the objective and subjective tests are not always in agreement.

An infant who fails to respond to normal environmental sound (whose behavior is that of a deaf child) and who is found to have decreased objective response is probably deaf (or hard of hearing, depending on the degree of impairment). As such a child matures and is able to cooperate, he will probably also show decreased auditory acuity on standard audiometer testing. The disorder is probably in the external, middle, or inner ear.

Another infant who also behaves like a deaf child may be discovered to have normal objective response to sound; such a child is then suspected of having a disorder in the central nervous system, of suffering from sensory aphasia rather than end organ deafness (Hardy, 1956).

The problem of distinguishing the child with end organ deafness from the child with central nervous system aphasia is unfortunately more complicated than this. Some children who do not learn to talk can apparently *hear* and *understand* speech. They get normal scores on objective tests, and if old enough they can get normal scores on subjective audiometer tests (provided they are not requested to give verbal cues as answers to whether or not they hear the tone of the audiometer), and yet they cannot talk. If such children are educated as deaf children, it is found that they do not respond. They fail to learn to lip read; they fail to learn to talk.

Not many years ago it was assumed that some "deaf" children were unable to learn to lip read because they lacked the special talent required for the skill. It seems probable now that such children may have been suffering from aphasia, either alone or in combination with end organ deafness.

Distinction between these various kinds of auditory impairment is of utmost importance in planning a remedial program for the child. The child whose difficulty is in the end organ of hearing—the deaf child—can usually be benefited by a hearing aid. However, even in the extreme cases of deafness, such a child can be taught to understand symbols, to lip read, and ultimately to speak and to write. The aphasic child presents a greater problem. In some cases of central auditory defect, loudness does seem to be a factor, and hearing aids are of benefit. In others, the defect is a central language disorder, and the increased volume of the sound does not help. Such children need very special training aimed at helping them comprehend symbols and ultimately express these symbols meaningfully in speech (Monsees, 1959).

Distinction between the various kinds of disorders in the entire auditory apparatus is often difficult to make. Not infrequently several types of conditions coexist in the same child.

Interpreting the Audiogram

Sound waves are produced by vibrating objects. The frequency of the vibration is recorded subjectively by man as pitch; the more cycles per unit of time, the higher the pitch, and, conversely, the fewer the cycles, the lower the pitch. The human ear is capable of responding to frequencies as low as 20 cycles and as high as 20,000 (Myklebust, 1956). Speech, however, does not make use of frequencies in either extreme of the range. A

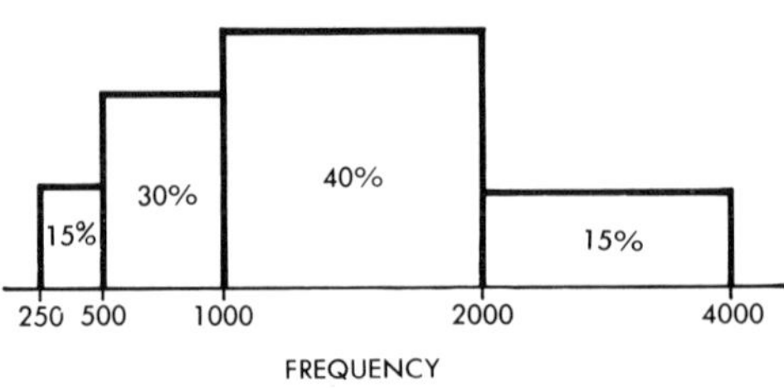

Fig. 23-4. Percent of speech tones by frequency. *(Drawn from data in Psychology of Deafness, by Helmar Myklebust, Grune & Stratton, Inc., New York.)*

median range between 250 and 2,000 cycles is about the outside limit of human speech, and the great majority of speech sounds fall within the narrower range of 500 to 2,000 cycles. Myklebust quotes the following figures of the relative importance of various frequencies within the speech range: approximately 15 per cent of the speech sounds fall between 250 and 500 cycles; 30 per cent, between 500 and 1,000 cycles; 40 per cent, between 1,000 and 2,000 cycles; and 15 per cent, between 2,000 and 4,000 cycles (Fig. 23-4).

Intensity of sound varies with the amplitude of the sound waves. It is a measure of the amount of energy expended in the vibrations. The human ear records intensity as loudness. Intensity and loudness, however, are not synonymous. Intensity is a physical absolute, but loudness is a subjective human quality and varies with the frequency of the sound. A tone in the middle frequency range is heard as louder than a tone in either the low or high frequency ranges, even though all sounds have the same degree of physical intensity. The human capacity to respond to the physical quality of intensity is greatest in the middle range of frequencies—the speech range.

Sound has a quality besides frequency and pitch, and besides intensity and loudness: timbre. Physically this quality is measured by the overtones in the frequencies. It is timbre that provides much of the quality of the individual human voice. Even though pitch and loudness are the same, the voice of one person can be distinguished by its timbre from that of another. It is timbre that contributes much of *phatic* vocal communication (p. 451).

The measurement of hearing involves pitch and loudness. Except in very special tests timbre is not measured. The aim of hearing tests is to determine how well an individual hears sounds of varying pitch and especially those sounds in the speech range. In hearing tests pitch is equated with frequency, and sounds produced in the audiometer are measured in physical units of frequency.

Loudness creates more problems in measurement. The physical intensity of a sound can be measured in energy units. However, it is not energy units but audibility that is of interest in testing hearing. The unit devised for this purpose is the decibel. One decibel (for practical purposes) is the amount of energy required to make a sound of any frequency audible.

The actual amount of physical energy involved in increasing the loudness of a sound rises in a logarithmic progression; a sound of 10 db requires 10 times (10^1) the energy of 1 db, but a sound of 100 db requires 10 billion times (10^{10}) the physical energy of a 1-db sound (Fig. 23-5).

On the decibel scale ordinary conversation has an intensity between 50 and 65 decibels. Sounds are felt as loud at a decibel strength of 80. At 100 db, sound becomes painful to the normal person.

The audiogram records the just audible loudness of a sound. The audiogram of an individual with normal hearing therefore shows a value of 1 db at each sound frequency tested. An audiogram showing a 10-db loss in one frequency means that sound must be increased by 10 db to be just audible. A person with hearing loss of between 30 and 70 db in the speech range is usually classified as one who is hard of hearing. Such an individual will have difficulty in hearing ordinary conversation and will benefit by the use of a hearing aid. Hearing loss of 90 or more db is usually classified as deafness.

In addition to determining the amount of hearing loss in specific frequencies, the audiometer is an aid in locating the site of the pathologic condition in the hearing mechanism. If the audiogram shows normal hearing by air conduction, no further testing is needed, but if a hearing loss is found, a further test of hearing by bone conduction is called for. If bone conduction hearing is normal, it can be assumed that the lesion is in the middle ear; if bone conduction hearing is impaired, it is in the inner ear.

VISION

Human vision is dependent upon a highly complex aggregation of structures—muscular, optical, sensory, and neural. Optical organs focus light rays on the retina, the light receptor tissue. From the retina, neural pathways extend to the visual cortex, where the sensations are received and transmitted to other areas of the cortex for interpretation. The complex and delicate eye is surrounded by protective and supportive structures (Fig. 23-6).

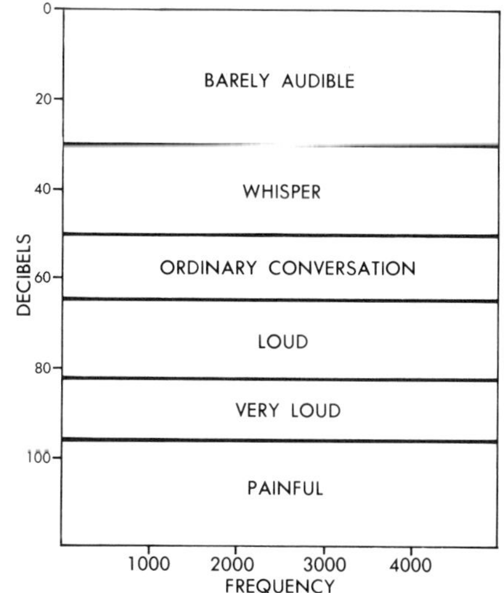

Fig. 23-5. Audibility of speech sounds by decibel strength. (*From Psychology of Deafness, by Helmar Myklebust, Grune & Stratton, Inc., New York.*)

The Visual Apparatus Before Birth

Developmentally, the eye is different from all the other organs of special sense. The retina, which contains the sensory cells, is part of the wall of the brain, pushed out early in embryonic life to form, first, a vesicle, and, later, the optic cup, the lining of which becomes the pars optica of the retina (Davson, 1962).

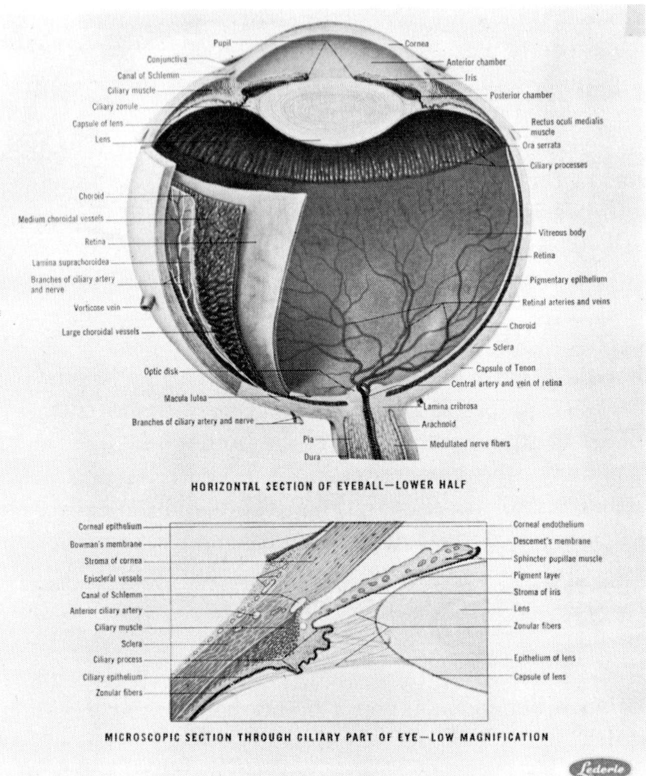

Fig. 23-6. Diagram of the eye. (*Courtesy of Lederle Laboratories, A Division of American Cyanamid Company.*)

In the embryo, the eye begins to form very early. By the third week, depressions in the still open neural plate foreshadow the formation of the optic cup, and soon thereafter the lens begins to make its appearance. Surrounding the optic cup, mesenchymal cells form a coat which differentiates into two layers, foreshadowing the choroid and the sclera. The retina arranges itself into characteristic layers, but only rod cells and visual purple appear in it prior to birth. The complicated development of the many structures forming the visual apparatus has been described by Mann. In spite of the early start in the embryo, the eye is not mature by the time of birth.

The Visual System at Birth

The immaturity of the eye of the neonate is evidenced in both optical and neural sensory structures. The eyeball of the newborn is less spherical than that of the adult because of the bulging of the temporal posterior segments and a greater anteroposterior diameter. The cornea is large at birth and has a greater curvature than later in life. The anterior chamber is shallower, the lens more spherical than that of the adult. The retina of the newborn is thicker than in the adult; the macula is not differentiated, and there are almost no cone cells.

The lacrimal gland is not functional at birth; the eye is kept moist only by the small mucous glands within the conjunctiva of the eyelids (Fig. 23-7).

The striated muscles which move the eyeballs are not under voluntary control in the neonate. Cerebral neural pathways are not myelinated beyond the midbrain.

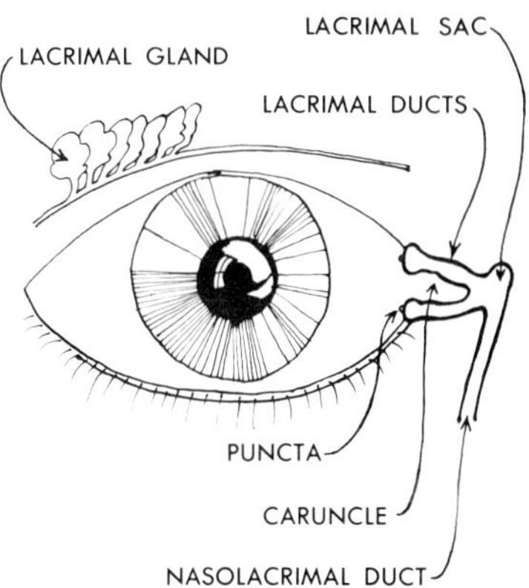

Fig. 23-7. Lacrimal apparatus.

Postnatal Development of the Visual System

The eye, like the brain, achieves a larger proportion of its total growth before birth than does the rest of the body. Total body weight increases about 20 times from birth to maturity; brain and eye size increase only about 3½ times. Most of the postnatal growth that does take place in the eye takes place rapidly in the first half-dozen years of life. At puberty, there is a slight additional growth in the size of the eye. The ciliary body and the crystalline lens, unlike the rest of the eye, continue to grow throughout life. The growth of the lens contributes to the developmental changes in the refractive power of the eye. Corneal curvature changes as the shape of the face matures.

Optimal vision at the human level requires (1) good visual function in the periphery of the retina and also in the macula of each eye, (2) the ability to focus a sharp image on the macula of each eye, (3) the ability to use the two eyes coordinately to obtain binocular vision, (4) the ability to fuse the two retinal images together in the brain and appreciate stereopsis, and (5) the ability to interpret the meaning of visual images.

The visual system of the newborn is not capable of any of these functions except part of the first, that is, peripheral vision. The changes that take place postnatally will be discussed in relation to the mechanism of seeing (Gesell, 1949).

Light Perception, Sharp Vision, and Color Perception

All the sensory cells which respond to the stimulation of light lie within the retina. The retina, however, is not a homogeneous structure; in fact, its anatomic organization and its functions are so different in different areas that it can be considered as consisting of two different sense receptor organs, the periphery and the macula.

The periphery of the retina is by far the larger part of the organ; the macula is only a 15° area at the posterior pole. The periphery contains visual purple, rod cells, and a few scattered cone cells. At the time of birth, while this area of the retina is a little thicker than in the mature eye, nevertheless, the sensory cells are present and show but little histologic difference from those of the mature eye. The periphery of the retina records light and dark and dim outlines of objects, and provides some awareness of color. It provides visual awareness of the surroundings in an area about 60° on the nasal side and 90° on the temporal side. This type of vision is usually spoken of as peripheral vision, the term applying both to the area of the retina recording the sensation and the part of the visual fields recorded.

The neonate possesses peripheral vision which is mature and undergoes little if any further maturation as life advances.

The macula is the part of the retina which provides central vision. It is not present at birth. It begins to differentiate within the first month of life. The retina thins out over this area, and cone cells squeeze between the sparsely placed rod cells, which are pushed farther and farther to the periphery. Cone cells are light-sensitive cells with two special attributes: they record sharp, clear images and are sensitive to color. By 4 months of age the macula is well organized, and by 8 months it is histologically mature. At this age, if the rest of development is adequate, the infant becomes more interested in tiny objects than in large ones. With his newly acquired prehensile grip (p. 402), he can be observed to pick up the most minute crumbs, which he is now able to see clearly with the use of his macula.

Also at about 8 months an infant may demonstrate a preference for certain colors, which he can now distinguish with the cone cells in his macula. Color discrimination in the infant is often difficult to distinguish from brightness discrimination.

Colorblindness is the result of some failure in development of the cone cells. Achromatopsia, or total colorblindness, is a rare sex-linked genetic defect and is associated with other visual defects presumably related to absence of cone cells or with failure of cone cells to function normally. Individuals with total colorblindness have visual acuity of 2/200 or less. They usually show nystagmus and photophobia (Walsh, 1957).

Partial colorblindness is a relatively common condition, occurring to some degree in about 8 per cent of the male population. The most frequent defect is inability to distinguish red and green. Not more than one-fourth of those affected have complete inability to distinguish these colors. The condition is therefore better termed a deficiency than an absence of red-green discrimination. In partial colorblindness, visual acuity is not affected (Sloan, 1954). This raises the question (unanswered at the present time) of whether or not there may be several types of cone cells, some for recording sharp images and others for recording color. It is even conceivable that colors in different parts of the spectrum are recorded in different cone cells.

Colorblindness, complete or partial, is a genetic defect for which no treatment is available. While the condition cannot be cured, awareness that a child has such a defect is necessary to protect him from failures over which he has no control (p. 551).

Depth Perception

A macula develops in each eye, and accurate vision is possible with one eye alone. However, two eyes, each recording a sharp image, are important for fine distinctions in perception of depth. When two normal eyes look at an object, each receives on its macula an image, but the two images are not identical, since light rays come to each macula at a slightly different angle. These two images are fused in the brain in such a way that a perception of depth is obtained.

Depth perception is therefore a cerebral function rather than a visual one, though of course it depends upon the adequate functioning of the visual apparatus. It begins to develop at about 9 months of age but matures slowly. At 18 months a child bumps into objects he sees, because his judgment of their distance is still poor. By the age of 6 years depth perception is usually mature.

Refraction and Accommodation

Light rays entering the eye are bent in such a way that they are brought to a focus on the retina. While all the transparent substances between the outer edge of the cornea and the retina contribute to the bending of light rays, actually only two are of significance, the cornea and the lens. The aqueous and the vitreous humor have refractive powers so similar to that of the cornea that they exert little additional effect on light that has penetrated the cornea (Fig. 23-8).

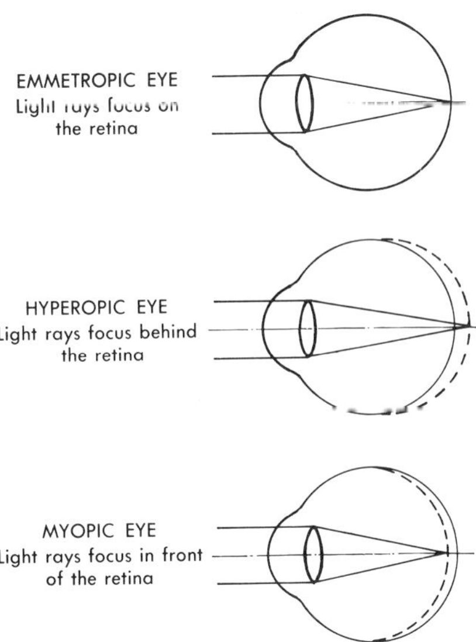

Fig. 23-8. Refraction, long eyeball and short eyeball.

When the eye looks at an object 20 ft or more away the light rays it receives are, for practical purposes, considered parallel, and the ability to bring them to focus on the retina depends upon the physical refractive powers of the cornea and lens, and the length of the eyeball.

The physical refractive power of the eye can be modified by the process of accommodation. This is accomplished by contraction of the ciliary muscles, which increases the curvature of the lens and thereby increases its refractive power. There is no mechanism for decreasing the refractive power of the eye.

With an eye at rest (that is, with no accommodation functioning) the adequacy of the physical refractive power to focus light on the retina depends largely upon the length of the eyeball. When the eyeball is overlong, the refractive power in cornea and lens are inadequate, and the light rays come to a focus in front of the retina. This is synonymous with myopia. Myopia is therefore universally found in individuals with overlong eyeballs. When light rays come to a focus behind the retina, the individual has hyperopia, a condition present when the length of the eyeball is short.

While long and short eyeballs are associated with myopia and hyperopia, respectively, lesser amounts of eyeball length are not universally associated with these refractive errors. The capacity of the cornea, and especially the lens, to bend light varies independently of eyeball length. This means that an individual with a moderate increase in eyeball length could be emmetropic, hyperopic, or myopic, depending upon the refractive capacity of his lens and of his cornea (Slataper, 1950).

The eye of the newborn is characteristically hyperopic; that is, the eyeball is too short for the refractive elements to bring parallel rays of light to a sharp focus on the retina. The eyeball grows rapidly for the first 8 years of life (roughly from about 16 to 24 mm). After the age of 8 there is very little further increase in length of the eyeball. An increase of approximately 8 mm in length of the eyeball would produce a severe degree of myopia if it were the only factor operating. Actually, Brown has found that during the first 8 years, the normal eye, hyperopic at birth, becomes increasingly hyperopic (at a rate of about +0.18 d per year) in spite of the increase in length of the eyeball. This comes about by changes in cornea and more particularly in the lens. The lens becomes flatter, and its structure alters as growth proceeds, lessening its refractive power. At about the age of 8 years, when the eyeball has reached its adult size, a reversal of the trend toward hyperopia takes place, again because of refractive changes in cornea and lens. The trend toward myopia is rapid in the years immediately prior to puberty (about −0.23 d per year). With the onset of puberty, the trend toward myopia continues, but at a decreased rate (−0.14 d per year). In the immediately postpubertal years, the eye tends to be emmetropic; the early trend toward hyperopia and the later trend toward myopia have evened out.

After the age of 20, myopia increases very slowly until the midthirties (−0.04 d per year), after which myopia begins to decrease slowly (+0.03 d per year), possibly because of weakening of accommodation.

While degrees of myopia and hyperopia are thus seen to be a normal part of development, there is a limit beyond which these conditions are sufficiently severe to require treatment (Fig. 23-9). Hyperopia is to be expected in the preschool and early school years. If this hyperopia is less

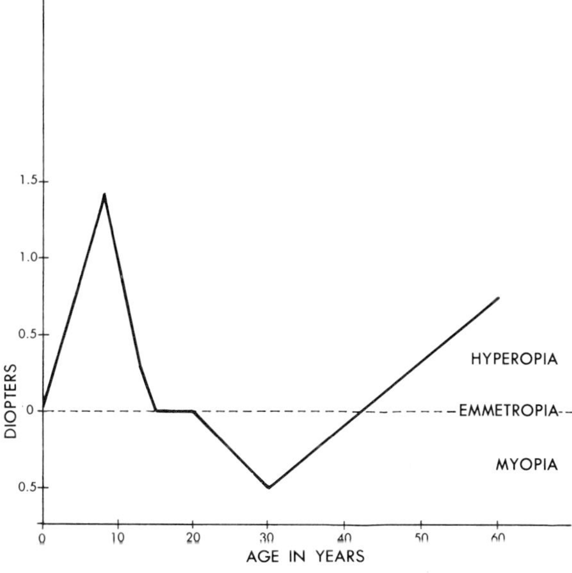

Fig. 23-9. Age trends in refractive power. *(From Brown, Net Average Yearly Changes in Refraction of Atropinized Eyes from Birth to Beyond Middle Life, Arch. Ophthal., 19:719, 1938.)*

than 2 d in each eye, it rarely needs correction. The powers of accommodation are sufficient to supplement the refractive powers of the eye, and so the child has good distant and near vision with but slight help from accommodation. If the hyperopia is over 4 d in each eye, the child will probably need glasses. If the refractive power of the two eyes is not equal, a condition called *anisometropia,* glasses may be needed, even though the hyperopia is less than 4 d in either eye. Constant use of excessive accommodation may cause headaches, eye pain, and other symptoms of eye strain and occasionally convergent strabismus (see below). When hyperopia is 4 d or more, accommodation is likely to be insufficient, and the child will have poor distant and near vision. Close work requires the greatest degree of accommodation and intensifies symptoms of eye strain. Since the developmental trend after the age of 8 is away from hyperopia and toward myopia, the child with hyperopia may improve as he gets older and be able to discard the glasses he needed as a small child.

Myopia, on the other hand, is not normal in the young child. Myopia present before the age of 8 is likely to increase during the next half-dozen years, because of the normal developmental shift toward myopia. A child with myopia will need glasses to enable him to see clearly objects at a distance. He will not outgrow the condition; in fact, as stated above, it is likely to increase in severity up to and beyond puberty.

Myopia does not produce symptoms of eye strain as does hyperopia. In myopia the refractive power is greater than it need be to focus the image on the retina, the sharp image falls anterior to the retina, and distant objects are seen as a blur. Powers of accommodation are of no help. The human being's ability to change the refractive power of his lens works only in one direction. He can contract his ciliary muscles and increase the curvature of his lens, thus increasing his refraction, but there is nothing he can do to decrease the curvature of his lens. Since the myope does not use accommodation, eye strain does not occur. He can usually see near objects adequately, though he may bring them closer to his face than is normal. The child with myopia does not bring his condition to the attention of his adults as does the child with hyperopia. Since he has always seen distant objects as a blur, he takes this as normal and makes no complaint. Since he sees near objects relatively well and does not suffer from eye strain, his condition can be detected only by objective tests. In a child in whom myopia has not been detected and corrected prior to school, academic failure may be a sign that the eyes are not functioning adequately. As stated above, myopia increases normally in the years before and during puberty. Frequent testing is essential to detect those children whose developmental shift toward myopia has exceeded the normal range.

Myopia is most frequently a gene-determined condition. Children of myopic parents should therefore be watched carefully by the physician for evidence of this condition (Kerby, 1958).

Refractive errors can be suspected from the results of testing a child's vision on the Snellen eye chart (see below), but for accurate determination of refractive power, accommodation needs to be eliminated by the use of a cycloplegic agent (Getman, 1959).

Binocular Vision

Optically, binocular vision is dependent upon the coordinated activity of the ocular muscles. The eyes must be so moved that each focuses an image on its own macula.

Immediately after birth the eye muscles seldom operate coordinately, and the normal infant can frequently be observed moving his eyes randomly, in much the same way as he moves his extremities. Within the first week of life, the extremely bizarre eye movements cease, and the infant's eyes move more or less coordinately. By the third month of life most normal infants use their eyes coordinately, although occasional squints may be observed in normal infants as late as the eighth month, especially when a nearby object is focused upon. It can therefore be said that mature adult function of the eye muscles is attained normally before the end of the first year.

Strabismus

Failure in eye muscle coordination results in strabismus, or squint. Strabismus can be due to paralysis of one or more eye muscles—paralytic squint, or it can be due to functional imbalance of the muscles—nonparalytic squint. It is also classified as convergent or divergent, depending upon which way the deviant eye moves. Squint may be constant or transient. True squint may be present at birth (congenital squint), in which case it does not disappear with normal development, or it may develop later (acquired squint). While acquired squint can develop at any time, its most frequent time of appearance is between 18 months and 4 years of age.

When the two eyes do not create the same image in the corresponding areas of each retina, the brain records two images, and the individual suffers from diplopia. A child with squint and subsequent double vision usually suppresses the vision from one eye—he looks with the deviant eye, but he does not see with it. An eye which is not used soon fails to be capable of seeing, and the child develops a condition known as amblyopia, or dimness of vision in one eye not due to any organic impairment in the retina. Amblyopia is a reversible condition if it has not existed for too long a time. Ultimately, however, the vision in an unused eye becomes permanently impaired. Adequate vision in both eyes is essential for the finer judgment of depth perception, so that a child with strabismus grows into an adult whose vision lacks an important aspect of optimal human sight.

In a young infant, paralytic squint is suspected if one eye is always deviant in the same direction. Such a child should be seen by an ophthalmologist within the first half year of life, and efforts must be made to preserve the sight in the deviant eye and to correct the muscle imbalance —usually by surgical treatment. An infant with transient squint, especially if there is no fixed pattern of deviation, can safely be watched throughout the first year, with the expectation that normal maturation of the eye muscles will correct the deviation.

After the first birthday a child who develops strabismus needs an ophthalmologic examination. The squint may be convergent or divergent, and while it may be transient in the beginning, it will soon become permanent. The most frequent cause of squint at this age is an excessive degree of hyperopia. To focus on a nearby object the child must use his powers of accommodation; when this requires considerable effort, the ciliary muscles become fatigued. The effort required is frequently more extreme in one eye than in the other. This is especially true in anisometropia. The child seems to concentrate his diminishing ability to accommodate on one eye and "forgets" about the other one, which then wanders away from the image being looked at. The earlier the condition can be detected, the better is the prognosis for optimal vision. If amblyopia has not developed, correction of the refractive error with glasses may be all that is necessary to bring the two eyes into coordinate use. If amblyopia has developed, a period of patching the good eye may be needed in order to restore the vision in the unused eye. Frequently orthoptic exercises are needed to strengthen eye muscles and establish the ability to fuse the images from the two eyes. If squint goes untreated for some years, surgical intervention may be needed to improve eye muscle balance before orthoptic exercises are effective.

Glasses which are required to correct an excessive degree of hyperopia may need to be worn constantly or only during close work. It is often possible to abandon glasses later in childhood as the normal developmental shift toward decreased hyperopia takes place. Needless to say, frequent ophthalmologic examinations are mandatory, since the refractive ability of a child's eyes changes appreciably as a result of normal maturation.

TABLE 23-1
Résumé of Maturation of the Visual Apparatus

Retina	The periphery is mature at birth. The macula is mature before the end of the first year.
Refractive power	Goes through a developmental cycle (see Fig. 23-9).
Eye muscles	Function at a mature level before the end of the first year.
Fusion	Begins to mature at about 9 months of age but not fully mature until the age of about 6 years.
Interpretation of visual experiences	Begins during the first year of life, reaches a peak during early school years when reading is acquired, and continues to mature for the duration of life.

Vision Testing

A great many visual defects are remediable if diagnosed and treated soon after their occurrence. This is especially true of refractive errors and errors of muscle balance. Therefore vision tests are a mandatory part of care of young children (Roper, 1964).

Vision, however, like other sensory abilities, is not a thing apart but constitutes an integral part of total development. Visual behavior matures as the total child develops. Vision can be thought of as a motor skill which is learned and improved through experience (Apell and Lowry, 1959). Keeney has formulated a chronology of ophthalmic development which in abbreviated form is given in Table 23-2. Failure in the normal progression of visual behavior can be due to impairment in ability to see; it can, of course, also be due to other failures in total development. In either case the child needs an accurate diagnosis and treatment tailored to his needs.

Muscle balance needs watching. In the first year of life, inspection alone, as the child uses his eyes to fix on a moving object, may be all that is needed. Later, in the preschool years, the cover test is a help in detecting slight muscle imbalance. This test is performed by covering one eye while the child is asked to look at a nearby object. The covered eye, which is not being used, assumes a position of rest. If, when the cover is removed, this eye shifts its position more than 2 or 3° to fixate on the object the other eye is looking at, it can be assumed that a muscle imbalance exists. The presence of strabismus of any degree after the age of 1 year calls for examination of refractive power.

Visual acuity is difficult to test objectively until the child is old enough to name objects which he sees. The Snellen test is the most widely used test. The Snellen chart consists of letters, pictures, or the E symbol in

TABLE 23-2

Chronology of Ophthalmic Development

Age	Level of development
Birth	Awareness of light and dark. The infant closes his eyelids in bright light.
Neonatal	Rudimentary fixation on near objects (3–30 in.).
2 weeks	Transitory fixation, usually monocular at a distance of roughly 3 ft.
4 weeks	Stares indefinitely at windows, follows large conspicuously moving objects.
6 weeks	Moving objects evoke binocular fixation briefly.
8 weeks	Following moving objects with jerky eye movements. Convergence is beginning to appear.
12 weeks	Visual following now a combination of head and eye movements. Convergence is improving. Enjoys light objects and bright colors.
16 weeks	Inspects own hands. Fixates immediately on a 1-in. cube brought within 1–2 ft. of eye. Vision 6/100 to 6/70.
20 weeks	Accommodative convergence reflexes all organizing. Visually pursues lost rattle. Shows interest in stimuli more than 3 ft. away. Becoming shy of strangers.
24 weeks	Rescues a dropped 1-in. cube. Can maintain voluntary fixation of stationary object even in the presence of competing moving stimulus. Hand–eye coordination is appearing.
26 weeks	Will fixate on a string. Grabs with both hands; only crudely engages object.
28 weeks	Binocular fixation clearly established.
36 weeks	Depth perception is dawning.
40 weeks	Marked interest in tiny objects. Approaches pellet with extended index finger. Tilts head backward to gaze up. Vision 6/70.
52 weeks	Fusion beginning to appear. Discriminates simple geometric forms, squares and circles. Looks intently at facial expressions. Vision 6/60.
12–18 months	Associates visual experience. Looks at pictures with interest.
18 months	Convergence well established. Localization in distance crude—runs into objects which he sees.
2 years	Accommodation well developed. Vision 6/12.
3 years	Convergence smooth. Fusion improving. May show tremor of hands when fine hand–eye coordination is required. Vision 6/9.
4 years	Vision 6/6.

SOURCE: Abbreviated from Arthur H. Keeney, "Chronology of Ophthalmic Development," Monograph, Charles C Thomas, Publisher, Springfield, Ill., 1951.

graded sizes so arranged that each line of the chart should be visible at a prescribed distance. The child who can read the 20 line at 20 ft with each eye is considered to have 20/20 vision. After the age of 8 years normal children should have 20/20 vision in each eye. Under the age of 8, when mild hyperopia is frequent, 20/30 vision can be accepted as adequate. A marked difference in visual acuity in the two eyes suggests amblyopia.

Tests for muscle imbalance and for visual acuity serve as screening tests to select those children who should be referred to the ophthalmologist for further investigation. In addition to those children who show objective indications of visual impairment, any child who has symptoms of eye strain (see above) and any school child whose academic work is unaccountably below his capacity should have his eyes examined by an ophthalmologist.

SENSATION IN DEVELOPMENT

In monitoring the development of children it is scarcely possible to overemphasize the importance to the child of his ability to receive and comprehend the afferent stimuli that are constantly bombarding his sense organs (p. 504).

Sensation is integrated into total development. In infancy and the early years what a child does with his hands, his body, his voice, is influenced by what stimulation he receives from his environment. Not only what he does but how he comprehends himself is affected by what his sense organs tell him.

The adequacy of sensory perception can be judged to some extent by the child's behavior. It must not be forgotten that adequacy of the sense organs alone is not enough to ensure that a child is taking in the phenomena about him. Failure of ego development can produce symptoms of withdrawal from the environment as profound as actual loss of a sensory receptor.

Every precaution needs to be taken to make sure that no remedial defect in any sense organ goes unattended. It is also essential to know very early in life whether a child has a defect in any sense modality with which he must live. At best it is difficult to help a blind or a deaf child grow up normally. It is impossible if his handicap is not recognized early enough to avoid the child's obtaining a distorted view of the world and of himself.

BIBLIOGRAPHY

Apell, Richard J., and Ray W. Lowry, Jr.: "Preschool Vision," American Optometric Assn., Inc., St. Louis, 1959.

Arey, L. B., M. J. Tremaine, and F. L. Monzingo: The Numerical and Topographical Relations of Taste Buds to Human Circumvallate Papillae throughout the Life Span, *Anat. Rec.*, **64**:9, 1935.

Bordley, John E., and William G. Hardy: A Study in Objective Audiometry with the Use of Psychogalvanometric Response, *Ann. Otol. Rhin. & Laryng.*, **58**:751, 1949.

Börnstein, Walter S.: Cortical Representation of Taste in Man and Monkey. II. The Localization of the Cortical Taste Area in Man and a Method of Measurement of Impairment of Taste in Man, *Yale J. Biol. & Med.*, **13**:133, 1940.

Brown, E. V. L.: Net Average Yearly Changes in Refraction of Atropinized Eyes from Birth to Beyond Middle Life, *A.M.A. Arch. Ophth.*, **19**:719, 1938.

Cohen, Jozef, and Donald P. Ogdon: Taste Blindness to Phenylthiocarbamide and Related Compounds, *Psychol. Bull.*, **46**:490, 1949.

Davson, Hugh (ed.): Vegetative Physiology and Biochemistry, vol. 1, The Visual Process, vol. 2, Muscular Mechanisms, vol. 3, Visual Optics and Optical Space Sense, vol. 4, in "The Eye," Academic Press, Inc., New York, 1962.

Fox, Arthur L.: The Relationship between Chemical Constitution and Taste, *Proc. Nat. Acad. Sc. U.S.*, **18**:115, 1932.

Geldard, Frank Arthur: "The Human Senses," John Wiley & Sons, Inc., New York, 1953.

Gesell, Arnold, Frances L. Ilg, and Glenna E. Bullis: "Vision: Its Development in Infant and Child," Paul B. Hoeber, Inc., New York, 1949.

Getman, G. N.: Techniques and Diagnostic Criteria for the Optometric Care of Children's Vision, Optometric Extensive Program, Duncan, Okla., 1959.

Goldschelder: Quoted by Geldard (see above reference).

Guilford, Frederick R., and C. Olaf Haug: Diagnosis of Deafness in the Very Young Child, *Arch. Otolaryng.*, **55**:101, 1952.

Hardy, W. G.: "Problems of Audition, Perception and Understanding," The Volta Bureau, Reprint 680, Washington, D.C., 1956.

Hirsh, Ira J.: "The Measurement of Hearing," McGraw-Hill Book Company, Inc., New York, 1952.

Keeney, Arthur H.: "Chronology of Ophthalmic Development," Mono. American Lectures in Ophthalmology Monograph, Charles C Thomas, Publisher, Springfield, Ill., 1951.

Kerby, C. Edith: Causes of Visual Defects in 7,310 Partially Seeing Children, *Exceptional Children*, **19**:137, 1952.

———: Causes of Blindness in Children of School Age, *Sight-Saving Rev.*, **28**:10, 1958.

Kronfeld, Peter C.: Gross Anatomy and Embryology of the Eye, in Hugh Davson (ed.), "The Eye," vol. 1, Academic Press, Inc., New York, 1962.

Mann, Ida C.: "Development of the Human Eye," Grune & Stratton, Inc., New York, 1950.

Monsees, Edna: Aphasia and Deafness, *Exceptional Children*, **25**:395, 1959.

Myklebust, Helmar R.: "Auditory Disorders in Children, A Manual for Differential Diagnosis," Grune & Stratton, Inc., New York, 1954.

———: Changing Concepts in Audiology, *Laryngoscope*, **66**:437, 1956.

———: "The Psychology of Deafness, Sensory Deprivation, Learning and Adjustment," Grune & Stratton, Inc., New York, 1960.

Nafe, John Paul, and Kenneth S. Wagoner: The Nature of Pressure Adaptation, *J. Gen. Psychol.*, **25**:323, 1941.

Newby, Hayes A.: "Audiology," 2d ed., Appleton-Century-Crofts, Inc., New York, 1964.

PFAFFMAN, CARL: Taste Mechanisms in Preference Behavior, *Am. J. Clin. Nutrition*, **5**:142, 1957.

ROPER, KENNETH L.: Referral to the Ophthalmologist. When and Why?, *Clin. Pediat.*, **3**:451, 1964.

SLATAPER, F. L.: Age Norms of Refraction and Vision, *A.M.A. Arch. Ophthal.*, **43**:466, 1950.

SLOAN, LOUISE L.: Congenital Achromatopsia, *J. Optic. Soc. Amer.*, **44**:117, 1954.

SMYTHE, R. N.: "Animal Vision. What Animals See," Charles C Thomas, Publisher, Springfield, Ill., 1961.

STIRNIMANN, F.: "Psychologie des Neugeborenen Kinder," Rascher-Verlag, Zurich and Leipzig, 1940.

TURK, AMOS: Some Basic Odor Research Correlation, *Ann. New York Acad. Sc.*, **28**:13, 1954.

WALSH, FRANK B.: "Clinical Neuro-ophthalmology," The Williams and Wilkins Company, Baltimore, 1957.

WEDDELL, G.: The Anatomy of Pain Sensitivity, *J. Anat.*, **81**:374, 1947.

24

Immune Mechanisms

The existence of living beings on this planet is predicated on the fact that one form of life obtains its subsistence from other forms. Creatures must grab and devour to live; all must protect themselves from being devoured. Through the evolutionary process many techniques—both aggressive and defensive—have come into existence.

In man's highly sophisticated society he has emerged from some of the more overt evidences of the law of the jungle, but man, like other creatures, continues to be the prey of microscopic organisms—organisms struggling, as is man himself, to maintain a place on the planet.

In the last few decades there have been enormous strides in the understanding of man's invisible enemies and of his inherent defense mechanisms against them.

While man's intelligence has helped him to avoid the onslaught of disease-producing microorganisms, the microorganisms themselves are not devoid of the ability to counteract man's attack against them. Nature has techniques other than cerebral capacity to help all her creatures survive. Some microorganisms have acquired the ability to cope with DDT and with chemotherapeutic agents, and to survive under conditions their less adaptable forebears found lethal. Perhaps in time man's brain will outstrip the defense mechanisms of the disease-producing microorganisms, and future generations will live as free from the terror of being pounced upon by a bacterium as by a tiger.

Man's techniques for reducing his hazards from infectious disease have taken two different directions. One is the elimination of the pathogenic agents from his environment; the other is the augmentation of his own resistance to attack. Purification of food and water supplies in some societies has virtually wiped out typhoid fever, cholera, and amebic dysentery. Eradication of disease-carrying insects has, in certain parts of the world, been successful in eliminating malaria, yellow fever, and plague. Where adequately used, immunizations have made smallpox and diphtheria rare diseases.

INHERENT DEFENSES AGAINST DISEASE

Man's body is fertile soil for the growth of some microorganisms, though by no means all. Even among parasites that require an animal host, not all find human tissues acceptable. Bacteria and viruses have specific requirements for their growth and reproduction. The virus of hoof-and-mouth disease finds conditions suitable in a cow but is unable to maintain itself in a human. Hog cholera and canine distemper, to mention but two, are diseases caused by microorganisms that do not find, within human tissue, a milieu suitable for their existence. Resistance to such diseases is called *native immunity* and is doubtless a genetic endowment. Native immunity in some cases is a specific characteristic and is absolute—no member of a species is susceptible to a specific microbe. In other cases native immunity is relative—some individuals within the species possess greater degrees of resistance than others.

Man, like other species, has several types of defense mechanisms to protect him from the ravages of microorganisms that seek him out. Three types of defense are recognized:

1. The first line of defense is mechanical and chemical; microorganisms are physically barred from entrance into the host, and at possible ports of entry subjected to conditions unfavorable for their survival. In some cases, specific enzymes which destroy microorganisms are present; in others, essential requirements of the microorganism are not met.
2. The second line of defense, in case the first fails, consists in engulfing and then isolating the microorganism—phagocytosis.
3. The third line of defense comes into play after the microorganism has penetrated the tissues. It is the mechanism whereby the microorganism is rendered innocuous either by being combined with a specific antibody or by some nonspecific inhibitor within the blood serum.

THE FIRST LINE OF DEFENSE: MECHANICAL AND CHEMICAL

The most favorable soil for the growth of many disease-producing organisms is the physiologic interior of the body. The various orifices of the body lead into channels, which, though lying deep within the body, are nevertheless part of the physiologic exterior. The body is covered with skin, which is directly contiguous with the mucous membranes lining the gastrointestinal, respiratory, and urogenital tracts.

Although but a few millimeters in thickness, the skin provides a formidable barrier to many disease-producing agents. The ease with which bacteria gain access to the physiologic interior when a cut or other abrasion renders the skin barrier impotent gives evidence of the effectiveness of the paper-thin epidermis. The protective quality of the skin is due to the presence of keratin and the secretions of the sweat and sebaceous glands (Chap. 22).

Mucous membrane, which lines the surfaces of the various body channels, is devoid of keratin; nevertheless the moist mucous films have considerable bactericidal power.

In the eye, tears wash out particulate matter mechanically and are capable of destroying many bacteria. The ear is protected by wax, which, through its mechanical and chemical properties, keeps the ear canal free from infection.

In the mouth, the saliva has bactericidal properties which aid the mechanical barrier of the oral mucous membrances. In the stomach, gastric secretions destroy many swallowed bacteria, so that chyme passed beyond the pylorus is, for the most part, sterile. Many bacteria enter the rectum and large intestine through the anus. Large numbers of these bacteria are not only harmless but beneficial; they synthesize organic compounds which are absorbed through the mucosa of the large bowel. There is little or no bactericidal action in the rectum.

The male and female urinary tracts and the reproductive tract in the male under normal conditions remain sterile. Bacteria are dealt with at the urethral meatus and in the healthy individual do not penetrate beyond the sphincter. The vagina, on the other hand, having no sphincter at its distal end, is open to bacterial invasion. It copes with pathogenic organisms by means of the chemical composition of its secretions and thus protects the upper reproductive passageways from infection.

The respiratory tract, of all areas in the body, has the greatest contact with the hostile sea of the environment. The surface area of the alveoli is roughly twenty-five times that of the skin. With each breath the surrounding air is brought into the deep recesses of the respiratory passages. Numerous mechanisms extract harmful substances from the incoming air. The nasal passages contain hairs which strain out gross particles; mucus traps bacteria and other solid matter; the tonsils as well as the lymphoid tissues at the distal end of the trachea extract some bacteria. These defenses protect the lower parts of the respiratory tract; nevertheless, the air breathed reaches the upper respiratory tract with a considerable fraction of the bacterial flora with which it entered the nose. It is not surprising that bacterial and viral invasion of the upper respiratory tract is the cause of the most frequent infections of man (p. 27).

THE SECOND LINE OF DEFENSE: PHAGOCYTOSIS

Once some particulate matter, be it living bacteria or viruses, inanimate organic or nonorganic matter, penetrates the barrier of skin and mucous membrane and enters the physiologic interior of the body, an immediate local response is activated. The tissues of the body are able to differentiate self from nonself, and the mere presence of nonself mobilizes defense mechanisms. Both fixed cells and wandering cells take part in this initial defense.

The cells of the body which engulf particulate matter are the *phagocytes.* Phagocytes are of two kinds, each with different origins. The first are the granular leukocytes of the blood and are made in the hematopoietic areas of the body. They constitute about 70 per cent of the total white cells of the blood in the adult. Their proportion is somewhat less in the child

(p. 178). Such phagocytes are referred to as *microphages.* The second type of phagocyte, the macrophage, originates from the mesenchyme. Mesenchymal cells line lymph and blood channels and are part of all lymphoid tissue—lymph nodes, the spleen, and the thymus. Altogether these widely disbursed mesenchymal cells comprise the reticuloendothelial system. The phagocytes of the reticuloendothelial system are both fixed and wandering cells. The fixed cells remain in the sinusoids of the lymph nodes, in spleen, in the liver, in bone marrow, and in the finer blood and lymph channels. Wandering cells of the reticuloendothelial system are found in connective tissue. Whether the monocytes of the blood are true macrophages from the reticuloendothelial system or cells from the hematopoietic system is a disputed point.

As soon as an injury occurs, the endothelial cells immediately begin making repairs, especially of damaged blood vessels. Fibroblasts aid by forming scar tissue. The fixed macrophages begin to engulf foreign material. Simultaneously with the action of the fixed cells, wandering cells, both macrophages and microphages, accumulate in the injured area and, like the fixed phagocytes, engulf foreign particulate matter.

Local inflammation occurs at the point of injury. The capillaries increase in diameter; their walls become more permeable than usual, permitting blood plasma and leukocytes to leak out into the damaged tissue. Phagocytic cells accumulate and ingest the foreign material. The area becomes swollen with the plasma and cells poured into it. Soon, fibrin clots form thrombi in the local lymphatic channels, which results in restriction of drainage and further swelling. All this slows transportation of the invading bacteria to other parts of the body. The local fibroblasts produce a capsule of connective tissue around the phagocytes, which by this time contain the invading foreign substance. Isolated and rendered incapable of multiplying by the unfavorable environment within the phagocytes, the bacteria succumb to digestion. This is the chain of events in conditions in which the local defenses of the host are more competent than the ability of the invading microorganism to survive.

When the original invasion of the foreign substance is confined to a small area, the resulting inflammation is a warm spot of local redness and swelling, which finally subsides as the bacteria are destroyed. On the other hand, if the original foreign material penetrates a wide area, such as the respiratory tract, local inflammation may take place, but alone local inflammation is not an adequate mechanism with which to cope with the invading microorganism. The response of the body is widespread instead of local inflammation. Reflexes which are set into action restrict the flow of blood to the surface of the body and thus reduce the heat loss that would normally occur. This causes a rise in body temperature, which speeds up phagocytosis and enzymatic processes generally. Fever is one aspect of the body's defense against infection and is basically similar to the local heat in a circumscribed inflammation. The illness of the host resulting from a widespread infection can be thought of as a whole-body reaction instead of a local one, but one in which the basic mechanisms of phagocytosis and enzymatic destructions of the invading microorganisms are similar.

In the newborn, and even more in the premature, phagocytosis is much less efficient than in the older person. The very young baby may succumb to an infection with almost no manifestation of defense action on his part. Inflammation involves mechanisms which must mature before they are operative. The nature of this maturity is not understood at the present time. Not only in the very young but also in the aged phagocytosis is not as effective a weapon as it is during the rest of life. Old persons and infants weather infection poorly.

Before a microbe can be digested, it must be killed. It is assumed that the interior of the phagocyte is unfavorable for the existence of the microbe and, once it is dead, enzymes digest it. However, some pathogenic organisms are able to withstand the intraphagocytic conditions and even multiply after they have been engulfed. Under such disastrous conditions the phagocytes actually spread virulent organisms throughout the body. The gonococcus and the meningococcus are diagnostically identified *within* the pus cells.

THE THIRD LINE OF DEFENSE: ANTIBODY FORMATION

Mechanical barriers and the ability to phagocytize and digest foreign substances are innate defense mechanisms, presumably transmitted in the genetic code. As such, they are species-characteristic and are designated as native immunity. All vertebrate animals have evolved an additional defense mechanism. Each individual animal is capable of making antibodies against certain pathogenic agents. An antibody is a specific protein which appears in body fluids, particularly in the blood serum, in response to exposure to a foreign protein—the antigen. An antibody is characterized by its affinity for its own antigen.

Antibodies are formed in response to the protein of microorganisms, a phenomenon which is part of the body's defense against infection. Antibodies are also formed in response to a variety of other proteins and to certain nonprotein substances, a phenomenon which brings about the state of hypersensitivity (p. 301).

Unlike native immunity, which is common to all members of a species, immunity based on antibody formation is an individual defense and depends upon the particular foreign protein with which the individual has had contact. Antibody formation is responsible for acquired immunity.

THE NATURE OF ANTIBODIES

Antibodies appear in the γ-globulin fraction of the serum proteins. Within the last few years new techniques have stimulated an upsurge of interest in γ-globulin. Biochemical, biophysical, and immunologic characteristics of γ-globulin are providing elucidating information about what appeared previously as bizarre and unpredictable reactions.

It now appears well documented that at least three moieties of the γ-globulin molecule exist. On the basis of electrophoretic mobility γ-globulin is divided into γ_1-globulin (fast) and γ_2-globulin (slow). On the basis of sedimentation constant γ-globulin is divided into 7S γ-globulin (small) and 19S γ-globulin (large) molecules. The 7S γ-globulins have a molecular weight of about 165,000 and are termed *microglobulins.* The 19S γ-globulins have a molecular weight of about 1 million and are termed *macroglobulins.*

γ_2 is usually (if not always) present as 7S; γ_1 can be either 7S or 19S. Thus the macroglobulin is usually (if not always) γ_1, while the microglobulin may be either γ_1 or γ_2.

In the adult about 90 per cent of the γ-globulin exists as 7S γ_2. The remaining 10 per cent is γ_1, about half of which is 7S and the remainder 19S.

Gamma-globulins have a life cycle. Not only does the total amount of γ-globulin change with maturity, but the various moieties of this substance have different capacities for responding to antigenic stimulation.

ONTOGENY OF ANTIBODY FORMATION

Mammals in utero do not normally synthesize γ-globulin. Under certain circumstances the fetus is able to manufacture some macroglobulins—19Sγ_1. The fetus apparently never synthesizes γ_2.

The placenta permits the transfer of 7S γ_1 to the fetus but selectively withholds the 19S γ_1 (Florman et al., 1963). The bulk of the transfer of γ-globulin from mother to fetus takes place in the last trimester of pregnancy; hence the blood levels of γ-globulin are greater in the full-term infant than in the premature.

Attempts to increase the resistance to infection of premature infants with injections of γ-globulin have not been successful (Amer et al., 1963; Hodes, 1963).

In the early months of postnatal life, the infant, by means of his passively acquired store of γ-globulin, possesses some immunity to diseases to which the mother is immune but only diseases whose antibodies are carried in 7S γ_2. Maternal immunity carried solely in macroglobulins is not passed on to the child.

The neonate usually possesses some immunity to many viral diseases, to the toxins of diphtheria and tetanus, and to the Gram-positive pathogens but has relatively little resistance to the Gram-negative enteric pathogens (Smith and Eitzman, 1964). It is now evident that this variability in resistance is a result of the selective placental transfer of immune globulins.

The passively transferred 7S γ_2 gradually disappears from the infant's circulation during the early weeks of life. The time of lowest levels of γ-globulin varies from 15 to 80 days (Good et al., 1957).

The neonate's supply of γ-globulin is thus characterized by a relatively high level of 7S γ_2 (passively transmitted) and an absence or marked deficiency of 7S and 19S γ_1 (Rosen, 1964).

The neonate has the capacity to respond to the type of antigenic stimulation which brings forth the production of 19S γ_1. Both the neonate and the fetus have been shown to be capable of synthesizing 19S γ_1 (Silverman, 1963). The fetus is usually sterile and hence has no antigenic stimulation; but when the fetus is invaded by certain pathogens, he is capable of responding by forming macroglobulins (Edds, 1958).

Smith and Eitzman demonstrated that newborns were able to manufacture antibodies against the flagellar antigen of Salmonella as early as 7 days of age. In adults similar antibodies appeared in 4 to 5 days after immunization. This suggests that the newborn's capacity to manufacture macroglobulins is but very slightly inferior to that of the adult. By the end of the first year of life, the child is as capable as the adult in 19S γ_1 synthesis (Osborn, 1952).

On the other hand, Smith has demonstrated that the newborn is unable to synthesize the 7S γ_2 globulin. In fact, if certain antigens are introduced into the newborn, not only is no antibody produced but the antigen remains in the circulation for prolonged periods. This phenomenon is known as *tolerance*. Smith has produced a similar immunologic paralysis in adult animals by total body radiation. He postulates that both the neonatal pattern of immune response (tolerance to specific antigens) and the induced adult immunologic paralysis depend either upon the absence of a type of cell which expresses its responsiveness by 7S γ_2 production or failure of a phase of differentiation of a single cell line to become capable of this type of expression.

In the normal adult the presence of 19S γ_1 is followed within a period of 5 to 15 days by the appearance of 7S γ_2 (possibly from a reduction of the macroglobulin). In the infant relatively little 7S γ_2 appears subsequent to 19S γ_1 formation.

Present knowledge suggests the undesirability of immunizing infants very early in life. Prior to 2 or possibly 3 months of age antibody mechanisms are too immature to enable the infant to build optimal defenses.

THE SITE OF ANTIBODY FORMATION

Gamma-globulin may be manufactured in more than one type of cell (Cushing and Campbell, 1957). Those at present given consideration for this synthesis are (1) the cells of the reticuloendothelial system, (2) the lymphocytes, and (3) plasma cells. Regardless of the exact type of *cell*, the *tissues* responsible for most of the synthesis of γ-globulin are lymph nodes, spleen, and bone marrow. Connective tissue, skin, brain, cornea, and even subcutaneous fat have all been thought to contribute γ-globulin, although Raffel believes that the presence of γ-globulin is due to the migration into them of one of the cells mentioned above.

Burnet has recently postulated that the thymus is the "first level" immunologic organ. He presents data which suggest that lymphoid cells first appear in the thymus and then proliferate to produce "second level" immunologic organs in spleen, lymph nodes, and bone marrow. Smith and Eitzman (1964) suggest that the γ_1 and γ_2 moieties may be synthesized in different types of cells.

The exact mechanism of antibody formation is far from clear at the present time. However, it is known that the lymph node plays an important role in antibody formation. When foreign material gains access to tissues, that which is not immediately dealt with locally is swept along in the lymph to a regional lymph node. In the lymph node the foreign material is filtered out and engulfed by phagocytes. The lymphocytic cell itself does not phagocytize, but its presence appears to increase the rate of phagocytosis of other cells. Some of the foreign material invades the lymphocytes. In this cell antibodies develop as γ-globulin is synthesized. One suggestion is that the foreign protein enters the locus of the globulin synthesis and influences the final folding together of the polypeptide chain, thus imposing its specific configuration on the globulin molecule, a configuration complementary to that of the original foreign protein, i.e., the antigen. γ-globulin synthesized in response to a given antigen is specific for that antigen. It unites with it, altering the invading protein and rendering the microorganism incapable of multiplication. As the microorganism dies, the patient recovers. It has, however, taken time for the host to manufacture antibodies, and it is during this interval that the clinical manifestations of the disease have been apparent.

After an antibody has been formed in the body of a host in response to a specific antigen, one of three things can happen:

1. The host continues to manufacture that particular γ-globulin configuration. In this case, the antibody can be detected in the blood long after the disease caused by the original microorganism has subsided. Apparently, some antigen has remained in the body and acts as a constant stimulus to antibody production.

2. The host does not manufacture the antibody constantly, and no antibody can be detected in the blood. By some unknown mechanism, however, the host can produce the antibody quickly when again stimulated by a reintroduction of the antigen. It is as though the body had "learned how" to cope with that antigen.

3. The host stops manufacturing the antibody after the stimulus provided by the antigen has ceased, and the body "forgets" how to make it. If the antigen is reintroduced, the host must start anew to manufacture antibody.

The individual will present the clinical signs of the disease, as he did on his first contact with the microorganism.

In the first two cases the individual has built up a specific defense. Should his body again be invaded by that particular microorganism, the microorganism would immediately be rendered innocuous, and the individual would not succumb to the disease: he would be immune. In the third case a second invasion by the same microorganism would produce disease just as it did the first time: the individual would not be immune.

AGAMMAGLOBULINEMIA AND HYPOGAMMAGLOBULINEMIA

In 1952 Burton described the first case of almost total lack of γ-globulin. His case was that of an 8-year-old boy who suffered from 19 serious respiratory infections in 4 years. Burton found that this boy was unable to build antibodies against pneumonococcal antigens, typhoid vaccine, or diphtheria vaccine. He had mumps three times.

Good et al. studied two infants born successively to a mother with agammaglobulinemia and found that only minute amounts of γ-globulin could be detected in the serum of either infant at birth. At 42 days of age in one infant and at a slightly earlier age in the other γ-globulin began to appear in the blood. Both infants developed into immunologically normal infants, though at birth they were virtually devoid of γ-globulin.

Another infant, also studied by Good, born to an immunologically normal mother had, at birth, the expected concentration of passively transmitted γ-globulin, which fell in the usual way during early infancy. The infant's γ-globulin, however, failed to rise during later infancy. This infant proved to have agammaglobulinemia, though in the neonatal period he was indistinguishable from a normal infant.

Agammaglobulinemia is a rare congenital disease which does not become obvious until the infant is 3 to 4 months of age, at which time the passively transferred antibodies from his mother have disappeared and his failure to make his own γ-globulin becomes apparent. Good et al. believe the disease is a sex-linked recessive trait found only in males and is due to an inborn error in protein metabolism. One case of Good et al. showed an even greater number of infections than Burton's original case. Good et al. observed, in one patient over a 6-year period, two episodes of pneumonococcal meningitis, 15 attacks of bacterial pneumonia, several episodes of septicemia, and innumerable episodes of otitis media, pharyngitis, and purulent sinusitis. Fortunately the response to antibacterial therapy is good in this condition.

Hypogammaglobulinemia is much more common than agammaglobulinemia. The two diseases may represent varying degrees of the same condition and be due to similar inborn errors in protein metabolism.

Acquired deficiency of γ-globulin is also a recognized disease. The acquired form can occur at any time in life and is equally frequent in either sex. Acquired hypogammaglobulinemia can appear for reasons that are quite unknown, and it can also disappear for equally unknown reasons. It can also appear as part of a more general abnormality in protein metabolism, such as nephrosis, multiple myeloma, nutritional failure, or failure of general protein manufacture. The prognosis under such circumstances depends upon the underlying pathologic condition.

Individuals with hypogammaglobulinemia may have a near-normal blood level of lymphocytes, but there may be a deficiency of these cells in the blood as well as in the cortices of the lymph nodes. Lymphoid tissue throughout the body is apt to be sparsely developed.

Gitlin et al. have reported a case of a patient with thymic alymphoplasia with lymphopenia and generalized paucity of lymphocytes in the tissues. The patient died at 15 days of age from overwhelming bacterial infection.

Intramuscular injections of γ-globulin can provide individuals with low levels of γ-globulin with usable antibodies and thus reduce the incidence of bacterial infections.

NATURALLY ACQUIRED IMMUNITY

The immunity any child develops depends upon (1) the adequacy of his antibody-building mechanisms and (2) the particular antigens with which he comes into contact.

The ability to manufacture antibodies is a gene-directed phenomenon. It is probable that more than one gene is responsible; hence different aberrant genes may be responsible for some of the clinically distinguishable disorders of the immune mechanisms.

The specific nature of the antibodies any child manufactures depends upon the particular antigens he meets. This means that the antibodies circulating in the body of any person are a highly individual matter. Since each individual has to build up his own immunologic defense, each person must live through many diseases to acquire resistance to the pathogens common in his environment.

Some clinical syndromes are caused by a single pathogen. A child comes in contact with the virus that causes measles; the symptoms characteristic of this disease develop, and simultaneously the child builds antibodies against the virus. The next time this virus reaches him, his body is able to render it harmless by virtue of the antimeasles antibodies he formed during his first encounter with this virus, and clinical symptoms of the disease do not develop.

Other clinical syndromes are not caused by a single pathogenic agent but by a whole host of different agents. The common upper respiratory tract infections are caused by perhaps a hundred different agents. In order for a child to acquire resistance to these common infections by natural means, he must live through a great many infections which appear clinically indistinguishable. Eventually, if his experiences are sufficiently varied, he acquires a store of defenses against the hazards common in his environment. For this reason young children succumb frequently to upper respiratory tract disease; as they grow older, they accumulate resistance against many agents capable of producing upper respiratory tract diseases, and ultimately they have fewer attacks of these diseases. It is possible also that the efficiency of their immunologic mechanisms improves with increasing maturity.

Not only the common upper respiratory tract diseases but also gastrointestinal diseases, pneumonia, kidney infections, and other infections are caused by many different bacteria and viruses; again, resistance is built up to the specific pathogen, not to the clinical illness.

Many infections leave in their wake a highly effective and durable resistance. In this class can be listed the organisms that produce an exotoxin, as in diphtheria and scarlet fever; bacteria, as in typhoid and pertussis; viruses, as in smallpox, chickenpox, mumps, measles, poliomyelitis, yellow fever; and *Rickettsia*, as in typhus and spotted fever. Second attacks of these diseases can occur but are rare. Whether second attacks are due to failure in antibody formation or to a variant in the pathogen is not known.

Some disease agents appear to produce but a short-term immunity. Second and even repeated attacks of pneumonia from presumably the same type of pneumonococcus are common. Failure of the development of the immune state may reflect failure of antibody formation or may reflect the development of antibodies which slowly disappear. It is also possible that apparent failure may be due to variations in strains of the organism. Seventy-five strains of the pneumonococcus are known at present. Bacillary dysentery is caused by any one of 19 known strains, and there well may be variants within these strains, each of which constitutes a different antigen.

ARTIFICIALLY ACQUIRED IMMUNITY

Techniques are available for artificially producing immunity against certain pathogenic agents. Artificial immunity is basically of two kinds: passive and active.

Passive Immunity

Passive immunity involves the transfer into a host of preformed antibodies—antibodies manufactured in the body of another animal. Passively transferred antibodies do not remain in the body of the host but are slowly dissipated, and no more are formed. The immunity, therefore, is transient. The immunity of the infant at birth is a passive immunity acquired by the transfer to the fetus of antibodies manufactured by the mother.

After birth, passive immunity can be induced by injecting into an individual antibodies produced in another host. These antibodies can be in serum from a patient who has recovered from the disease or in hyperimmune serum produced in man or in an animal. In either case the whole serum can be used or a concentrate of the γ-globulin fraction. When serum from an animal is used, hypersensitive reactions may occur because of the foreign protein of the animal serum.

Passive immunity, under certain circumstances, is a useful technique for avoiding an illness either after exposure has taken place or when exposure seems imminent (as in institutionalized children in time of epidemic) (see Table 24-1).

TABLE 24-1

Available Passive Immunization Procedures

Infection	Immunization
Diphtheria	10,000 units antitoxin (horse). Should be given all non-immunized exposed children.
Infectious hepatitis	0.04 ml/kg γ-globulin (human) should be given any exposed person.
Measles	0.25 ml/kg γ-globulin (human) immediately after exposure to prevent infection. 0.05 ml/kg γ-globulin (human) 6 days after exposure to modify infection.
Mumps	5–7.5 ml hyperimmune mumps γ-globulin (human). Seldom desirable for children, but may be used for exposed non-immune post-pubertal males or women in first trimester of pregnancy.
Pertussis	2.5 ml hyperimmune pertussis γ-globulin (human). Should be given all non-immunized exposed children.
Poliomyelitis	0.3 ml/kg γ-globulin (human) may be used for household contacts.
Rabies	0.5 ml/kg hyperimmune anti-rabies serum immediately after bite of animal suspected of rabies, followed by active immunization.
Rubella	20 ml γ-globulin (human). Seldom desirable for children, but may be used for women in first trimester of pregnancy.
Tetanus	5,000–10,000 units antitoxin (horse). Should be used in non-immunized persons with potentially contaminated wounds.

SOURCE: Report of the Committee on Control of Infectious Diseases, 14th ed., American Academy of Pediatrics, Evanston, Ill., 1964.

Active Immunity

Active immunity is produced by the injection of an antigen into the body of the host, who then responds to it by the manufacture of antibodies. The antigen has "taught" the host how to make antibodies against itself. Active immunity develops slowly but remains for prolonged periods. Artificially induced active immunity is seldom as effective or as durable as immunity acquired naturally by having the disease. Nevertheless, when vaccines are used at the right time in proper doses and suitable stimulating doses are given at appropriate intervals, the resulting immunity has proved so effective that some diseases have been virtually eradicated (Smith, M., 1963).

Antigens used to produce active immunity are of several kinds depending upon the nature of the metabolic processes within the microorganisms.

Soluble toxins. Some bacteria elaborate exotoxins, which thus become the substances that stimulate antibody production. For such pathogens, the toxin itself can be used as antigen, and since it is nonliving, it does not duplicate itself within the body of the host. Diphtheria and tetanus are bacteria of this kind.

Dead microorganisms. Some pathogens stimulate antibody production by the protein of their bodies. The whole organism is the antigen. Such organisms can be killed by physical or chemical means in such ways that the protein is unchanged and the dead organism used as antigen. Killed bacteria capable of producing immunity are those which cause typhoid fever, pertussis, cholera, plague. Viruses in this class are those causing rabies, influenza, poliomyelitis, and mumps, and certain of the adenoviruses.

Living attenuated microorganisms. Other pathogens stimulate antibody production through the products of their metabolism. As the organism multiplies, it elaborates a soluble product against which the host builds antibodies, or the organism, in the course of its metabolism, may produce substances in the cells of the host, which are the stimulus to antibody production. In either of these cases, a dead organism is incapable of inducing immunity; only the living organism has antigenic capability. Vaccines from such pathogens must be viable organisms so attenuated that they produce but mild symptoms in the host. Vaccines of this type are those against smallpox and yellow fever, the Sabin vaccine against poliomyelitis, and measles vaccine.

In the United States today immunizations against smallpox, diphtheria, pertussis, tetanus, and poliomyelitis are mandatory for the adequate care of all children. Now that the measles vaccine has been perfected, it has been added to this list. These procedures are safe and effective. Their widespread use has all but wiped out the diseases they are designed to prevent. However, the elimination of the clinical diseases means that children growing up today have no opportunity for the minute exposure from which some of those of past generations often built up immunity without actually acquiring the disease. Maintaining an immunized population is the only way to safeguard the next generation from the ravages of these diseases.

The schedule of immunizations recommended by the American Academy of Pediatrics is given in Table 24-2. This publication discusses also the contraindications for various immunologic procedures.

The Academy suggests beginning the schedule with the combined DTP vaccine, because pertussis is a most serious disease in young babies. This is desirable if there is any pertussis in the community, but when, as is so often the case, there are no cases of pertussis, it is safe to start the immunization schedule with smallpox vaccine. The practical advantage is that a 3-month-old baby is not sufficiently coordinated to pick at the pustule made by the vaccine, whereas a year-old baby often cannot be persuaded to leave it alone.

TABLE 24-2

Recommended Schedule for Active Immunization of Infants and Children

Age	Preparation	Alternate polio schedule
2 months	DTP*	
	Type 1 OPV†	IPV‡
3 months	DTP	
	Type 3 OPV	IPV
4 months	DTP	
	Type 2 OPV	IPV
9 months	Measles vaccine	
12 months	Smallpox vaccine	
	Tuberculin test	
15 months	DTP	
	Type 1 & 2 & 3 combined OPV	IPV
2 years	Tuberculin test	IPV
4 years	DTP	IPV
	Tuberculin test	
6 years	Smallpox vaccine	IPV
	Tuberculin test	
8 years	DTP	IPV
10 years		IPV
12 years	TD§	IPV
	Smallpox vaccine	
14 years		IPV
16 years	TD	IPV

* DTP = diphtheria–tetanus–pertussis.

† OPV = oral poliovaccine of the Sabin type.

‡ IPV = inactivated poliovaccine of the Salk type. If IPV is used, separate injections of DTP and the poliovaccine may be given or quadruple preparations may be used.

§ TD = tetanus-diphtheria toxoids, combined (adult type). After 16 years of age, smallpox revaccination and tetanus toxoid booster doses should be repeated every 5 years.

SOURCE: Report of the Committee on Control of Infectious Diseases, 14th ed., American Academy of Pediatrics, Evanston, Ill., 1964.

Immunizations against gastrointestinal diseases are necessary only under special conditions. Water and milk supplies are so well supervised in this country that routine immunizations against water and food-borne diseases are not called for.

Likewise immunizations against insect-borne diseases are not needed in this country, except possibly against Rocky Mountain spotted fever in those people whose work or habits bring them in contact with infected ticks.

Immunization against influenza is effective and can profitably be used in selected cases.

Immunizations against the upper respiratory tract infections and the common cold are at present not practical. Some of the adenoviruses lend themselves to preparation of vaccines which will protect the individual from these particular viruses; however, they represent but a small number of the many microorganisms that produce the clinical symptoms of upper respiratory tract disease. Whether or not the future holds the possibility of a vaccine capable of producing an immunity to the many pathogens affecting the upper respiratory tract is problematic.

NONSPECIFIC FACTORS INFLUENCING RESISTANCE TO INFECTION

From a common sense point of view, it would seem that an individual in buoyant health would be better able to resist the inroads of pathogenic agents than one in a constant state of fatigue. However, there is a negative side to the interaction between the growth potential of the microorganisms and the powers of resistance of the host. Bacteria and viruses flourish on the tissues of a host who can supply them with optimal conditions for their metabolism; they too become apathetic when they are undernourished. The better the general well-being of the host, the more vigorous is the growth of those microorganisms which invade the body. The other side of the coin is that the better the general well-being of the host, the more vigorous is his ability to cope with pathogens. In the healthy body, invaded by a pathogen, fever develops, phagocytes are poured out, and antibodies are vigorously synthesized. The individual may become acutely ill, but as he rapidly mobilizes his defenses, he is apt to recover quickly (Boycott, 1926).

When the host's body is undernourished, skin and mucous membrane barriers may have less than optimal ability to resist inroads of pathogens. If protein intake is so low that edema results, the invading microorganisms grow slowly. But in the poorly nourished host both phagocytes and antibody production are apt to be decreased. Body temperature rises only slightly, if at all. The patient may not appear ill, but his disease is apt to linger for a longer period than in the healthy person. During such periods, spread of infection may take place and complications result. There is little evidence that optimal health reduces the *incidence* of attack by pathogens.

It must be pointed out that while optimal health is a goal to be sought, the superabundance of any or all vitamins or of proteins does nothing to increase resistance to infection.

HYPERSENSITIVITY

In discussing immunity, attention has been focused on the antigen. The antigen which produces immunity comes from pathogenic microorganisms or their metabolic products. The goal (teleologically) is the neutralization and detoxification of the potentially injurious antigen by its union with antibody. The product of the mechanism is a new substance, antigen plus antibody, or antigen-antibody. Under most circumstances and in most people this new substance induces no reaction in and of itself (Criep, 1962).

In some individuals and under some circumstances, materials other than those derived from pathogenic microorganisms have antigenic ability. The variety of substances that can, at times, act as antigen is very great. Food proteins, pollens, animal danders, dust are frequent offenders. Some drugs and some products derived from microorganisms can also act as antigens under certain circumstances. Unlike the antigen that produces immunity, all these substances have in common an initially harmless character. The first time one of them gains access to the body of a host, no adverse reaction takes place; nevertheless, the hypersensitive host builds antibodies against this substance. On second or subsequent exposure to the same antigen, the now sensitized host immediately forms antigen-antibody. This substance is capable of inducing injury. The point is worthy of reiteration: the hypersensitive or allergic reaction is due to the presence of antigen-antibody, not to the presence of either antigen or antibody alone (Table 24-3). The hypersensitive reaction serves no useful purpose as far as known (Raffel, 1961).

TABLE 24-3

Comparison of Immunity and Hypersensitivity

	Immunity	Hypersensitivity
Prevalence	100% except relatively few individuals with a- or hypogammaglobulinemia	10% of total population
Value to host	Protective	Harmful
The antigen	Pathogenic microorganism or product of their metabolism	Many proteins and some non-protein substances
Toxicity of antigen	Toxic	Non-toxic
Symptoms on 1st contact with antigen	Infectious disease	None
Symptoms on subsequent contact with antigen	None	Allergic reaction
Route of absorption of antigen	Any route	Any route
Induction period	Yes	Yes
Reaction of host to presence of antibody	None	None
Reaction of host to presence of antigen + antibody	None	Allergic reaction

Antigen-antibody can injure tissue directly, but it has to be present in large amounts to do this. This direct reaction, the Arthus phenomenon, is a relatively infrequent occurrence and seldom occurs spontaneously. It is usually the result of injections of relatively large doses of antigen into sensitized individuals.

A more frequent mechanism by which deleterious effects are produced is by means of an intermediary product released when antigen-antibody is formed. Histamine is thought to be the most important of these substances, although serotonin, acetylcholine, heparin, and some others have been implicated. Hypersensitive reactions involve smooth muscle, blood vessels, and collagen.

Once a hypersensitive reaction has taken place, eosinophils make their appearance. These cells are abundant in local lesions in hives, in nasal secretions during hay fever, in mucus from the gastrointestinal tract during allergic diarrhea. They are also increased in the blood during attacks of asthma and atopic dermatitis. The role of the eosinophil is not well understood, though it is assumed to be significant in destroying the histamine produced by the antigen-antibody.

Some hypersensitive reactions are iatrogenic, the result of injections of antigen into sensitized individuals. If the injection is of a small amount of antigen and it is placed in the skin, the reaction is a local one *in situ*, consisting of edema and blood vessel dilation—the hive. This reaction is the basis of skin sensitivity tests and is a means of determining the specific antigens to which a particular individual has already built antibodies. If the injection is of a larger amount of antigen, the reaction may be an immediate systemic one, especially if the injection is intravenous. The reaction may consist of generalized edema and blood vessel dilation alone, or smooth muscle spasm may also occur. Such reactions can be life-threatening. In a highly sensitive individual intramuscular or even intradermal injection can be enough to produce systemic reactions. Some of the most serious hypersensitive reactions are the result of injection of drugs. In a nationwide survey in 1959, Welch et al. found over a thousand cases of life-threatening hypersensitive reactions and almost two thousand serious but not life-threatening cases. Penicillin injections were the culprit in a startlingly large number of these reactions.

Naturally occurring hypersensitive reaction (atopy) develops in some people as a result of casual exposure, by inhalation, by ingestion, or occasionally by epidermal contact. The most frequent symptoms produced by subsequent exposure are asthma, hay fever, urticaria, angioedema, and eczema. A great many other symptoms, referable to almost every organ system in the body, have been considered from time to time to be the result of hypersensitive reactions.

Atopic sensitivity has been thought to be confined to man, although a few exceptions have been found. It occurs in almost 10 per cent of the total population and is without doubt a gene-directed phenomenon. The allergic constitution is an inherited quality and is found much more frequently in some families than in others. While the ability to form unwanted antibodies is inherited, the specific atopic disease (asthma, hay fever, eczema, etc.) depends upon the organ system utilized as a target area and is, to a large extent, an individual matter.

Age is a factor in determining which organ system will take the brunt of the allergic reaction. In infancy eczema is a frequent manifestation of the allergic constitution and asthma an infrequent one. After the age of about 3 years eczema becomes less frequent and asthma more frequent. Gastrointestinal allergy seldom occurs after infancy. Hay fever tends to develop in later childhood.

The infant who inherits an allergic constitution must become sensitized to specific antigens before he will demonstrate atopic disease. Whether or not the human fetus becomes sensitized in utero by transmission of antigen through the placental barrier is a disputed point.

During infancy the immaturity of mucous membranes and particularly those of the gastrointestinal tract predispose the infant to sensitization. Whole proteins penetrate the intestinal wall in healthy infants more readily than after the age of 2. After bouts of diarrhea, the infant's gastrointestinal tract is even less able to hold back unsplit proteins than is the healthy intestine. Foods are therefore the most important sources of sensitizing antigens in infancy.

Potentially allergic infants, that is, those whose families contain many allergic individuals, can often be protected from the development of atopic disease by careful management of their dietaries. Breast feeding eliminates the need to introduce the foreign protein of cow's milk. When breast milk is not available, the use of a soybean milk substitute which is less antigenic than cow's milk can be considered. Introduction of food known to be highly antigenic, such as eggs, citrus fruits, or wheat, can be delayed until the gastrointestinal tract has achieved a greater degree of maturity. All foods are less antigenic when well cooked, and care can be exercised to see that the potentially allergic child receives no raw or partly cooked foods.

Not only foods but also inhalants can sensitize the potentially allergic infant. Care to see that he has a minimal exposure to dust, feathers, or animal danders can help prevent his sensitization.

Emotional states play a significant but little understood role in atopic disease. No amount of emotional stress produces these diseases unless the allergic constitution is present. But given the capacity to synthesize antibodies against allergens, anxiety, fear, and tensions seem able to precipitate an attack of atopic disease or to accentuate an existing attack.

TONSILS, ADENOIDS, AND OTHER LYMPHOID TISSUES

The lymphoid tissues comprise the lymph nodes, thymus, spleen, tonsils, adenoids, and lymphocytes of the blood. All these tissues share a growth pattern quite different from that of the body as a whole. They increase rapidly in size for the first decade of life, reaching approximately twice the dimensions they will occupy in the adult (Fig. 11-8, p. 126). Beginning at about the age of 10 to 12 these tissues shrink rapidly and reach adult size by the end of the second decade. This growth pattern of lymphoid tissue parallels the development of immunity, and doubtless one is dependent upon the other (Scammon, 1934).

Lymphoid tissue is responsive to infection. Already large, it increases still more during invasion by microorganisms. There is an absolute lymphocytosis in the blood during childhood (p. 178). The lymphoid tissues in the mesentery are large in childhood and atrophy as life advances. This fact is significant in the outcome of a ruptured appendix at different times of life (p. 192). The thymus is a large structure in infancy but becomes so small that it is hard to detect in older people. Lymph nodes throughout the body are large, and those in superficial areas are often palpable in childhood.

Children with hypogammaglobulinemia who do not develop immunity in response to infection have less lymphoid tissue, and what they do have does not hypertrophy in response to infection.

Of all the lymphoid tissues the tonsils receive the most attention. The faucial tonsils are the showcase of lymphoid tissue—on display every time a child opens his mouth for medical inspection. The pharyngeal tonsils (the adenoids) are not so readily seen.

At birth, the faucial tonsil is barely visible on inspection of the infant's mouth. It lies flat against the wall of the pharynx. None of the other tonsillar tissue is visible.

The rapid growth of tonsillar tissue, which begins in the last month of intrauterine life, continues without interruption after birth and is so much more rapid than that of the rest of the body that the tonsils occupy a larger and larger proportion of the throat as the child grows. It is during the years of early childhood that tonsil masses are seen so large that they meet in the midline when the child gags. By the end of the first decade tonsillar tissue begins to atrophy and continues to shrink as the rest of the body is responding to the pubertal growth spurt.

The tonsil, like the rest of the lymphoid tissues in the body, is sensitive to infection and hypertrophies when pathogenic agents lodge in it. Usually the tonsil shrinks back to its normal size when the infection subsides, but when infection becomes chronic, tonsils may remain hypertrophied.

There are times when the mere mechanical size of the tonsils, especially the pharyngeal tonsil (the adenoids), causes interference with normal function. When the pharyngeal tonsil increases sufficiently to interfere with passage of air through the nose, the child breathes with his mouth open and is apt to snore while asleep. Persistent mouth breathing calls for investigation of possible mechanical obstruction by enlarged adenoids.

The adenoids will shrink by the normal process of growth a little before puberty, but if they become so large that they interfere with breathing some years before puberty, it is seldom wise to allow a child to struggle along for years with this obstruction.

The faucial tonsil also increases greatly in childhood but almost never to the point of mechanically interfering with either breathing or with swallowing. However, this tonsil can encroach on the opening of the eustachian tube, which is very near it. If the eustachian tube is blocked, hearing is interfered with (p. 268); this may be remedied by surgical removal of the tonsils.

While mechanical size of the tonsil can, as in the above situations, cause untoward symptoms, in the vast majority of children large tonsils are a normal phenomenon of childhood and need no treatment.

In addition to hypertrophy of tonsil tissue these organs sometimes become so overwhelmed by their constant battle with infection that they not only do not aid in protecting the respiratory tract from infection but actually feed pathogenic agents into it. Under these circumstances, their removal releases the body of a constant source of infection. Indications for tonsillectomy are a history of frequent sore throats (to be distinguished from frequent colds) or attacks of otitis media, combined with the appearance of the tonsils when no acute infection is present. Overwhelmed tonsils appear dull and cryptic, and exude a foul-smelling pus when pressed with a tongue stick. In addition, the chain of lymph nodes in the cervical area which drain the tonsils remains large and tender after acute infection has subsided. In contrast, while a healthy tonsil may be large, its surface is smooth and glistening, and it does not harbor pus.

BIBLIOGRAPHY

AMER, JULES, ESTHER OTT, FRANK A. IBBOTT, DONOUGH O'BRIAN, and HENRY KEMPE: The Effect of Monthly Gamma Globulin Administration on Morbidity and Mortality from Infection in Premature Infants During the First Year of Life, *Pediatrics,* **32**:4, 1963.

American Academy of Pediatrics: Report of the Committee on Control of Infectious Diseases, 14th ed., Evanston, Ill., 1964.

BOYCOTT, A. E., and C. PRICE-JONES: Experiments on the Influence of Fatigue on Infection, *J. Path. & Bact.,* **29**:87, 1926.

BURNET, F. MACFARLANE: The Pattern of Disease in Childhood, *Australasian Ann. Med.,* **1**:93, 1952.

———: The Immunological Significance of the Thymus, *Australasian Ann. Med.,* **11**:79, 1962.

BURTON, OGDEN C.: Agammaglobulinemia, *Pediatrics,* **9**:722, 1952.

COLLINS, SELWYN D.: Age Incidence of Common Communicable Diseases of Children, *Pub. Health Rep.,* **44**:763, 1929.

CRIEP, LEO H.: "Clinical Immunology and Allergy," Grune & Stratton, Inc., New York, 1962.

CUSHING, JOHN E., and DAN H. CAMPBELL: "Principles of Immunology," McGraw-Hill Book Company, New York, 1957.

EDDS, MAC. V., JR.: "Immunology and Development," The University of Chicago Press, 1958.

EDSALL, GEOFFREY: Passive Immunization, *Pediatrics,* **32**:599, 1963.

FLORMAN, ALFRED L., GERTRUDE H. LAMBERTSON, HELEN ZEPP, EUGENE AINBENDER, and HORACE L. HODES: Relation of 7S and 19S Staphylococcal Hemagglutinating Antibody to Age of Individual, *Pediatrics,* **32**:501, 1963.

GITLIN, DAVID, and JOHN M. CRAIG: The Thymus and Other Lymphoid Tissues in Congenital Agammaglobulinemia, *Pediatrics,* **32**:517, 1963.

———, Gordon Vawter, and John M. Craig: Thymic Alymphoplasia and Congenital Aleukocytosis, *Pediatrics,* **33:**184, 1964.

Good, Robert A.: Immunity and Resistance to Infection in Early Infancy, in S. J. Fomon (ed.), Report of 29th Ross Pediatric Conference, Columbus Ross Laboratories, 1959, p. 13.

———, Richard L. Varco, Joseph A. Aust, and Solomon J. Zak: Transplantation Studies in Patients with Agammaglobulinemia, *Ann. New York Acad. Sc.,* **64:**882, 1957.

Hodes, Horace L.: Should the Premature Infant Receive Gamma Globulin?, *Pediatrics,* **32:**1, 1963.

Osborn, John L., Joseph Dancis, and Juan F. Julia: Studies on the Immunology of the Newborn Infant. 1. Age and Antibody Production, *Pediatrics,* **9:**736, 1952.

Raffel, Sidney: "Immunity," 2d ed., Appleton-Century-Crofts, Inc., New York, 1961.

Rosen, F. S., and C. A. Janeway: Immunological Competence of the Newborn Infant, *Pediatrics,* **33:**159, 1964.

Scammon, Richard E.: The Measurement of the Body in Childhood, in J. A. Harris, C. M. Jackson, D. G. Patterson, and R. E. Scammon (eds.), "The Measurement of Man," The University of Minnesota Press, Ann Arbor, Mich., 1930.

Silverman, Arthur M., E. B. Thornbecke, Keith L. Kramer, and Robert J. Lukes: Fetal Response to Antigenic Stimulus. III. Gamma Globulin Production in Normal and Stimulated Fetal Lambs, *J. Immunol.,* **91:**384, 1963.

Smith, David T., and Norman F. Conant: "Microbiology," 12th ed., Appleton-Century-Crofts, Inc., New York, 1960.

Smith, Margaret H. D.: Active Immunization: Current Considerations, *Pediatrics,* **32:**444, 1963.

Smith, Richard T.: Immunological Tolerance as a Developmental Phenomenon, *Pediatrics,* **34:**14, 1964.

———, and D. V. Eitzman: The Development of the Immune Response, *Pediatrics,* **33:**163, 1964.

———, J. James, and D. V. Eitzman: Production of Type 19S Gamma Globulin Antibody by Neonatal Infants in Response to Typhoid Immunization, *J. Dis. Child.,* **98:**644, 1959.

Thornbecke, G. J., H. A. Gordon, B. Wostman, M. Wagner and J. A. Reyniers: Lymphoid Tissue and Serum Gamma Globulin in Young Germ Free Chickens, *J. Infect. Dis.,* **101:**237, 1957.

Vahlquist, B.: Transfer of Antibodies from Mother to Offspring, *Advances Pediat.,* **10:**305, 1958.

Welch, Henry, C. H. Lewis, H. I. Weinstein, and B. B. Boeckman: Severe Reactions to Antibiotics: A Nationwide Survey, *Antibiot., Med. Clin. Therapy,* **4:**800, 1957.

Werne, Jacob, and Irene Garrow: Sudden Apparently Unexplained Deaths During Infancy, *Am. J. Path.,* **29:**633, 1953.

Section V

LIFE PATTERNS OF SLEEP AND NUTRITION

25

Sleep

The physiology of sleep is not fully understood. A center in the reticular formation is thought to be significant in the states of sleep and wakefulness. This hypothesis gains support from the fact that tumors or inflammatory diseases of this area produce disturbances in the sleep-wakefulness periodicity (Kleitman, 1963; Oswald, 1962).

Arousal stimuli can be afferent stimuli from sensory nerves—a noise, a light, a touch, even an odor (as of something burning)—or they can be proprioceptive—a cramped leg, a full bladder, a pain. They can be emotional stimuli, especially anxiety or stimuli from a dream. The physical intensity of the stimulus is not the factor that causes arousal. One can sleep through the loud banging of a loose shutter but be instantly awake at the sound of footsteps in the front hall. The effectiveness of arousal stimuli varies according to the emotional meaning of the stimuli (Cruden, 1960).

PHYSIOLOGY OF SLEEP

During normal sleep the body appears to rest, and most of the physiologic functions slow down. Muscles relax, the facial expression is peaceful, the skin is flushed and usually warmer than during wakefulness, although the internal body temperature is lower. The metabolic rate is lowered, the pulse slows, the blood pressure drops, the respiratory rate slows, and respirations are deeper. The muscular movements of the gastrointestinal tract are slowed, and its secretions are reduced; formation of urine decreases; secretion of sweat, however, is usually increased. Reflexes are sluggish but are not lost. The sleeper can cough, sneeze, vomit, or scratch an itch without waking up. The sphincter muscles do not relax as do the somatic muscles but remain closed, even in deep sleep, once toilet training has been established.

SLEEP DEPRIVATION

It is, of course, common knowledge that everyone must sleep. After a night's sleep the normal healthy individual awakens refreshed; the feeling of fatigue he had when he went to bed has disappeared. His feelings, however, are subjective; objective data to demonstrate the effects of sleep are difficult to disentangle from data that record other bodily states. Individuals deprived of sleep show their fatigue in derangements of behavior. Morris et al. kept a group of young men awake for periods of 72 to 98 hours and found that as the period of sleep deprivation increased, these young men had increasing degrees of failure both in visual tests and temporal relationships. They also had hallucinations, complained of feelings of depersonalization, were unable to think clearly, and were restless and irritable. These symptoms disappeared after they were permitted to sleep. However, this does not mean that similar symptoms in other people can be cured by sleep. Sleep deprivation is probably but one cause of symptoms similar to those Morris's subjects demonstrated.

NECESSITY OF DREAMING

There is evidence that dreaming is an essential part of normal sleep. Wolpert has shown that brain waves, eye movements, and electroencephalographic potentials in the extremities are correlated with periods of dreaming. Dement found that in a typical night's sleep there are four to five periods of dreaming and that dreaming time constitutes about 20 per cent of normal sleeping time. Dement demonstrated that waking a sleeper every time he started to dream produced symptoms quite different from those produced by waking him the same number of times during nondreaming periods. Dream-deprived subjects showed increasing agitation and anxiety as their sleep was deprived of dreaming. After five nights of such deprivation, Dement's subjects, when allowed to sleep without interruption, made up their lost dream time by dreaming more than during their control baseline period. Not until his subjects made up their lost dream time did their symptoms disappear. Dement concluded that a certain amount of dreaming each night is a necessity. The relation between the symptoms produced by dream deprivation and those produced by sleep deprivation is in the realm of speculation.

OPTIMAL AMOUNT OF SLEEP

There is little objective data on how many hours of sleep any individual needs. Lewis and Masterson permitted a group of men on an expedition to Greenland to sleep as much as they liked, when they liked, over the 2-year period of the expedition. They found that 7.9 hours per man per 24 hours was the average. Eight hours of sleep per twenty-four is frequently quoted as about average for adult man. Variations are considerable. Some people appear to do very well with 5 or 6 hours of sleep per 24 hours; others feel they must have between 9 and 10.

In his study of narcolepsy, Yoss concluded that, under some circumstances, this disease is but an extreme variant of the normal.[1] Yoss suggested that narcoleptics suffer from hypoactivity or perhaps hypoplasia of the reticular activating system and that the disease is probably a genetically determined condition. It is usually present from the time of birth and neither improves nor progresses as age advances. The existence of some individuals with genetically determined hypoactivity of this brain area suggested to Yoss that there might be other individuals with hyperactivity of their reticular systems—people who require less sleep than the average.

The amount of sleep any individual needs must be his own subjective decision. In the case of a child it is the mother who must often make the decision. There is no objective criterion which points specifically to need for more sleep. Symptoms called fatigue—irritability, emotional instability, poor intellectual performance, inadequate weight gain during the growing years—*may* be due to lack of sleep, but may also be due to nutritional inadequacies, physical illness, emotional tension, and perhaps other things. Any or all such symptoms call for a full appraisal. It must be kept in mind that lack of sleep *may* be a significant factor.

The question so frequently asked by a parent, "How many hours should my child sleep?" is quite unanswerable in terms of a specific number of hours. Like the adult, the child should sleep until he is rested.

LIFE PATTERNS IN SLEEP

Although there are differences in the amount of sleep different individuals need, there is a lifetime pattern. Whether an individual is one who needs much or little sleep, he will need more sleep as a child than he will need as an adult (Fig. 25-1).

During childhood the number of hours per day spent sleeping roughly follows the growth increment curve. During the rapid growth of infancy, more sleep is required than during the slow-growth middle years of childhood; at adolescence, concomitantly with the pubertal growth spurt, more sleep is required than during the middle childhood years. Once mature size is reached, adult sleeping patterns become established.

Parmelee found the mean of the number of hours asleep for 75 healthy newborns during the first 3 days of life to be 16.6 hours with a range of 10.5 to 23 hours. By 3 months of age the average sleeping time is reduced by about 2 hours, and by 6 months by another 2 hours with an unbroken 12-hour night and two daytime naps. By 1 year of age, total amount of sleep averages 12 to 14 hours, and the number of daytime naps is often reduced to one. During toddlerhood and the preschool years, the total amount of sleep has dropped to 10 to 13 hours with one daytime nap. Some children, who require less sleep than the average, abandon daytime naps early in

[1] There may be other forms of narcolepsy in which the somnambulance is a seizure equivalent.)

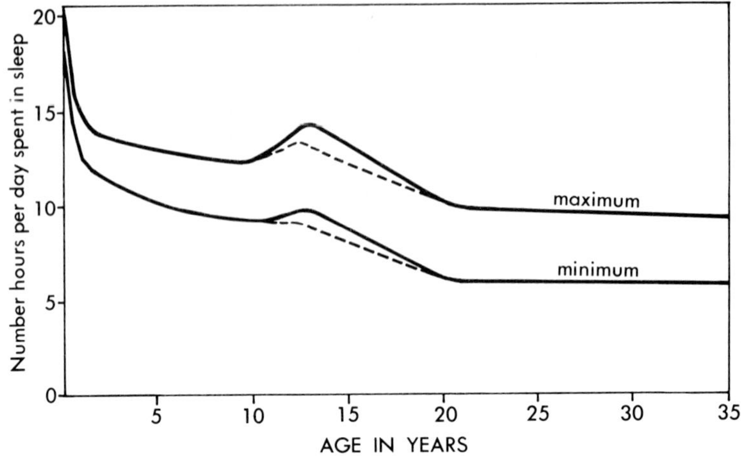

Fig. 25-1. Life patterns in sleep. There is much individual variation at all ages. Except during the pubescent growth spurt, there is little difference attributable to sex.

this period; others may need to continue them up to the beginning of first grade. During the school years daytime naps are abandoned, and an unbroken night's sleep of 9 to 12 hours suffices (Hellbrügge, 1959).

In puberty the need for sleep jumps up. Pubescent boys, whose weight gain is greater than that of girls, may need from 10 to 14 hours of sleep for a year or two; pubescent girls, from 9 to 13 hours. When adulthood is finally reached, the need for sleep declines; the average figure for adults is about 8 hours, though individual needs may be for any amount between 6 and 10 hours. There appears to be no consistent sex variation in amount of sleep needed in adulthood.

Any individual may at times need more sleep than usual. It is common knowledge that unusual physical exertion makes the individual more tired than usual. Dement's data on dreaming tempts the speculation that at certain times the need for additional dreaming may necessitate more sleep.

There are other problems, however, besides the *need* for sleep, which will be taken up below at specific age periods.

Sleep in Early Infancy

Young babies *want* to sleep. When an infant's needs are met, he sleeps. This means *all* his needs—for food, for physical comfort, for warm interpersonal relations.

Occasionally a young infant will cry because he wants sleep, just as he will cry when he wants food or mothering. He does not know what he wants; he has an awareness of an unmet need, so he cries. If he is placed in a comfortable spot, he will go to sleep. Crying a few minutes before sleep is not the same thing as screaming for a prolonged period and then finally falling asleep out of pure exhaustion (Kleitman, 1953).

Young infants sleep at any time during the 24 hours. They wake when they have needs, sleep when all their needs are met. Quite early in life an infant responds to conditioning, and his sleep pattern can be pushed into one that fits the family schedule. A baby who is made comfortable and prepared for bed for the night at roughly the same hour and put into his own crib learns to go to sleep under these conditions. On the other hand the infant who is allowed to go to sleep in a variety of places and at various hours and then later moved to his crib is less likely to associate his crib with sleeping. Likewise, the baby whose crib is used for play periods as well as sleeping is less motivated to go to sleep when laid in his crib.

By about 3 months of age many babies can be conditioned to sleep for a 12-hour stretch at night; others hang on to one night feeding for several months longer.

Even in early infancy individual differences in sleeping patterns become obvious. Some infants sleep soundly immediately after a meal; others feel sociable then and want to sleep only after they have had their fill of companionship as well as food (Fig. 25-2).

In early infancy sleeping problems are related to physical discomfort (especially colic (p. 193)), inadequate or indigestible food, illness, or emotional tensions. They are *not* related to any desire on the part of the infant to stay awake.

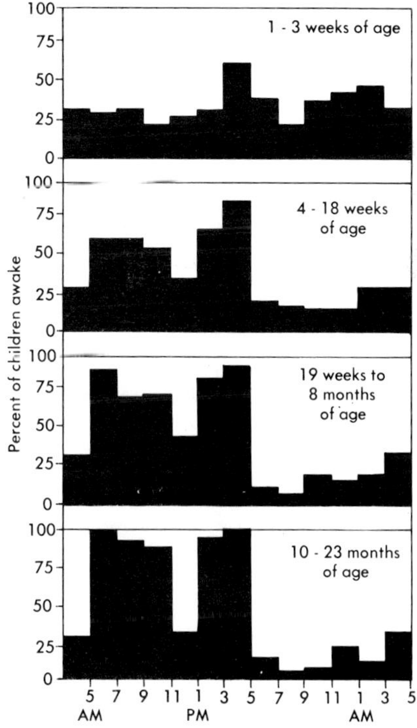

Fig. 25-2. Development of diurnal sleep rhythm in the infant. (*From Helbrügge and Lange, The Characteristics of Childhood Sleep, Med. Klin., 54:946 and 954, 1959.*)

Sleep during the Early Years

There comes a time when a normal, healthy child no longer *wants* sleep as he did when he was an infant. The usual time for the appearance of "sleep fighting" is in toddlerhood, but it may occur earlier. Sleep fighting has two aspects, one a part of normal maturation, the other a manifestation of anxiety. The borderline between normal and abnormal development here, as in many areas, is not clear-cut (Huse, 1960).

As the normal child becomes aware of himself as an independent person, he becomes simultaneously aware of the interesting and exciting things in the world about him. He plays incessantly, not to amuse himself, but to satisfy the unquenchable thirst for knowing (p. 490). A child continues to play even when exhausted. Sleep is an intolerable interruption in his life occupation.

Compare the attitude of an adult and that of a toddler to the question of going to bed. The adult *knows,* intellectually, that he needs sleep. He has had plenty of experience with dragging himself about when his sleep has been short-changed. He anticipates the day ahead of him. The adult goes to his bedroom, undresses, gets ready to retire, opens his window, climbs into bed, turns off the light, and settles himself to sleep.

The toddler, however, does not know he needs sleep; tomorrow is an infinite distance away; his world is made up of *now,* and now he wants to play. This is normal sleep fighting. It comes along in the lives of most children. It takes firm (though gentle) handling. Whether he wants to or not, the child must go to bed at the prescribed time.

Rituals often help. If one thing follows another in a predictable way, the child finds himself in bed: supper, quiet play with Dad, bath, tooth brushing, hair combing, putting on pajamas, pulling down the bedspread, climbing into bed, a story or a song, a goodnight kiss, and, finally, lights out. Sleep is the next item on the agenda, and many little children will peacefully go to sleep; however, there are times when nothing seems to work. The ruses of the little child are many. He wants one more story, he wants a drink of water, he needs to go to the bathroom, he wants a toy to sleep with. But while he will do his best to find reasons for staying awake, nevertheless he needs sleep and will respond to firm, consistent insistence that he stay quietly in bed.

The situation most difficult for the little child to cope with is unpredictability. If sometimes he is allowed to stay up late, sometimes allowed to get up after he is in bed, sometimes yelled at, sometimes cuddled, he feels that if only he can hang on, something more interesting than sleep will happen.

Anxiety creeps into normal sleep fighting. The child finds it scary to be all alone in his bed. If he goes to sleep, will mother be there when he wakes up? Will mother disappear because he cannot see her or feel her? Some anxiety is usual; it is impossible for a child to live so that he feels absolutely safe all the time. He can cope with small amounts of anxiety. Taking a favorite toy or blanket to bed may help (p. 395). A night light helps some children realize that the physical surroundings have not disappeared because he cannot see them. Thumb sucking and rhythmic rocking are comforting habits and help the child accept separation from his mother at bedtime.

There will be times in the lives of normally contented children when bedtime anxiety is greater than at other times. It takes sensitivity on the part of grownups to distinguish anxiety that needs a little extraparental attention from normal reluctance to cease the day's activities. One little fellow, at the end of an exciting day, insisted his mouth was so full of words he could not go to sleep. After an extra time of quiet talk, he finally opened his mouth wide to demonstrate that it was now empty of words and he could go to sleep.

Anxiety or separation may become panic. A child in panic screams, kicks, clutches his mother frantically. Such a child needs comfort and reassurance, not punishment, but he also needs an appraisal of why bedtime separation causes him such agony. Sometimes the answer is not hard to find. Perhaps Mother has been away; perhaps the child has awakened in a strange bed with only a strange grandmother near by, and he is in a panic lest it should happen again. Sometimes a child's panic is due not so much to an experience of physical loss of his mother as to a chronic fear of loss of her love.

Night Terrors and Nightmares

Waking up in the night screaming with fear is also often a manifestation of separation anxiety. Night terrors can occur in children too young to talk. The child probably has some dream, awakens, screams, but almost immediately becomes quiet when he can clutch his mother. A slightly older child may have a similar experience, but, being verbal, he may relate what it was that terrified him. However, regardless of the story he relates, the most basic fear of the little child is fear of loss of his mother. This fear may take many forms in a dream. Night terrors can occur occasionally in the life of any normal child; it is only when they are frequent that they constitute a danger signal.

Television and horror stories are often blamed for children's disturbed sleep. While stories of violence may not be the best intellectual diet for children, it is probable that they cause far fewer nightmares than do harsh punishments, parental indifference, parental separation, or a generally chilly home climate.

Sleep in the Middle Years of Childhood

The school-age child knows he has to go to bed and to sleep. He may not want to, but the exercise of consistent firm and friendly discipline is usually sufficient to produce reasonable conformity. A certain amount of ritual often helps the schoolchild get to bed, although he is far more able than the toddler to accept with equanimity deviations in his routine. A quiet private talk with a parent after he is tucked into bed is often an excellent anodyne for sleep.

The Adolescent and Sleep

With the onset of puberty sleep looms large as a problem in our society. The unvarnished physiologic truth is that an adolescent during the years of rapid growth actually needs more sleep than he did a few years earlier when he was not growing so rapidly.

Sleep constitutes one of the major problems of early adolescence. There is a head-on clash between physiologic needs and our cultural pattern. As children grow up, they want the privileges of their increasing maturity. They want, and should have, the recognition that they are soon to be members of adult society. Sitting up at night is something that adults do, and so the pubescent youth wants to do it, too. The fact that his body needs more sleep than that of a younger brother or sister is certainly not acceptable to him, although it is the physiologic truth.

There is no way of meeting this problem except through understanding. Both child and parents have to understand all the implications of the clash between body needs and cultural needs. The child must understand that he needs more sleep, not because he is a baby, but precisely because he is an adolescent. Nobody wants to keep him a baby—this is quite naturally his interpretation of his parents' efforts to get him to bed at night. An adolescent who really understands this will be far more cooperative in getting to bed on school nights. He does not enjoy being tired, and when he can be relieved of (1) the fear that his parents cannot accept his maturity and (2) the fear that there is something wrong with him because he wants to sleep so much, he will go to bed at a reasonable hour with some degree of inner peace—at least on school nights.

If, combined with early bed through the week, the youngster is permitted to stay up as late as he wants to on weekend nights, he will know that his growing up is acceptable to his parents. But when he does stay up on weekend nights, he needs to sleep late the next morning. The child is usually more than willing to do this. It is the parent who often objects. Many a parent cannot bear to see a big hulking adolescent lolling around in bed until noon on Saturday or Sunday mornings, especially when there is so much work the parent would like to see him do. But when a parent can be made to understand that the sleeping adolescent is working hard on his assignment to grow, he can often come to accept it. Like the enormous appetite at this time of life (p. 381), the need for extra sleep is temporary. It is not a developing permanent pattern of laziness.

An adolescent allowed to sit up late on weekend nights, allowed to sleep in the morning until he is slept out, and then greeted pleasantly and offered a good and plentiful meal is apt to be such a contented and pleasant person that he might even *offer* to scrub the kitchen floor for Mom or cut the lawn for Dad!

BIBLIOGRAPHY

Burns, Charles: Sleep: Physiology, Pathology, and Groups of Therapeutic Agents, *New Zealand M. J.*, **58**:584, 1959.

Cruden, W. V.: Sleep and Wake, *Brit. J. Clin. Pract.*, **14**:475, 1960.

Dement, William: The Effect of Dream Deprivation, *Science*, **131**:1705, 1960.

Hellbrügge, T. H., and J. Lange: The Characteristics of Children's Sleep, *Med. Klin.*, **54**:946, 954, 1959.

Huse, Betty, and Mildred January: Sleep Disturbances in Young Children, *Clin. Proc. Child. Hosp.*, **16**:297, 1960.

Kleitman, Nathaniel, and Theodore G. Engelman: Sleep Characteristics of Infants, *J. Appl. Physiol.*, **6**:269, 1953.

———: "Sleep and Wakefulness," The University of Chicago Press, Chicago, 1963.

Lewis, H. E., and J. P. Masterson: Sleep and Wakefulness in the Arctic, *Lancet*, **1**:1262, 1957.

Morris, Gary O., Harold L. Williams, and Ardie Lubin: Misperception and Disorientation during Sleep Deprivation, *Arch. Gen. Psychiat.*, **2**:247, 1960.

Oswald, Ian: "Sleeping and Waking, Physiology and Psychology," Elsevier Publishing Company, Amsterdam, The Netherlands, 1962.

Parmelee, A. H., Jr.: Sleep Patterns in Infancy. A Study of One Infant from Birth to Eight Months of Age, *Acta Pediat.*, **50**:160, 1961.

———, H. R. Schulz, and M. A. Disbrow: Sleep Patterns of the Newborn, *J. Pediat.*, **58**:241, 1961.

Pavlov, I. P.: Lectures on Conditioned Reflexes, translated by W. H. Gantt, New York International Publishers, 1928.

Wolpert, Edward A.: Studies in Psychophysiology of Dreams, *Arch. Gen. Psychiat.*, **2**:231, 1960.

Yoss, Robert E., and David D. Daly: Narcolepsy, *Med. Clin. North America*, **44**:953, 1960.

26

Nutrition

Adequate food is, of course, essential for good health, but what constitutes adequate food varies as biologic requirements change. The life pattern of food needs is the topic of this chapter.

Food supplies the energy needed to maintain life processes and the raw materials from which body substance is built and maintained. It consists of protein, carbohydrate, and fat as well as vitamins, inorganic elements, and inert ingredients. Water is an essential dietary ingredient. Energy requirements are supplied by the first three substances—protein, carbohydrate, and fat; and body substance is built and maintained from protein, fat, minerals, vitamins, and minimal amounts of carbohydrate.

The amount of food needed increases as the body becomes larger. However, size is not the only criterion. At different times in the life cycle the need for both energy food and building-material food per pound of body weight varies.

SOURCES OF NUTRIENTS

The ultimate source of all energy for life on this planet comes from the sun. Green plants capture sun energy by synthesizing carbohydrates from carbon dioxide and water in the presence of chlorophyll. Plants also use nitrogen from the air and synthesize protein, although most plants manufacture much more carbohydrate than protein. In the process of converting inorganic carbon and nitrogen into carbohydrate, fat, and protein, plants incorporate other inorganic elements, such as sulfur, phosphorus, iron, and copper, into the organic compounds that constitute plant tissue.

No animal can use elemental carbon or nitrogen to manufacture organic compounds as can plants. To a limited extent, most animals can use elemental metals and electrolytes.

Herbivorous animals consume huge quantities of plant material. They use some of it for energy, and from some of it they concentrate enough protein to build their bodies. Carnivorous animals consume herbivorous ones and thus obtain a concentrated supply of protein, fat, and vitamins. Herbivorous animals are equipped with copious gastrointestinal tracts for processing the large volume of food they must consume. Carnivorous animals, on the other hand, have relatively small, short gastrointestinal tracts adequate to cope with their concentrated dietary. A cow could not manage on a carnivorous diet, nor could a wolfhound live by grazing. It is worth noting, in passing, that the carnivorous animal, in a state of nature, always consumes the entrails of his prey. It is in these metabolically active organs that valuable nutrients are concentrated.

Man is an omnivorous animal. His intestinal tract is designed to receive both plant food and animal food. While some individuals, and some human races, do exist on strictly vegetarian diets, it is difficult, though not impossible, to maintain optimal human nutrition without the use of animal products. The human infant, like the young of all mammalian species, lives during the nursing period on a diet consisting entirely of animal products, that is, milk.

In broad outline, man, after weaning, obtains his carbohydrate from vegetable food, much of his protein from animal sources, and his fat from both plants and animals. As long as man consumes food as nature provides it, he obtains not only protein, carbohydrate, and fat but also the accessory substances—vitamins and inorganic elements—accumulated by the biologic processes of the plants and animals he consumes. However, civilized man discovered how to modify natural foods; he learned how to remove the outer covering and the germ of grains and how to refine his sweets. Man has "educated" his taste so that he not only prefers the flavor of milled cereal and refined sweets but has come to prefer muscle meats almost to the exclusion of organ meats.

The science of nutrition can almost be considered an evolutionary adaptation to the human ingenuity of altering natural dietaries. There are two alternatives if civilized man is to maintain buoyant health: he must either return to natural foodstuffs, or he must replace from artificial sources those accessory substances that have been eliminated in the refinement of foods.

Food manufacturers in the United States aware of nutritional needs, have

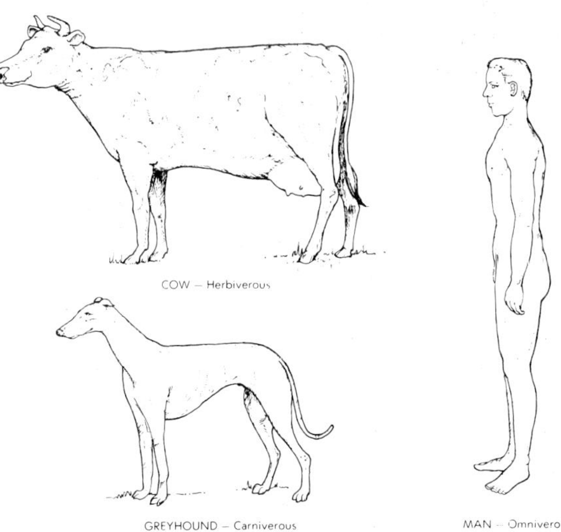

Fig. 26-1. Man is an omnivorous animal. His nutritional needs lie between those of a cow (herbivorous) and a greyhound (carnivorous.)

fortified many of the refined foods with synthetic vitamins and with essential inorganic substances (enriched cereals). They have added to refined foods those substances which either were not present at all or were present in minimal amounts in the natural food (iodized salt, vitamin D milk, bread fortified with milk). It is only the refined sweets which contribute little but calories to the diet. When they are used to excess, recourse must be had to concentrated synthetic vitamins and mineral preparations. Even then the diet containing excessive sweets may be inadequate in protein.

NEEDS FOR ENERGY

Energy is needed for five different purposes in the animal economy. In some of these categories the amount needed per pound of body weight remains more or less constant throughout life; in others it changes as age advances. Energy needs are based on:

1. Basal metabolism. Energy is required to maintain body heat and to carry on the vital functions. Every cell in the body has work to do, and to accomplish this work it must have energy. Gland cells must secrete, muscle cells must contract, kidney cells must excrete. Energy is required to keep the organism alive. The needs for basal energy per pound of body weight are high at birth and gradually decrease to puberty, at which time there is a moderate rise followed by a continuation of the downward trend.

2. Specific dynamic action of food. It costs the body energy to digest and use food. Protein costs more than carbohydrate, which in turn costs more than fat. The energy required to use the food consumed therefore varies with the diet, but on a normal mixed diet it remains relatively constant throughout life.

3. Energy lost in excreta. On an ordinary mixed diet about 10 per cent of the ingested food is lost in the stool. This is largely in the form of fat, but some protein is lost also. In infants this loss may be slightly greater than later in life; nevertheless, the amount of energy that must be supplied to take care of this loss remains more or less constant throughout life.

4. Growth and maintenance. Getting bigger represents work done; it takes energy to grow. The calories needed are in direct relation to the amount of growth. Hence, in early infancy and during puberty the need for calories to supply the energy to grow is greater than during the slow period of middle childhood. After adult stature is finally reached, energy is no longer needed for the purpose of adding new body substance (Fig. 26-2). While growth ceases after mature size is reached, there is, throughout life, a need for calories to repair and maintain tissue. Calories for such maintenance constitute a small part of the total at all ages.

5. Activity. The above energy needs go on night and day, awake or asleep, but in addition to these staying-alive needs, energy is needed to do things.

When energy requirements are added up, it becomes obvious that the amount of food needed per pound of body weight goes down quite steadily from infancy to old age, with the exception of the brief rise during the pubertal growth spurt. As body size increases, the total amount of energy needed daily increases; once adult size is reached, energy tends to decrease slowly as activity becomes less strenuous. Thus the need for energy has a life pattern. Four of the five energy needs (basal, cost, lost in excreta, and growth) might be spoken of as the inherent needs. These needs are roughly similar in all human beings of the same age, size, and sex. The fifth need is the big variable (Mayer, 1961).

Some people hold their muscles, even at rest, tauter than others. They move more and faster, and as children they wiggle more.

These differences in people are individual characteristics; they may be related to body build. Such differences make it difficult to prescribe the total caloric requirement of any individual person, and also account for the fact that one person may be lean and another obese when they consume virtually isocaloric diets.

The animal organism has no excretory process for ridding itself of excess calories as it has for eliminating excess sodium chloride or organic acids. Excess calories result in synthesis of fat, which leads to obesity. The only control is limitation of input. The body does possess a mechanism which alerts to hunger and satiety (p. 366), but when good food is abundant, this biologic mechanism is not always adequate to adjust caloric input to energy needs (Prugh, 1961).

The obese child (or adult) needs fewer calories per pound of body weight than the average child, because some of his pounds are inert adipose tissue which requires fewer calories for maintenance than active tissue.

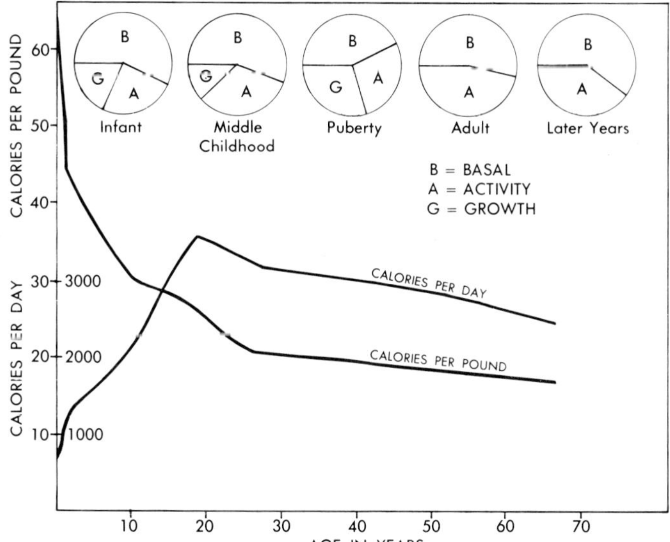

Fig. 26-2. How calories are used through the life span.

Conversely, the malnourished child or adult needs more calories per pound than the average, because more of his pounds are made up of active tissue.

In illness calorie needs change. If the illness is without fever, basal needs remain about the same, but reduced activity decreases total needs. Therefore, in a long-continued afebrile illness, total calories should be reduced, or else considerable excess adipose tissue will be deposited. On the other hand, when fever accompanies an illness, basal needs go up, and the whole body works at a faster rate—the pulse rate increases, the respiratory rate goes up, and more energy is needed to maintain the body economy. Often in illness, in spite of greater need, increased or even normal food cannot be tolerated. The body must live on its own reserves, and weight is lost. This may be true in any illness, but it is especially true in disorders of the gastrointestinal tract. Extra food must be supplied during convalescence to restore the depleted reservoirs.

This points up the fact that any child with fever should be kept as quiet as possible so that he will not burn up what calories he is able to ingest for activity but will preserve them for maintaining his body under the stress and increased load caused by fever. The goal is decreased activity, not bed rest per se. Not infrequently a small child is quieter sitting on the floor playing with his toys than he is fussing and crying in his bed.

PROTEIN

Protein is the mainstay of animal life. Not only does every living cell in the animal body consist of protein, but most of the extracellular fluids, too, contain large amounts of protein. There are thousands of different proteins in the human body, and each serves its own unique function (Burton, 1959).

Proteins consist of huge molecules of the basic units, amino acids. The many proteins achieve their individuality by various combinations and permutations of 22 different amino acids. While the amino acids vary from one to another, they all have in common the presence of the amino group NH_2.

Of the 22 amino acids, nine cannot be synthesized in the human body and must be supplied preformed in the diet. These nine are: histidine, tryptophane, methionine, valine, phenylalanine, tyrosine, lysine, leucine, and isoleucine. The body is capable of building the other 13 amino acids from these nine. Therefore, in planning dietaries one must consider not only the total quantity of protein but also its quality so that the essential amino acids are supplied in adequate amounts. In general, animal protein has a greater biologic value than vegetable protein, and mixtures of proteins are considered superior to a single protein, since a deficiency of one amino acid in one protein is likely to be compensated by its presence in another.

The Food and Agriculture Organization of the United Nations (FAO) has scored dietary proteins according to their amino acid content and established minimum standards of protein intake. More work is needed to determine precisely the optimal pattern of amino acids for human beings at various ages; nevertheless, the standards of the FAO have practical value in determining protein adequacy.

Egg protein is at the top of the list of proteins of high biologic value; it is closely followed by milk protein. These two proteins can furnish all the amino acids essential for optimal nutrition. Meat, fish, and poultry are also high in biologic value. Plant proteins of wheat, corn, rice, beans, and nuts are distinctly lower in biologic values. While most of these proteins contain all the essential amino acids, the amounts of some of them are so low that they cannot supply optimal needs in the human being when any one is the sole source of protein. The human being, not being a herbivorous animal, finds it difficult to consume a large enough quantity of a single plant protein to obtain sufficient amounts of the essential amino acids.

Whenever protein intake is inadequate, skeletal muscle is sacrificed to protect more essential tissues. Growth failure is an early manifestation of protein deficiency in the growing organism. If the deficiency is long-continued, wasting of previously formed tissues takes place, followed by disturbance in fluid balance due to inadequate serum proteins, and edema becomes manifest.

The intestinal mucosa of young infants is more permeable than that of older infants. Occasionally undigested whole proteins instead of amino acids penetrate from the intestine into the bloodstream. When this happens, the foreign protein, circulating in the bloodstream, sets up allergic reactions which can be manifested by symptoms related to the gastro-intestinal tract, the respiratory tract, or the skin (p. 301).

The child needs more protein per pound of body weight than the adult. Part of this protein is needed for growth and part for what Holt et al. call "maturation." The more rapid his growth, the greater is his daily protein need. Thus the premature infant needs more protein per pound than the term infant, and the child in puberty needs more protein than the school-age child (Fig. 26-3). During growth, more nitrogen is consumed than eliminated, and the child is in a state of positive nitrogen balance. After growth has been completed, the organism is maintained in a state of nitrogen equilibrium—as much nitrogen is eliminated as is consumed.

During the period of growth, the amount of nitrogen retained varies, within limits, with the amount of protein in the diet (Holt et al., 1955). That is, the higher the protein intake, the faster the child will grow. There is a limit beyond which this increase in size cannot be pushed, a limit presumably determined by the genes. On high-protein diets both the liver, which must deaminate excess protein, i.e., remove the nitrogen radical from the amino acids and form urea, and the kidney, which must excrete the increased amount of urea, increase in size to take care of their extra load.

In our enthusiasm to push nutrition to its maximum effectiveness, we

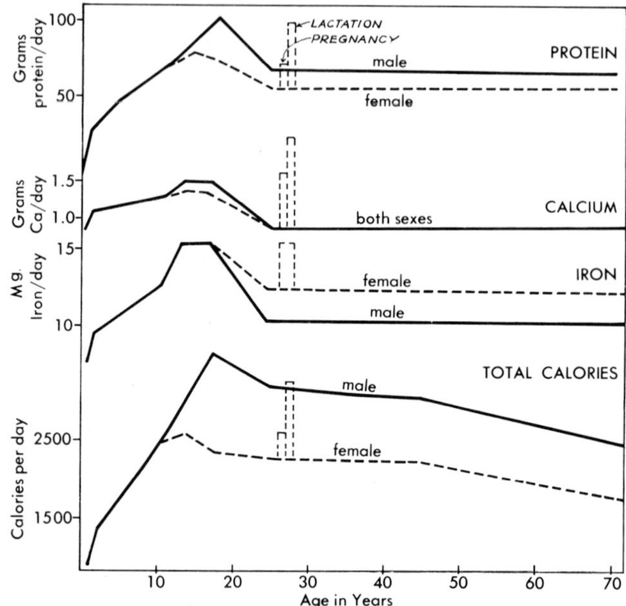

Fig. 26-3. Daily requirements for calories, protein, calcium, and iron throughout the life span for both sexes. (*From Recommended Dietary Allowances, A Report of the Food and Nutrition Board, 6th ed., National Academy of Sciences, National Research Council Publication 1146, Washington, D.C., 1964.*)

must not lose sight of the quite unanswered question: Is faster growth necessarily better? There is some evidence that bigger children, bigger presumably because of high-quality nutrition, are not *ipso facto* healthier (Forbes, 1961). There is also evidence from animal nutrition studies that animals whose growth has been pushed in youth by high-protein diets do not live as long as those permitted to grow at a more leisurely pace (Silberberg and Silberberg, 1955). Maximum and optimum limits of protein intake are not clearly defined at present.

Protein needs cannot be determined without considering the amount of fat and carbohydrates in the diet. Both these food elements are used to supply energy, but if they are deficient, protein is used. Energy needs come first—the organism must stay alive before it can grow. Thus fat and carbohydrates act as protein savers. When they are abundant, all the protein can be used for body-building activities. When they are deficient, the minimum energy requirements must be met before new tissues can be laid down or old tissues repaired and maintained.

On the other hand, if more calories are available than needed for energy requirements and more protein than needed for growth and maintenance, the excess amino acids are deaminized, the nitrogen is excreted as urea, and the rest of the molecules are transformed into glucose and then fat and stored in the adipose depots of the body.

CARBOHYDRATE

Fruits, vegetables, and cereals constitute the source of the majority of carbohydrate food after weaning. The sugar of milk contributes an important source of animal carbohydrate. Glycogen, also an animal carbohydrate, is a minor source of carbohydrate in human dietary.

Lactose

The infant at birth does not possess the ability of the mature individual to digest carbohydrate, because his salivary digestion is skimpy and he lacks pancreatic amylase (p. 187). He is, however, competent to digest and use lactose, the disaccharide of all milks. In fact, the infant is endowed with a greater ability to use lactose than is the more mature individual. Wasserman has demonstrated a high content of the enzyme lactase in the cells of the infant's intestinal mucosa. This enzyme begins to increase before birth, reaches its peak concentration in the early weeks of life, and then decreases until it reaches mature levels soon after weaning.

Not only is the infant able to absorb lactose efficiently, but there is evidence that lactose stimulates the absorption of calcium in some way not presently understood.

On hydrolysis lactose yields glucose and galactose. Lactose is almost the sole source of galactose. The function of galactose is not well understood at present. A rare disease, galactosemia, exists in which the specific enzyme which converts this monosaccharide to glucose is absent. In this disease, galactose accumulates in the tissues and produces a chain of symptoms, chief among which is mental retardation. Platt thinks it is possible that galactose is essential in the synthesis of cerebrosides and that deficiency of galactose in early life might lead to disease in later life involving structural or nervous tissue substance. This hypothesis has some support from animal experiments in which Maier and Longhurst showed that rats reared without lactose were less able to solve a maze than their milk-fed controls. On the other hand, Stanbury et al. deny that galactose has any function in the normal individual other than as a precursor of glucose. Certainly no evidence at present suggests that children allergic to milk protein and raised on soybean milk substitutes free of lactose as well as of cow's milk protein suffer neurologic damage.

FAT

Classified with fats are several groups of compounds, all of which have the common property of being insoluble in water and soluble in the so-called fat solvents (ether, benzine, and others). This group of compounds is referred to as *lipids*.

Lipids significant in nutrition are of several kinds:

Simple fats. Esters of various fatty acids with glycerol.
Waxes. Esters of various fatty acids with alcohols other than glycerol.
Compound lipids. Simple fats in which one unit of fatty acid is replaced by another chemical group. Important in this group are the phospholipids and cholesterol.

The fatty acids vary with respect both to the length of their carbon chains and to the number of double bonds within the carbon chain. Those with no double bonds constitute the saturated fatty acids; those with double bonds, the unsaturated fatty acids. Saturated fats in general have higher melting points than unsaturated ones. Fats, if liquid at room temperature, are referred to as oils.

Sources

Dietary fats are of both vegetable and animal origin. The vegetable fats come from corn, peanut, soy, olive, and cottonseed oil and small amounts of fat in many fruits, vegetables, and grains. Animal fats come from dairy products, eggs, meats, and fish. There are exceptions, but in general vegetable fats are more unsaturated than animal fats. While the saturated fatty acids can be synthesized in the animal body from glucose, some of the unsaturated linkages must be supplied preformed.

Linoleic acid, considered an essential fatty acid, is widely distributed in animal fats and especially in the fat of milk. It is present in some vegetable oils. Cholesterol is an animal sterol and therefore is present only in foods of animal origin. It is, however, not a dietary essential, since it can be synthesized in many tissues in the body. Cholesterol is not used as a source of energy. It is widely distributed in the body, and its functions are multiple. It is used in the syntheses of bile salts, adrenal and sex hormones, and vitamin D in the skin. It also plays a role in the absorption of fatty acids from the intestines and their transportation in the bloodstream. The role of cholesterol in relation to the cardiovascular system is discussed elsewhere (p. 169).

The phospholipids, like cholesterol, are widely distributed in the body and are an essential component of all cells; in addition they play a role in the transportation and utilization of the fatty acids. The phospholipids are not used, as such, as a source of energy, although they constitute a reservoir of fatty acid which can be called upon in times of stress.

Fat is a desirable constituent of the human diet. It is a concentrated source of energy and thus reduces the bulk of the necessary food. Fat is digested hardly at all in the stomach; thus fat-containing meals remain over a long period in the stomach and delay the feeling of hunger. This fact is useful in reducing regimes that call for a normal fat intake. Fat and fat-soluble substances account for much of the taste and smell of food and are needed to make food attractive to the palate. Fat-soluble vitamins are obtained from fatty foods, and the essential unsaturated linkages of linoleic and arachidonic acids are needed for optimal nutrition. The work of Burr and Burr indicates that the human being is dependent upon preformed linoleic acid. Infants deprived of linoleic acid have been shown by Hansen to develop skin disorders which are cured by administration of this fatty acid. As with other dietary ingredients, natural foodstuffs offer greater quantities of the accessory nutritional needs than do highly purified ones.

The human infant's ability to digest, absorb, and utilize dietary fat is not as great as that of the older child and adult. The infant can handle the fat of breast milk adequately, but he often has difficulty with cow's milk fat. The fat of breast milk is highly emulsified; it contains more unsaturated fatty acid than cow's milk (55 per cent against 42 per cent) and a higher concentration of linoleic acid (8.5 per cent against 2.7 per cent). Many manufacturers of the prepared infant formulas on the market take cognizance of this difference in fat between human and cow's milk and substitute an emulsified vegetable oil for butterfat in their preparations. By the time the infant is 3 or 4 months old, he can tolerate cow's milk adequately, although throughout childhood homogenized cow's milk is easier for him to handle than milk with large globules of fat.

VITAMINS

Vitamins are accessory food factors necessary in small amounts for normal tissue metabolism. None of them can be synthesized by the animal body, and therefore they must all be supplied preformed in the diet. Most of the vitamins of the B complex can be synthesized in small quantities by the bacterial flora; this supply, however, is not of significant value, since absorption from the large intestine is limited. With respect to vitamin K, however, this source is significant.

Thirteen vitamins are now known. Each has been isolated in pure crystalline form, and biochemical roles have been identified for almost all. It is customary to divide the vitamins into two major groups, the fat-soluble ones and the water-soluble ones. Fat-soluble vitamins include:

Vitamin A
Vitamin D (calciferol)
Vitamin E (α-tocopherol)
Vitamin K (menadione)

Water-soluble vitamins are those of the B complex and vitamin C.

Vitamins of the B complex:
- Thiamine (vitamin B_1)
- Riboflavin (vitamin B_2)
- Niacin (nicotinic acid)
- Pyridoxine (vitamin B_6)
- Cyanocobalamin (vitamin B_{12})
- Folic acid
- Pantothenic acid
- Biotin

Vitamin C (ascorbic acid)

Fat-soluble Vitamins

Fat-soluble vitamins are ingested and absorbed along with dietary fats; hence any condition which interferes with normal fat digestion tends to interfere with the availability of this group of vitamins. Long-continued diarrhea from any cause, disorders that involve bile or pancreatic secretions, and celiac disease all impede the ability of the body to make use of whatever fat-soluble vitamins are ingested. The frequent use of mineral oil for the relief of constipation also interferes with absorption of fat-soluble vitamins, because these substances dissolve readily in the non-digestible oil and are carried from the body in the feces.

The liver has the capacity to store, to a limited extent, a supply of fat-soluble vitamins. This capacity increases with age as the liver matures. The young infant has virtually no such ability, but the adult can build up a reserve of fat-soluble vitamins that can last him over a period of several months of dietary deprivation.

While digestion and absorption of all the vitamins of this group are roughly similar, each vitamin has a specific metabolic function.

Vitamin A has three main functions: (1) It is essential for the normal metabolism of epithelium. Since epithelium is an essential part of many organs, deprivation of vitamin A results in widespread derangements. (2) Vitamin A plays a role in vision; it is essential for the formation of the visual purple in the retina. (3) Vitamin A is also essential for growth of bone and teeth.

Vitamin D is necessary for normal bone growth and maintenance. It aids in the absorption of calcium and phosphorus from the small intestine and has an action at the site of actual bone formation, possibly that of aiding in the conversion of organic phosphorus to inorganic phosphorus. Vitamin E has been proved to be a human dietary essential, although its precise function is not understood. It is necessary in some animals, notably the rat, for normal function of the germinal epithelium. Vitamin K is essential for the normal clotting of blood.

Dietary Sources

Fat-soluble vitamins are not present in all dietary fats. Since the animal liver concentrates these accessory food factors, it is not surprising that dietary liver offers an excellent source of all the fat-soluble vitamins. Fish liver, especially that of the halibut, has an unusually high concentration of vitamins A and D. This oil was formerly used as a source of these vitamins, but today it has been replaced by synthetic sources.

Vitamin A is present in eggs and whole milk. A precursor of vitamin A, carotene, is present in appreciable amounts in the oil of dark green leafy vegetables, yellow fruits and vegetables, and tomatoes.

Vitamin D is not widely distributed in common foods except liver and eggs. It is also manufactured in the skin of human beings exposed to sunlight. However, the supply of vitamin D in foods other than liver is so skimpy and so subject to variability that this vitamin is most efficiently supplied in concentrated medicinal forms. It must be pointed out, however, that all evaporated milk on the United States market, some fluid milk, and many prepared infant foods are fortified with added vitamin D.

Vitamin E is present in eggs and in the oils of whole grains. Vitamin K is widely distributed in common foods. It is present in green leafy vegetables, whole grains, eggs, and milk. In addition to dietary sources of vitamin K normal bacterial flora synthesize this vitamin.

Water-soluble Vitamins

This group consists of the B complex vitamins and vitamin C. Eight separate entities have to date been identified in what was originally called vitamin B. Gross deficiencies of some of these factors are associated with specific diseases. Lack of thiamine is related to beriberi; lack of niacin, to pellagra. Minor deficiencies of riboflavin result in fissure at the angle of the mouth, glossitis, seborrheic dermatitis, and sometimes photophobia. Lack of B_6 produces symptoms somewhat similar to those due to lack of riboflavin. Folic acid deficiency is associated with anemia. Vitamin B_{12} also plays a role in erythrocyte synthesis and in the metabolism of nervous tissue.

Vitamin C (ascorbic acid) is necessary for normal function of the connective tissue. It is needed for the intercellular matrices in bone, cartilage, teeth, and connective tissue. Walls of the small capillaries are dependent upon ascorbic acid to maintain their integrity. Since wound healing is dependent upon the laying down of a suitable connective tissue matrix in the traumatized tissue, vitamin C plays a role in recovery from local trauma. This vitamin is also thought to be important in the final oxidation of some of the amino acids. Severe deprivation of vitamin C results in scurvy.

All the water-soluble vitamins are absorbed from the gastrointestinal tract and transported to the liver. From the liver they are transported to the necessary tissues. The body has little ability to create a reservoir of any water-soluble vitamins; those supplied in excess of immediate needs are excreted in the urine.

Dietary Sources

While most of these vitamins are widely distributed in natural foodstuffs, many of them are destroyed by heat, sunlight, and oxidation. Because of their solubility in water, they are readily leached out if the food is soaked in water or cooked in a large volume of water.

All the factors of the vitamin B complex have a more or less common source in the normal dietary. Most of them are present in organ meats, lean muscle meat (thiamine is especially high in pork), leafy vegetables, eggs, milk, and whole grains. The milling of cereal removes certain of the B vitamins, especially thiamine. Most of the B group of vitamins are synthesized to a limited extent by the bacterial flora.

Vitamin C is abundant in citrus fruits; it is found in somewhat less concentrated form in melons, tomatoes, cabbage, green peppers, and potatoes.

INORGANIC ELEMENTS

Almost all the inorganic elements listed in the periodic table have been found in the bodies of healthy human beings. However, only 14 are known to be essential for health. These are calcium, phosphorus, magnesium, sodium, potassium, sulfur, chlorine, iron, copper, cobalt, iodine, manganese, zinc, and fluorine.

The inorganic elements are constantly excreted by the human body and therefore must be constantly replenished by the diet. However, there are reservoirs within the body which provide temporary protection against transient deficiency of intake. The extracellular fluids, and to some extent the blood plasma, serve as reservoirs of sodium and chloride, and the intracellular fluids contain potassium, magnesium, and phosphorus. The bones and teeth provide reservoirs of calcium and phosphorus and, to a lesser extent, fluorine; the thyroid contains iodine. in the early months of life the liver contains stores of iron, copper, cobalt, and manganese.

Inorganic elements are ubiquitously supplied in nature, so that only four are of concern from the point of view of normal dietary intake, namely, calcium, iron, iodine, and fluorine.

Calcium

Ninety-nine per cent of the body calcium is present in the bones and teeth. The remaining 1 per cent is in the blood and soft tissues, where it is needed for the clotting of blood, for the normal metabolism of nerve tissue, and for muscle contraction.

Calcium is absorbed in the bowel, and its absorption into the bloodstream is increased by adequate amounts of vitamin D. Calcium is utilized by the bones and teeth at a rapid rate during periods of skeletal growth and to some extent at all ages. It is excreted through the kidney, where the parathyroid hormone regulates the renal threshold for this substance (p. 325), and through the feces. Calcium deficiency is one cause of rickets in children, although vitamin D is also an important factor in this disease.

No deleterious effects have been reported from overabundance of dietary calcium. The serum calcium values do not rise, nor have calcifications of soft tissue been reported.

The most important sources of dietary calcium are milk and other dairy products. Eggs, shellfish, and certain saltwater fish are fair sources of calcium. Soybeans and some of the leafy green vegetables contain appreciable quantities of calcium.

Iron

Iron is essential for the production of hemoglobin, the respiratory protein in the blood, and myoglobin, the respiratory protein in muscles. Iron serves a function also in intracellular energy metabolism by means of the cytochrome enzyme system.

Only about 10 per cent of dietary iron is absorbed from the gastrointestinal tract. Absorption is facilitated by the presence of vitamin C. More of the dietary iron is absorbed if the body is deficient in iron; less, when an abundant supply is present. Iron in the blood, circulating in a complex protein molecule, is absorbed by the bone marrow and used for the synthesis of hemoglobin.

The body conserves a large part of its iron. Nevertheless, small amounts of iron are lost daily in sweat, desquamated epidermis, and feces. The normal adult male loses only approximately 1 mg iron daily and can maintain an iron equilibrium on only 10 mg dietary iron daily (since but 10 per cent of dietary iron is absorbed). Women during their reproductive life lose an additional 10 to 30 mg with each menstrual flow. In the later half of pregnancy the mother contributes 30 to 500 mg iron to the fetus.

Children, in contrast to adults, must build their iron reserves. The daily dietary requirement per pound of body weight is therefore appreciably greater during childhood than during adult life, and the greater the growth rate, the greater the iron requirements. The infant at term has iron in his hemoglobin, iron in the myoglobin in his muscles, and storage iron in his liver.

During the first year of life, storage iron is mobilized to synthesize hemoglobin to keep pace with blood volume, which more than doubles. Dietary iron is necessary to restore iron in the storage depots. The amount of iron in the storage depots of the infant at birth varies greatly. There is a correlation between the weight of the infant and the amount of stored iron, the larger infants having greater stores. However, a more significant factor than weight is the length of time in utero. Premature infants have much less stored iron than term infants. Probably maternal diet is also a factor in the amount of iron deposited in the infant's iron store. If maternal iron is inadequate, most of the available iron is used to manufacture hemoglobin, and little is left over for iron store. Hemoglobin in the blood at birth, therefore, gives but little information concerning the amount of storage iron in the liver. Sturgeon has pointed out that even among normal term infants, whose initial hemoglobin values are approximately equal, there may be as much as a 300 per cent difference in the amount of iron available for hemoglobin synthesis. Thus infants who at birth appear to have adequate hemoglobin levels may become severely anemic during the first year.

Guest found that hemoglobin levels at the end of the first year were significantly higher in firstborn children than in those born after subsequent pregnancies, especially if the pregnancies were closely spaced.

The amount of daily dietary iron needed during the first year of life thus may vary from 0.5 mg per kg to 2 mg per kg. For a 10-kg baby at 1 year this would mean a daily iron intake ranging from 5 to 20 mg. The latter figure is more than twice that of the requirements of an adult male (Table 26-1).

Deficiency in iron leads to hypochromic anemia, in which the circulatory hemoglobin is below optimal levels. The blood is unable to carry a normal amount of oxygen or of carbon dioxide, and as a result the individual tires easily, his muscles are weak, he suffers from dyspnea on exertion, and he often complains of headaches. The child fails to grow at a normal rate. Iron deficiency anemia may result from dietary iron lack. This is relatively uncommon in adult man, though it may develop in children or in women with frequent closely spaced pregnancies. The chance of iron deficiency anemia is, of course, increased if blood is lost by hemorrhage or if intestinal parasites are present. Normal hemoglobin formation is dependent not only upon adequate dietary iron but also upon adequate dietary protein, calories, vitamin C, and the B vitamins.

The dietary sources of iron are highest in liver, eggs, and red muscle meat. Shellfish, legumes, beans, nuts, green vegetables, and whole grains contain fair amounts of iron. Milk is almost devoid of iron.

Iodine

The sole function of iodine in the human being, as far as is known, is the manufacture of thyroglobulin, the active principle of the thyroid hormone. During fetal life, iodine is passed through the placenta, and the fetus combines it with the amino acid tyrosine to manufacture hormones in its own thyroid gland. The human body conserves its iodine supply, but it needs additional iodine to take care of the increase in size. If it receives more than an adequate supply, the excess iodine is eliminated by the healthy body. This element is needed during infancy and childhood; its need jumps up with the pubertal growth spurt and then subsides during adult life. The most spectacular need for iodine is during pregnancy and lactation, when the basic supply for the fetus must be established (Table 26-1). Deficiency of iodine has its most disastrous sequelae during fetal development, because both physical growth and central nervous system maturation are dependent upon the thyroid hormone.

The main natural source of iodine is the sea. Marine food is universally high in iodine, and coastal areas, enriched by iodine-containing rain, produce vegetation with fair amounts of iodine. As noted in Chap. 20, in the

TABLE 26-1

Recommended Daily Dietary Allowances—Age and Sex Trends

Age, yr	Calories	Protein, Gm	Calcium, Gm	Iron, mg	Vitamin A, I.U.	Vitamin D, I.U.	Thiamine, mg	Riboflavin, mg	Niacin, equiv. mg	Ascorbic acid, mg
Both sexes										
0–1	kg × 115 ± 15	kg × 2.5 ± 0.5	0.7	kg × 1.0	1,500	400	0.4	0.6	6	30
1–3	1,300	32	0.8	8	2,000	400	0.5	0.8	9	40
3–6	1,600	40	0.8	10	2,500	400	0.6	1.0	11	50
6–9	2,100	52	0.8	12	3,500	400	0.8	1.3	14	60
Male										
9–12	2,400	60	1.1	15	4,500	400	1.0	1.4	16	70
12–15	3,000	75	1.4	15	5,000	400	1.2	1.8	20	80
15–18	3,400	85	1.4	15	5,000	400	1.4	2.0	22	80
18–35	2,900	70	0.8	10	5,000		1.2	1.7	19	70
35–55	2,600	70	0.8	10	5,000		1.0	1.6	17	70
55–75	2,200	70	0.8	10	5,000		0.9	1.3	15	70
Female										
9–12	2,200	55	1.1	15	4,500	400	0.9	1.3	15	80
12–15	2,500	62	1.3	15	5,000	400	1.0	1.5	17	80
15–18	2,300	58	1.3	15	5,000	400	0.9	1.3	15	70
18–35	2,100	58	0.8	15	5,000		0.8	1.3	14	70
35–55	1,900	58	0.8	15	5,000		0.8	1.2	13	70
55–75	1,600	58	0.8	10	5,000		0.8	1.2	13	70
Pregnant 2nd & 3rd trimester	+200	+20	+0.5	+5	+1,000	400	+0.2	+0.3	+3	+30
Lactating	+1,000	+40	+0.5	+5	+3,000	400	+0.4	+0.6	+7	+30

SOURCE: "Recommended Dietary Allowances," National Research Council Publication 1146, 6th ed., 1964.

United States the use of iodized salt has almost eliminated iodine deficiency disease. Commercially iodized salt contains 0.01 per cent of potassium iodide. Assuming an average consumption of roughly 60 Gm salt per day, an iodine intake of 0.48 mg, which is ample even during pregnancy and lactation, is assured. In iodine-poor areas the main source of this element comes from iodized salt, and restriction of salt intake during pregnancy may deprive the fetus of an adequate supply.

Fluorine

Fluorine is present in the bony skeleton and in the teeth. It has been shown that fluorine has a specific effect on the teeth. When small amounts of fluorine are ingested, the teeth are much more resistant to caries than when this substance is absent. The exact mechanism of this action is unknown, but the presence of fluorine apparently reduces the solubility of the enamel in the products of bacterial action normally present in the mouth. Small amounts of fluorine are effective; larger amounts, while not deleterious, nevertheless produce a cosmetically undesirable mottling of the enamel.

Fluorine is distributed widely but in very uneven amounts in nature. Water normally contains traces of fluorine, but in some areas, where drinking water seeps through rocks and soil with a high fluorine content, the water may contain excessive amounts of fluorine. On the other hand, drinking water may be almost devoid of fluorine. Aside from water, the most significant human source of fluorine is sea food and vegetables grown in fluorine-rich areas (Schelsinger, 1963; Zipkin, 1961).

In some areas of the United States where drinking water is low in fluorine, sodium fluoride has been added to municipal water supplies in such amounts that the total fluorine in the water is 1 ppm. This amount contributes roughly 1.0 to 1.5 ppm to the diet of the average adult and 0.4 to 1.1 ppm to that of children. This amount, if ingested by the mother throughout pregnancy when the fetus is forming his deciduous teeth and by the child throughout the early years when permanent teeth are forming, has resulted in marked reduction in dental caries without any deleterious side effects (Shaw et al., 1961; Tank and Starvick, 1961; Paynter, 1961).

Table 26-2 and Fig. 26-2 summarize the trends of nutritional needs throughout the life span. A few of the following generalizations are so obvious as to be clichés; a few others are somewhat more subtle.

1. The need for all nutrients, except vitamin D, increases as the body increases in size.

   a. Women during their reproductive life (not considering pregnancy) need more iron than men because of the periodic loss of iron in the menstrual blood.

   b. Children in puberty need more of all nutrients than adults, even

TABLE 26-2

Three Meals a Day for All Ages

	6 mo–12 mo	Childhood	Puberty	Adult	Pregnant woman	Lactating woman	Middle-age and more
Breakfast	Fruit[a] Cereal Egg yolk Milk	Fruit[b] Cereal[c] or Egg[d] Toast Milk	Fruit[b] Cereal[c] Eggs[d] Bacon Toast Milk[e]	Fruit[b] Eggs[d] Toast Coffee	Fruit[b] Cereal[c] Eggs[d] Bacon Toast Milk[e] Coffee	Fruit[b] Cereal[c] Eggs[d] Bacon Toast Milk[e] Coffee	Fruit[b] Egg[d] Coffee
Mid A.M.	Juice	Juice					
Lunch	Meat[a] Vegetable[a] Milk	Soup or Vegetable Salad or Sandwich[c] Milk	Meat[f] Vegetable[g] Salad Bread and butter[c] Fruit Milk[e]	Soup or Salad or Sandwich[c] Milk[e]	Meat[f] Vegetable[g] Salad Bread and butter[c] Fruit Milk[e]	Meat[f] Vegetable[g] Salad Bread and butter[c] Fruit Milk[e]	Salad Milk[e] Coffee
Mid P.M. or after school	Juice	Juice Fruit	Cheese or Deviled egg or Cold meat Fruit Cookie Milk[e]	— —	Milk[e]	Milk[e]	Tea
Dinner	Fruit[a] Cereal[a] Milk	Meat[f] Vegetable[g] Salad Milk or fruit dessert Milk[e]	Meat[f] Vegetable[g] Vegetable[g] Salad Bread and butter[c] Milk or fruit dessert Milk[e]	Meat[f] Vegetable[g] Salad Fruit Coffee	Meat[f] Vegetable[g] Vegetable[g] Salad Bread and butter[c] Milk or fruit dessert Milk[e] Coffee	Meat[f] Vegetable[g] Vegetable[g] Salad Bread and butter[c] Milk or fruit dessert Milk[e] Coffee	Meat[f] Vegetable[g] Salad Fruit Coffee
Bedtime snack	—	—	Milk[e] Cookie			Milk[e]	

[a] Pureed foods.

[b] Fruit high in vitamin C—citrus or citrus juice, berries, melons in season.

[c] Cereals, breads, or muffins made from whole grain or enriched grains. Pancakes or waffles may be substituted for cereal but should be served with applesauce or other fruit, not with syrup.

[d] One or two eggs, depending upon size and appetite. When calories need to be restricted, eggs should be boiled or poached and eaten without added butter.

During times of nutritional stress, bacon or ham can be included with eggs.

When eggs become tiresome to the palate, other protein food can be served for breakfast—chipped beef on toast, creamed codfish, French toast, cheese, or even a hamburger (especially for the teen-ager).

[e] When calories need to be restricted, skim milk can be substituted for whole milk.

[f] Meat or other high protein food—fish, poultry, cheese, eggs. Liver, kidney, or other glandular meats should be used once a week. Shellfish or other marine fish are a good addition.

[g] Vegetables should be of many kinds—roots, legumes, leafy, seeds, green and yellow varieties.

NOTE: Tea and coffee can be used as desired after puberty.

Meats, vegetables, cheese, rice, noodles, and spaghetti may be combined in many ways in stews, soups, casseroles, salads.

Size of portion and number of portions will vary with size of appetite and caloric needs.

though of the same size. Here growth rather than size is the determining factor.

2. The larger the body, the greater the need for calories. Exceptions:

   a. Active people need more calories than sedentary people of the same size. They need but minimal additional amounts of other dietary essentials.

   b. Older people need fewer calories than younger people. The need for total calories decreases as people slow down with the increasing years; however, the need for almost all other nutrients used for maintenance remains relatively constant during all the adult years.

3. Growth calls for all nutrients. A healthy body cannot be built unless all its nutritional needs are met. The infant has limited capacity to store essential nutrients and therefore must have an adequate supply on a day-to-day basis. As maturity advances, storage capacity, especially in the liver, becomes greater, so that older children are better able than infants to withstand brief periods of nutritional deprivation.

4. Pregnancy is the most crucial of all times from the nutritional point of view. During fetal life the child's body must be built up from scratch, and in general this is accomplished by means of the nutrients in the mother's diet. If the mother's intake of essential nutrients is insufficient for both her needs and those of her unborn child, more often than not it is the fetus who suffers. A glance at Fig. 26-3 indicates the rather spectacular increase in almost all nutrients needed for optimal fetal development.

The pregnant woman's need for additional nutrients is a qualitative one. She needs more of specific foods, not just more total food. While her caloric need does go up, it is undesirable for her to consume so many more calories that she gains excessive weight. It has been demonstrated that the toxemias of pregnancy, and especially eclampsia, are more frequent in obese women than in those with a normal weight. Women in the United States, normally a weight-conscious group, have been so terrorized at the prospect of gaining excessively during pregnancy that it is not infrequent to see a pregnant woman try to maintain herself on a diet not only low in calories but inadequate in nutriments needed by the fetus for optimal development.

Diet during pregnancy needs careful professional supervision. Total calories should be so adjusted that a gain of not more than 15 to 25 lb is permitted. At the same time protein, calcium, iron, iodine, and vitamins need to be increased.

Failure to achieve optimal diets during pregnancy has been correlated with fetal aberrations. If failures are considerable, stillbirth, premature births, and gross abnormalities result (p. 63). Minimal deficiencies probably are related to the birth of infants poorly equipped for life—inadequate iron stores, poorly calcified bones, and muscles with poor tone.

5. Lactation, like pregnancy, requires additional nutriments. The needs for protein, calcium, vitamins, and calories increase. Inadequate breast milk results from failure to supply the dietary essentials for lactation.

DIETS AT ALL AGES

For the first 2 to 3 months of life an adequate diet consists entirely of milk, with the addition of vitamins (see below). Ideally the milk should be breast milk, although one of the many modified infant foods on the United States market can supply adequate nutrition (Table 26-3). After this age additional foods are needed, the chief of which is iron, and often added calories. They can be given in the form of iron-enriched cereals and egg yolk (p. 304 for diets for potentially allergic infants). Milk, both human and bovine, has a precarious supply of vitamins A, D, and C. It is nutritionally sound practice to supplement the diet of infants with a concentrated source of these three vitamins.

By 4 to 6 months of age, the infant can be given a general mixed diet to which pureed fruits, vegetables, and meats are added to the cereal and egg yolk he is already receiving. Milk is still the main source of his nutriments.

From 6 months on through life an optimal diet consists of foods selected from each of the major groups of foodstuffs with quantities adjusted to individual size and growth needs (Table 26-2).

When food is supplied by natural foodstuffs, it is virtually impossible for an individual to obtain an excess of any nutrient (with the exception of fluorine), although it is possible for him to obtain an overabundance of total calories. Nutrients are never in such excessive quantities in natural foodstuffs as to cause toxic symptoms. Diets can be so ill-chosen even from natural foodstuffs or consumed in such large quantities that excessive calories are taken.

In the United States today the diets of infants are usually good, nutritionally speaking. Most infants are fed the prepared infant foods manufactured by a nutrition-conscious industry. Cereals are enriched, and fruits and vegetables are prepared by techniques that preserve almost all the original minerals and vitamins.

However, once the infant graduates to "table food" and has access to the refrigerator and the pantry, his nutrition may suffer. While there are an enormous number of delectable and nutritious foods on the market, so are there an even greater number of tasty, sweet, and rich foods that contribute almost nothing but calories. The little child who munches between meals on cookies, candies, and cakes washed down with sweet drinks has little desire for meat, vegetables, eggs, and milk at his meals.

Another factor militates against optimal nutrition even in our abundance. Cooking techniques can destroy the thermolabile and oxidation-sensitive

TABLE 26-3

Composition of Various Prepared Infant Foods[f]

	% Protein	% Fat	% Carbohydrate	Vitamin A, units/qt	Vitamin D, units/qt	Vitamin C, mg/qt	Vitamin B_1 mg/qt	Niacin	Riboflavin	B_6, mg/qt	Iron, mg/qt	CA : P ratio
Human milk	1.25	3.5 Human	7.0 Lactose	1,750	0	30	0	5	0.4	0.1	trace	2.2-1
Cow's milk	3.3[g]	3.7 Butter	4.8 Lactose	1,100	0	0	0.4	8	1.5	0.4	trace	1.3-1
Baker's Modified Milk	2.2[g]	3.3 Coconut Corn	7.0 Lactose Glucose Maltose Dextrine	2,500	800	50	0.6	10	1.0	0.4	7.5	1.3-1
Bremil (Borden)	1.5[g]	3.5 Palm Coconut Peanut	7.0 Lactose	2,500	800	50	0.4	9	1.0	0.4	0[a]	1.5-1
Carnalac (Carnation Co.)	2.8[g]	3.2 Butter	7.1 Lactose	950	400	0	0.3	6	1.3	. . .	0	1.3-1
Enfamil (Mead Johnson	1.5[g]	3.7 Oleo Corn Coconut	7.0 Lactose	1,500	400	50	0.4	7.5	1.0	0.3	trace[b]	1.3-4
Lactum (Mead Johnson)	2.7[g]	2.8 Butter	7.8 Lactose Maltose Dextrins	800	500	0	0.3	6	1.2	. . .	0	1.3-1
Modilac (Gerbers)	2.0[g]	2.6 Corn	7.7 Lactose Glucose Maltose Dextrins	3,000	600	45	0.55	5	1.0	0.7	0	1.3-1
Olac (Mead Johnson)	3.4[g]	2.7 Corn	7.5 Lactose Maltose Dextrins	2,500	400	0	0.4	7	1.5	. . .	0	
Similae (Ross Lab)	1.7[g]	3.4 Butter Olive Coconut Corn	6.6 Lactose	2,500	400	50	0.65	4	1.0	. . .	0[c]	1.3-1

S.M.A. (Wyeth)	1.5[g]	3.6 Oleo Corn Soy Coconut	7.2 Lactose	2,500	400	50	0.67	8	1.0	0.4	5	1.3-1
Mulsoy (Borden)	3.1[h]	3.6 Soy	5.2 Soy Starch Dextrins Maltose Glucose Sucrose	2,000[d]	400	30[d]	...	...	...	...	5[d]	
Sobee (Mead Johnson)	3.2[h]	2.6 Soy Coconut	7.7 Soy Starch Maltose Dextrins Sucrose	2,500	400	0	...	...	...	...	0[d]	
Soyalac (Loma-Linda)	2.0[h]	4.0 Soy	6.0 Soy Starch Glucose Maltose Sucrose Dextrins	2,500[e]	400[e]	0	...	...	...	...	10[e]	

[a] Powdered Bremil contains 8 mg iron per quart. Liquid Bremil contains no iron.
[b] Enfamil with iron contains 18 mg iron per quart.
[c] Similac with iron contains 12 mg iron per quart.
[d] Powdered Mulsoy contains no vitamins or iron. Liquid Mulsoy contains Vitamin D and iron.
[e] Powdered Soyalac contains no vitamins. Liquid Soyalac contains Vitamin D and iron.
[f] All of these foods in normal dilution contain 20 Cal per oz.
[g] Cow's milk protein.
[h] Soybean protein.

accessory factors; washing, soaking, and boiling in large quantities of water can leach out water-soluble nutrients, which, if poured down the sink, do not contribute to optimal nutrition.

The menus suggested in Table 26-2 provide optimal nutriment at all ages—the kind of nutrition that contributes to buoyant well-being. In the United States, the land of abundance, nutritionally good foods are available and are within financial reach of the vast majority of the population. Nevertheless, as a nation, we are not free from health problems that could be improved by better nutrition. Frank deficiency diseases are seldom seen here, as they are in less fortunate parts of the world, but poor nutrition is frequent. Fatigue and irritability due to low hemoglobin, inadequate calcium, or poor protein are seen at all ages; overweight has become a national problem; chronic constipation and dental caries unnecessarily detract from health. Education in nutrition is mandatory—education for the mothers who plan the menus and education of the palates of children so that they enjoy food that is good for them all life long.

From the basic menus, selections can be made to provide for individual needs. Caloric intake can be varied by proper selection. If calories need to be kept low, milks should be skimmed instead of whole, lean meats and fish selected, low-calorie vegetables and fruits used, and fat consumed sparingly. Cooking should be with very little added fat, fruits eaten without cream or sugar. If calories need to be increased, the above selections are reversed, and, in addition, moderate amounts of pastry and sweet breads can be added (Wohl, 1960).

Optimal diets are expensive, but intelligent selection can greatly reduce the cost. Organ meats, such as liver, kidney, tripe, and heart, are not only less expensive than muscle meat but more nutritious. Inexpensive cuts of meat provide as much nutriment as filet mignon at a quarter of the price. Fish, cheese, eggs, and poultry can replace meat for less money and at no nutritional sacrifice. Careful buying of vegetables and fruits—fresh, canned, or frozen—can reduce costs. Good cooking, with an imaginative and subtle use of herbs, can make the most inexpensive food delectable and, at the same time, preserve its nutritional value. Good food, attractively served, helps convert eating into dining (Chap. 28).

Food bills can be reduced and nutrition improved by avoiding expensive pastries, bottled sweet drinks, and candy. When adequate amounts of nutritious food are consumed, money need not be spent for expensive vitamin concentrates.

BIBLIOGRAPHY

Bacigalupo, F. A., J. R. Couch, and P. B. Pearson: Effects of Sucrose, Lactose, Galactose and Fructose on Fecal Excretion of Biotin, Riboflavin and PGA in Mature Cotton Rat, *Am. J. Physiol.*, **162**:131, 1950.

Boothby, Walter M.: Basal Metabolism, *Physiol. Rev.*, **4**:69, 1924.

BURKE, B. S., R. B. REED, A. S. VAN DER BERG, and H. C. STUART: Caloric and Protein Intake of Children between 1 and 18 Years of Age, *Pediatrics*, **24**, supp. 5, 1959.

BURR, GEORGE R., and MILDRED M. BURR: A New Deficiency Disease Produced by the Rigid Exclusion of Fat from the Diet, *J. Biol. Chem.*, **82**:345, 1929.

———: On the Nature and Role of the Fatty Acids Essential in Nutrition, *J. Biol. Chem.*, **86**:587, 1930.

BURTON, BENJAMIN T. (ed.): "The Heinz Handbook of Nutrition," McGraw-Hill Book Company, New York, 1959.

"Evaluation of Protein Nutrition," National Academy of Sciences, National Research Council, Publication #711, Washington, D.C., 1959.

FORBES, GILBERT B.: Overnutrition for the Child: Blessing or Curse? *Nutrition Rev.*, **15**:193, 1957.

———: Symposium on Overnutrition, *J. Clin. Nutrition*, **9**:525, 1961.

GUEST, GEORGE M.: Hypoferric Anemia in Infancy in Symposium on Nutrition, vol. 1, "Nutritional Anemia," The Robert Gould Research Foundation, Inc., Cincinnati, 1947.

HANSEN, ARILD E., and HILDA WEISE: Tissue Lipids in Child with Chylous Ascites Maintained on Low Fat Diet, *Fed. Proc. Fed. Amer. Soc. Exp. Biol.*, **5**:233, 1946.

———, HILDE WEISE, A. N. BOCLSCHE, MARY E. HAGGARD, D. J. D. ADAM, and HELEN DAVIS: Role of Linoleic Acid in Infant Nutrition, *Pediatrics*, (Supp.), **31**:171, 1963.

HOLT, L. EMMETT, JR., PAUL GYÖRGY, EDWARD L. PRATT, SELMA E. SNYDERMAN, and WILLIAM M. WALLACE: "Protein and Amino Acid Requirements in Early Life," New York University Press, New York, 1960.

MAIER, NORMAN R. F., and JOAN U. LONGHURST: The Effect of Lactose-free Diet on Problem-solving Behavior in Rats, *J. Comp. Physiol. Psychol.*, **43**:375, 1950.

MAYER, JEAN: Obesity: Physiologic Considerations, *J. Clin. Nutrition*, **9**:530, 1961.

PAYNTER, KENNETH J., and ROBERT M. GRAINGER: Influence of Nutrition and Genetics on Morphology and Carias Susceptibility, *J.A.M.A.*, **177**:306, 1961.

PLATT, B. S.: Human Nutrition and the Sophistication of Foods and Feeding Habits, *Brit. M. J.*, **1**:179, 1955.

"Protein Requirements," F.A.O. Nutritional Studies, no. 16, Food and Agriculture Organization of the UN, Rome, 1957.

PRUGH, DANA E.: Some Psychologic Considerations Concerned with the Problem of Overnutrition, *J. Clin. Nutrition*, **9**:538, 1961.

"Recommended Dietary Allowances," 6th rev. ed., 1146 National Academy of Sciences, National Research Council, publication 1140, Washington, D.C., 1964.

SCHELSINGER, EDWARD R.: Dental Caries and the Pediatrician, *Am. J. Dis. Child.*, **105**:1, 1963.

SHAW, JAMES H.: Symposium on Nutrition in Tooth Formation and Dental Caries, *J.A.M.A.*, **177**:304, 1961.

SILBERBERG, MARTIN, and RUTH SILBERBERG: Diet and Life Span, *Physiol., Rev.*, **35**:347, 1955.

STANBURY, JOHN B., JAMES B. WYNGAARDEN, and DONALD S. FREDERICKSON:

"The Metabolic Basis of Inherited Disease," McGraw-Hill Book Company, New York, 1960.

STURGEON, PHILLIP: Iron Metabolism. A Review with Special Consideration of Iron Requirements During Normal Infancy, *Pediatrics*, **18**:267, 1956.

TALBOT, FRITZ B.: Basal Metabolism in Children, *Physiol., Rev.*, **5**:477, 1925.

TANK, GERTRUDE, and CLARA A. STARVICK: Dental Caries—Experience of School Children in Corvallis, Oregon, after 7 Years of Fluoridation of Water, *J. Pediat.*, **58**:528, 1961.

WALLERSTEIN, RALPH O., and STACY R. METTIER: "Iron in Clinical Medicine," University of California Press, Berkeley, 1959.

WASSERMANN, R. H., and F. W. LENGEMAN: Further Observations on Lactose Stimulation of Gastrointestinal Absorption of Calcium and Strontium in the Rat, *J. Nutrition*, **70**:377, 1960.

WOHL, MICHAEL G., and ROBERT S. GOODHART: "Modern Nutrition in Health and Disease," Lea & Febiger, Philadelphia, 1960.

ZIPKIN, ISADORE: Chemical Agents Affecting Experimental Caries, *J.A.M.A.*, **177**:310, 1961.

Section VI

DEVELOPMENT OF BEHAVIOR

27

On Being Human

MAN'S PLACE IN EVOLUTION

Human beings share with the rest of the animal kingdom an integrated system of organs which must work smoothly together to maintain life. Human beings, like other animals, move about, breathe, eat, urinate, defecate, sweat, and procreate their kind. They also smell, taste, feel, look, and listen. Human bodies function in more or less the same ways as those of other species.

A brief backward glance helps to establish the human species in the hierarchy of living things on this planet. Evolutionary principles are overwhelmingly demonstrated in organic structure. From the single-cell organism which emerged from the primordial ooze, the march of events has been toward greater complexity and specialization of structure. Millions, probably trillions, of modifications have appeared through haphazard mutations, and only those forms have survived whose structural alterations gave the animal an edge over his peers. Countless millions of forms have appeared for an evolutionary moment, only to disappear because of their inability to compete in the relentless struggle to maintain themselves and their progeny. Once a species evolved a refinement that aided its survival, development pushed ahead in that direction. The huge variety of animal organisms in the world today gives ample evidence that survival can be achieved in a multitude of ways.

The human being has emerged from the group that took the path of rearing its young, in the earliest stages of development, within the maternal organism. Many of the bodily processes of man are virtually identical with those of other mammals. The breathing mechanism, for example, is essentially no different in a human being, in a cat, or in an elephant. The process is under reflex and hormonal control and goes on night and day for the duration of life. It speeds up with physical exertion, with anger, with fear; it slows down during sleep. Once this mechanism was discovered in evolutionary progression, it remained, with only minor refinements, in subsequently developed mammals. Likewise, digestion, circulation of the blood, formation of urine, and many other bodily activities are essentially the same in man and in other mammalian species.

Survival, however, depends not only upon a system of organs capable of assuring the maintenance of the animal, both as an individual and as a progenitor of his species, but also upon a coordinated system of behavior which achieves the potential inherent in the structure. No matter how fleet of foot an animal may be, unless he runs away at the approach of danger, he will be devoured by his enemy. He has to *act* as well as possess the structure capable of performing the act (Kubie, 1948).

Throughout evolution, behavior, as well as structure, is built into the organism and transmitted from generation to generation in the genes. Such predetermined behavior is called *instinct.* In simple forms virtually all behavior is instinctive; nothing is left to the whim of the animal. He survives, or he fails to survive, as a species, because his genes determine not only structure and function but also behavior—all of which are in balance with his environment.

The animal acts as he does because he is made that way. However, as the evolutionary scale is mounted, instinctive patterns become capable of some modification. The animal still possesses the urge to maintain himself, but he becomes capable of choosing one method of behavior over another. He learns through experience which actions are most useful to him (Beach, 1955).

Learning necessitates the making of a choice and is dependent upon a nervous mechanism that provides the possibility of alternative pathways. Halstead and also Renech have shown that the larger the percentage of nervous tissue in the total organism, the greater is the ability of the animal to find a variety of ways of responding. The basic instincts provide the motive force, but the specific action resulting from the instinctive push is of increasing variety as the evolutionary ladder is mounted.

However, it is to be noted that only certain functions are alterable by learning. The workings of the viscera remain in man, as in lower species, under control of autonomic mechanisms. Man does not *learn* how to produce urine, how to breathe, how to digest his food. These acts are carried on in man, as they are in lower species, without conscious control. Man does, however, learn how to manipulate his voluntary musculature, not only the muscles which move his body in space, but also the muscles around his excretory sphincters, the muscles of his vocal apparatus, the muscles that move his eyes. He is able to exercise a choice in performing many acts—a choice which depends upon impulses generated in his higher cerebral centers. The ability to make choices has contributed to the quality of humanness. Man shares his structures, his functions and his instinctive drives with his evolutionary ancestors, but, unlike lower forms, man has broken away from much of his inborn patterned behavior, and his instincts have become to a great extent only a motive power which each individual human being must channel in ways characteristic of himself. There are indications of this breaking away from gene-directed behavior in lower forms, but in man the break is sufficient to have produced changes so great that they appear as new qualities of life. Man has broken the sound barrier, as it were, and, having freed himself from automatic behavior, he has become human (Washburn, 1958).

THE QUALITIES OF HUMANNESS

What are the qualities that separate man from even his closest simian relatives—his species characteristics which set him apart, not only from his evolutionary predecessors, but from all other forms of life on the planet?

First is man's ability to comprehend himself as a unique entity in the universe. Man develops self-awareness. He has come to understand that within his own skin he is something different and apart from all else. He has a personal identity. He knows who he is. No mouse knows he is a mouse. Lower species fuse with their surroundings. For an animal, the environment has meaning only as it relates to him; only as it is useful or dangerous to him does the world have existence. Man, having become aware of the unique core within him, has simultaneously come to appreciate the essential corollary—the world about him exists apart from himself. Some aspects of the world may be useful or dangerous; some may have no bearing on him, but they nevertheless exist. Not only things but people have an existence apart from him. As man understands the *I* within him, he also understands the *you* within another person. Each little human capsule of individuality lives his life among other equally unique capsules.

Man's ability to understand his own separate and unique existence and its corollary, the independent existence of external reality, confers on him alone, among all animal species, the capacity to appreciate the esthetic quality of a sunset, grief in a stranger, or the binomial theorem.

However, humanness has its hazards as well as its assets. Man not only has the capacity of knowing "Who and what am I," but he must achieve some degree of satisfaction with his own identity. A dog does not worry about whether he is good or bad, strong or weak, worthwhile or useless, but a man, if he is to live successfully as a human being, not only must know *who* he is but must be able to accept that *who* as a person worthy of a place on the planet. Failure to achieve a satisfactory identity is an important aspect of mental illness.

The possession of an individual identity, even a relatively satisfactory one, has the further hazard of creating a sense of aloneness. Within his own skin, man is absolutely all by himself, one tiny entity in the whole universe. This aloneness is terrifying. It implies responsibility for his own feelings, thoughts, actions. The terror of aloneness, the panic of overwhelming responsibility for the *I*, are the price man must pay for his achievement of self-awareness.

To mitigate the fear of aloneness, man has evolved an additional quality. He can relate to other human beings. When the *I* in one person can make contact with the *you* in another person, the fear of utter aloneness is dissipated. The coming together of *I* and *you* Sullivan calls interpersonal

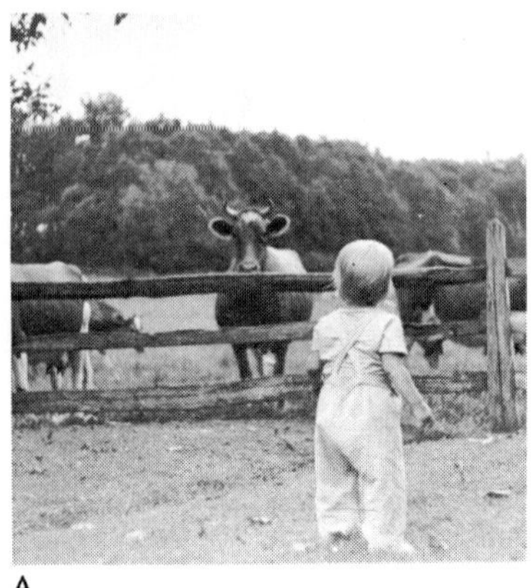
A

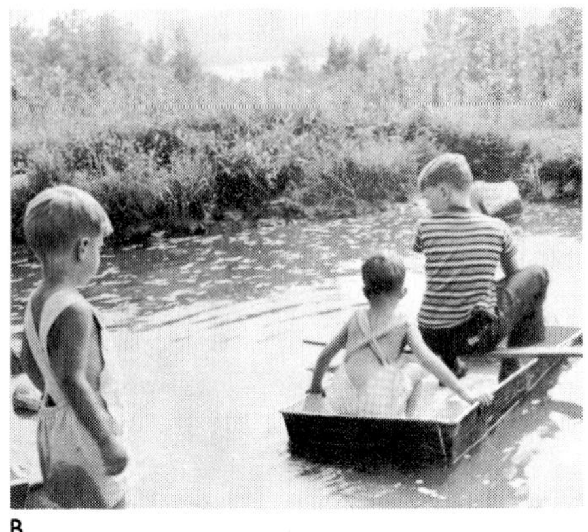
B

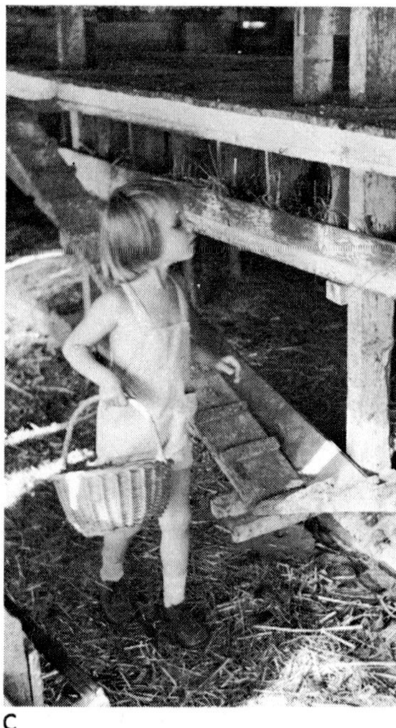
C

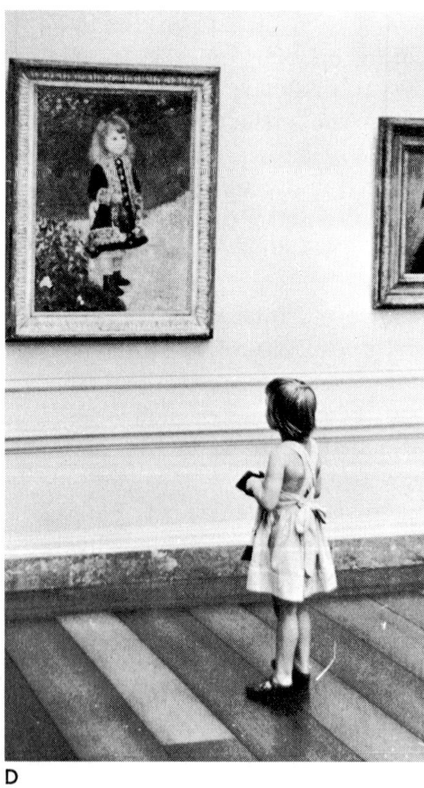
D

Fig. 27-1. Qualities of humanness emerge in the early years. A. Taking in the wonders of the world. *B.* Courage comes with human relations. C. Self-confidence comes with learning and doing. *D.* Absorbing the culture of the race. (*Photographs A, C, and D by Robert Wood.*)

contact; Fromm calls it love; Buber speaks of an *I-thou* relationship. Whatever its name, it is not only a human achievement, but a human necessity. Human beings not only are able to relate to each other, but they must achieve a mutuality with others for survival on a human level. Like failure to establish a satisfactory identity, failure to establish human contacts is a component of mental illness.

THE MATURE ADULT

These qualities of being human—self-awareness and awareness of external reality, combined with a relatedness to other human beings—constitute the unique core of each human being by means of which he is able to experience his own thoughts, feelings, and wishes, and through which he expresses his responsibility. When these qualities are satisfactorily developed, the resulting human being is what is called a *mature adult.* A mature adult, by one definition, is an individual who has been able to achieve a reasonably accurate evaluation of himself, an evaluation which is fairly close to that which others have of him. He knows what kind of person he is; he recognizes his strengths, accepts his limitations. When this has been accomplished, his energies can be directed toward developing and improving his strengths. They are not consumed in a constant and futile attempt to prove to himself and to the world that he is what he is not. The mature person, who can accept himself and then explore the world, can also understand other people. He is capable of relating in true mutuality with others perhaps because he is willing to show his naked self without consciously or unconsciously trying to gloss over his bad qualities or magnify his good ones.

MENTAL DEVIANTS

When the self fails to mature adequately, the resulting individual suffers from varying degrees of what is called *mental illness.* His development becomes arrested, he fails to progress step by step, and as a physically grown person he manifests evidence of childish behavior. The extreme forms of mental illness make life in society impossible, and the victim must be separated from the group; lesser forms of mental illness do not make group life impossible, but they interfere with the full and complete functioning of the individual.

Mental illness has doubtless been a problem through all of man's history. Some individuals suffering from mental illness have, in spite of their illness, been capable of great creative achievement: Van Gogh, Nijinsky, Schumann, Dostoevski, Swift, Poe, Rimbaud—the list is long. Though their illnesses may well have contributed to their achievements, each of these men paid an enormous price in misery and unhappiness. Other mental deviates, instead of benefiting mankind with their gifts, have caused untold havoc to the race—Hitler, for example. Man's vastly increased knowledge of the physical environment and his ability to produce weapons of destruction demand a greater understanding of what makes human beings act as they do.

Mental illness looms large as a problem in society today. By providing scope for more individual freedom and self-direction, modern "affluent" society demands more maturity. Neurotic functioning, which was latent to a degree in autocratic and feudal societies, has become visible in present-day United States and Western European cultures. In a sense our society may breed mental illness at the same time that it provides greater opportunities for creative expression. Increased awareness of mental deviates means that more and more people are classified as pathologic who in times past would have existed without a label. Probably many factors play a role in the mounting toll of mentally ill people.

MAN'S EARLY CONCEPT OF HIMSELF

Self-awareness has been with man ever since he evolved into man. It is what has made it possible for him to speculate on the mysteries of life, both those in the external world and those within himself. The nature of his own inner core has been one of man's earliest and most persistent concerns. Unable to locate his thoughts, feelings, wishes in any part of his body, primitive man conceived the idea of a spirit within him, separate from his physical organism. His body he could touch and see; it was real and comprehensible. His spirit, on the other hand, was invisible, powerful, and mysterious, but although he could not see his spirit, he felt it controlled him, that it made him and his fellows act as they did.

This concept of a dichotomy within himself of body and spirit led primitive man to extend this idea to those aspects of the external world that he was unable to explain; he endowed objects of nature with spirits similar to those he felt existed in himself. He came to think that anthropomorphic spirits resided in the wind, the rain, the sun, the moon, the trees, and animals.

Through the centuries, in his insatiable quest for understanding, man has been a good deal more successful in probing the mysteries of his physical environment than in learning to know himself and how he came to be what he is. He no longer explains a physical phenomenon by attributing it to an unknown spirit. He understands, more or less, how wind and rain and clouds are produced. Man has grasped the way matter is put together. He can conceive of the immensity of the universe and can break the links in the atom. He can also grow a wheat that ignores the evolutionary enemies of the plant. He can build airplanes that surpass the evolutionary accomplishments of any bird. Man can even tinker with his own physical organism; he can prevent many diseases, cure others, repair faulty structures. Man's accomplishments in understanding and subduing his physical environment are indeed impressive.

But when it comes to understanding what man himself *is* and how he came to be what he is, his knowledge is still fragmentary. He knows little more than that there is a central core in a human being that separates him from other animal species.

There have been many theories to account for man's human capacities. The central core of a human being has been thought to be a God-given spirit deposited preformed in a child, either at conception or at some time thereafter. More recent concepts postulate that the central core of a human being—call it what you will: spirit, self, ego, psyche—emerges slowly after birth and is the product of the gene-directed potential inherent in the organism and the milieu in which it develops.

If the inner core of a human being is not miraculously deposited preformed in man but, rather, matures as his physical body matures, it may or it may not achieve the full potential inherent in the genes. Its development will depend upon whether or not the milieu in which it grows is conducive, at each developmental level, to optimal development. This idea that human characteristics are modifiable during life puts upon the adults in any society the responsibility of understanding, insofar as possible, the factors of the milieu which foster or hinder the optimal development of man's human qualities.

THE CONTRAST IN DEVELOPMENT OF PHYSICAL STRUCTURE AND OF THE SELF

It is now a generally accepted hypothesis that, in contrast with most of the basic physical structure which develops in utero the self emerges after birth. This brings about a profound difference between the nature of development of the physical organism and that of the human qualities of self.

The human zygote has no choice. It grows and develops in utero according to the impetus inherent in its genes and without any exercise of will. It is protected not only from itself but also from the whims of its mother. The mother protects and nourishes her unborn child because her body is so organized that these processes go on automatically. During intrauterine life, the fetus constructs not only the structures he shares with lower forms, but he also manufactures those special aspects of his structures with which he will ultimately be able to fulfill his human potential. Before birth there is no exercise of the qualities of humanness, either from the emerging human being himself or from his mother. While the intrauterine environment cannot be influenced by the *will* of the mother, there is evidence that her nutritional level, certain toxic conditions, some diseases which she may contract, or her emotional state may all have an influence on the environment within her uterus (p. 63).

But once the fetus emerges from the uterus and becomes a neonate, he is subject not to an automatic milieu but to one controlled to a great extent by the human will of the adults who care for him. He has left behind him the security of his automatic evolutionary past. Here is where the conditions of life of the human newborn differ greatly from those of all other species. The environment after birth for all mammals except man is almost as automatic as that before birth. The mammalian animal mother has rigid instinctive patterns to guide her in the care of her young, but the human neonate is at the mercy of a mother whose instinctive patterns are far less rigid and who, in the main, decides what manner of care her infant is to receive. He is subject to the hazards of individually directed, instead of instinctively directed, external factors. How the human mother cares for her infant depends on her instinctive drives modified by her emotional health and the dictates of the culture in which she lives. If the child is to achieve the magnificence of the human potential which was initiated during the automatic development in utero, the care he receives after birth must be carried out in such a way that, as far as possible, his needs are met in their totality (Schachtel, 1959).

MODERN THEORIES OF PERSONALITY DEVELOPMENT

Freud developed the basic concepts from which stem much of our understanding of the developmental processes of the human personality. Much of the detail of Freud's concepts has been altered over the years, but his original tenets and penetrating insights have paved the way for recent elaborations and refinements. Two of Freud's contributions are significant to the present discussion:

1. Human personality develops after birth and is the result of the interaction of the basic instinctive drives within the child and the forces of the milieu. Prior to Freud, little scientific attention was given to childhood. Children just grew up. When they finally put away childish things, philosophers found them subjects worthy of study. That they acted as they did was considered to be "human nature." The adage that human nature cannot be changed was shown by Freud to be far from an absolute truth. Human nature, or at least human personality, is malleable in youth and ultimately takes the shape into which its own organism and life experience mold it.

2. The earliest years of life are the most important ones in forming personality. It is then that the individual gets his essential concept of himself, and it is this concept that he carries through life. Freud showed that development could stagnate at various critical points and that when it did, the individual carried childish traits to adulthood. Freud discovered and demonstrated the child in adult man.

These two concepts of Freud are basic and are accepted by all modern schools of psychologic theory.

Since Freud opened the doors of understanding, innumerable scholars have entered those portals and explored deeper and deeper recesses of human personality development. It is beyond the scope of this book (and well beyond this author's capacities) to trace or evaluate these many contributions.

Erikson's work has been selected as representative of modern thinking on the development of human personality, and while it does not represent the sum total of knowledge, it is a most useful schema with which to trace the stages through which the ego passes, as the human being travels the road between neonate and mature adult.

ERIKSON'S EGO EPIGENESIS

Erikson uses the expression *ego-identity* to designate the core of the individual personality. His theory assumes that each human child is endowed with autonomous drives to react to his environment in such ways that ultimately an ego emerges. While the drives are common to all human beings, each individual reacts to the milieu in which he grows up, especially to the persons who look after him.

The neonate has no sense of his ego; it emerges as life goes on. However, the progression is not in a straight line but in a series of jumps—"phases," Erikson calls them. He outlines a series of phases which he considers universal in all men of all cultures. In each phase the emerging ego is confronted with a task. Some resolution of each age-specific task must be found before a new phase begins and a new task is presented to the developing ego.

While the major solution must be arrived at during the specific phase, nevertheless, preparations for the task are laid in earlier phases, and refinements of solution take place later.

In a somewhat analogous way, the task of the first grader is to learn to read, but prior to first grade the child learns to recognize shapes and configurations; after first grade, he extends his vocabulary. Nevertheless, the basic concept of learning to understand the printed word is acquired in first grade.

And so with the tasks of the ego. The individual must achieve some resolution of each task as it is presented. If a task is poorly handled, the individual, as it were, goes to second grade a poor reader and will probably remain a poor reader unless he is given special help. Ego scars too occur. If conditions are not favorable for an adequate solution of each stage-specific ego task, the individual carries a bruised ego into the next phase. Unless he is given help to heal the damage to his ego, it is likely that the ego scar will remain and affect subsequent development.

Erikson describes eight phases of personality development.

Basic Trust versus Basic Mistrust: Infancy

Since the human infant must have physical care to survive, there is always a caretaking person, usually, of course, the mother. As the months go along, a relationship builds up between the infant and his mother—a mutuality. It is the quality of this relationship which is significant in personality development. Through his contacts with the mother the young infant either establishes a basic feeling that the world is a place in which his needs will be taken care of more or less as they arise, or he comes to feel that the world is a threatening place not to be counted upon. Later in the first year the infant must cope with the anxiety engendered by separation from his mother and thus learn to accept aloneness as part of mutuality. The balance between the positive and negative feelings is critical at this stage. It is inevitable that there will be some frustrations, precipitating fear and rage, but if the balance tips toward the positive side, the infant emerges from this stage with the feeling that the world is a safe place and that since he is able to cope with minor infringements on this safety, he has qualities of worthiness. However, if the balance is on the negative side, the infant will carry with him to subsequent stages a sense of fear and dread of the world plus a fundamental sense of his own inabilities to obtain what he needs. Later in life these feelings will interfere with his zeal to explore his world, and with his ability to relate intimately with other people.

Autonomy versus Shame and Doubt: Toddlerhood

During toddlerhood, the child learns to master his body. He learns to control his motor apparatus, including his sphincters. The relation of motor maturation to personality development has to do with the feelings engendered in the child by his new-found powers.

Ideally, the child who enters this phase with a firmly established basic trust as a heritage from the first phase tackles the problems of bringing his body under the control of his will with enthusiasm and with relative freedom from the negative feelings of shame and doubt. The acquisition of each new skill slowly builds up in the child a feeling of his own strength and worth. He comes to feel that he is the master of himself. In his enthusiasm for self-mastery the toddler often appears stubborn, willful, aggressive.

Sphincter control, while part of motor control, adds special features, since it includes the ability to hold on and let go at will. Holding tight or giving freely, experienced most vividly in relation to the anal sphincter, are feelings extended to other ways of holding and giving, both in motor actions—hoarding and throwing away—and ultimately in total personality—stinginess and generosity. Other factors later in life have an influence on these qualities; nevertheless the twig is bent during the development of sphincter control.

The toddler learns to control his body in the milieu of his family. The way the people with whom he lives react to his new-found abilities and his self-mastery determines how the child feels about himself. Prohibitions are essential; the toddler has no capacity to judge the physically dangerous nor the socially unacceptable. Prohibitions need to be firm, gentle, and above all free from sadism.

The crisis in personality development at this stage comes about through the resolution of satisfactory and frustrating experiences. While the actual techniques used by a family to guide a toddler have a bearing on how he feels about himself, more important than mere techniques are the integrity, maturity, and confidence of the adults. These qualities are what ultimately get across to the child.

Ideally, the child emerges from toddlerhood with a body he takes pleasure in manipulating in ways that conform to the mores of his family. This is autonomy. If this ego crisis is met less well, the child goes on to the next stage with doubt about the capacities of his body and shame in his accomplishments.

Initiative versus Guilt: Preschool Years

The child enters the preschool years with a body he "owns" and with the knowledge that he is an independent person. If the crises of the early phases of personality development have been weathered satisfactorily and he is reasonably content with the discoveries he has made so far, during the next years the child will devote himself to sharpening his focus on just what kind of a person he is.

An essential part of himself is his gender. The preschool child becomes interested in sexual matters. This is the period Freud called the "genital phase"—the phase of infant sexuality. Sexuality is not the preschooler's only interest by any means, but it is apt to produce more problems, at least in our society, than the many other aspects of the child's curiosity.

The preschooler knows he is a boy or girl, but what does this signify? He asks questions, he explores himself and, if he gets the opportunity, the bodies of his playmates. How his curiosity is met by his adults determines how he feels. He can come to feel he is a good, worthwhile person all over, including his genitals, or he can be made to feel uneasy and guilty about his sex. This is the age when castration fears develop if guilt is pronounced (p. 428).

Part of the little child's sexual interest extends to identification with the parent of the same sex. This identification quite usually is so all-encompassing that the child, in fantasy, takes over the role of his like-sex parent. This precipitates him into the oedipal triangle (p. 429).

The crisis of personality development for the preschooler revolves around gaining a comfortable feeling about his sex role and thus fostering his curiosity and initiative in continuing his explorations, not only of his body, but of all aspects of his surroundings. If he comes through well, he has an inner conviction that he is a worthwhile person and that explorations are valuable enterprises. His enthusiasm to find out, to learn, is undampened; he has the initiative to go on. On the other hand, if he has been made to feel uneasy, especially about his sexual interests, he develops a sense of guilt about the kind of person he is; his guilt plus his fears that further explorations will lead to deeper guilt consume much of his energy. Therefore his enthusiasm is dampened, he holds back, he lacks initiative.

Industry versus Inferiority: School-age Child

At the end of the preschool years, the child's interest in sexual matters subsides. He enters what Freud calls the "latency period." This is a uniquely human period of development (animals enter puberty soon after infancy). The child during the school years, having discovered in earlier phases (however satisfactorily) what sort of a person he is, turns his attention away from himself to the world of things and people about him. He is granted time to learn human culture before he is beset with the problems of full maturity.

The crisis of personality development at this time revolves around his attitude toward learning, making discoveries, understanding the phenomena in the world about him. An important part of these discoveries is that of his relation to people, especially people outside the immediate environs of his family.

Much depends upon the resolution of the tasks of previous stages. The child who enters the school years firmly convinced that the world is trustworthy and that the *I* he has so far discovered is competent wastes little energy in guilt and shame and doubt. He forges ahead with insatiable curiosity and zeal.

The learning of the school-age child includes "book learning," motor skills, and knowledge about people. The attitude of his important grownups —family and teachers—can either foster or thwart his zeal. There will, of course, be frustrations as he tackles the impossible, but if there are also successes, he can take his failures in stride. It is when the whole climate of adult judgment is indifferent or antagonistic that the child slumps into despair. While the school-age child makes a great show of independence as his horizons widen out, nevertheless, the attitude of his home is of paramount importance to him. Indifference on the part of his parents is, perhaps, the greatest trauma. If the important people in his life do not care what he does or thinks, the value of his deeds and thoughts is less significant to him. On the other hand, if he is nagged at, overprotected, held up to impossible standards, he becomes convinced of his own inability to measure up. He feels nothing is worth the effort, and he ceases to try. His zeal to learn and his curiosity about the world die on the vine.

School-age children thrive on interest, success, and praise, but the articles must be genuine. Interest must be sincere and long-continuing, not feigned or spasmodic. Praise for a job the child knows was poorly done not only destroys his confidence in himself but creates contempt for the praiser.

Consistent reasonable discipline, with coercion now and then, are essential and contribute to the child's feeling that he is important enough to be of concern to his adults; restraints also help the child feel protected from his own often unmanageable desires.

During the school years a child develops his first true equal relations with other people—a buddy of his own sex and age. The warmth and outgoing qualities of such relationships stand in contrast to even the best of relationships to adults, which can never have the equality that exists between child and child. Acceptance and tolerance from the child's significant adults for these intense buddy friendships lay the groundwork for later mature interpersonal relations.

The child who weathers well his school-age ego crisis emerges not only with confidence in himself but with an enthusiasm to tackle the unknown. Failure at this stage is usually compounded with previous failures, although even a well-integrated ego at the onset of the school years can fail to solve satisfactorily the tasks of this stage if beset with insurmountable obstacles. Failure is evident in a sense of inferiority and willingness to exist within the narrow confines of that which is safe.

Identity versus Identity Diffusion: Puberty

With the onset of puberty enormous changes take place in somatic growth—rapid increase in size and also genital maturity. The changes in size alone are so rapid and extensive that in themselves they create a loss of the sense of sameness to which the individual has become accustomed. He has to get used to his body all over again; simultaneously, genital maturity floods him with powerful new drives and new flights of fancy. All these new experiences must be incorporated into his concept of *I*. "Who and what am I" is the dominant preoccupation of the pubescent youth. It is not surprising that the child's attention is directed back to his body in his struggle to achieve what Erikson calls egoidentity.

The integration that takes place is the heritage of all the previous tasks the developing ego has had to meet and solve in one fashion or another. It is a synthesis of the basic drives, endowment, and opportunities. What emerges is an identity the youth can recognize and accept as himself. The identity must be his own; it cannot be handed out to him preformed. To achieve it, the youth may question his parents' (and society's) values on sex, religion, ethics, and social and political questions. Ultimately as he accepts this, rejects that, he establishes values he feels are his own. Self-confidence, confirmed in each previous step, becomes so firm that the individual is convinced that he, as an entity, has an intrinsic value in the society to which he belongs.

Failure to establish an egoidentity results in what Erikson calls "ego diffusion," in which the image the young person had of himself prior to puberty disintegrates under the stress of the new body, new feelings, and fears of approaching maturity. In our society, a great many young adolescents encounter some ego diffusion as they try to establish a place for themselves. With some, a temporary group identity in a gang supports them until they can come to further grips with their individual identity. In others, the need for some kind of gang—some group identity—becomes permanent. In still others the failure to arrive at personal identity pushes them into neurotic or psychotic behavior.

Intimacy versus Isolation: Postadolescence

After egoidentity is established, the young person once again turns his interest outside himself. He has passed the crisis of doubting what and who he is; he has energy now to push on toward the world. Puberty, as it were, is a moratorium in personality development during which time the drives to the outside slow down while the youth gathers together the threads of his childish ego and weaves them into his concept of his grownup ego. Once this is accomplished, he can then push on in study, in a career, and in relations with others. It is only when he is convinced of his own identity that he can seek intimacy with another, not only sexual intimacy, but friendship, a true mutuality. Establishment of identity does not imply uncritical acceptance of the self as it is. Rather, it includes an ability to oppose the devalued in self and in others as well as an ability to confirm the valued.

Failure at this stage results in inability to establish a truly mutual relation, in work, in friendship, in marriage. Such people are constantly changing jobs, establishing new friends, seeking new marital partners. Seldom do the changes help; their need is to establish integrity within themselves before they have anything that can be shared with a partner.

Generativity versus Stagnation: Maturity

"Generativity" is the term with which Erikson expresses the desire of two mature people who have found a satisfying mutuality in their relationship to combine their personalities and energies in the production and care of offspring. This is a stage in personality growth. While many people express the qualities of this stage by becoming parents, the ego energy used for creating children can be diverted into other forms of creativity—artistic, scientific, political.

During the mature years the individual develops an increased empathy for others, not only in family life, but in his work, in his community, and in the world at large. His sense of responsibility grows as his understanding grows. He acquires qualities of leadership and ability to influence others. His judgment, imaginative creativity, and intelligence are able to function at peak capacity during this phase of life.

The mere fact of having children does not necessarily mean that the stage of generativity in personality development has been reached, any more than experiencing the sex act means that the preceding stage has been successfully met, or the mere fact that a toddler finally learns to use the bathroom means that he has succeeded in establishing autonomy. While ideally there is a correlation between ego and somatic development, nevertheless it is possible that an individual's physical organism can reach somatic maturity even though his ego has failed to reach a mature ego-identity. The very fact that the bearing of children is dependent only upon physiologic (and not psychologic) maturation gives our society many parents unfit for the responsibilities of parenthood.

Integrity versus Despair: Postmaturity

Unlike physical development, personality development does not stop with physical maturity. The ego can go on developing to the end of life. Each age has its tasks, its problems, its solutions. The individual who has, with reasonable success, met life head on, lived through exaltation and despair, been the originator of ideas and children, destroyed as well as created can finally accept himself as a member of the human race and feel a sense of oneness with other human beings, even those in distant cultures and distant times. He is able to accept his own limitations without despair. He does not spend his energies wishing he had had other opportunities. He has verve to go on, to continue, to create, to do.

HUMAN DIMENSIONS OF FUNCTION

Erikson has outlined the tasks of the ego and discussed the social milieu in which these tasks must be solved. There remains to be discussed the contribution to personality development made by the biologic equipment of the developing individual.

There is no new organ which takes over the functions of the ego. The human being must put to new human use his ancestral functions. Adapting structure or function originally designed for one purpose to serve the needs of another form of life is an oft-repeated technique in evolution.

The ego develops through the way the individual *feels* about what he does and what goes on within and about him. By *feelings* is meant an emotional response, what the psychiatrists call *affect.*

Erikson and other contributors to the psychoanalytic literature, as well, concentrate on certain areas of the body which, it is claimed, have preeminence at different times in the life cycle. In early infancy it is the mouth through which the infant takes in not only food but also much of the care given him by his mother; later the focus shifts to the anal region, and still later to the genitals. Organ modes—oral, anal, and genital—are considered the important tools with which the child reacts to his milieu and through which his ego develops. In addition to feelings generated in his mouth, anus, and sex organs, the maturing child gains experiences and feelings through his motor apparatus, his sense organs, his ability to play and to talk.

Each of the organ modes is related to a function. Man eats with his mouth, eliminates through his sphincters, and exercises his sex functions with his genitals. Eating, elimination, and sex have overtones in man in addition to their biologic functions. They are all functions which man shares with his mammalian ancestors but which man has put also to uniquely human use.

These overtones create what the author calls *human dimensions of function.* Each of these functions is carried on through life, but the needs of the developing ego have molded the manner in which man eats, eliminates, and exercises his sex function to meet the needs of his ego. In other words, each of these functions has a life cycle. Therefore the author has elected to discuss personality development in terms of those functions of man which have acquired human dimensions, rather than in terms of organ modes. This does not mean that the concept of organ modes is abandoned; organ modes are a significant description of the relation of parts of the body to human development.

All through life man eats as a human being; his manner of eating has a human overtone that contributes more to his ego development than merely the oral mode. Eating is a continuum from birth to old age; its human dimensions contribute to the ego throughout life.

Man also exercises his sexuality throughout most of life. His genitals make an important contribution to ego development in childhood (the genital mode), but sexuality in man is more than a means of procreation, more than an organ mode. From infancy to old age sexuality has a human dimension.

Muscular activity is another function which man shares with lower species but which in man has acquired a human dimension. In infancy instinctive motor patterns constitute a human technique of ensuring for the child close proximity to his mother (Bowlby, 1958). This proximity has a bearing on the infant's ability to establish basic trust. Other motor activities provide the means by which the child gains a feeling of self-competence and ultimately achieves autonomy. Motor skills contribute throughout life to the ego.

The voluntary control of the eliminative sphincters is a special aspect of motor control which, during the period of toilet training, makes a profound contribution to the ego.

The human being uses his sense organs to comprehend himself and the world about him. In early life sensations produce only feelings within the child; the child is egocentric. As maturity advances, sensation develops its truly human dimension of providing knowledge of the inherent traits of things in the external world. Both egocentric and world-centered sensation mold the developing ego.

Play is a combination of motor and sensory abilities. It has, however, special overtones in man.

Communication, like play, is accomplished by the use of motor apparatus and sensory powers. The ability to talk is essential for the full development of the ego, and in our society the ability to read and write is necessary for optimal development.

In the following chapters of this section, the life cycle of each of the functions of man which have acquired human dimensions will be discussed. This approach to total development is a pragmatic one, related to the role of a pediatrician in guiding normal children in healthy growth. Ego development is only a part of a total picture and is woven into total care.

BIBLIOGRAPHY

Buber, Martin: "Pointing the Way," collected essays translated from the German by Maurice Friedman, Harper & Row, Publishers, Incorporated, New York, 1957.

Beach, F. A.: "The De-Sent of Instinct," Presidential Address, Eastern Psychological Assn., 1955.

Bowlby, John: The Nature of the Child's Tie to His Mother, *Internat. J. Psychoanalysis,* **39**:350, 1958.

Erikson, Erik H.: "Insight and Responsibility," W. W. Norton & Company, Inc., New York, 1964.

———: "Childhood and Society," 2d ed., W. W. Norton & Company, Inc., New York, 1963.

———: "Identity and the Life Cycle," Psychological Issues, vol. I, Monograph I, International Universities Press, Inc., New York, 1959.

———: "Young Man Luther," W. W. Norton & Company, Inc., New York, 1958.

Freedman, L. Z., and Anne Rae: Evolution and Human Behavior, in Anne Roe and George C. Sampson (eds.), "Behavior and Evolution," Yale University Press, New Haven, Conn., 1958.

Freud, S.: "Basic Writings of Sigmund Freud," Vintage Books, Random House, Inc., New York, 1938.

Fromm, Eric: "Escape from Freedom," Holt, Rinehart and Winston, Inc., New York, 1941.

———: "Man for Himself," Holt, Rinehart and Winston, Inc., New York, 1947.

———: "The Forgotten Language," Holt, Rinehart and Winston, Inc., New York, 1951.

———: "The Art of Loving," Harper & Row, Publishers, Incorporated, New York, 1956.

Halstead, Ward C.: "Brain and Intelligence, A Quantitive Study of the Frontal Lobes," The University of Chicago Press, Chicago, 1947.

Kubie, Lawrence S.: Instincts and Homeostasis, *Psychosom. Med.,* **10**:15, 1948.

RENECH, BERNARD: Increase of Learning Capacity with Increase of Brain Size, *Am. Naturalist*, **90**:81, 1956.

SCHACHTEL, ERNEST G.: "Metamorphosis," Basic Books, Inc., Publishers, New York, 1959.

SULLIVAN, HARRY STACK: "The Interpersonal Theory of Psychiatry," W. W. Norton & Company, Inc., New York, 1953.

WASHBURN, S. L., and VIRGINIA AVIS: Evolution and Human Behavior, in Anne Roe and George G. Sampson (eds.), "Behavior and Evolution," Yale University Press, New Haven, Conn., 1958, p. 421.

28

Eating through Life

NOURISHMENT, EATING, AND BEING HUMAN

All living organisms must be nourished. They must take in raw materials from the environment and transform them into structures characteristic of the species and of the individual. Human beings share with the entire plant and animal world this need for nourishment.

In the simplest forms of animal life, nourishment is merely absorbed from what is available. As the evolutionary ladder is ascended, special organs for taking in, storing, and processing of food make their appearance. The organs of taste and smell combine with powers of locomotion to give greater ability to select and reject potential sources of nourishment. The higher animals not only are nourished; they eat. They exhibit hunger, they seek food, eat, cease eating.

In man, nourishment and eating take on a new dimension. Man savors his food. He prepares it, cooks it, arranges it, combines this with that. Man enjoys the tastes, the smell, the consistency of what nourishes him; and most important of all, he enjoys the company of his fellows while he eats. The human being not only eats; he dines. It is his capacity to dine that constitutes the human dimensions of eating. Many of life's gratifications and frustrations are related to the biologic necessity of obtaining nourishment. During all of life, food, eating, dining are part of the armamentarium with which man achieves not only bodily integrity but also the means of realizing some of his inherent human potentials.

The pleasures of dining have a definite developmental progression. The good things that go with eating are dated in the life cycle. A toddler no more enjoys dressing up and having a fancy meal than a grownup enjoys a martini from a nursing bottle.

In early infancy the pleasures of eating are obtained from the warmth and comfort of the mother's tender care of the infant as he sucks in the milk. It is through food that the newborn human infant makes his first contact with another person. The infant dines, and as he does so, his personality begins to emerge.

In later infancy the developing awareness of self makes the infant desirous of adding new skills to his eating repertory. Throughout toddlerhood the emerging independence shows itself in the little child's desire to "do it myself." Dining at this stage is largely a matter of the joy of getting the food into the mouth "by myself."

As the years pass, the child, now competent at negotiating the trip from plate to mouth, is eager for companionship and obtains pleasure from association with family or peers at mealtime. All through childhood dining pleasures are part of many activities—tea parties, picnics, or the special treat of a meal in a restaurant. No childhood is complete without the ice cream and cake at birthdays.

In adolescence dining pleasures are great indeed—partly because of the growth spurt at this age which demands an increased food intake but also because of the companionship offered in such places as the drugstore snack bar.

In adult life dining continues to be one of the joys of life. The tête-à-tête in an offbeat restaurant with a special companion, an occasional breakfast in bed, a clambake with a big crowd, dinner parties, cocktail parties, banquets—food is part of the social contacts of modern man. Dining looms large in the good things of life—all life long.

HUNGER AND SATIETY

The central nervous system initiates the desire to eat and alerts the animal to the fact that he has eaten enough. Brobeck and his coworkers discovered that destruction of a small area in the hypothalamus destroyed the animal's ability to know when he had had enough. Animals with such lesions gorged themselves and became grossly obese. This tiny area in the brain stem, the satiety center, through some unknown mechanism, sends out nerve impulses which make an animal stop eating.

Anand and Brobeck demonstrated that other small areas slightly lateral to the satiety center were involved in initiating eating. When these areas were destroyed, the animal refused to eat, in fact violently objected if food were forced upon him. Animals with lesions in this area starved to death in the presence of adequate food.

Many animals in their natural habitats seem to possess a greater ability than civilized man to select an adequate diet from an array of available foodstuffs. No animal could have long survived if he were not able to select his food and avoid poisonous substances. Man's inability to nourish himself adequately under civilized conditions may of course be a cultural rather than a biologic phenomenon.[1] Again it may be that his eating controls are not as keen as those of lower animals. It is also possible that man's need to dine, as well as to eat, may exercise a supercontrol over the biologic mechanism.

[1] Clara Davis's experiment with children on an orthopedic ward indicated that when only natural foodstuffs were available, the children selected for themselves an adequate diet. The crucial point of this experiment was that none of the refined foods (sweets, milled cereals) were available.

APPETITE

Appetite and hunger have been much confused, but they are not the same thing. Hunger is a biologic call for fuel; appetite, a desire to enjoy the pleasures of eating. In this sense it is only man who has true appetite: appetite is the urge to dine. While examples can be found which indicate that some animals apparently savor their food, nevertheless these are but faint shadows of the dining pleasures which flower in the human being.

Appetite develops through the years of infancy and childhood, and what emerges in adult life is a complicated combination of desires for specific foods under culturally controlled conditions, all tied into the personality. Other hungers besides the need for fuel are not infrequently confused in the growing personality with appetite for food. The child whose hunger for love and warm interpersonal relationships has not been adequately met may confuse this with hunger for fuel and try to eat his way to satisfaction.

Appetite is not controlled biologically as is hunger, and not infrequently the needs of the personality are stronger than the biologic needs; some people eat too much, while others do not eat enough for their biologic requirements.

NUTRITION PRIOR TO BIRTH

The fetus is nourished constantly, every heartbeat picks up the essential nutrients and propels them to all cells of the body. The phenomenon of hunger does not exist, nor does the gastrointestinal tract participate in the preparation of food. The fetus does not eat; it is nourished. It develops no tensions because of lack of food; therefore neither are there satisfactions and gratifications connected with food.

EATING IN INFANCY

When the infant wakes up from his first big sleep after birth, he is apparently uncomfortable. He cries. His discomfort is probably due largely but not entirely to hunger. Some infants wake up, cry, but are not interested in sucking at this very early age. All they need is a sensation of warmth, a little rocking, and they will go back to sleep.

Eventually, however, the pinch of hunger becomes more demanding; the infant's eating center is being stimulated.

Occasionally it takes an infant 2 or 3 days to become interested in sucking. This may be due to the amount of sedation he received during the birth process or to some innate slowness within the infant himself.

However, eventually every healthy infant does suck. The infant cannot be fed by food alone; he needs to dine. For an infant to dine, he needs to experience total body pleasure. This consists of whole body contact—of a

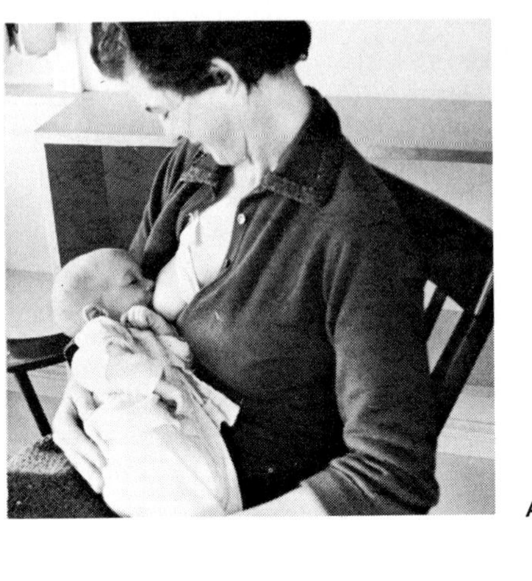

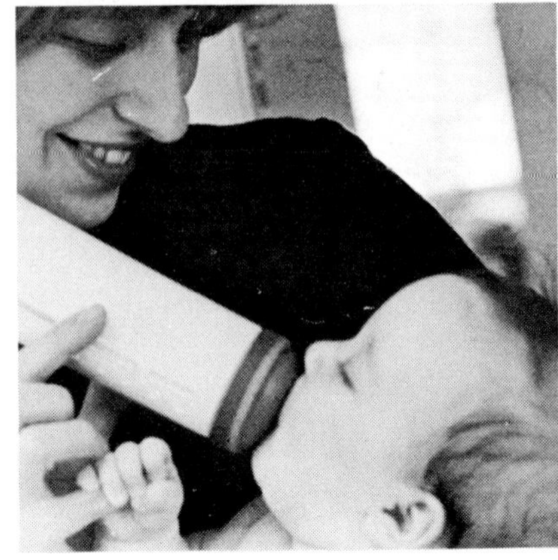

A

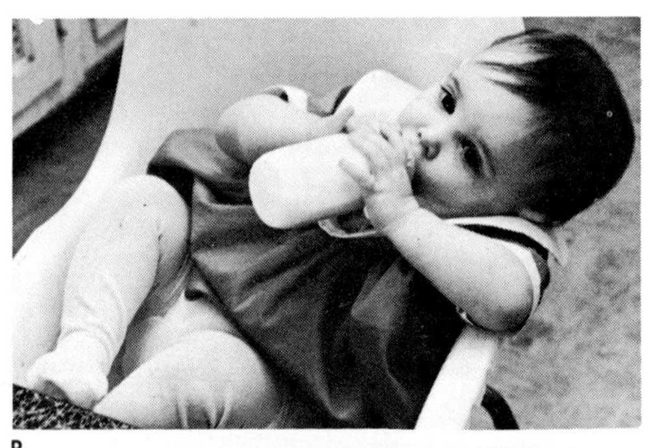

B

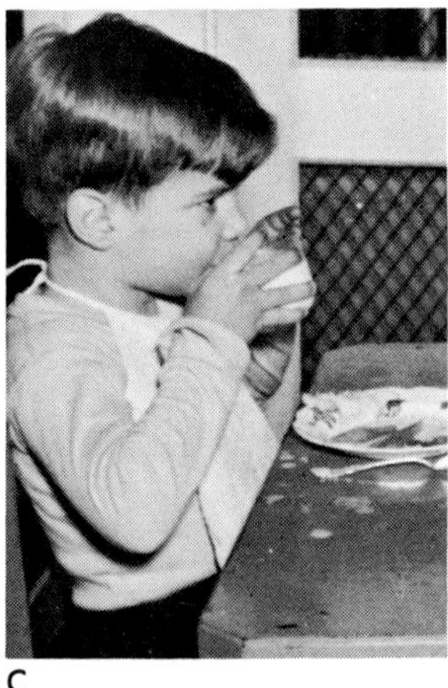

C

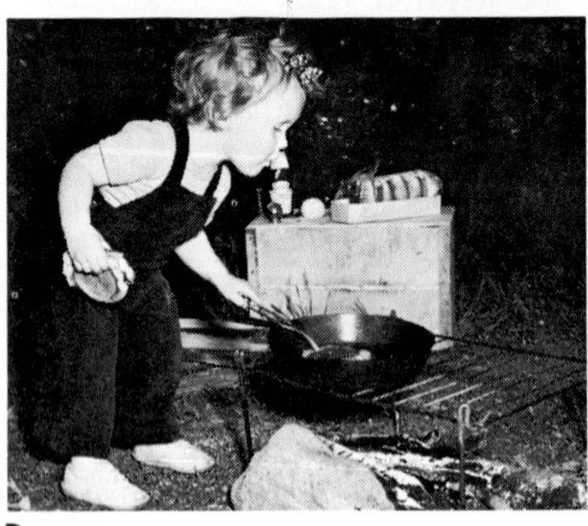

D

Fig. 28-1. Dining in early life. *A.* The young infant dines from the breast or from the bottle. *B.* The older infant dines as she holds her own bottle. *C.* Dining pleasures for the toddler consist of negotiating the trip from plate to mouth. *D.* Picnics add joy to eating.

sensation of warmth and motion and also of a nipple on which the lips can suck. In other words the infant needs to be picked up, held, rocked, and allowed to suck. In the last months of prenatal life, while nourishment is supplied through the umbilical circulation, the fetus is busy perfecting its equipment for existence outside the uterus. This equipment includes not only the apparatus for sucking but also all the sensory mechanisms by means of which the infant can appreciate the sensations of warmth, of motion, of snugness. For the first few months of life the pleasures of being mothered dominate the eating experience.

In each eating experience the cycle is similar to that of the very first need for nourishment after birth. There is a mounting biologic need for nutrients throughout his body tissues, a falling blood sugar level, gastric contractions, pain, general discomfort. All this adds up to a mounting tension sufficient to arouse the infant from sleep. He cries; the longer he cries, the more uncomfortable he becomes, and the more his whole body participates in the sensation of displeasure. Before he can successfully eat, he needs his general body sensations quieted. Once this is accomplished by his mother's ministrations, he can settle down to sucking, which brings relief to his gastrointestinal tract. The relaxation of the infant's muscles is obvious as he is rocked and cuddled prior to sucking. As his stomach fills up, his relaxation continues, and finally he falls asleep.

A young infant is very sensitive to the quality of the care he receives from his mother. If a mother is tense and jittery, if she is trying to rush through a feeding, the infant feels her agitation and will not suck. Her emotional state is probably transmitted to the infant through the muscular tension in her arms, perhaps through the shrill quality of her voice. But whatever the exact mechanism through which the infant absorbs his mother's emotional state, he does react to it. He becomes agitated, restless, and anxious if his mother is upset. He cannot eat until the conditions for dining have been met. Contrariwise, the infant relaxes and is eager to eat when picked up by gentle, warm, comfortable arms. Sullivan describes this as the "good nipple" and the "bad nipple."

Breast or Bottle Feeding

For some mothers breast feeding is the epitome of joy, a true fulfillment of their maternal function. Such women have plenty of breast milk and feed their babies successfully and easily. In our culture, however, many young mothers do not feel this way about breast feeding. To be satisfactory to the infant, breast feeding must also be pleasurable to the mother. While it may be that feeding the infant from the breast is a more totally satisfactory experience for the infant than bottle feeding, it is not breast feeding per se that produces the good experience. A young woman who breast feeds her child because she has been forced into it because she feels it is her duty but who objects to the process and may even be revolted by it will not be able to convince her infant that her breast is a comfortable source of nourishment. Such a mother may be able to give her child more genuine warmth and comfort when she holds a bottle for him.

But successful bottle feedings cannot be done with a bottle propped up for the infant to suck lying alone in his crib. An infant can accept a rubber nipple instead of a human nipple without much difficulty, provided the whole eating experience carries with it the same tender care which is almost automatic with breast feeding. This does not mean that occasionally an infant cannot accept a propped up bottle with equanimity. In a household where there are several young children, especially if there are twins, one lone woman cannot always supply all the children with all their needs simultaneously. But if the quality of care is good, an infant can cope amazingly well with occasional reductions in its quantity.

During the early months a good eating experience for the infant lays the groundwork for a personality relatively free from anxiety. The basic trust of Erikson's terminology (p. 356) is developing. During the infant's brief waking periods he can reach out to explore his world with his sensory equipment (p. 510).

The infant whose eating experience is less satisfactory may be given an adequate supply of milk, but he is not given the total body comfort he needs. His unsatisfied valences make him apprehensive and dampen his desire to explore his world during his waking periods. He does not suck, when the opportunity comes, with the same expectation of total satisfaction as does the better-fed baby. He probably will not eat as much or gain weight as rapidly, though he may gain enough to get by. Emotionally catastrophic situations, in which institutionalized infants were severely deprived of human contact, have been shown by Spitz to result in refusal of food so extreme that the infants died.

Sucking: Nipple, Thumb, Pacifier

In the early months all the infant's eating is accomplished by sucking. The need for nourishment and the need to suck are two different needs. Ideally they "come out even"—when the infant has had enough food, he has also satisfied his sucking need. But this is not always the case; some infants appear to need more sucking than others. An infant with a strong sucking urge may take all the milk his body requires but still want to suck. If he is breast-fed, he may satisfy himself by sucking a little longer on the relatively empty breast; if bottle-fed, he may be satisfied if his milk is given him through a nipple with a smaller hole. A fed infant who still wants to suck but has no nipple (either breast or bottle) on which to suck is likely to find his thumb or finger and "finish up" on them. It is desirable for the infant to satisfy his sucking urge, and his instinctive technique is adequate.

Many parents in our society dislike to see a baby suck his fingers. It is possible to use a pacifier with some babies. Pacifiers can be used intelligently, but they are often abused. Intelligent use means giving a clean pacifier after the baby has had enough milk if he still seems to need to suck. Many babies will accept the pacifier under these conditions, suck vigorously for a time, and then let it slip from the mouth. A few babies completely refuse the artificial sucking device and insist upon finishing up on their fingers. They had best be permitted to do so.

Abuse of a pacifier comes about when it is popped into a baby's mouth every time he whimpers, in order to "shut him up." Under such conditions the baby is being conditioned to overuse of sucking for comfort. When this happens, he is apt to continue to want a pacifier long after the normal sucking urge of early infancy should have abated.

Introduction of the Spoon

In the United States a milk diet alone is not considered adequate nutritionally beyond the first few months. Therefore new foods are introduced by new methods of eating. For a discussion of specific foods, and for techniques to use for infants who may have inherited an allergic constitution, see pp. 339 and 340.

Eating from a spoon is quite different from sucking, and the infant must learn a new skill. The tongue, cheeks, and palate are used in one way to suck fluid from a nipple and in quite a different way to push a spoonful of applesauce to the back of the throat where it can be swallowed.

The infant's first attempts are clumsy and often unsuccessful. He feels the food with his tongue and lips, moves it around, and is apt to push it out of his mouth. The first time he tries a spoon he is apt to be slow in actually getting any food into his stomach.

If the infant is ravenously hungry, he will become frustrated and angry if he is offered food he does not yet know how to get readily. He is in no mood to learn a new eating skill when he is in agony from hunger. If given about half his quota of milk, "burped," put in a comfortable position, he will be interested in trying this novel method of eating. Handled well, the infant gets considerable pleasure as he masters his new skill in eating; before long he opens his mouth in anticipation as he sees the spoon approach.

The age at which the spoon is introduced has some significance. Sucking time is automatically reduced by spoon-fed food, since calories are absorbed from the more concentrated pureed food. Sucking time may be so much reduced that the infant either begins sucking on his fingers or increases the finger sucking he was already doing. While this subsidiary sucking does little harm, it is on the whole a more satisfactory experience for the infant to suck food than extraneous objects. Contrariwise, his body's nutritional demands can be quite satisfactorily met with milk in the early months, so that there is little real need for spoon-fed food until such time as milk ceases to supply his nutritional needs.

From Passivity to Participation

As the months pass the infant begins to take a more active interest in the eating part of his life. Instead of lying back comfortably in his mother's arms, he begins grabbing with his hands toward the food. The breast-fed baby uses his hands to pump on the breast, the bottle-fed baby reaches up to try and hold the bottle. The 5- or 6-month-old baby grabs for the spoon, or he may dive into the bowl with his whole hand, bypassing the spoon entirely. The look of food is now attractive to him.

The infant is learning to bring his body under the control of his will. He needs to become independent, to develop confidence in his ability to do for himself. Therefore (within limits, of course), his slowness and messiness must be endured (p. 492).

Chewing

Some time after the half-year mark of the first year is passed, the child develops a new feeding interest—chewing. It is at this time that his teeth are beginning to make themselves evident. He wants to gnaw on everything he can get hold of. The gnawing and the biting are soothing to his often irritated gums, and they help push the teeth through.

While the baby at this stage is chewing on everything, he needs to be introduced to the fact that food is good to chew. He is now competent at swallowing smooth food introduced by spoon. But if there should be a lump in the spoon-fed food, he is confused. He is accustomed to pushing spoon-fed food back to his throat and slipping it down. Lumps do not go this way, so not knowing how to manage a lump, the baby spits it out. However, if this same baby picks up an object in his fingers and puts it in his mouth, he will immediately begin to chew on it.

Once he gets the idea that he can chew food as well as bedposts, toys, and fingers, he quite quickly discovers that he can pick up small bits of food and manage them satisfactorily. The skill of chewing has been learned. He cannot yet handle hard food or big lumps, and such food is dangerous, because the baby may well choke on them.

The infant denied the opportunity to chew by being fed only liquid and smooth pureed food beyond the time when teeth have come in may later on refuse to chew. He has passed the point where he wants to chew, and his desire to learn the skill is greatly diminished. Ultimately such a child will learn to chew but with much more difficulty than if he had learned it at the optimal point for the development of the skill.

Biting

Another ramification of chewing is biting. Biting may constitute a big problem when the infant is breast-fed beyond the time the teeth come in. In the United States today relatively few infants are breast-fed this long, so the problem is seen less in our culture than in times and places where prolonged breast feeding is customary.

An infant with a few teeth, interested in chewing on whatever he can, tries out his accomplishments on his mother's breast. This is an extraordinarily painful experience to the mother. She jumps, pulls her breast away, and is apt to give the infant a slap, an automatic reaction to a sudden sharp pain. To the infant this behavior on the part of his mother is astonishing and frightening. The experience can be very traumatic for an infant. From his point of view he was only trying out a new accomplishment, but as a result the very foundation of his security was suddenly pulled out from under him.

Different babies react differently to this experience. Occasionally, a child seems to learn from one time that biting results in maternal behavior he does not like, and he ceases to bite her breast. Some babies, however, will have nothing to do with the mother's breast after such an experience. Such a child cries when put to the breast and refuses to nurse. This usually results in immediate weaning. Other infants continue to experiment with biting the breast from time to time, usually each time with disastrous results to infant, to mother, and to their relationship. Fear, anger, rage, hostility, and finally guilt can be built up. It is not inconceivable that these strong emotions at this early age have lasting effects on the infant's emerging self-awareness. Much emphasis has been placed on this trauma of the biting phase in Freudian literature, which describes biting as a primary aggressive instinct rather than a mere experimentation with a newfound ability.

Early Desire for Independence

Toward the end of the first year, the baby has outgrown his early desire to be cuddled while eating. He now wants to sit at a table and take an active part in feeding himself. His joy in eating has shifted to his joy in his own emerging powers of independence. Dining now is doing, and all of it with the comforting presence of mother nearby.

If his enthusiasm for eating is to be maintained and his confidence in himself developed, he must be encouraged to do as much as he can. He will be slow and messy but full of joy. With a little ingenuity some of the messiness can be reduced. He can be offered ground-up meat, soft pieces of vegetables and fruit, egg either hard-cooked or scrambled until firm, pieces of dry cereal. He can be offered enough food at each meal to satisfy his desire to help himself. When he gets tired of his effort, he will often accept some help from his mother. So long as the child is doing his best to feed himself, he needs encouragement even if he is messy. This is a *constructive* mess. However, as soon as he begins just playing with the food, stirring it up, deliberately throwing it on the floor, he needs to be stopped. This is a *destructive* mess, and the child is better off if it is never tolerated. Food is to eat and to enjoy eating. Food is not to play with. Firm, gentle, and, above all, consistent discipline, combined with a casual attitude, are essential. Scoldings, don'ts, screams are ineffective methods of discipline. When food is not eaten, it is taken away. A child learns quickly that if he is hungry, he had better get busy and eat, or else he will be uncomfortably hungry before the next meal (see Chap. 33).

Drinking from a Cup

Infants vary a good deal in the age at which they are willing to graduate from sucking to drinking in the adult fashion. However, all children go through somewhat the same phases. Long before a baby will have anything to do with milk in a cup he will be interested in experimenting with water or juice from a cup. Sucking milk is a more fundamental satisfaction than sucking juice. Therefore a few tentative offers of juice from a cup can be made when the mother thinks the baby is interested. If he refuses completely, the cup had best be put away for a later date. If he accepts a few swallows, he is beginning to be ready. Little by little he can be offered more water or juice from the cup. Before long he will become quite competent. He may even be able to pick up a glass of juice by himself and drink the contents down. He is about ready then for a few swallows of milk in the cup along with his solid foods. The first few times he will probably only take a little bit and want to finish his milk from the bottle. But if he is developmentally ready, he will progress rapidly and soon be taking his full quota of milk from a glass. He should never be rushed. Provided he is slowly increasing his cup drinking, he should be allowed to finish his milk in a bottle for as long as he wants to.

It must be mentioned here that the total daily quota of milk should not be influenced by the technique of its consumption. A child who is loath to give up sucking completely may be permitted to have some of his milk in a bottle, but he must not be allowed to increase his milk intake. Excessive milk intake leads to failure to consume nonmilk foods and results in nutritional anemia.

Avid and Lackadaisical Suckers

Sucking never seems as vital to some children as it does to others. The avid sucker is violent about his desire to suck. He sucks a nipple with vigor and power. When he is not especially hungry, he goes after his fingers or whatever else he can find. He obviously gets much satisfaction from his lips and his sucking apparatus. He is always more interested in sucking his milk than he is in his solid foods. Mothers of such children report that the bottle must be kept out of the child's sight while he eats his solids. Once the child spies the bottle, he will have nothing more to do with a spoon. These avid suckers are not eager to hurry along to the next stage of eating development. They usually hang onto the bottle well beyond their first birthday, refusing the cup almost completely. When they do finally accept the cup for some of their milk, they may want to have some sucking pleasure well beyond the second birthday. They do, of course, ultimately take the big step and abandon the bottle completely.

The lackadaisical suckers, on the other hand, do suck in early infancy. They get hungry, have a good appetite, and are eager to suck down milk, but it never seems quite as important to them. Such children seldom suck their fingers. When solid foods are introduced, they often show a great deal more interest in the solids than in the milk. Such children must be fed the bottle before their solids, or they will not be interested in taking any milk. A baby to whom sucking is not too vital usually weans himself early. He likes the cup, even prefers it to the bottle, and may give up sucking for good in his seventh or eighth month.

Thus the age at which any one child is willing to give up sucking can vary anywhere from 7 months in a lackadaisical sucker to 3 years in an avid sucker.

There are environmental factors as well as innate differences between avid and lackadaisical suckers which influence the age at which different children are willing to abandon sucking milk. To all babies sucking is part of earliest gratification. The more completely the infant is satisfied in his earliest experiences, the more ready he will be to go on to the next step. His confidence in himself is growing, he has found his world dependable, and he is willing to forge ahead apparently with the expectation that new experiences will have their satisfactions, too. The infant who has never had quite enough of the subsidiary pleasures that go with the early eating experience, the infant who has not dined well, is the infant anxious to hang on to his infantile ways. He seems reluctant to give up the familiar for the uncharted sea of new experiences.

Babies who are slow to give up the bottle completely need careful appraisal. The reasons for delayed weaning are subtle. One slow weaner may be an avid sucker and an emotionally sturdy baby whose need to suck is part of his biologic makeup. For him permissiveness in weaning time is most desirable. Another slow weaner may hang onto a bottle not because of an innate sucking drive but because he is emotionally reluctant to take a step forward. Such a child needs encouragement, even coercion to abandon his infantile ways. Permitting him to prolong bottle feedings will not help him mature. Forced weaning when the baby is not ready for it has serious repercussions. It is important that a baby give up infantile ways for more grownup ways with enthusiasm. He will then accept his maturity with pleasure and confidence. On the other hand permission to hang on to infantile behavior because of anxiety tends to prolong the anxiety.

GROWTH RATE, APPETITE, AND MATERNAL ATTITUDE

Toward the end of the first year the infant's growth slows down (p. 108), and fewer calories are needed. The mother's first awareness of her child's growth comes to her during the early months of his infancy. This is the period of most rapid growth. The mother is pleased and proud of the large gain her baby makes each month. But no baby is destined to keep up a gain at the rate at which he starts off. The baby himself "knows" about the inherent human growth pattern; he is doing his best to follow. His tissues are not grabbing for as much food; he is just not as hungry at 10 months or at a year as he was at 3 months. He takes as much as he needs to meet the nutritional requirements of the gain in weight he is foreordained to make.

The baby "knows"—his tissues "know"—but unless someone tells his mother, she does not know that this is normal and expected behavior (Fomon, 1964). With explanation mothers can accept a normal growth pattern. They do not want obese children. They can reduce the amount of food offered and feel confident and secure in the fact that they know what to expect.

THE TODDLER EATS

By the time the child is toddling about under his own power, he is also sitting at a small table for his meals and managing most of his feeding himself. Eating at this age is a fascinating, all-absorbing occupation. The very act of getting the food into the mouth is interesting. Fingers are often far handier tools than the forks and spoons of adult life. The toddler will try to use the tools to some extent, often using his fingers to put the food into the spoon, and then, with the one hand guiding the other so the food does not fall off, the whole bite will get to the mouth, and the child will give an overall wiggle of satisfaction in his accomplishment. He is dining; he is getting joy from the act of eating.

He can drink his milk from a cup or a glass. He loves the added accomplishment of pouring it into his own cup from a small pitcher. If his food is arranged for him so that he can manage reasonably well, he will eat his entire meal by himself. He may resist help with the familiar refrain, "No—me do it." Occasionally, if he is more than normally tired, he may slip back into more baby ways and say, "You feed me." It does not hinder developing independence to resort to baby ways once in a while, when the inevitable fatigues and tensions of life make independence not worth the effort for the moment.

The toddler, however, has abandoned for good any desire to be cuddled while he eats. He loves to eat partly because he loves to do. He is in the second phase of ego development, during which he is establishing mastery over his body. Eating is an important tool in the development of autonomy.

The toddler will be discouraged if he is held up to standards of neatness and niceness of table manners beyond his capacity. If he is jumped on every time he spills something, every time he uses his fingers instead of a fork or spoon, he will soon lose his pleasure in his own efforts, since they get him nothing but scoldings. If he is not permitted to dine in the ways a toddler enjoys dining, he loses much of his interest in eating. Dining is more important to him than nourishing his body. When eating no longer gives him satisfaction in itself, the toddler is apt to dawdle and just not eat very much, perhaps not as much as his body really needs. Hunger may be there, but the biologic demand for fuel is not enough by itself to make the child eat.

To a toddler, eating is a full-time operation, and he needs no diversion during mealtime. In fact, a toddler will stop eating completely if something interesting is happening nearby. He cannot eat and talk, or even eat and listen very satisfactorily. He needs a quiet place for his meals with a minimum of outside distraction. He needs good food in small amounts attractively and interestingly put before him. Then he needs to be left alone with mother not far away so that she can lend a hand, if necessary.

Eating with the Family

At what age the little child comes to the family table depends upon the circumstances. Sometimes a young couple with a first baby enjoy pulling the baby's high chair up to their table and letting the baby eat with them. This works well if the parents can quietly enjoy the baby's enthusiasm for eating without interfering, if his inevitable messiness does not bother them, if he can be permitted to eat as much as he wants without urging him to consume more than he needs. Oftentimes, the food on mother's plate adds new attraction to the baby. He wants to copy his adults and will be eager to try new foods purloined from his parents. This is often a most successful way to introduce new foods. Needless to say it must be combined with a firm denial of foods unsuitable for the baby's as yet not fully mature digestive apparatus.

When eating with the family is not a pleasant experience, the small child will be better off if he has his meal in peace and quietude by himself. Nagging—"Eat this," "Don't spill," "Hurry up"—does not do anybody any good, and it does the baby a good deal of harm.

THE PRESCHOOL CHILD EATS

There comes a time when the mechanics of eating are fairly well mastered and the child is ready for the next step in the maturation of eating behavior. He is now ready for companionship during eating. He can eat and talk at the same time. He can think about something more than how the next bite is going to get to his mouth and how it will feel to his tongue and cheeks. He wants to eat with others, especially with his family; he wants to talk; he wants to feel he is one of the group. Dining now includes association with other people. In ego development the preschooler is trying to establish what kind of person he is. The family dinner table can make a contribution to his sense of inner worth.

Family conversation needs to include the child. It needs to be at his level of understanding. The child wants to talk of his day's activities, of the events that interest him. He enjoys stories told by his parents, little episodes within his comprehension. In such a setting the child participates, feels happy and comfortable, and feels that he belongs. He will eat as the family eats. His table manners may not be perfect, but they are reasonably acceptable. He has a good appetite. His body is ready for the food and takes it in as readily as his personality takes in the warmth of family participation. He is dining.

On the other hand, if the family table conversation is over the child's head and he feels left out, he is apt to take matters in his own hands and find a way of directing attention to himself. His hunger for personal relations is greater than his hunger for food, and he may mess with his food, use table manners which are well below his capacity, and fail to eat. This behavior is pretty apt to direct attention to him. He gets scolded, yelled at perhaps, but he most effectively brings himself into the group's attention. If he does eat, if he does behave more acceptably, once again he is ignored. He soon learns that eating and behaving acceptably does not get him what he craves—participation. He would rather be scolded than ignored.

The family who understands the little child's emerging needs in connection with eating seldom has many "eating problems." Small portions of good food served attractively and eaten in a congenial atmosphere of family participation usually result in acceptable eating behavior on the part of the child. The actual foods which the child eats will of course be those of the culture in which he lives, and they are apt to be the ones he will most enjoy all his life.

Some small children do very well on three meals a day with nothing but water between meals. However, an appreciable number really need a little nutritional boost in the long interval between breakfast and lunch, and between lunch and dinner. The blood sugar level drops, and as it does the youngster becomes restless and irritable. His disposition is often improved with a little quickly available carbohydrate. Nursery schools recognize this fact, and almost all of them have a "juice time" in midmorning and midafternoon. Juice time, however, should be a meal, even though a small one. The child puts on his bib, sits down at the table, eats his crackers, drinks his juice. Having these snacks in a meal situation controls the nutritional adequacy of the food offered, avoids the desire to munch sporadically, and may make the child a pleasanter person to live with.

Young children play incessantly; fatigue and dirt are an inevitable result. A little washing up and a brief quiet period before meals are a desirable prelude to a peaceful meal.

THE SCHOOL-AGE CHILD EATS

Once the child has entered the world of school, his eating habits become influenced by his new-found independence from home. As in other realms of life, he wants to conform to the ways of his age-mates. He eats his basic meals with his family, but he also loves odd kinds of eating. Boys build a hut, and part of the joy is eating in the hut. Girls play house and want to serve each other food as part of the play. Both boys and girls love picnics and cookouts and food eaten in places other than at the family dining table. The joy of eating is the companionship that goes with it. Dining at this age is far more a quality of people and places than of food.

During the school years the family table is a most important part of eating, too. Good table talk geared to the interests of the children makes for good eating habits. Nowhere is the atmosphere of a family more obvious than around the dinner table. It is here that the family gathers, and mealtime is often the only time when the family is together for an activity. Word games, talk of the days' activities, and jokes make dining out of eating and provide the subsidiary pleasures so necessary for full development of the children. Also enjoyment of their children provides dining pleasure for the parents. On the other hand, a family dinner table where the adults talk over the children's heads gives the school-age child such a leftout feeling that like the preschooler he may well resort to various undesirable techniques to bring himself into notice and participation. For an adult it is quite an uncomfortable experience to sit at a table where others are talking a foreign language, especially if it is known that they can speak the common language. An adult in such a situation probably behaves properly, but he feels angry and annoyed. A child with similar feelings, when dinner table conversation is not understandable to him, is apt to express his emotion in unpleasant behavior. Among adults, table conversation that needlessly leaves out a member of the group is considered rude and discourteous. Children are people and are entitled to the same courtesies accorded adults.

Before the child ventures outside the home, he may have eaten only the foods served in his home. He has accepted the cultural pattern of his family. Once he begins eating at school and at his friends' homes, he broadens his eating horizons. The type of food served in the home, however, is the food the child will best accept and enjoy. Because lifetime food patterns are likely established during the early years, nutritional patterns are of great importance. If the food served in the home is limited in variety, even

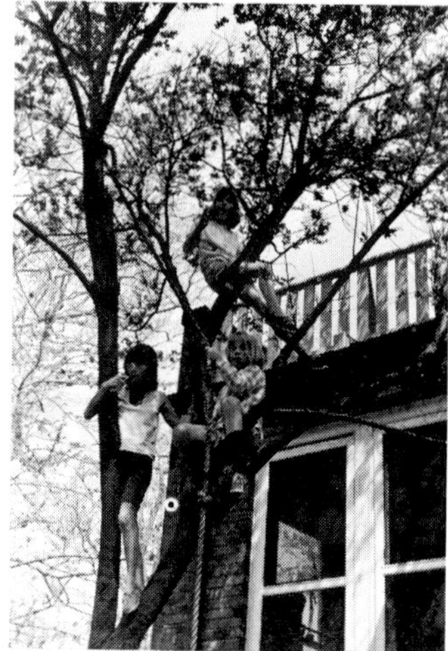

School age children love eating in odd places

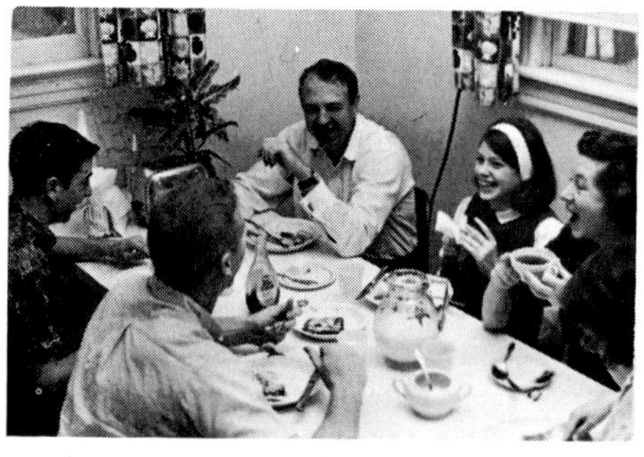

The family table provides dining pleasures for children and parents

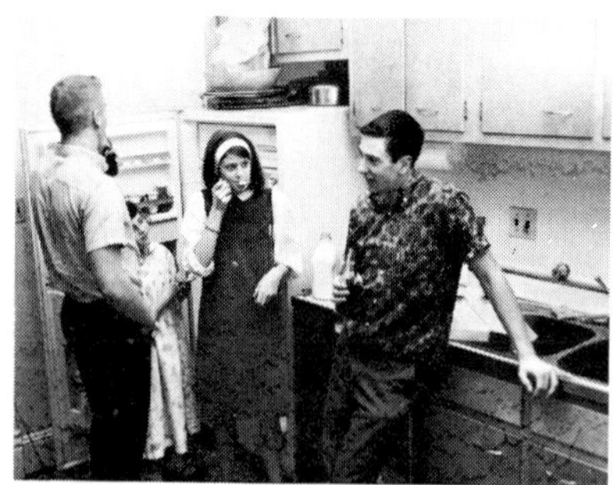

Refigerator raiding is part of the dining pleasures of the adolescent

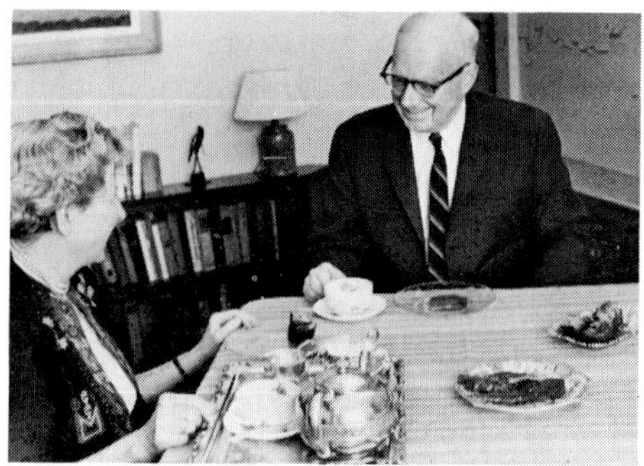

Throughout the years dining is part of the good life

Fig. 28-2. Dining after the early years.

though adequate in amount, the child's repertory of food will be small, and he may have difficulty in accepting a more varied menu later in life. On the other hand, a family with a constantly changing menu conditions the child to the excitement of trying something new, especially if the adults of the family are interested in gustatory delights. This does not mean that young children will relish many varieties of exotic food, but they will be less resistant to them if they have grown up in an atmosphere in which food is appreciated.

THE ADOLESCENT AND FOOD

When children enter the rapid growth of early adolescence, eating looms large as one of the joys of life. The need for food suddenly spurts up in puberty to take care of the added call for fuel needed for the rapid growth of this age. The young adolescent wants food. Some boys put on 20 lb in a year; girls do not gain quite as much, but a girl can easily gain 10 to 15 lb in a year (p. 87). Rather obviously this body substance cannot be made unless the building stones of growth are provided. Appetites soar. These are the years when a boy can consume four portions of everything at dinner and be raiding the refrigerator an hour later.

The insistent demands of hundreds of thousands of growing cells craving energy to fulfill their biologic destiny drive teen-agers to some source of food whenever there is a lull in the day's occupations. After school the corner drugstore draws them as a magnet draws iron filings. The drugstore provides ice cream, lush sundaes, soft drinks, and the company of their equally starved peers. Peanuts and popcorn eaten in the movie house are as much a source of pleasure as the movie itself.

The adult who tries to guide an adolescent must be ever mindful of the significance of these pleasures. The inseparability of the hungers for food and for love is at no time more apparent than during the adolescent period of rapid growth. Denial of enjoyed foods is interpreted as denial of love and augments the often shaky feeling adolescents have about themselves. All too often adult supervision consists of threats, nagging, and prohibitions from which the independently minded young adolescent rebels and goes his own way, depending as far as food is concerned upon the demands of his taste buds and the dictates of his companions.

Adolescents are, in general, very body-conscious. They are concerned about themselves and their physical well-being. If talked *with*, not to, and given some straightforward facts about bodily needs, it is not too difficult to get their cooperation on the matter of diet. The friendly discussion dispels the fear of loss of love. An opportunity to take over responsibility on the basis of knowledge gives the adolescent a feeling of self-confidence, because he knows his adults respect him. Thus his hunger for love is appeased, and his hunger for fuel can more easily be diverted toward the kind of food his growing body needs.

Adequate breakfasts are often a big problem. The adolescent needs more sleep than the younger child (p. 317), just as he needs more food. He is sleepy in the morning, hates to get up, puts it off to the last second, then does not have time for breakfast. If he is tired of the conventional bacon and eggs, there is no reason why he cannot have a hamburger. It is good, both nutritionally and gustatorily. Adequate, good-tasting food with enough time to eat it with pleasure and enjoyment is the goal. Mother's job is to prepare the food; the child's responsibility is to arrange for the time.

Adolescents *must* eat after school. They are ravenous; they would simply fall apart if made to starve until dinner time. But their bodies need good food—fruit, meat, milk—not candy, cakes, soft drinks, and cookies.

A shelf in the refrigerator labeled with the child's name and stacked daily by mother with something good—deviled eggs, cold meat, cheese, fruit, milk—can do wonders to improve an adolescent's diet. Not only does this service by mother improve the child's diet, but her willingness to do the extra work helps build up a rapport with her youngster. He feels that his mother does real things for him and does not fuss or nag. This gives him the feeling that he is a worthwhile person.

In adolescent girls the desire for a slim figure may be so strong that nutritionally inadequate reducing regimes sap the strength of the growing body. Again sympathetic understanding from a perceptive adult can go a long way toward maintaining good eating habits, good nutrition, and a stable personality.

In adolescence much of the harvest of the early years is reaped. The child whose eating experience has been good and whose emerging personality is not overburdened with anxieties is in a position to weather the turbulence of adolescence. Many things besides eating are significant at this age (Chap. 40), but food and dining can help establish relationships on all fronts.

MATURE JOYS OF EATING

After they have grown up, human beings still love to eat. They eat not just to supply fuel but because they enjoy eating. Good food attractively served, eaten in pleasurable surroundings and with congenial people, continues, as in childhood, to constitute an important aspect of the good life. The child who has had good eating experiences throughout most of his life becomes the adult who can maintain satisfaction from this most biologic of necessities.

In the *mature* adult the hypothalamic regulation of food intake dominates the amount of food consumed (p. 366). Hunger for food is not confused with hunger for emotional satisfaction, and the individual's appetite becomes a fairly accurate gauge of his fuel requirements. He dines with pleasure and satisfaction and finds other appropriate gratifications for other emotions.

The actual dietary ingredients consumed are closely related to the type of food eaten during the growing years. Whether an adult's diet is good or bad depends in large measure upon the nutritional adequacy of the food served him as a child. Cultural patterns formed in childhood are changed only with difficulty.

EATING TOO MUCH

There are a host of factors that cause overeating and resulting obesity. They can be divided into those due to some organic pathologic condition and those due to genetic, environmental, and emotional factors (Mayer, 1955).

Organic conditions probably account for but a small proportion of human obesity. Excessive intake of food may be due to errors in the central regulating mechanism or to abnormalities in the metabolism of fat and carbohydrates. It has been found (Prugh, 1961) that animals with a hyperglycemic syndrome synthesize more fat than normal animals when both are on isocaloric diets.

There are gene-determined factors related to the amount of fat deposited. In a study made by Prugh, obese children were found in only 8 to 9 per cent of families in which both parents had normal weight, in 40 per cent where one parent was obese, but in 80 per cent where both parents were obese.

Familial obesity, while doubtless partly related to common constitutional factors, is related also to the type of food served in the home. People with an endomorphic body build, with a predominant gastrointestinal tract, enjoy eating (Sheldon, 1940). By definition a woman with this type of constitution is a good cook. A family table planned by an endomorphic woman is apt to be one in which high caloric foods predominate. A child coming to maturity in this gastronomic environment learns to prefer this type of food. Obesity developing under these conditions may be both genetic and environmental. Such a person may truly dine at each meal.

Emotions can play a role in obesity which may begin early in life, most frequently in families with a history of obesity (Prugh, 1961). The mother may express an abnormal concern for the child, possibly in compensation for guilty feelings because she once rejected him (Bruch, 1958). She lavishes him with physical attention in the form of food, and simultaneously she curtails his physical activity lest he injure himself. The child grows up realizing that food consumption is the one activity that gets him maternal approval. The resulting obesity compounds his feelings of inadequacy. Later in life the memory of the satisfactions accompanying a full stomach cause him to eat whenever he faces the tribulations of life, and he may have many such tribulations since his home climate has not been conducive to normal personality development. Such a person seldom dines, the hunger that prompts his eating is hunger for love and appreciation, not the hunger for body fuel.

EATING TOO LITTLE

Just as there are some people who tend to eat too much, so are there others whose dining pleasures are so few that they tend not to nourish their bodies adequately. (It should be pointed out that the obese person is not necessarily well nourished.)

In early infancy failure to eat (in the absence of a gross abnormality) is closely related to failure in interpersonal relations. An infant cannot eat until his dining needs are satisfied (p. 370). In late infancy and early childhood poor eating habits may result from the overzealous efforts of parents to get more food down his gullet than a child needs. This may produce a disgust for food which lasts for years.

The child who gets greater pleasure from not eating than from eating is apt to have a body with a large ectomorphic potential and a minimum of the endomorphic. His gastrointestinal tract and the normal urges that go with it are a small proportion of his total makeup. He is better able to forgo the pleasures of eating than is the child with dominant gastrointestinal mechanisms.

The senses of smell and taste are clearly related to the consumption of enough food. If these senses are lost, much of the physiologic pleasure in eating disappears. The decrease in the anticipatory salivary and gastric secretions (p. 191) may interfere with digestion. The pleasures of dining then become almost entirely those of social contact. The individual who has lost his sense of smell or taste forgets to have a meal if he must eat it alone.

Minor degrees of anorexia are encountered frequently. Occasionally such severe forms of self-induced starvation are seen that life itself is threatened. Anorexia nervosa has been considered a manifestation of a suicidal tendency in adolescent girls who become obsessed with self-denial of eating pleasures.

BIBLIOGRAPHY

ANAND, BALK, and JOHN R. BROBECK: Hypothalamic Control of Food Intake in Rats and Cats, *Yale J. Biol. & Med.*, **24**:123, 1951–1952.

BEST, CHARLES H., and NORMAN B. TAYLOR: "The Physiological Basis of Medical Practice," The Williams and Wilkins Company, Baltimore, 1955.

BROBECK, JOHN R.: Neural Control of Hunger, Appetite and Satiety, *Yale J. Biol. & Med.*, **29**:565, 1956–1957.

BROZEK, JOSEF: Nutrition and Behavior, An Epilogue, *Am. J. Clin. Nutrition*, **5**:332, 1957.

BRUCH, HILDE: Psychological Aspects of Obesity in Adolescence, *Am. J. Pub. Health*, **48**:1349, 1958.

———: Transformation of Oral Impulses in Eating Disorders: A Conceptual Approach, *Psychiat. Quart.*, **35**:458, 1961.

———: Obesity, *Ped. Clin. North America*, p. 613, Aug., 1958.

DAVIS, CLARA M.: Self-selection of Diet by Newly Weaned Infants, *Am. J. Dis. Child.*, **36**:651, 1928.

ERIKSON, ERIK H.: "Childhood and Society," 2d ed., W. W. Norton & Company, Inc., New York, 1963.

FOMON, SAMUEL J.: Factors Affecting Food Intake, *Pediatrics,* **33**:135, 1964.

MAYER, JEAN: The Physiological Basis of Obesity and Leanness, *Nutrition Abst. & Rev.*, **25**: part I, 597, part II, 871, 1955.

MINER, ROY W. (ed.): The Regulation of Hunger and Appetite, *Ann. N.Y. Acad. Sc.*, **63**:1, 1955.

MOORE, HARRIET BRUCE: The Meaning of Food, *Am. J. Clin. Nutrition,* **5**:77, 1957.

PRUGH, DANE E.: Some Psychological Considerations Concerned with the Problem of Overnutrition, *Am. J. Clin. Nutrition,* **9**:538, 1961.

SHELDON, W. H.: "The Varieties of Human Physique," Harper & Row, Publishers, Incorporated, New York, 1940.

SPITZ, RENÉ A.: Hospitalism, The Psycho-analytic Study of the Child, **1**:53, 1945.

SULLIVAN, HARRY STACK: "The Interpersonal Theory of Psychiatry," W. W. Norton & Company, Inc., New York, 1953.

TALBOT, NATHAN B., EDNA H. SOBEL, JANET W. MCARTHUR, and JOHN B. CRAWFORD: "Functional Endocrinology from Birth through Adolescence," published for the Commonwealth Fund, Harvard University Press, Cambridge, Mass., 1953.

29

Motor Behavior

Motor behavior is dependent upon physical structure and passes through an orderly series of changes as muscles, nerves, and sense organs mature. Human behavior is dependent also upon the ego; how the individual feels influences how he uses the equipment under his control.

Motor behavior can be divided into three main categories: first, that which remains for life under involuntary control, including visceral functionings and reflex activity; second, instinctive behavior; third, behavior which becomes truly voluntary.

MUSCULAR BEHAVIOR AT BIRTH

All the muscles in the body, both those under control of the autonomic nervous system and those under control of the central nervous system, exhibit a phenomenon called *tonus*. This is a condition of tension independent of activity. It is a sustained partial contraction that increases when movement takes place; it decreases during sleep, but it never disappears until life ceases. Tonus is the main source of heat generated in the body.

Tonus develops during fetal life. By the end of a normal gestation period the fetus has built up enough tonus to maintain body posture. The prematurely born infant lacks sufficient tonus, as is evidenced by his limp body and unsustained movements.

The entire muscular apparatus and most of the sense organs are present in the full-term infant, but the immaturity of the cortex precludes truly voluntary behavior. Below the cortex the central nervous system, the peripheral nerves, and the autonomic system are mature enough to function adequately. The neuromuscular action of the viscera is somewhat more labile than it will be later and less able to cope with adversity, but essentially it is functional. The striated musculature exhibits reflex activity at the time of birth.

REFLEX ACTIVITY AT BIRTH

Reflex activity develops during fetal life as muscle and nerve form. As early as 2 months of fetal life, the trunk flexes, the head retracts. By 4 months the extremities move about quite actively, and the tongue begins to practice sucking movements. By the time of birth several reflex patterns are well established.

The *Moro reflex* has recently been subject to critical evaluation by Parmelee. He found that the most effective and reliable stimuli for eliciting the reflex were (1) allowing the baby's head to drop back suddenly and (2) slapping the examining table near the baby's head. Contrary to rather common belief Parmelee found that a loud noise was an ineffective stimulus.

The response of the Moro reflex is predominately an outward and upward extension of the arms and opening of the fingers. Extension of the legs occurs in many but not all babies. The reflex terminates by return of the arms and a clasping maneuver of the hands. The face shows some contortion, and often the baby cries. Parmelee found the movement of the arms to be the most reliable aspect of the Moro reflex; the secondary movements, while usually present in the neonate, faded more quickly than the arm movements.

The Moro reflex develops some time between the sixth and seventh month of fetal life and is therefore not present in early prematures. It is present in all neurologically healthy newborn infants after the seventh month of fetal life. Absence of the reflex or an asymmetric reflex suggests a pathologic condition. The Moro reflex gradually fades and cannot be elicited after 12 weeks of postnatal life. Its persistence after 4 months of age is considered an indication of delay in neuromuscular maturation. Although the full-blown Moro reflex disappears, a remnant of this reflex persists throughout life as the jump, or startle, reaction.

In the *seeking reflex* the hungry neonate turns his head sideways when he receives tactile sensation on his cheek. At the same time he opens his mouth, apparently seeking a nipple on which to suck.

The *tonic neck reflex* is one of the earliest true reflexes to develop. By the twentieth week of gestation, the beginnings of this reflex are evident. From then on it becomes stronger and more pronounced until it finally fades out between the seventh and eighth month of postnatal life. At birth this reflex is very pronounced. When the infant turns his head to one side, the arm on that side extends, and the arm and leg on the opposite side flex. Most newborns, when lying on the back, prefer to keep the head turned to one side or the other (most often to the right side). The tonic neck reflex is most clearly shown when the head is forcibly moved either to the midline position or to the opposite side. The infant quickly moves the head back to the position he prefers and goes through the movements of the whole reflex.

Clonus is a quivering motion seen especially in the jaw, although the feet and also the hands often show clonus spontaneously or in response to sudden flexion. This reflex is quite normal in the newborn and gradually fades out by about 6 months of age. Its persistence or its recurrence later in life is a pathologic sign.

The *grasp reflex,* like the Moro reflex, is an evolutionary hangover. If a bar or a finger is placed across the infant's hand, he immediately closes his hand and grasps what touches it. The flexion is so forceful that the fingers blanch. His grip is strong enough to support his whole weight; he can be lifted from a supine position to an upright one by the strength of his own grasp. This reflex gradually fades out and is gone by 3 or 4 months of age.

Tendon reflexes are present in the newborn and are similar to those found throughout life. They are somewhat difficult to elicit, because the newborn is seldom sufficiently relaxed.

The *Babinski's sign* is elicited when the plantar surface of the foot is stroked. In infancy the toes extend and fan upward. Later in life the same stimulus produces flexion of the toes, so that they curl downward. The extension response, normal in infancy, later in life suggests a lesion in the postpyramidal tract.

Chvostek's sign is a contraction of the muscles of one side of the face when an area in front of the ear on the same side is tapped. It is a normal reflex of the first few months of life, after which it disappears in most healthy children. Its appearance after 6 months of age is a diagnostic sign suggestive of tetany (increased muscle irritability). Chvostek's sign, however, can sometimes be elicited in a small proportion of quite healthy older children, and therefore its presence in older children must be interpreted with caution.

The *stepping reflex* is an odd reflex of the newborn. If an infant is held upright, he will move his feet as though walking. He cannot, of course, support his weight, but he coordinates his legs and feet as though he were walking with his feet on a firm surface. This reflex fades out toward the middle of the first year, and when the child is ready to learn to walk, he must learn the coordination which he apparently possessed unlearned at birth.

The *swimming reflex* is similar to the walking reflex. A newborn suspended in a bath of warm water will execute coordinated swimming movements, almost sufficient to keep himself afloat. This reflex too disappears, and swimming ultimately has to be learned.

All these reflexes are part of the activity of the newborn infant, but none of them except perhaps the seeking reflex has survival value at the human level. Their presence, however, is indicative of normally functioning neural and muscular systems.

INSTINCTIVE BEHAVIOR

Bowlby has advanced some strong arguments for the existence of instinctive motor patterns. He has suggested that the human infant is equipped with five instinctive patterns which serve the purpose of getting for him the care necessary for his survival. These instinctive patterns are, according to Bowlby, crying, sucking, clinging, smiling, and following.

Sucking, clinging, and following are each drives which accomplish their

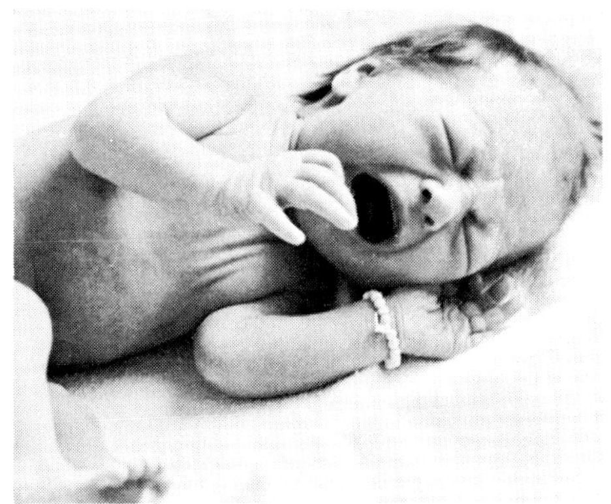

Crying

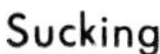

Sucking

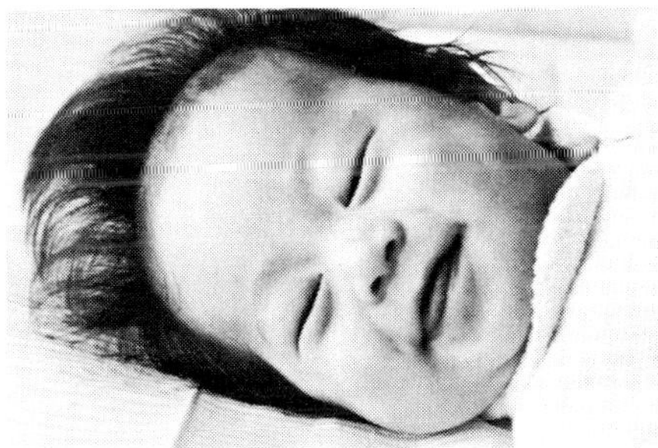

Smiling

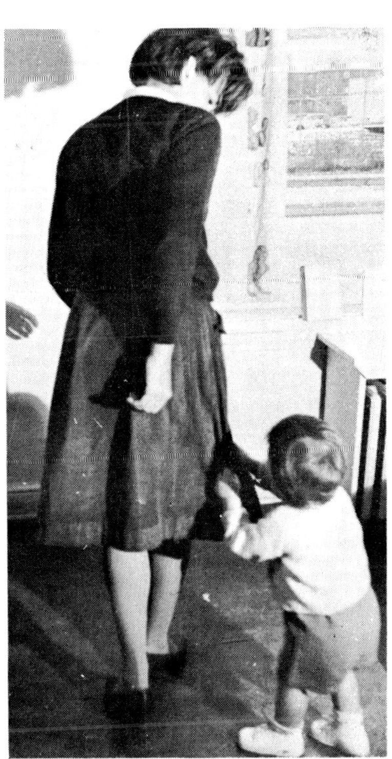

Following

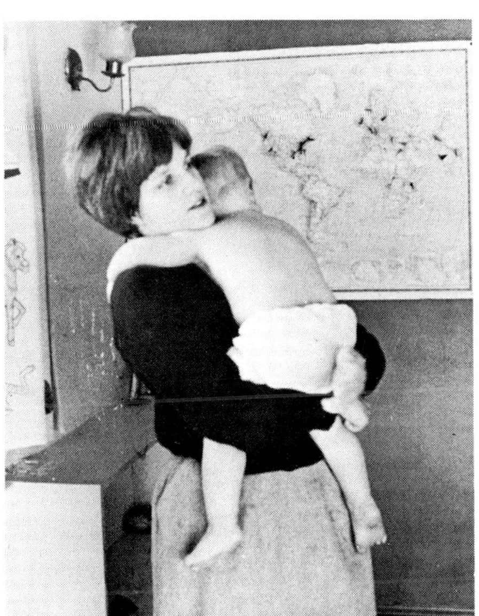

Clinging

Fig. 29-1. Basic instinctual patterns.

own ends: the first, food; the other two, close proximity to the mother. The mother must cooperate in achieving the ends, but the main activity comes from the infant. Crying and smiling, on the other hand, are forms of infant behavior which, in and of themselves, accomplish nothing; both depend upon activity in the mother for accomplishment of their ends, which again are close proximity to the mother.

Crying

Crying is elicited by discomfort, any kind of discomfort, whether it be hunger, cold, posture, pain, or any amorphous disequilibrium. Crying is more fully developed in the human being than in any other species. The young of many species are able to bleat or whimper or peep—sounds which bring the mother—but no species can put up the lusty bellow of a distraught human infant. Perhaps this is because the human newborn is more dependent upon his mother than any other species, dependent both for his physical survival and for the development of his human qualities.

Crying is a maternal activator. It brings the mother to the side of her infant. A mother is attuned to her infant's cry; she reacts differently to this sound than to other sounds of the same intensity. A mother can sleep through a thunderstorm and yet be alert to the first whimper of her baby. Similarly, there is a difference between the response of the mother to a baby's cry and the response of another person. A nurse or a father may be able to ignore or perhaps even not hear a cry that alerts the mother into activity. (*How* a mother responds to the cry of her own infant may well be intellectual or cultural behavior. She may decide to do this or do that or decide to do nothing, but the fact that the sound alerts her in a peculiarly intense fashion is part of *her* instinctual equipment.)

The crying is terminated when the infant feels the mother pick him up, hold him, rock him, give him tender care. If the discomfort which produced the cry was largely hunger, the mother's presence will terminate the crying only briefly, until further needs are satisfied. But hunger or pain are not the only stimuli which set the cry into operation. Human infants have a need for tenderness, for human warmth, and they cry for the satisfaction of these needs as well as for the opportunity to suck and relieve hunger. The human mother, while perhaps also endowed with instinctual neural pathways, has lived long enough in a human society to have acquired an overlay of sophistication which may exert a stronger influence on her overt behavior than any inborn patterns. In other words, the baby can be counted on to ask for what he needs, but more often than not the mother needs instruction in how to meet those needs.

If the normal infant's needs are met as they arise and as he calls for help, trust develops in him; he confidently expects gratification. Not only has he faith that he is safe, but also he is becoming more and more able to take care of his own needs and less and less in need of summoning help.

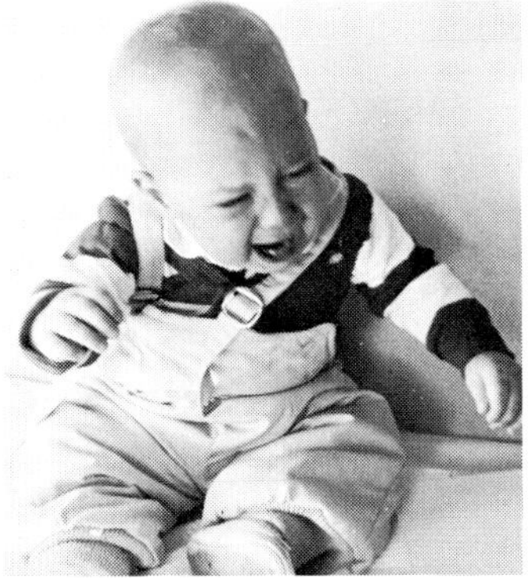

Crying is useful throughout infancy

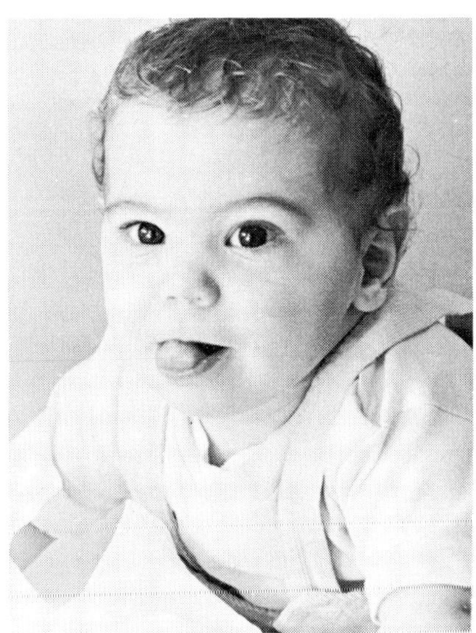

Some infants suck their tongues

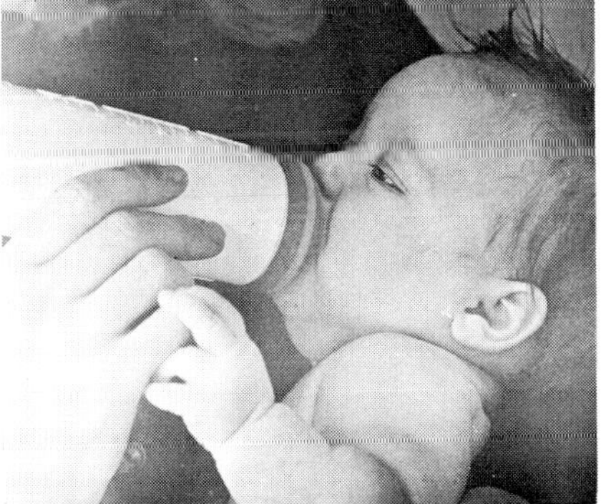

Infants suck a rubber nipple as readily as the breast

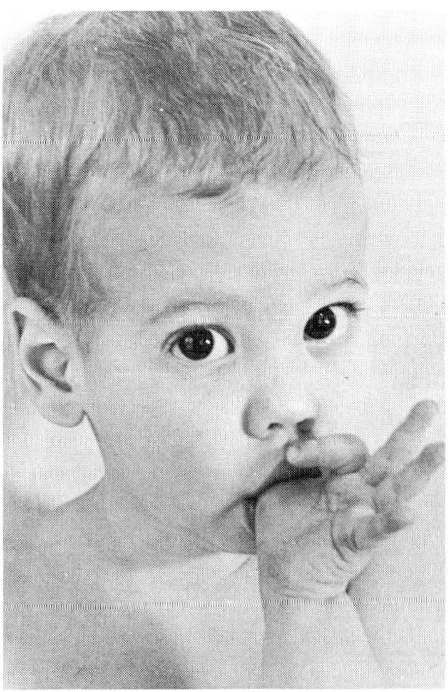

The thumb gives comfort in time of stress

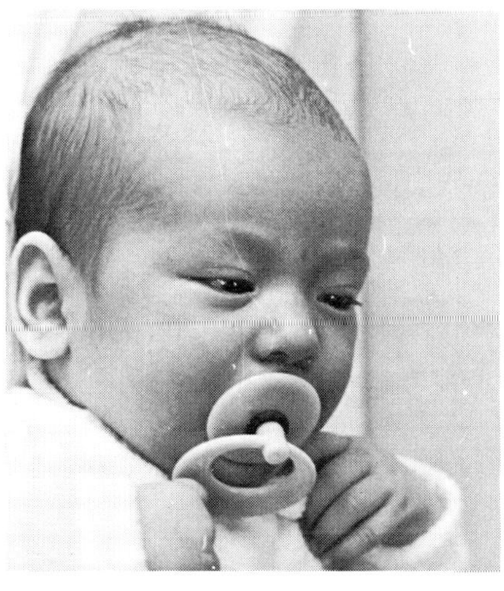

A pacificer satisfies some sucking urges

Fig. 29-2. Patterns derived from basic instinctual patterns—crying and sucking.

He no longer needs to cry and, gradually, as the months pass he cries less and less. He still has the crying equipment, and it will be brought into use in times of distress (Aldrich et al., 1945).

On the other hand, if the infant's needs are attended to only sporadically, if he frequently has to live through long periods of mounting panic, he will continue to cry at the first manifestation of discomfort. He has no inner conviction that good things will come if he waits a few minutes.

Throughout all of childhood a youngster will cry when he is physically hurt or emotionally distressed—whenever life poses problems with which he cannot cope. Those children who have not found life trustworthy continue to demand satisfaction by crying and by other modes of behavior which, in a more ideal situation, would have been outgrown. The severely rejected infant may discover that crying does not bring him relief from his discomforts, and ultimately he abandons it and sinks into apathy (Spitz, 1946).

There is little, if any, sex difference in the amount of crying during the early years. Trust, contentment, self-assurance, as well as bodily pain, are the dominant factors which determine how often a child cries. In our culture, a sex difference manifests itself after puberty. Girls and women cry under duress more easily than men.

Sucking

This subject is discussed in Chap. 28.

Smiling

At birth the only technique at the infant's disposal to get his mother is to cry. The neonate is unable to smile. The neural pathways to the facial muscles acquire their myelin sheaths during the early postnatal weeks. Between 3 and 4 weeks of age an infant begins to squinch the muscles around his mouth and eyes, practicing, as it were, his new-found ability to work these muscles. At about 1 month of age the mechanism is sufficiently mature to respond to stimuli. The stimulus that activates the smile, says Bowlby, is two bright dots in the infant's visual field. These dots are usually the mother's eyes. At all events, at about 1 month of age, the infant beams his toothless grin at his mother.

The smile is a powerful stimulus to the mother. She is already there beside him when he smiles, since it is her eyes that set off the behavior. The appealing nature of the baby's smile stimulates the mother to pick him up, hug him, croon to him, give him the tender care he needs.

The infant soon learns to associate his smile with the tender care it elicits, and he uses it. At first the human infant smiles because he has an instinctive pattern that responds to a given stimulus, but he continues to smile because he has learned that his smile brings him what he needs. He

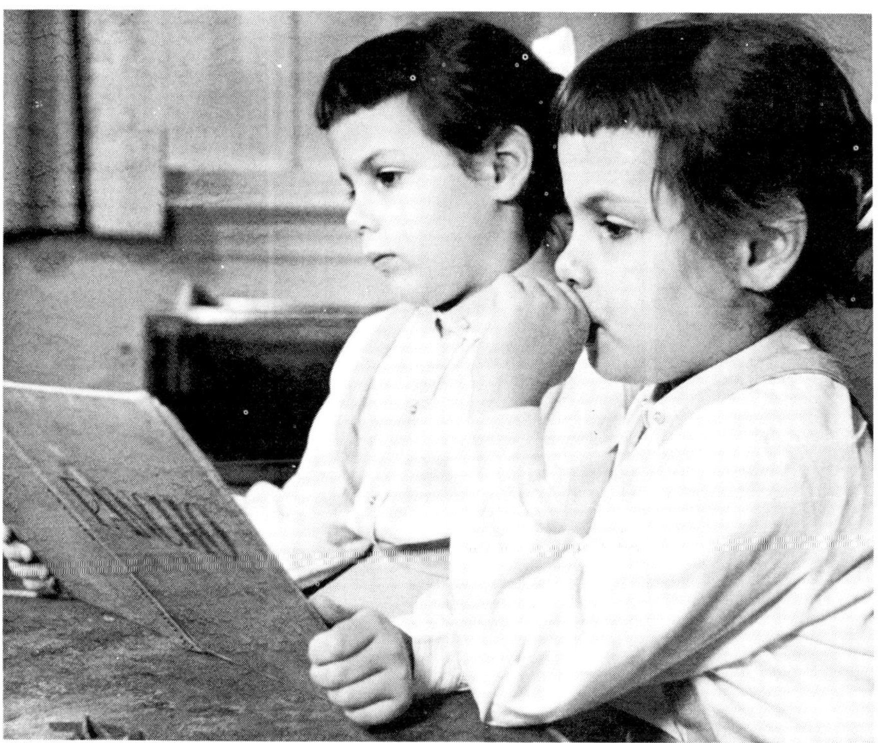

Only one twin sucked her thumb

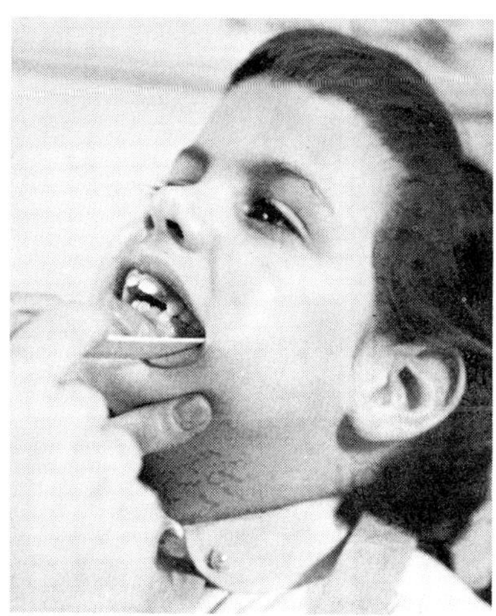

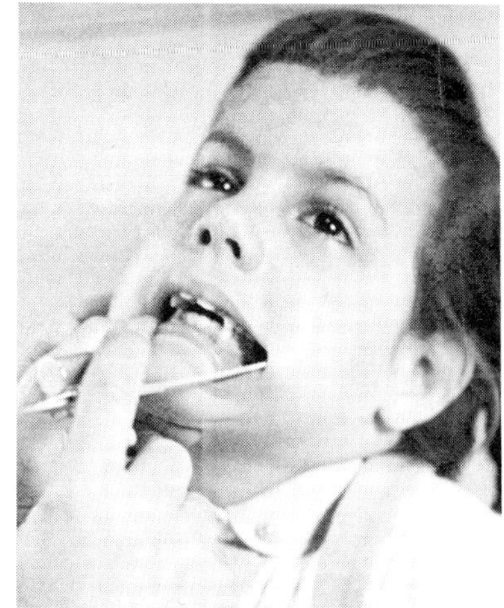

Both needed orthodontia

Fig. 29-3. Thumb sucking.

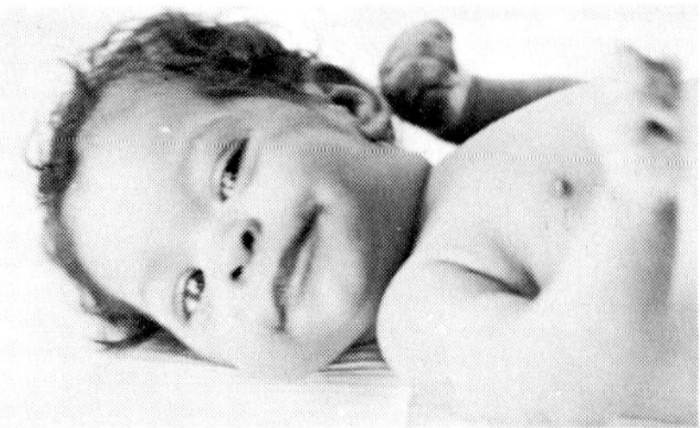

The first tentative smile

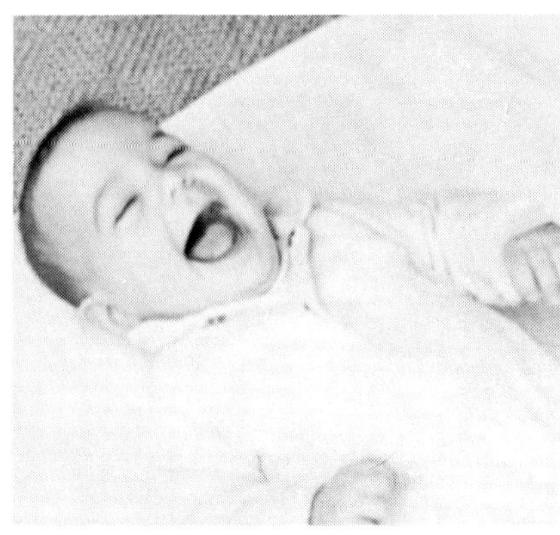

Soon develops into a belly laugh

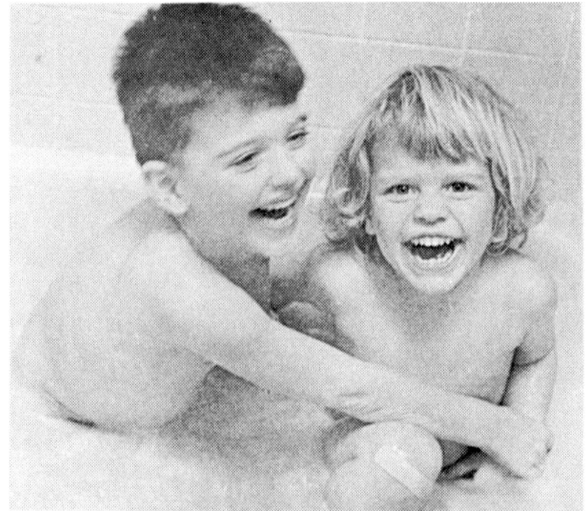

Laughing is part of the early years

Fig. 29-4. Derived patterns—smiling and laughing.

is beginning to take an active part in establishing the interpersonal relations with his mother so essential to his human development. The more an infant finds satisfaction accompanying his smile, the more he smiles. Those infants who are not given tender care soon cease to smile; they *can* smile, but they have not found the smile useful, so they seldom try it (Spitz, 1946).

From the age of 1 month, when the smile first appears, on through infancy, the normal child smiles a great deal. He improves his techniques, and at 3 or 4 months he adds a rollicking laugh. As times goes on, when an infant smiles and laughs, his whole body partakes in his expression of pleasure. He extends his legs, straightens his trunk, perhaps reaches up with his arms in invitation to be picked up. He smiles with his toes as well as with his face. It is in infancy that the smile reaches its maximum. Toddlers still smile and laugh, but less so than the infant, and by the time school age is reached, the child is a good deal more solemn than in the earlier years (Bowlby, 1958).

The smile and the laugh are human evolutionary accomplishments. No other species has the ability to smile or to laugh, nor does any other species need the warmth and tender care essential for the human.

Clinging

Like smiling, the clinging reaction is dependent upon maturation of neural pathways. It cannot be activated until the necessary muscles respond to cortical stimulation.

Clinging behavior makes its first appearance when the infant is about 4 to 5 months of age. It is most pronounced when the infant is distressed or fearful. He cries and extends his arms and legs in a gesture which clearly indicates his desire to be picked up. When clinging first becomes evident, the infant will accept any comfortable arms and hang on tight to any neck, but by the time the infant is 6 to 8 months old, he is able to distinguish his mother from everyone else, and it is only she whom he wants when distressed; no other person, no matter how kind, how warm, how considerate, will do if his mother is present. Even if the mother is a cold unresponsive person, she is the one the infant wants (Burlingham and Anna Freud, 1944). Occasionally one sees an infant who clings with all his might to a mother who actually scolds him and even rejects him. The mother's behavior seems not to dim the infant's desire to cling, although the mother's rejection may well alter the quality of comfort the child receives from the total situation.

Although the mother is the most desired of all, should she not be present, the infant will cling to the next most familiar person—the father, the grandmother, a nurse, or anyone else whom the child knows. Not only can the clinging response be transferred from the most desired to a less desired person, but it can even be transferred to an inanimate object. Bowlby has suggested that the attachment of many children for a favorite toy or a blanket is a manifestation of the clinging desire. A blanket or a toy can be more ever-present in case of danger than the mother. The toy or the blanket may be most essential at bedtime, when our culture demands that the child be separated from his mother to go to sleep.

Clinging is a human pattern which motivates the mother to comfort her baby and protect him from fear. The more the infant is permitted to cling and the more often it is the mother or some equally familiar person he can reach, the more easily does the infant build up his sense of trust in his world.

Clinging reaches its zenith at about 8 or 9 months of age, when anxiety in strange situations is also at its height (p. 543). Clinging gradually fades from the picture, and it fades more quickly and completely in those children who have been given the opportunity to cling whenever they needed it. A subtle distinction must be made between the *infant's* need to cling and the *mother's* need to have her infant dependent upon her (p. 444). Indul-

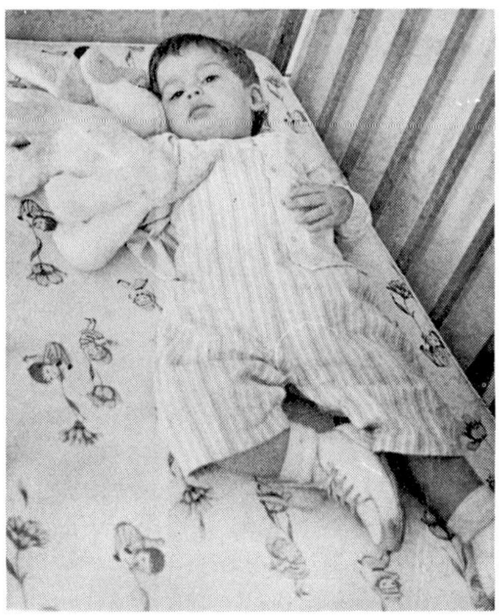

The yearling feels safe clutching a soft toy when he must be alone to sleep

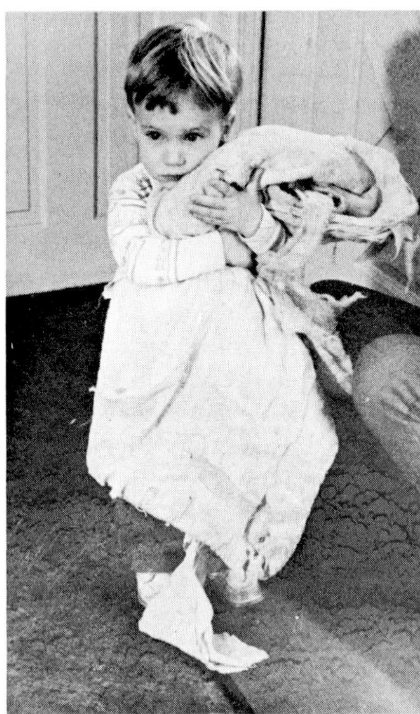

The toddler clings to a blanket when mother is not available

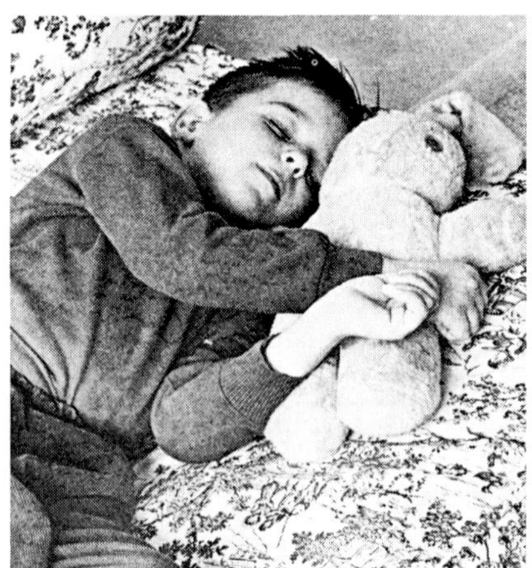

The five year old still falls asleep more easily with the company of his teddy bear

Fig. 29-5. Derived patterns—clinging.

gence of an instinct for reasons other than its basic purpose, as well as deprivation of expression of an instinct, can accentuate and prolong the expression of that instinct.

Following

Following has its rudimentary beginnings as early as the eyes mature adequately to permit the infant to watch his mother, between 3 and 5 weeks of age. At this age babies will often cry to bring the mother back where they can keep an eye on her, or at least an ear on her whereabouts. But the following pattern really comes into full bloom when the child becomes mobile enough actually to go after his mother, by any means of locomotion available to him. When he finally begins to walk, the toddler follows his mother about constantly. He will play briefly by himself, but frequently he must "go see Mommie." This behavior, like the clinging behavior, is especially evident in times of stress. A fearful child runs to his mother, clutches her skirt or her legs, and runs right along with her if she moves. It is during these years that the child is struggling with the ego task of establishing his autonomy, but the following pattern is more closely related to the ego task of the first stage—establishing basic trust—than it is to establishing bodily independence.

Unlike clinging, following requires but passive participation of the mother. She does not need to *do* anything, only to *permit* the child to act. Perhaps this is the reason so many mothers, at least in our culture, react with irritation to the child's desire to grab their skirts and remain underfoot. Many mothers need intellectual understanding of the significance of the child's action.

Environmental conditions can alter the natural history of these instinctive patterns. Since fear and anxiety are seen to intensify clinging and following in the short term, so long-continued anxiety tends to perpetuate the behavior. Bowlby is impressed by the correlation between the degrees of emotional disturbance seen in older children and the degree to which mothers permit these instinctive patterns to run their course. He feels that the need of the little child to exercise his desire to follow his mother is so deeply inherent in the child that frustration of this pattern leads to an undue amount of anxiety.

VOLUNTARY BEHAVIOR

The distinction between instinctive and voluntary behavior is not sharp. Some of the instinctive patterns described above depend upon the use of voluntary muscles and for this reason are not as stereotyped as many of the instinctive patterns of lower species. Nevertheless, if Bowlby is correct, which seems plausible, the drive that initiates such patterns as clinging and following is gene-directed.

Behavior that is usually considered voluntary consists of postural control, locomotion, manipulation, and sphincter and vocal control.

Posture and Locomotion

At birth the infant remains in more or less the position in which he is placed; he has very little control of his posture. When on his back, he does, however, prefer an asymmetric position which he can achieve for himself. He will lie with head turned to one side, the arm on that side extended, the other arm flexed. When in the prone position, many infants can raise their heads a little from the bed. Following the cephalocaudal law, the infant's first abilities to alter his position are evident in the head.

Head Control

By 1 month the normal infant in supine position can rotate his head from side to side, and in the prone position he can raise his head so that his face is at right angles with the bed. By 3 months he can support his head on his shoulders unaided when he is held in a sitting position. By 4 months, he can push his body up from the prone position, rest his weight on his extended arms, and rotate his head from side to side.

By 4 months of age the baby has his head pretty much under his own control. He can move his head this way and that; he can also move his eyes coordinately (p. 276), smile (p. 392), swallow or spit things out of his mouth voluntarily, make guttural sounds with his vocal apparatus (p. 464), and suck and cry (these last two he could, of course, do from the beginning). Refinements will come later, but by 4 months his head is beginning to belong to him. Since as yet he cannot control his back, the 4-month-old is very appreciative of being propped up so that he can take full advantage of his capacities to use the equipment he can control.

Sitting Posture

Up to 3 months, when the youngster is supported in a sitting position, his back is rounded from cervical to lumbar regions. By 4 months, when the head has become steady on the shoulders, the back is straighter, and the curvature is confined to the lumbar regions. At this age the infant cannot support his own weight unaided in a sitting position. By 7 months, most infants can hold the trunk erect for short periods, and by 8 months, for indefinite periods. At this time the infant can usually lean forward and return to the erect sitting position. By 10 months he can pull up from either prone or supine position to sitting and can pivot about.

He "owns" himself down to his waist now. His eyes have matured so that his focus is sharp (p. 276); his hands are becoming useful tools; he has a large repertory of sounds; he can chew as well as swallow soft food.

Locomotion

By about 5 months the infant lying in the supine position can roll over on his side by rotating the upper part of his body, then flexing his hips and throwing his legs to that side. In another few weeks he is able to get himself in a crawling position, but he has trouble raising his abdomen. Few babies actually crawl around much before 8 months, and the first attempts are often by means of pivoting with the arms; soon, however, the infant is able to coordinate hands and feet and really get himself about. Crawling is a highly individualistic skill. Each infant develops his own method. Some use hands and feet; some, hands and knees; some, two hands, one knee, and one foot; and some, other variations with their extremities or abdomen. But whatever the particular technique, the ability to get from one place to another opens up a whole new world to the baby. He can now get himself across a room and feel, mouth, shake, an attractive object, instead of just gazing at it from a distance. The exercise of the ability to crawl, however, requires more than neuromuscular maturation. The infant must muster the courage to separate himself from his mother voluntarily. The more adequately he has established trust, the more ready he is to expand his physical horizons.

At about 10 months most infants will pull themselves up, first to their knees, then to their feet, by means of the bars of the crib or playpen, supporting the weight on the entire sole of the foot. Once an erect posture has been accomplished, the infant is so entranced with himself that he wants to be on his feet every waking moment. Sitting he tolerates briefly, but he cannot abide the supine position even long enough to have his diaper changed. Soon after standing has been achieved, the infant begins to cruise around, at first with both hands firmly grabbing some support; later, as he gains more confidence, he lets go with one hand; ultimately he lets go with both hands and toddles across the open space of a room completely alone. His equilibrium is shaky; he flexes his hips and knees, keeps his legs far apart, often elevates his arms for balance, and thrusts his head and the upper part of his trunk forward.

Walking is a milestone in development. With the ability to go places on his own two legs the child has taken a leap in independence. He prepared for this leap by creeping, which involved voluntary separation from his mother, but walking takes still more courage. Walking upright, with nothing to hang on to, with nothing to support him but his own two legs, gives the child a sense of bodily aloneness, a sensation that can be coped with only by confidence and inner security. Most children have adequate neuromuscular maturation to enable them to walk alone before they have the inner strength to give up that one-hand clutch still needed for emotional support.

Once the courage has been mustered and the child discovers that he can venture out into free open space with nothing to hold on to, walking becomes an all-absorbing occupation. Other interests are often dropped for a time while the child concentrates on perfecting his walking skills. He wants to walk, walk, walk.

The child's balance on his legs is unsteady for a year or more after he takes his first step alone, and walking continues to require conscious effort; nevertheless he is constantly trying out variations of his walking skills. He walks backward and sideward; he runs; he kicks a ball and usually does not fall over. He does fall many, many times a day, but nothing dampens his enthusiasm for more trials.

By 3 years most children have achieved an ability to walk without conscious effort—walking has finally become automatic. The child can then run, jump, skip, stand on one foot, walk on tiptoe, and walk more or less along a straight line.

The 4-year-old has left behind him the clumsiness of the toddler; he is lithe and graceful and, if he tries, can carry a glass of water without spilling.

The urge to become a biped is profound. The child gains a sense of mastery over himself; he can make his body do what he wants; his independence is growing. His satisfaction comes largely from his own accomplishments, but here, as elsewhere in child development, the appreciation of his adults for his feats cements his inner feelings of worthiness.

Manipulation

Simultaneously with the development of posture and locomotion, the infant brings his eyes, arms, and hands under his control. The sequence of development is looking, reaching, contacting, grasping, handling, and, finally, exploitation of objects.

Looking constitutes the infant's first "reaching" movements. The eyes, according to the cephalocaudal law, come under voluntary control before the arms and hands. At birth eye muscles are not coordinated, the expression is vacant, the gaze vague. By 1 month, eye movements are better coordinated, and the infant looks at a nearby object, following it in the midline of his vision. By 3 months, his expression is alert; he looks actively and follows a moving object a full 180°, turning his head to do so. Close vision is not as yet distinct (p. 276); the 3-month-old looks at his total surroundings more than at objects. By 4 months vision is more accurate, and the infant begins truly to look at individual objects; he prefers large and bright-colored ones.

The arms and hands play little part in the infant's explorations until about 3 months. At this age the sight of an object stimulates a massive body reaction in which the arms tense and make a global lunge toward an object. The infant may or may not succeed in touching the object.

By 4 months the lunge is better directed, and he usually makes contact with the object; by 5 months he manages a two-hand grasp, using a whole-hand approach. At this age his arms are held flexed at the elbow most of the time, which keeps them more or less within his visual range. He spends long periods of time inspecting his hands visually and grabbing one hand with the other. The hands are kept close to his chest within easy access of his mouth; his hands and any object he may be holding are frequently carried to the mouth, where the sensitive tactile receptors of this organ aid the hands in further explorations. These manual, oral, visual, tactile, and auditory manipulations are the beginning of sensorimotor play (p. 490).

By 7 months of age the infant begins to grasp with one hand instead of both hands; his bidexterity is giving way to the permanent pattern of unidexterity. A 7-month-old grabs for an object as soon as he sees it. He

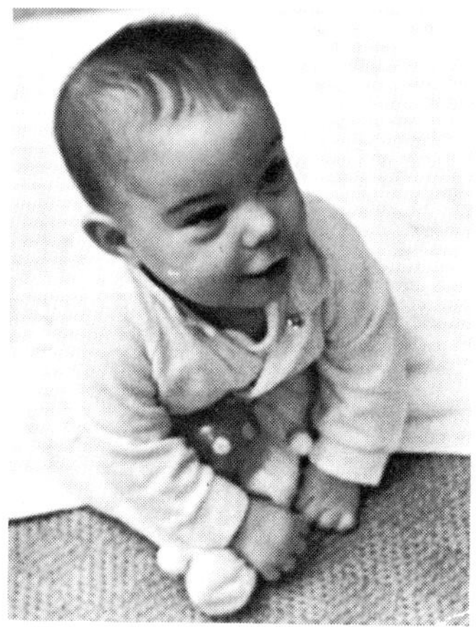

Lunge

One hand grasp

Two hand grasp

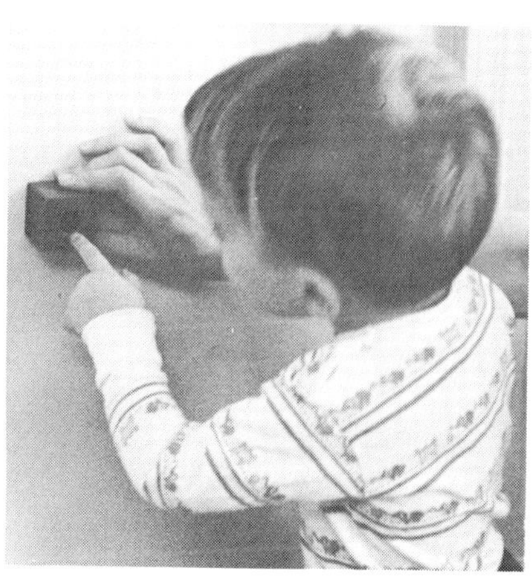

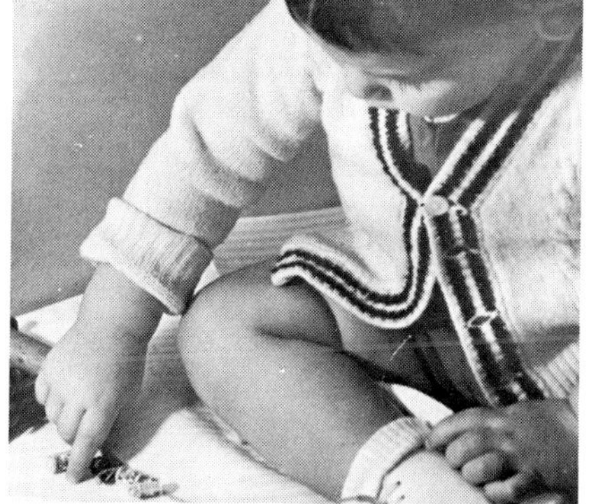

Prenhensile grip

Exploring with the index finger

Fig. 29-6. Maturation of hand skills.

feels it with his hands, takes it to his mouth, where he mouths it, takes it out of his mouth, looks at it again, shakes it, listens to it if it makes a noise, transfers it to the other hand, turns it over, bangs it, shakes it, gives it another "mouth feel," drops it, gets it back if he can, and begins his explorations all over again. The 7-month-old uses his whole hand to grasp, and is unable to release voluntarily.

By 10 months of age dexterity has progressed considerably. Not only has an infant at this age a well-coordinated hand at the end of a well-coordinated arm, but he also has sharp and accurate vision. The 10-month-old has a definite preference for one hand; he has a good prehensile grip and has abandoned his earlier clumsy whole-hand approach to objects. He can release at will. By 10 months, voluntary control (following the cephalocaudal-proximodistal law) has extended all the way to the periphery—the fingertip, the tongue tip, the toes have become manageable. The baby is now on his feet, his busy hands exploring everything within reach. He approaches the world with his outstretched index finger. He no longer grabs; he pokes and picks up. His interest has shifted from big things to tiny ones. He will ignore a cup and go for a crumb. Gesell says that the 10-month-old begins to penetrate the third dimension with that outstretched inquiring index finger. He explores the insides of containers, dumps out their contents, understands the difference between solid and hollow, inside and outside, top and bottom. He combines two objects and gains a dim awareness of the quality of twoness. He feels with his hands, pokes with his finger, tastes and feels with his tongue. Meanwhile he is up on his feet, exhilarated by his vertical position. He is also using the muscles of his vocal apparatus to make a large repertory of sounds. He is using in play all his voluntary equipment to take in and assimilate sensory experiences.

The year-old child improves on the techniques of the 10-month-old. He sharpens his skills, develops greater dexterity. His ability to release voluntarily makes it possible for him to put small things into containers. He begins to imitate what goes on around him.

By 1 year of age a child's body is essentially organized. He will learn many more skills; he will acquire greater control of the small muscles of his hands; as his intelligence develops, he will be motivated to do as the people about him do.

THE LEARNING OF SKILLS

While all normal children learn neuromuscular skills, no two children learn them in exactly the same way. This is the essence of voluntary control. An infant discovers that he can use his arms and hands to prop himself up, but the exact technique he uses is his own particular pattern discovered through trial and error. He tries this way and that way, and with one particular way he is more successful than with another, and he repeats the pattern that worked for him. With repetition the pattern becomes fixed; he establishes a facilitated neuromuscular pathway (p. 146). Next time he wants to perform the same action, it is easier for the neural impulses to travel the previously used tract than to form a new one, and we say he has established a *habit* or a *conditioned response*. Thus while every normal child holds his head up, sits up, crawls, stands up, walks, uses his hands and fingers, each child develops his own individual ways of doing these things.

Children do things as quickly as they can. As soon as an act becomes possible, a child exercises his new-found ability to perform the act. Adults do not teach the baby to crawl or to sit or to walk; the child crawls because his ability to control his muscles has matured. But nevertheless he *learns* to crawl. The very performance of the act seems to give the child pleasure and satisfaction. He does it because he likes to do it. He enjoys the feeling of body mastery. He performs the same act over and over again. Each time he repeats, he increases his competence. It is also beginning to dawn on the child that he is the master of his body, that he can make it do what he wants, and with this knowledge comes the dim realization that there is an *I* within him that has power. He is developing autonomy. While the years of toddlerhood are the time when the urge for autonomy is most evident, nevertheless the desire to control the body begins in infancy and continues through all the years of childhood.

But the child is not developing in a vacuum; he is living in an interpersonal world in which his relation to his mother is of vital importance. The *I* who can make his body perform these fascinating acts must also maintain a warm and loving relation to his mother. The pleasure of doing is either enhanced or interfered with by the response his act receives from his mother. If his mother responds with smiles, hugs, and general approbation, the inherent pleasure of the act is multiplied by the feeling that it is a good and valuable and loved *I* that is acting. The child performs the act with ever renewed vigor and enthusiasm.

In early infancy most of the child's voluntary activity is approved of; there is not much the relatively immobile infant can do that meets with parental disapproval. In general, parents are delighted with each new thing a baby can do. They love to see him shake his rattle, bounce up and down, grab for the spoon, etc. There are a few exceptions—biting the breast (p. 373) and handling the genitals (p. 422).

But once the child becomes mobile, he is capable of a great deal of activity, some of which meets with parental disapproval. Love is withheld when he pulls on the table cloth, tears books, bangs on the furniture. He is entering the world of discipline (p. 490). If parental discipline can be consistent and reasonable, the child's ability to control his body in such a way that he can maintain parental approval enhances his feeling of his own competence.

On the other hand, the child whose life is a constant succession of no's, don'ts, and slaps has difficulty in appreciating himself as a person worthy of love and respect. His motor abilities are not helping him establish autonomy.

During infancy and toddlerhood the skills the child acquires are learned as a result of his own drives and the examples of the people with whom he lives. Later additional skills are more formally taught. However, whatever the specific skills, each can be learned only when structure is mature enough to make the act possible and when motivation from the child himself encourages sufficient repetition to translate conscious voluntary effort into conditioned responses.

The child himself gives the cues for the optimal time of much learning. When he is interested in learning to skate or to play baseball or swim, he will struggle to learn. Then is the time his learning can be enhanced by adult help and interest.

During the middle and adolescent years the child's enthusiasm to learn sometimes outstrips society's desire for him to be entrusted with the responsibilities inherent in the performance of some skills. Boys want to tinker with powerful machinery; girls may want to use stove or other household equipment the danger of which they are not mature enough to appreciate fully. Young adolescents, especially boys, often have an unquenchable urge to drive an automobile before adults feel they are ready to shoulder the responsibilities involved. Here, as in other areas of adolescence, there is a clash between physiology and culture. The young teen-ager is quite able to manipulate an automobile—his neuromuscular maturation is entirely adequate. What he lacks is judgment and experience. These come with greater maturity and training. However, while prohibitions are essential, it must not be forgotten that skills are most efficiently learned when motivation is strong. Adult guidance and understanding not only can help the youngster perfect skills but can encourage the maturation of responsibility necessary for participation in our mechanized society.

There are other motor skills which society deems necessary but which children are not always as eager to learn as those which result in immediate pleasure and stature with their peers. Reading and writing are prime examples, although playing a musical instrument and skills associated with the work of family living come in this group.

It is essential to remember that these skills cannot be learned until the child is mature enough in both neuromuscular and ego development to be able to accomplish the skill and to understand what it is about. Attempting to teach reading and writing too early only delays the time when proficiency will be acquired. Fortunately, readiness tests (p. 478) have been devised whereby the optimal time for beginning the learning of literacy skills can be determined.

From infancy through the adult years motor skills contribute to an individual's feeling of competence. Children need an opportunity to learn as many skills as possible when they are ready to learn. Sometimes they need coercion to perfect culturally necessary skills; sometimes they need prohibition against using skills that require greater degrees of responsibility than they are capable of.

DEVELOPMENTAL APPRAISAL

Development of motor behavior is an orderly process which follows the same general pattern in all normal human beings. While the overall pattern is universal, the speed with which any given individual travels the road to maturity varies within wide limits. While the tempo of motor maturity is dependent upon the integrity of the neuromuscular mechanisms, it can be influenced by the development of the ego (Bakwin, 1959; Cattell, 1940).

In order to appraise the development of a given individual for the purpose of attaining some measure of his normalcy, it is desirable to have norms against which to compare him. Gesell has devised a series of profiles of normal behavior at various ages by means of standardized examinations of a large number of healthy children. Gesell measured motor behavior, both gross body control and fine motor skills, language development, and some aspects of social adjustment. To compare a child to Gesell's norms, it is necessary to observe him in a test situation similar to the one Gesell devised. When this is done, a figure is obtained for the child's maturity age—his performance compared to that of the average of the normal children in the original series. Maturity age divided by chronological age gives a figure called the *developmental quotient* (DQ).

The DQ is useful; nevertheless, its use must be tempered with clinical judgment. Neurologic or sensory impairments certainly impede motor development and need to be assiduously ferreted out. Sensory loss can play havoc with development; such losses are sometimes amenable to treatment. Needless to say, the earlier in life visual or hearing defects can be corrected, the greater is the possibility of obtaining normal development. Neurologic impairments also prevent normal maturation. Such derangements can be due to gene-determined inadequacies or to environmental insults to the central nervous system. Treatment aimed at restoring normality to a brain-damaged child is not promising. However, awareness of a child's inadequacy early in life is helpful in arranging his milieu so that he has every possibility of achieving as much potential as he does possess. He can be protected from further handicaps imposed by anxiety and frustration (Bayley, 1958; Caldwell, 1964).

The deviations in development for which no explanations can be found pose the greatest problems in total appraisal. One child walks alone at 8 months; another, not until 18 months. The early walker is not necessarily a genius, and the later walker may grow up to be a Ph.D. Some children talk early and much; others are less verbal and take their time in adopting semantic communication. And so with manual dexterity: children with equal ultimate potential may not necessarily progress at the same tempo on all fronts. Slow or accelerated maturation *may* be criteria of poor or superior endowment, but also they may not be. There is still much we do not know about correlation of early behavior and ultimate attainments.

It is helpful in appraising the progress of any child to have in mind average performance against which to compare him. Deviations call for investigation of the causes, lest a remedial defect be overlooked. Where no defects are found, caution needs to be exercised in making a prognosis.

In Section VII normal profiles at key ages in all areas of maturation are compiled, together with the limits beyond which a pathologic condition must be suspected. This material is further summarized in Chap. 41.

BIBLIOGRAPHY

Aldrich, C. Anderson, Cheech Sung, and Catherine Knop: The Crying of Newborn Babies, *J. Pediat.*, **26**:313, 1945.

Bayley, Nancy: Value and Limitations of Infant Testing, *Children*, **5**:129, 1958.

Bakwin, R. M.: Office Evaluation of Intelligence of Children, *Pediatrics*, **23**:989, 1959.

Bowlby, John: The Nature of the Child's Tie to His Mother, *Internat. J. Psychoanalysis*, **39**:350, 1958.

Caldwell, B. M., and R. N. Drachman: Comparability of Three Methods of Assessing the Developmental Level of Young Infants, *Pediatrics*, **34**:51, 1964.

Cattell, Psyche: "The Measurement of Intelligence of Infants and Young Children," Psychological Corporation, New York, 1940.

Fletcher, Ronald: "Instincts in Man," International Universities Press, Inc., New York, 1957.

Freud, Anna, and Dorothy T. Burlingham: "Infants Without Families," International Universities Press, Inc., New York, 1944.

Gesell, Arnold, and Catherine S. Amatruda: "Developmental Diagnosis," 2d ed., Paul B. Hoeber, Inc., New York, 1954.

McGraw, Myrtle: "The Neuromuscular Maturation of the Human Infant," Columbia University Press, New York, 1943. Reprinted by Hafner Publishers Company, New York, 1963.

Parmelee, Arthur H.: Critical Evaluation of the Moro Reflex, *Pediatrics*, **33**:773, 1964.

Ribble, Margaret A.: "The Rights of Infants," Columbia University Press, New York, 1943.

Spitz, René A., and K. M. Wolf: The Smiling Response, A Contribution to the Ontogenesis of Social Relations, *Genetic Psychology Monographs*, **34**:57, 1946.

Thorpe, W. H., and O. L. Zangwill: "Current Problems in Animal Behavior," Cambridge University Press, London, 1961.

Timbergen, N.: "The Study of Instinct," Clarendon Press, Oxford, 1951.

30

Eliminative Function

Human beings eliminate their waste products by the same basic mechanisms as do other mammalian species. Human beings sweat, defecate, and urinate, and by so doing they rid their bodies of the unneeded by-products of their metabolism in such ways that homeostasis is maintained. Sweating has evolved no special human overtones (p. 254), but defecation and urination in the human being are more than a means of eliminating waste products and maintaining homeostasis. By means of the voluntary motor control of the acts of elimination and the sensations emanating from the sphincters these acts contribute to the development of motor and sensory autonomy.

THE PHYSIOLOGY OF DEFECATION

Defecation is periodic; digestion, on the other hand, is continuous as long as chyme is present in the bowel. Several times in 24 hours powerful peristaltic contractions in the large bowel move masses of intestinal contents distally. These mass peristaltic waves, which throughout life are below the level of consciousness, begin in the hepatic flexure of the large bowel, continue along the transverse and descending colon, and deliver fecal material into the pelvic colon—the reservoir of the lower bowel. As pressure in the pelvic colon mounts, the sphincter at its distal end opens and permits fecal material to enter the rectum. When the rectum becomes distended, sensory nerves in its walls send impulses to a spinal reflex center. The actual act of defecation requires the participation of abdominal muscles and diaphragm. The diaphragm is fixed in inspiration, the abdominal muscles contract and increase the pressure in the rectum, a peristaltic wave passes over the colon; the anal sphincter relaxes; and the stool falls away.

In normal children, sometime during the second year of life the voluntary component of defecation makes its appearance. Cortical neural pathways from the rectum mature; the sensory stimulus from a distended rectum then no longer initiates the act of defecation; it only alerts to the need for defecation. The child has a choice: he may bring his accessory muscles into operation and defecate, or he may choose to ignore the sensory alert and *not* defecate. How he acts depends in large measure on how he feels about his stools and about the act of defecation.

THE ELIMINATIVE PRODUCTS

Unlike other voluntary muscular activity, the eliminative acts result in the production of objects—urine and stool. As the child matures, he becomes interested first in the products of elimination and, later, in the acts of elimination.

Throughout early infancy, the child is unaware of the process of elimination and equally unaware that he produces either urine or stool. Long before the child acquires any voluntary control over the *acts* of elimination, he learns about these substances that pass from his body, and particularly about his feces.

Toward the end of the first year, when the baby is exploring his body and everything within reach, he is likely, one day, to come upon a mass of feces. At this early age, he may not be aware that he produced the stool himself. The material is new and interesting. He enjoys the feel of it. If he has the opportunity, he squeezes it in his hands. He plays with it. He may even taste it. To adults, the odor of fecal material is unpleasant, but not so to the baby; it is merely something new to be explored.

At this early stage it is most desirable for the mother to accept her infant's stool at his level of understanding. She, of course, wants him to have normal stools at normal intervals, and if she can express pleasure when she finds a stool in his diaper, the baby, as he grows a little older and is aware that he made his stool, comes to realize that his beloved mother is pleased with his accomplishments and the products of his body. On the other hand, the mother who makes a nasty face and in other ways shows her aversion to stools may inculcate in the child the notion that there is something evil about his body.

Of course, no mother can be expected to enjoy the job of cleaning up a crib smeared end-to-end with stool. However, if this does happen and the mother can accept the episode with equanimity, without punishment, and perhaps even with a bit of humor, she will reassure the child that his body is acceptable to her. The child who feels that his body and its products are pleasing to his mother accepts himself as a good and valuable person.

Later, after voluntary control of the sphincters is acquired, the child expresses a greater interest in his stool and his urine than he did as an infant. Now he definitely knows that he made these substances; they are his, almost as much so as his arms and legs. He is fascinated if his urine drips on the floor; he will want to get down and splash in it. He wants to look at his stool, to talk about it; he can be dissuaded from playing with it only by tactful firmness.

When he is content and pleased with his world and feels especially safe with his mother, he may carry his potty to his mother and offer his stool to her as a gift. The child is sharing with his mother something of great value to him. If such a gift can be accepted by the mother with an understanding on her part of what it means to the baby, the little fellow learns that giving is a pleasure in itself. He wants his mother to look at his stool, to admire it. Sometimes he hates to see it flushed down the toilet. However, his attention span is short at this age; the delay of a few minutes, during which time his stool is appreciated and he is assured that there will be another stool tomorrow, is usually sufficient to satisfy him; then the stool can be disposed of without offending him.

On the contrary the child who learns that his mother does not like his gift, is even revolted by it, and wants to flush the nasty, dirty thing immediately down the toilet discovers that there is no pleasure in the giving of this gift. What pleasure the child is able to obtain from this product of his body he gets by keeping his valuable possession all to himself.

THE ACT OF DEFECATION

According to the cephalocaudal law of growth, neural pathways to the caudal end of the body do not mature until the more cephalad structures have come under voluntary control. It can usually be assumed that by the time a child is walking well and easily, not just tottering across the room, he has developed some ability to control the events of his anal sphincter. He develops not only motor ability but also sensory awareness of events in his anal area. These capacities usher in what in the psychoanalytic literature is termed the *anal phase* of development.

Stages of Sphincter Control

Sphincter control has three distinct stages. It is not until the third stage is reached that the child has sufficient maturity for initiation into the culturally accepted techniques for disposing of fecal material.

The first stage is an awareness on the part of the child that he has just defecated. The process still takes place automatically, but the child now knows when he has done it and is aware of the sensations in his anal region. He will announce by word or gesture the fact that he has defecated. As his pants are changed, he will want to look at his stool and will enjoy his mother's appreciation of it. Since at this stage of maturity he is beginning to understand the symbolic value of words, this is an opportune time to help him establish a word for his stool.[1] The word is a handle which will facilitate later stages in toilet training. Teaching the word and participating in the child's interest constitute the parents' role in this first stage.

[1] "B.M." is easy to say. Whatever word is used should have no emotional overtone. Such words or phrases as "bad boy" or "nasty" or "dirty" or "doing your duty" are better avoided.

The second stage of sphincter control comes when the child is aware of what he is doing at the actual moment of defecation. His expression and his activity are not difficult for an observant mother to interpret. If she comments casually on the fact that he is defecating (using the word she has already established), she indicates to him her interest in his bodily activity, thereby increasing his own interest. This is no time to rush the child to the bathroom or to scold him for not telling his mother sooner. It gives the child a sense of triumph to recognize the signals that result in mastery of himself, and at this stage his ability is confined to telling his mother what he is doing *now.* In addition the sensations accompanying the act give him satisfaction, and he enjoys the pleasant empty feeling in his rectum. After he is finished he will be glad, as in the earlier stage, to have his mother change his pants, to inspect his stool, and to have her comment favorably on his accomplishment.

The third stage of sphincter control comes with a little more maturity, when the child knows a few moments in advance that he will soon defecate. He will run to his mother, use her word, and enjoy her interest. Now that there are a few minutes between the time he is alerted to the need for defecation and the actual act and now that he has a means of telling his mother what he is about to do, he is ready for an introduction to the culturally accepted place to perform the act. At this age, the little runabout is very observant of the activities of others. He tags around after his mother and has probably already discovered that she uses the bathroom. While he may know this, he may not be too enthusiastic about sitting on the big toilet himself. Its noisy, gushing waters, which make things disappear, may terrify him. Many a toddler is more amenable to sitting on a small, quiet potty chair and dropping his stool into this safe place. In addition to its safety, the potty provides an easier receptacle than the big toilet for inspecting and admiring the stool before it is disposed of.

Toilet training consists of letting the child know the culturally accepted place to defecate. A child is not *taught* to control his bowels; he matures so that he can do this. He is taught *where,* not *how.* When toilet training is carried out with these developmental stages in mind, the child matures with a maximum degree of self-mastery.

A few toddlers have their stools at nearly the same time every day. Such a child can be placed on the toilet at the expected time and may then defecate in the toilet even though he is not mature enough to have developed voluntary control. While this procedure avoids soiled diapers, it must be pointed out that this is not true autonomy. The child's defecation is controlled by his mother, who puts him on the toilet when *she* thinks it is time for him to perform. Many children do learn to use the toilet by this technique, but some have difficulty. A few children refuse to defecate as long as they sit on the toilet, only to let go immediately after they are taken off. Such a youngster insists on calling his own signals and refuses to accept his mother's control over him. Other children accept the mother's control but may have trouble later in taking over responsibility for their own actions.

Even though a little child may defecate in the toilet at times, he will also experiment with defecation in other places. The child is exploring his powers of control over himself. Ideally speaking, if defecation in the toilet gains for him both interest and approval from his mother and defecating in other places meets with no interest from her, he will discover that defecation in the toilet is altogether the most satisfying of all places, and he will more and more often choose this location. His success, both with himself and with his mother, gives him a sense of bodily competence. The self that is emerging is a totally good and worthy self.

Scoldings and punishments for "accidents" (they are seldom accidents from the child's point of view) frequently serve only to increase the child's desire to perform in the way that brings to him excitement and commotion. He would rather be scolded than ignored. One often hears the comment: "He knows better. He does it on the floor just to plague me." This is true; the child repeats acts which bring him the greatest satisfaction. If defecating on the floor brings the child greater excitement and maternal interest than defecation performed on the toilet, it is inevitable that the child will choose the socially undesirable behavior.

While carrying out toilet training according to the child's developmental abilities is desirable, it is nevertheless pertinent to mention that the child needs encouragement to conform and steady, firm, and unemotional discipline. Spock is impressed by the fact that some mothers (and especially educated ones) have become so fearful of producing neurotic symptoms in their children that they ignore the child's often obvious readiness to use the toilet.

Significance of Sphincter Control

Sphincter control consists of two opposing muscular abilities—that of squeezing the muscle tight, holding on and keeping the stool inside and that of relaxing the muscle, opening up the sphincter, and letting go the stool. While these two abilities, holding tight and letting go, are most obvious in relation to sphincter control, they are part of other muscular abilities. The child can clutch with his hands and throw away with those same hands.

These two abilities become woven into the fabric of the child's developing ego. Since in sphincter control there is a body product involved as well as muscular action, it is sphincter control that seems to exercise the most vivid and predominant influence on the child's ultimate reaction to his capacity to hold and let go. At least this is so in our culture, where so much emphasis is placed on toilet training.

The child who has been unable to gain parental approval from his ability to control his sphincter in ways that give *him* satisfaction may come to feel that his only recourse is not to have stools at all. He begins to use his new-found power over his sphincter to keep it tightly shut, because when he does let it go, his mother condemns him for producing a stool (so he feels) and in addition she may be revolted by the stool itself. What pleasure he is able to get comes from excessive holding and from holding his stool within himself. It is possible he obtains some sensory pleasure from his distended rectum, however, the child begins to suffer from emotional constipation.

It is only within rather narrow limits that most little children can control their sphincters. After a while the full rectum opens the sphincter against the child's will to keep it closed. He then defecates involuntarily.

Some children, perhaps those whose organic sensory mechanism in the rectum is less sensitive, are able to go a week or more without having a stool. These are the children who may occasionally soil themselves involuntarily from mucus that seeps over an impacted mass of fecal material (see below). Involuntary defecation, whether it be the whole rectal contents or just a small amount of seepage, is a devastating experience to a small child. His body has controlled him. His *I* is a weak, powerless thing that will not respond to his wishes. He is not pleased with what he is discovering inside himself. The sense of his own competency is in jeopardy.

Around toilet training there can develop the sense of autonomy, the mastery of bodily functions, the feeling that the power within, the *I*, is strong and capable, worthy of respect, or there can develop the feeling that the *I* lacks the ability to control, that it is weak, overwhelmed by external events and internal forces, and the child matures ashamed of himself.

Ideally the opposing forces of holding tight and letting go can mature into constructive forces; holding becomes related to care for the self and consideration for others, and letting go matures into an ability to give freely, to be generous. Under adverse conditions both these forces can become destructive. They can be directed against the outside world, in which case holding becomes hoarding, miserliness, stinginess, and letting go a hostile firing at the enemy. The destructive forces can also be directed against the self. Denied the gradual opportunity of manipulating by free choice, the child may turn all his urge to control on himself. He over-manipulates himself; he becomes ritualistic, excessively clean, excessively slow and dawdling.

Because sphincter control is crucial in ego development, toilet training is a critical stage in child development in our culture. If there is excessive pressure, if toilet training is attempted before the child can voluntarily control his sphincter, his development can become slowed down or even arrested at this stage. He ultimately learns to use the toilet, but the fear and anxiety experienced at this stage remain in the unconscious associated with the opposing muscular forces of holding and letting go.

During the actual months when toilet training is going on, the child may express in a variety of ways that he is having trouble with the difficult tasks of this period. Stubborn refusal to use the toilet at an age when the child understands what is expected of him is but one manifestation of his inner turmoil. His difficulties may be expressed more obliquely as temper tantrums, fastidiousness about keeping clean, refusal of food, sleeping problems, or other forms of undesirable behavior. Occasionally a child will show a sudden distaste for foods that remind him of feces—chocolate syrup or chocolate candy, or browned potatoes. Such behavior, especially during toilet training, constitutes a danger signal. Relaxation of the demands being made on the child not infrequently relieves this anxiety sufficiently so that he returns to normal behavior.

Constipation and Soiling

Constipation is the failure to expel the contents of the rectum at normal intervals. It can occur at any age. Constipation that occurs before voluntary control of defecation has been acquired is usually, if not always, due to organic causes. Sensitivity to rectal distention varies considerably from individual to individual even in infancy. Some young infants defecate after almost every feeding; others, even in early life, defecate but once in 24 hours. Occasionally an infant is seen who defecates so infrequently that the stool is hard, dry, and painful. Sometimes this condition can be relieved by increasing the bulk-producing ingredients in the diet, thus augmenting the stimulus to sensory nerves which are constitutionally sluggish in their responses.

Defecation requires not only a sensory stimulus from a distended rectum but also muscular propulsive force. This may be deficient in some infants. Such infants may need the administration of foods such as prunes which stimulate peristalsis. Rarely constipation in infants is due to more serious congenital defects, mechanical obstruction, Hersprung's disease, ileus.

After the age when voluntary control of defecation has been acquired, constipation may be the result of failure to use the new power to the best interest of the child's body. When an individual is alerted to the need to defecate and uses his voluntary control to refuse to empty his bowels, the barrage of sensory impulses from the distended rectum soon ceases. The rectum accommodates itself to its distention. Defecation cannot then take place until the next mass peristaltic wave moves additional fecal material into the pelvic colon and from there into the rectum, thus further increasing the distention of this organ. The increased distention serves to stimulate the spinal reflex, and the urge to defecate is again felt. If the alert is denied many times, the rectum ultimately becomes so overloaded that it is no longer sensitive to further stimulation. When the spinal reflex fails to function, no amount of voluntary muscular action can result in emptying the organ. Such a fecal impaction has to be removed mechanically before the normal spinal reflex can again function.

A large fecal impaction tends to irritate the rectum with the result of a flow of mucus from the rectal glands. This mucus seeps over the fecal mass and accumulates in the distal end of the rectum. The sphincter cannot maintain its competence over this liquid material, and before long involuntary seepage from the rectum takes place. This is the mechanism of the soiling that frequently accompanies prolonged constipation with a full rectum (Vaughn, 1961).

Defecation is a visceral function, but unlike most other visceral functions it acquires a voluntary component. Disorders of defecation can be organic or volitional. It is possible that children whose organic mechanism has borderline efficiency are more prone to demonstrate deviant ego development via their anal functions than children whose anal mechanisms function in optimal fashion (Kempton, 1961).

In appraising a child whose presenting symptom is constipation, a careful analysis of his past history and present milieu is essential. Constipation that predates voluntary control suggests organic inefficiency; constipation that has its onset soon after voluntary control has been established points toward failure in the development of the ego stage of autonomy and calls for an investigation of the child's milieu and especially of his parents' attitude toward soiling. As suggested above, both factors may be involved.

URINATION

Bladder control usually develops a little later than bowel control. In general, girls learn control at a slightly earlier age than boys. Perhaps because control comes later, perhaps because urine is a less fascinating substance than stool, perhaps for other reasons, bladder training never seems to present as difficult a task to the developing ego as does control of defecation.

The stages in bladder control are similar to those in anal control. The first glimmering that bladder control is on the way is shown when the child is aware that he has wet himself. He often announces the fact proudly. It is important that the mother accept this with interest and approval and not condemn the child for not having told her beforehand. He could not have told her—he did not know. The next step in control is the child's awareness that he is wetting right *now*, and this too he will announce. A few months more, and he will know a moment or two ahead of time and announce that he is going to wet soon. This is the time to suggest he go to the bathroom. Usually the child is already acquainted with the potty chair, because he is beginning to use it for his stools. Once in a while he will make it with dry pants. It will take some time after an initial success before regular urination in the toilet can be expected. Praise for success and ignoring accidents speeds the time of full control. Children at this age are very eager to take care of themselves. Training panties which the child can pull down himself and a low potty chair he can back into unaided spur him on to urinate in a desirable place.

Before the child has acquired the ability to hold his urine long enough to get to the toilet, he urinates many times a day. This frequency is still evident when control begins to make its appearance. Not only does the little child have to empty his bladder frequently, but once the organ is full, he must empty it immediately. He can wait but a moment. As maturation proceeds, urgency decreases; even when his bladder is full, the child is able to hold his sphincter tight and wait a time before he urinates. This ability to hold urine, Muellner believes, is an important factor in stretching the bladder and increasing its capacity. Muellner found that bladder capacity more than doubles between the ages of 2 and 4½ years.

Night control of urination can develop when the bladder is large enough to hold all the urine formed between bedtime and waking time. This stage in maturation comes along automatically. When the child can hold his urine in the daytime for relatively long periods, he is ready to begin keeping his bed dry.

The age at which normal children stay dry at night varies over wide limits. Muellner feels that 4½ is the critical age, and he relates it to his studies on bladder size. Bakwin speaks of enuresis after the age of 3, and Hill sets the age at 5. In a study of 800 children, Harper found that 66 per cent were dry at 3 years; 80 per cent at 5 years; and at 8½ years, when his study ended, 90 per cent were dry, but the proportion was apparently still rising.

Successful nighttime control depends upon the ability to hold the night's urine: the process is not speeded by limiting fluids in the evening or by picking up the child during the night to take him to the bathroom. He must grow up enough to establish automatic control by himself.

Enuresis

Some children are so slow in establishing night control that the subject of enuresis has attracted much attention, and many theories of its cause have been suggested.

As the word is usually used, enuresis means involuntary urination during the night in children who have attained some measure of daytime control. At what age a child is labeled enuretic is a matter of opinion (Hallgren, 1960).

Daytime control comes first. A child who fails to achieve daytime control should be investigated for organic causes. Diabetes mellitus, diabetes insipidus, and some urinary tract abnormalities are associated with round-the-clock frequency. These conditions are relatively rare; nevertheless, when they exist, they may be responsible for failure to keep the bed dry.

Physiologic maturation of a normal urinary tract is essential before a child can hold his urine all night, but this is not the only factor involved.

Muellner attacks the problem solely on the basis of bladder size. He suggests a simple test for determining the amount of urine a child should hold. He asks the child to urinate into a measured container and see how much urine he can produce at one voiding. When this volume reaches 10 to 12 oz, the child has achieved the capacity to hold a night's urine. If a child cannot accomplish this, Muellner suggests "training" him by asking him to drink as much water as possible, hold his urine as long as possible, and thus stretch his bladder. Muellner claims that a period of 3 to 6 months usually is adequate for increasing bladder size sufficiently to hold a night's urine.

Bakwin has been impressed with the familial incidence of enuresis. He found a high incidence of bed wetting in the parents, siblings, and near relatives of a bed-wetting child. In a carefully studied group of 25 families with an enuretic child he found a history of enuresis in one or both parents in 72 per cent (Bakwin defines enuresis as bed wetting after the age of 3). Frary (1935) has commented also on the familial incidence of enuresis. Bakwin comes to the conclusion that bed wetting is an inborn hereditary developmental lag in gaining control of urinary function. He found it often associated with daytime frequency and urgency in otherwise healthy children. Bakwin also states that enuresis is a self-limited condition, being outgrown by the age of 6 to 8 years in many and by the early teens in most children.

Both Muellner and Bakwin have come to the conclusion that enuresis is primarily an organic problem. In spite of this fundamental agreement, these two investigators have arrived at very diverse methods of treatment. Muellner tackles the problem by increasing fluids and trying to increase bladder size; Bakwin, on the other hand, limits fluids in the evening and uses drugs to decrease bladder flow and clocks or mechanical devices to awaken the child from sleep and make him empty his bladder.

It must be pointed out that the child who gets up during the night and goes to the bathroom may keep his bed dry but that he has not achieved the desired goal of holding his urine from bedtime to waking time.

In addition to their special techniques, both Muellner and Bakwin discuss the problem of enuresis with both parents and child. They try to relieve feelings of guilt and attitudes of shaming on the part of the parents. Both inspire the child with confidence in himself and secure his cooperation in a training program and assure him of ultimate success.

Both systems record a reasonably successful incidence of recovery in spite of their diametrically opposite concepts of how treatment can be beneficial.

The question arises as to how large a part the least common denominator in these two systems plays. Both systems relieve the child of guilt (and of nagging and shaming from his parents). They increase his self-confidence, encourage his independence, and assure him of ultimate success. Doubtless these supportive measures play a role.

Organic competency is not the sole answer to enuresis. Children sometimes achieve a dry bed for prolonged periods only to revert to bed wetting during periods of emotional stress. Bed wetting after the birth of a sibling is frequent, and many summer camps make special provision for the wet beds of anxious campers away from home for the first time. Such examples are clear indications that emotions play a role, since these children have previously demonstrated adequate organic competency. If temporary anxiety can cause bed wetting, it seems logical to assume that chronic anxiety can interfere with the initiation of staying dry at night.

In a study of 46 children referred to a psychiatric clinic because of enuresis, Gerard reported that neurotic symptoms were present in all these children. Anderson concludes that emotional factors constitute the largest group of factors in the causation and continuance of enuresis. The emotional conditions most frequently referred to are passivity and failure to assume responsibility in many areas of life. The parents of enuretic children have been described as, typically, an overprotective and dominant mother, who fosters dependency in the child, and a self-effacing father. Children whose enuresis seems related to various anxiety syndromes frequently show other symptoms related to nervous tensions, such as fear of physical injury, dawdling, dependency.

It would appear that enuresis is a symptom, not a disease entity, and can have multiple causes. In some, developmental delay, possibly on a hereditary basis, is dominant, in others, disturbed parent-child relationships are most significant; and possibly in others a combination of organic and emotional factors are involved.

In the treatment of any child with enuresis, an evaluation of the total situation is most important. Regardless of the particular cause, there is nothing to be gained by condemnation, punishment, and nagging. The elimination of these attitudes from the family scene can only be helpful; sometimes it is sufficient by itself. The addition of any positive program in which the child cooperates and assumes responsibility is apt to be helpful. In those children with many manifestations of emotional immaturity, only one of which is enuresis, further psychiatric treatment is sometimes needed.

BIBLIOGRAPHY

Anderson, Forrest N.: The Psychiatric Aspects of Enuresis, *Am. J. Dis. Child.*, **40**:591, 818, 1930.

Bakwin, Harry: Enuresis in Children, *J. Pediat.*, **58**:806, 1961.

Frary, Louise G.: Enuresis: A Genetic Study, *Am. J. Dis. Child.*, **49**:557, 1935.

Gerard, M.: Enuresis: A Study in Etiology, *Am. J. Orthopsychiat.*, **9**:48, 1939.

Hallgren, Berthil: Nocturnal Enuresis in Twins, *Acta psychiat. et neurol. scandinav.*, **35**:73, 1960.

Harper, Paul A.: "Preventive Pediatrics—Child Health and Development," Appleton-Century-Crofts, Inc., New York, 1962.

Hill, Lee Forest: The Enuresis Problem in Children, *J. Pediat.*, **58**:889, 1961.

KEMPTON, JOHN: Constipation and Encopresis, A Pediatrician's View, in Ronald MacKeith and Joseph Sandler (eds.), "Psychosomatic Aspects of Pediatrics," Pergamon Press, London, 1961.

MUELLNER, S. RICHARD: Development of Urinary Control in Children: Some of the Causes and Treatment of Primary Enuresis, *J.A.M.A.*, **172**:1256, 1960.

SPOCK, BENJAMIN, and MARY BERGEN: Parents' Fear of Conflict in Toilet Training, *Pediatrics*, **34**:112, 1964.

VAUGHAN, G. F.: Constipation and Encopresis: A Children's Psychiatrist's View, in Ronald MacKeith and Joseph Sandler (eds.), "Psychosomatic Aspects of Pediatrics," Pergamon Press, London, 1961.

31

Sexual Maturation and the Development of Loving

THE ABILITY AND THE NEED TO LOVE

Human beings, like all animal species, procreate their kind. But procreation is not the only function of the reproductive apparatus in man. Sexual function in man has acquired a human dimension. It is at least partly through his sexuality that man learns to love. The ability to love is human. Animals have instincts that make them protect their young, instincts that produce behavior that looks to us like love. Some animals have the rudiments of love and pets are not infrequently selected for this trait—but no animal is capable of the true mutuality that distinguishes human love. Not only does man have the ability to love, but man *must* love.

Sexual acts are possible in man without love, as they are in other species, just as eating in man is possible without dining (p. 365). But to reach the heights of which man is capable, he must climb the ladder by means of his bodily organism. The most totally satisfying, the most spiritual love to which man can aspire has its origin in his bodily organism.

This conception, that sexuality in man has acquired a human dimension, stands in contrast to the view that man achieves human heights by suppressing what have been called his "animal instincts."

Love does not spring full-blown into existence at maturity. It evolves slowly through all of life as the ego matures. The baby learns to love as a baby; as he grows a little older, his baby love evolves into childish love. Both baby love and childish love are directed primarily toward the child himself. Loving to the little child means to be loved. He has relatively little concern for the welfare of those who love him. A little later, when the child has reached the school years and after he has begun to discover himself, he turns his attention to his peers. His ability to love reaches a new height during these years. The love a child has for an age-mate includes a concern for his friend's welfare—it is his first truly outgoing love. After puberty the child becomes capable of extending his love beyond himself and his peers, and ultimately when he reaches a full maturity, love evolves not only into a true mutuality with a mate but also into a sympathetic relatedness with most people encountered through life. In the mature years, the capacity to love as a parent emerges as one aspect of the full human achievement. As in other areas of development, there are critical phases in learning to love. If the child is not adequately nurtured, during these phases, he may never realize his full capacity to love.

The reproductive apparatus has been used in the process of evolution as part of the means by which the human being achieves two basically human attributes, both of which are essential for the maturing of love. The first is an appreciation of his bodily self. It is through the sexual apparatus, at least in part, that the child gains an understanding of his own body—of how *it* feels and finally of how *I* feel. The second is a corollary of the first —when an individual can understand about the *I* within his own skin, he is capable of appreciating the *you* within another person's skin. The *I* within and the *you* in the other person are more complicated than merely their sexual aspects, but it is possible to distill out the sexual components, look at their developmental trends, and then weave them into the whole pattern of the emerging personality.

INFANCY: BABY LOVE—LOVE IS FREE

At birth the outline of the human being is all there. Much of his structure has more development on the agenda, but basically his body is organized. The infant is equipped to take in sensation and to react to it. The receptors for touch are spread over his entire body, and his tactile nerves are functional by the time of birth (p. 263). The newborn baby can feel "all over." At this very early period, the mouth is the most sensitive area of all. It is more richly endowed with functional nerve endings than any other part of the infant's body. For this reason, early infancy is often spoken of as the *oral phase* of development. But this does not mean that a newborn is nothing but a mouth with an appended body. All of him is important; he makes contact with his environment through his total organism.

A newborn infant appears to have needs for bodily contact. When distressed for almost any reason, he quiets down with apparent pleasure when he receives sensations of warmth, of human contact, of gentle motion, even before he has an opportunity to suck. When sucking is added to his other bodily pleasures, he expresses total contentment. Contrariwise, he is restless when bodily pleasures are denied him, although he is given the opportunity to suck. These early primitive pleasures of contact through the skin, and also through the mouth, remain all life long a part of human pleasures. Some become quite definitely sexual—kissing, the touch of another body; others invoke the contact of personalities rather than of the physical organism. It is the mouth that man uses for talking and dining—activities which help maintain his relatedness to others.

Thus, in the very beginning of independent life the infant experiences his body, and he does so in relation to another human being, his mother,

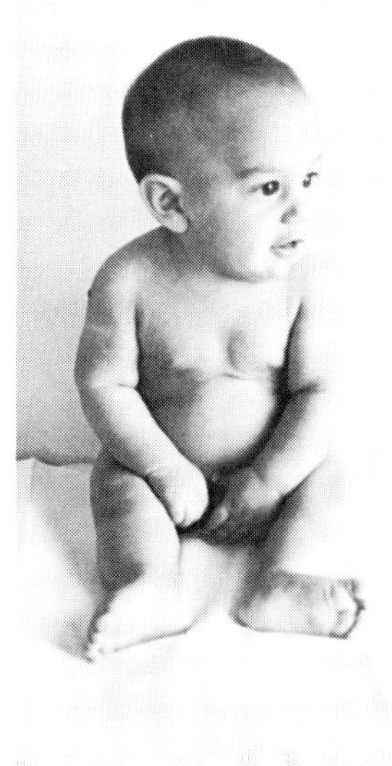

The infant clutches his genitals

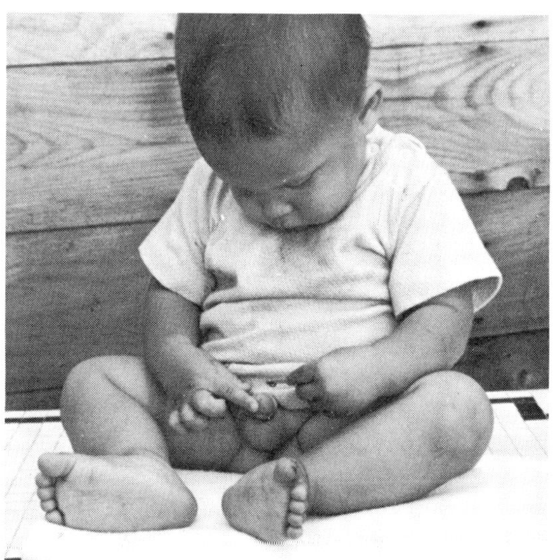

The toddler examines his genitals

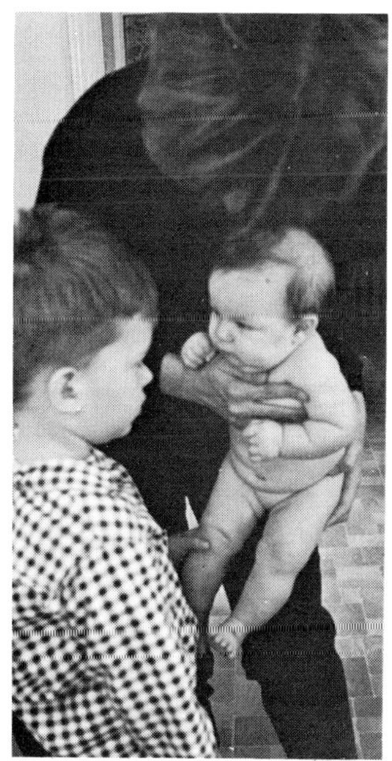

The older toddler is facinated with his baby sister

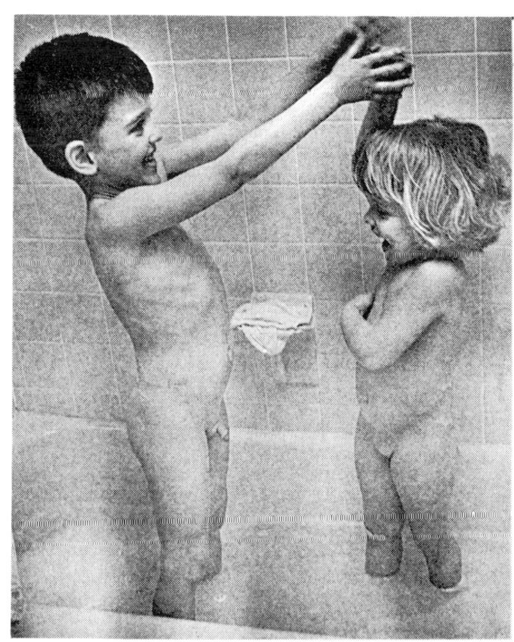

Preschoolers are interested in each other

Fig. 31-1. Sexual development in the early years.

who supplies or withholds the ministrations which provide gratifications. At this early period the infant has no awareness of himself. He does not distinguish between himself and his mother. When the infant is uncomfortable, the whole world is, to him, uncomfortable. When comfort comes, it is mother who *is* food and warmth and pleasure. What is meaningful to the baby are only those sensations within him; what is outside him has meaning to him only insofar as it relates to his own feelings (Harlow, 1958).

As the months slip along, the infant begins to get a glimmering of something "out there," something that supplies the pleasant feelings "in here." As this faint hint of awareness begins to dawn, the infant, instead of passively accepting his mother's care, begins to reach out to her with all the means at his disposal. He listens to her voice, he gazes at her face, snuggles his body next to hers, smiles and laughs at her approaches, and all the while he is taking in through all his sensory equipment the bodily gratifications she offers him. His ego is beginning to emerge.

As he grows a little older his diffuse whole-body gratifications become more localized. His body is beginning to come under his control; he can do things with it purposely.

As we watch the baby from the far horizon of our adulthood, it is possible to appreciate, be it but dimly, the enormous excitement that opens up as the first rays of humanness begin to penetrate the amorphous preconsciousness of a baby. His curiosity is insatiable; he touches, he feels, he bangs, he squeezes, he tastes, he looks, he listens to everything—and everything is new, full of surprises, full of excitement. Most of all the baby explores himself (Dearborn, 1961). He wants to know how he feels in all parts of himself. Those far-off toes have become part of him; when put in his mouth, they feel different from the previously discovered fingers-in-the-mouth. The middle part of him, his genitals, is capable of giving him pleasurable sensations quite different from those of other parts of him. Though his genitals are sexually immature, nevertheless their nervous connections are all intact. He or she has erectile tissue in penis or clitoris, which, when stimulated mechanically, exercises its power of erection and sends nervous impulses throughout the body—sensations of a pleasant character (Reevy, 1961). Throughout the whole period of infancy, the child is coming to know his body—how it feels, what he can do with it. It is a source of endless pleasure and excitement to him. It is at this time that he often discovers his feces (p. 408), which are also a source of interest. His genitals at this time are but one part of the whole, different from the rest of him but perhaps no more important to him than other areas. The baby is learning to love himself.

During all the time that the baby is exploring his body, coming to know and like himself, he is relating to both his parents, but especially to his mother. He is becoming more aware now that she is "out there." He needs and must have her approval. He wants from his mother an unconditional love, an acceptance of the total self he is coming to know. The baby is content when his mother is relaxed and loving, but if she is cold or disapproving, the baby becomes terrified. He is utterly dependent upon her, not only for his physical care, but for helping him appreciate that the *I* he is discovering is good. When she accepts him without reservation, he is confident of his intrinsic value. If she withholds her love, the baby is afraid of himself; he cannot feel sure of himself, of the *I* within him.

If the baby's explorations of his genital organs are met with reactions from his parents different from those which he experiences when he explores other parts of his body, he is aware of this. If either his mother or his father pulls his hand away from his genitals, frowns or scolds as they do so, but allows him to play with his toes, he soon realizes that the genital area is somehow different; he feels that this is a bad part of him. He still likes the feeling of touching his genitals, but the threat of parental withholding of love if he does so frightens him and overshadows his pleasure.

Very early in life a child can come to understand that his genitals are somehow taboo, that the self he is discovering has a rotten spot at its core. Or at this same early period he can come to understand that his genital area is a nice comfortable part of him, that he is a good *I* all over.

Thus the baby love that develops in infancy is the first stage of loving. It contributes to the basic trust the infant's developing ego is attempting to establish at this time of life. Ideally, baby love consists of unconditional acceptance from the parents and its counterpart in the baby—unconditional acceptance of himself. This mutuality is baby love—love of the fully mature adults for the baby and love of the baby for himself. In its totality, it is a transient stage but one which lays the foundation for all that is to come. Unconditional acceptance is of course an ideal. Like all ideals, it is a goal which may be captured once or many times but perhaps not always.

TODDLERHOOD: CHILDISH LOVE—LOVE HAS A PRICE

As the months mount up, the infant grows up into a toddler who can go places on his own momentum and who can communicate in the language of his parents. When a child becomes mobile, his horizons widen. His insatiable curiosity has not abated; he still wants to explore everything within reach, and his reach has now extended to every place his legs can carry him. He can go places and get things, and when he does, he runs into inevitable frustrations. His mother, who up to this time has accepted him unconditionally, now begins to accept him only when he acts as she wants him to act. Love is no longer free; it now has a price. "Behave acceptably and you will be loved; transgress and you will be deprived of love" is what the child feels. No matter how steady is the mother's love, the toddler has difficulty in feeling that love at the very moment he feels reproof.

The little child has to learn to conform to the demands of his society.

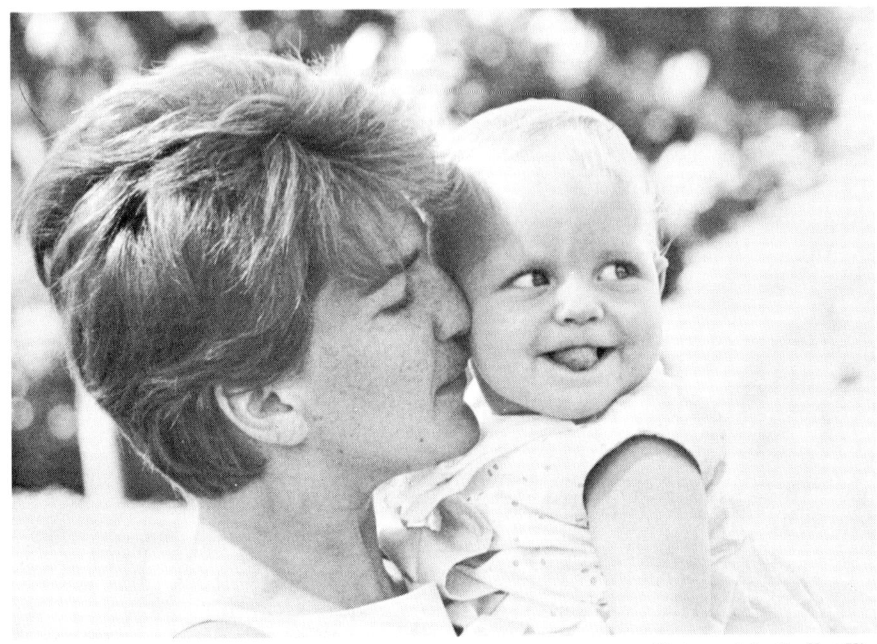

Photograph by Le Van Kim

Baby love is free and unconditional

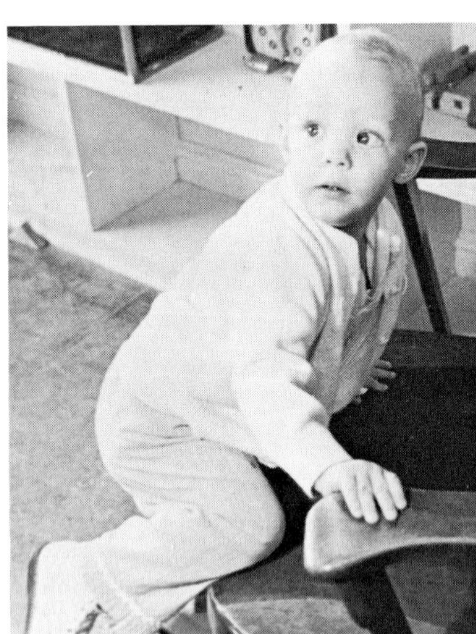

Love begins to have a price
"Don't climb up there."

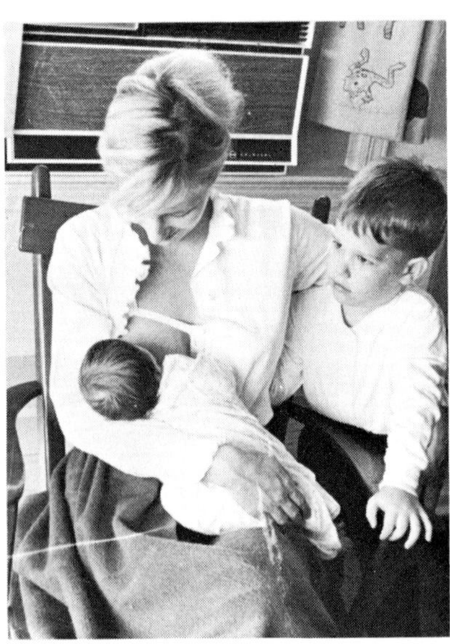

Sharing of love with a sibling

Fig. 31-2. Maturing of love.

If his first budding awareness of himself has established a reasonable amount of self-confidence, he can stand some frustration. He learns that he must leave some things alone, e.g., the books in the bookcase. If he does not, mother is cold and disapproving, and he does not feel comfortable with himself. Little children learn quickly what they can and cannot do. If discipline is relatively consistent and trustworthy, the child's confidence in himself and his feeling of acceptance by mother may be shaken now and then but not shattered (Chap. 33).

Sometime between the first and second birthdays, the child becomes able to control his sphincters, and the important cultural lesson of depositing his waste products in the bathroom is learned (p. 409). This phase of development helps the child discover the pleasures of giving. He will spontaneously make and give presents to his mother and his father. This givingness of the little child is only the embryonic beginnings of the true generosity it is hoped will ultimately emerge. The little child gives because he enjoys the experience, not because he is concerned about the well-being of the recipient of his gifts. Not only does the little child give, but he may also do many things that appear to be acts of consideration. It is important to understand, however, that these acts must not be viewed from the adult perspective. The child is polite, considerate, generous, because he feels good when he acts that way. He probably has a rudimentary feeling of pleasure toward the person who makes him feel good, but he is not yet mature enough to appreciate the fact that his behavior affects adults in any way other than their expressed approval of him. The little child is absorbed in establishing his own autonomy. Encouragement of the givingness of the little child by means of adult praise and appreciation helps establish patterns of behavior that, in years to come, will serve other purposes than mere self-satisfaction.

At the time when the little child is beginning to go places under his own steam and learning to conform, he is also learning to talk. He learns the names of things and people—*Mommy, Daddy, little boy, little girl.* He also learns the meaning of the pronouns *I, me, you, he, she, it.* With this knowledge comes the identification of himself as a boy or a girl. From the time of a child's birth the parents' reactions to a boy baby are different, often in quite subtle ways, from their reactions to a girl baby, their acceptance of his gender helps the child appreciate his identification. The child's acceptance of his gender role is primarily a semantic and cultural phenomenon and has surprisingly little to do with the configuration of his external or internal genitalia. Those rare children who are born with indeterminate sex can be brought up with equal ease as either male or female, quite regardless of which type of gonad is ultimately found to predominate.

In the second year of life, a child learns whether he is a boy or girl and begins to identify with the parent of his own sex and with the whole cultural pattern of maleness or femaleness. A child is often quite firm about

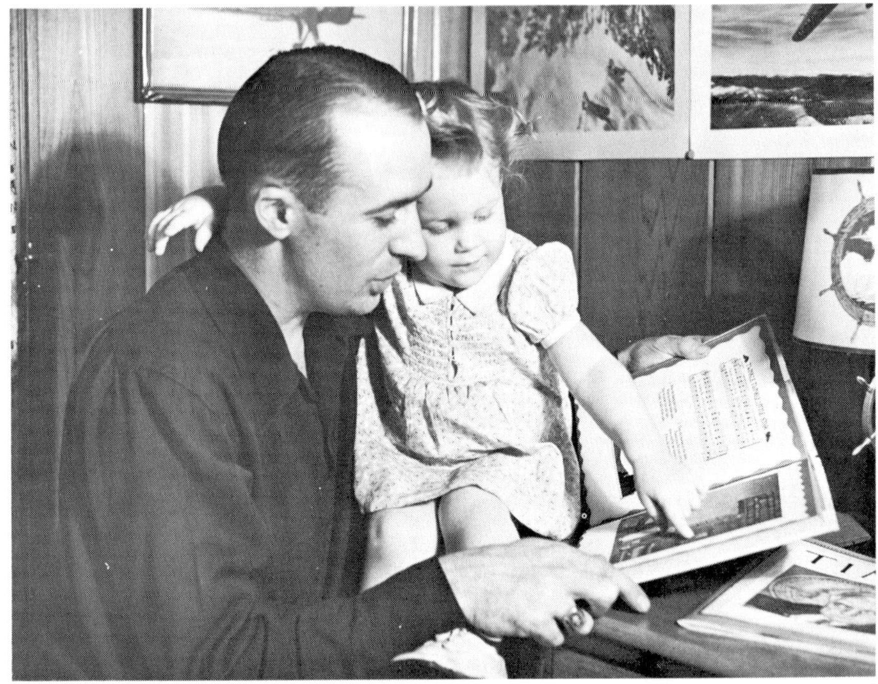

Photograph by Robert Wood

Father and daughter

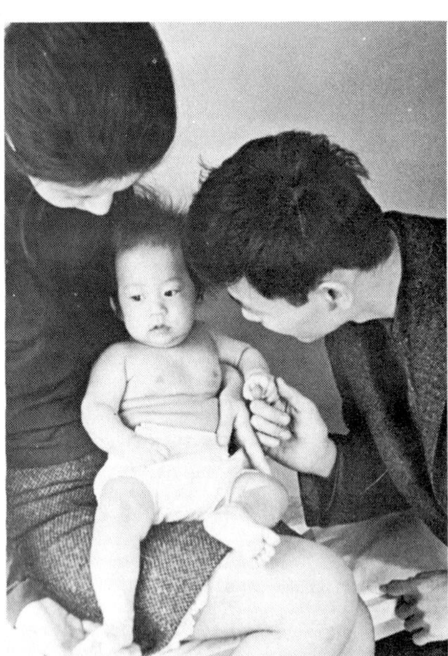

Both parents accept the infant

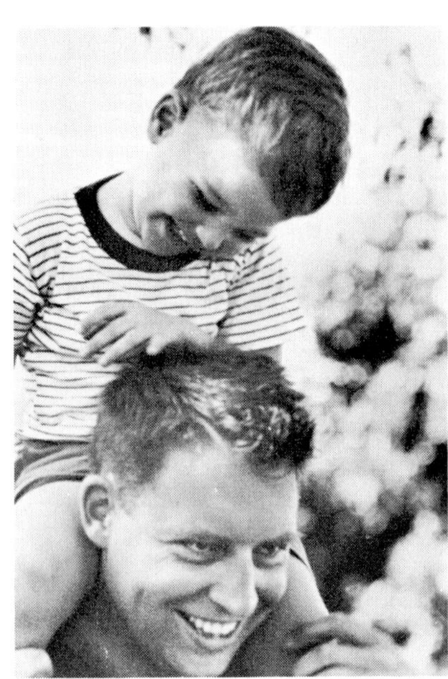

Photograph by Le Van Kim

Companionship

Fig. 31-3. Paternal love.

his own gender before he is aware of the difference in genital configuration of boys and girls. A child's sex role is important to him; it is part of his emerging concept of *I*. The *I* of the infant is neuter gender; the *I* of the 2-year-old definitely includes a concept of which segment of society he belongs to. The more wholeheartedly a child can accept his gender, the more competent he feels his emerging self to be. His acceptance depends upon the attitude of his parents. If Father considers Mother an incompetent fool, their daughter will not be too pleased to identify with Mother. Daughter will know how Father feels, not so much by his words as by the phatic communication of which children are such great masters (p. 451). Such a father may well treat his little girl as though she were his son. Though the child knows she is a girl, she nevertheless gets little pleasure from this knowledge and does her best to live up to her father's desire for a son. Since it is manifestly impossible for her to grow up to be a man, foundations are being laid for failure and frustration—not good qualities for that self that is trying to emerge.

By the age of 2 or 3 and sometimes as late as 4, a child is apt to show an increased interest in his genital organs (Conn and Kanner, 1947). By this time he is very definite about his own sex. He knows who he is; he can talk about all sorts of things. He is familiar with his body; he knows how it feels here and there. He is very familiar with his mouth, with his hands and feet, and with his genitals. He likes to touch them; he feels good when he does. He likes to talk about his genitals and about bathroom activities (Hattendorf, 1932). At this age the child is not aware of the functions of the reproductive organs. The only overt function he has experienced so far in this region of his body is elimination, and to him this is what these organs are for. Elimination is a part of the day's activities, a subject for conversation, a subject for play. While the little child has no knowledge from his own experience of reproduction, nevertheless he is now aware of the difference between boys and girls. He is interested in everything that comes his way, so he is interested in how children of the opposite sex are made. Left alone, he will explore himself and sometimes the genitals of his playmates. He will ask questions. He wants to know why boys and girls are different, he wants to know where babies come from, he wants to know why girls sit down to urinate (or why boys stand up). The small child's interest in his genitals is so universal that this stage is often spoken of as the *genital phase* of development (Kanner, 1957; Erikson, 1963).

The genital phase may be a difficult period for parents. Many adults are embarrassed by their children's questions, even horrified by children's curiosity and explorations. They fear that a child is "depraved" because he is interested in his genitals; they fear he will grow up to be a sexual pervert. They are not aware that this is a normal phase of development, and that the child will mature beyond it. All little children go through this genital phase, but what happens to them and their emerging concept of themselves depends on how their adults accept this phase of growth.

During infancy if a child learns that his genitals are a bad part of him, he may be very circumspect in any overt manifestation of his genital interest. A parent who has been unable to accept his infant's genital exploration is more than likely to continue the same attitude during the far more pronounced genital interest that comes along during toddlerhood. Even the child who has achieved a reasonably adequate infantile integrity may run into difficulties during his genital phase. If the child discovers, as much through phatic as semantic communication (p. 451), that his mother or his father disapproves of his genital explorations, he soon learns that this is a pleasure he must enjoy in private. He also learns it is better not to talk about it, not to ask questions. However, the knowledge of his parents' disapproval makes him feel guilty. He feels that his genitals are a bad part of him and therefore that the total *I* he is struggling to achieve is partly evil. He is not comfortable with himself.

It is during the genital phase that a child who has been made to feel guilty about his interest and pleasure in his genitals may feel that he is so bad that he should be punished for his secret transgressions. The punishment that many, many children spontaneously dread is that the genitals will be mutilated. If the child is a boy, he fears his penis may be cut off; if the child is a girl, she becomes convinced that she once had a penis that has been cut off.

It is easy to understand that a child at whom an angry parent yells, "Leave it alone, or I'll cut it off" could develop the fear of castration. But many a youngster who has never had such strong overt threats nevertheless develops the same fear. He senses his parents' disapproval, even if unspoken, and reacts to it with guilt and dread of punishment, and an enormous number of children seem to think up the same punishment: removal of the offensive part.

Castration fear has different overtones in boys and girls. It is perhaps at this time that we begin to see divergence in the development of the two sexes. While both boys and girls may be made to feel guilty about their genital pleasures and fear punishment, nevertheless the boy's fear is a dread of what might happen. He still has a penis, and it gives him sensations he likes. These feelings may be compounded with guilt, which is often expressed by the little boy as aggression. He becomes excessively active; he tries to conquer the world about him. Every 3- or 4-year-old is pretty active, but there is often a kind of belligerence which may well be a reaction to his deep fear that his parents may take away his precious penis.

The little girl, on the other hand, has to explain to herself why she does not have a penis. What did she do that made her mother or her father take this thing away from her? She is resentful, rather than aggressive. She is apt to turn her feelings inward, to feel incompetent because she has been denuded. The little girl whose feelings of guilt about her genitals are not too great may simply feel envious of boys, feel that somehow she has been cheated. These feelings vary greatly in intensity in different little girls, depending in large measure on how they are treated in this important phase of development, but some degree of genital trauma is quite universal. Deutsch feels that many of the characteristics of the feminine personality have their origin in the anatomic consequences of the genital phase.

Parental awareness of the universal interest of children in their genitals at this early age may help reduce both child and adult tension and provide parents with a chance to clarify children's common misconceptions.

The childish love that emerges during the years of toddlerhood is compounded, as was baby love, of the attitude of the child and that of his parents. The child is still primarily concerned with grappling with himself. The image of the *I* is becoming more definitive.

Under favorable conditions the child discovers a competence in himself: his body is good, he has power to make it do what he wants it to do, he has pleasure in its workings and all its feelings. The child is developing self-confidence and self-respect. He loves the *I* he is learning to know. His parents have expressed their love for him in acceptance and approval of his activities and his increasing ability to conform to their demands.

If the price of parental love is not too high, the child is capable of paying the price; he gets satisfaction from his ability to conform.

A child can withstand a storm or two. It is the constant repetition of traumatic events which is devastating. He can recover, if the prevailing climate is salubrious. He has no opportunities to recover if the weather is always inclement. The boy turns to aggressiveness, the girl to resentment. Both try to forget, and often they do forget at the superficial level. They stop genital play and interest, stop talking about bathroom activities, stop asking embarrassing questions. But they carry with them into later phases of development the repressed conviction that they harbor an evil core.

PRESCHOOL CHILD: OEDIPAL LOVE—LOVE MUST BE EXCLUSIVE

In the preschool years, there comes a new phase of loving. Up to this time the little child has accepted the love of his mother and his father, and so long as they were warm and loving toward him he did not much care what else they did or whom else they loved. But suddenly (so it seems) the child wants to be the exclusive recipient of the love of one parent. He becomes inordinately jealous of any demonstration of affection toward anyone but himself. Quite often the little boy wants to be his mother's sole object of love, and the little girl turns to her father. While this turning toward the parent of the opposite sex is frequent and is what has given this phase of development its name, *oedipal phase,* nevertheless, the fundamental characteristic of this period is not so much the person selected by the child as the desire for the exclusive affection of some one adult.

The fact that this phase of development comes along in the lives of most children is quite well established (Erikson, 1963), but the explanation of why it comes is far from clear. Its usual timing is toward the end of the genital phase and well after the child has a clear understanding of his own sex identity. His genitals are immature, they give him pleasant feelings, but most children at this age are vague about the role their genitals play in procreation. Whether the oedipal phase is truly genital is debatable. Freud considered oedipal love as the first true "falling in love" experience. It certainly shows the jealousy often associated with romantic love, but it has none of the giving qualities of mature love, and to call it "falling in love" is to give it an adultomorphic interpretation.

The child is 4 or 5 years old by this time. He has a distinct knowledge of his gender. In his play the child is learning about the innate attributes of things and people outside himself, by his special human technique of pretending to be that other person or thing (Chap. 33). He imagines himself grown big. He is Daddy (or Mommy if the child is a girl). To be Daddy, he wants to feel just the way he imagines Daddy feels. He tries to talk big, he walks like Daddy, he stumps around in Daddy's shoes, or puts on Daddy's hat. He calls his mother by her first name, the way Daddy does. Then, somewhere along the line, the idea dawns on him that Daddy has some sort of special relation with Mommy. They sleep in the same bed, though he is made to go to his own room. With the penetration of childhood he cuts through conventional overlays and gets to the heart of the matter. *Mommy is Daddy's woman.* To really feel like Daddy, the little boy also wants Mommy to be his woman. He would just love to have the exclusive attention of his mother. His imaginative play is being superseded by his wishes as a little boy. He no longer wants to pretend to be Daddy; he wants to be himself and yet have Daddy's prerogatives. But Daddy is very real and very much there. The little boy begins for the first time to feel a competition with Daddy. He would like to get rid of him, so he could have Mommy all to himself. He is quite likely to say he would like to marry his mother. He may want to get into his mother's bed and snuggle up next to her. While these may be his actions and his words, he is but a 5-year-old. He has no conception of adult sexual relations. He may like to snuggle because of the nice warm over-all-his-body feeling he receives; maybe he even feels special pleasure in his genitals along with his overall body pleasures, but that he has any desire for adult sexual acts seems most unlikely. He seeks pleasure as a little child—body pleasure and pleasure in an exclusive loving relation. He has no concept of loving his mother as a wife. He is still in an egocentric stage where love means to be loved.

However, he does feel a rivalry with his father which is quite ambivalent because he also wants his father's love and approval. The child is in a quandary. He wants his father, and simultaneously he wants to be rid of him. The little boy whose relation with his father has, up to this time, been loving and good is even more torn by conflicting emotions than the child whose father has been distant or even forbidding.

These are difficult feelings for a 5-year-old to resolve. He feels bad and guilty about his wishes to eliminate his father. At 5 years of age he is still not quite clear about the differences between his fantasies about his father and the actuality. Because he wants to get rid of his father, he feels a guilt as though he had accomplished the feat.

The 5-year-old in this dilemma needs help. He cannot control his feelings; they come to him willy-nilly. If either one of his parents can let him know that he is loved in spite of his feelings, he can make a step toward accepting himself. "You would like to get rid of me, I know, so you could have Mommy all to yourself. I know how you feel. It is all right to feel that way, but, you see, Mommy needs both of us." Suddenly the child feels better. Daddy can love him, bad feelings and all.

If handled with understanding and with sensitivity for the child's feelings, the oedipal stage does not last long. The child who can be helped from time to time as he passes through it emerges with a deeping awareness of what it really means to be a grownup man. He has played at being Daddy long enough to get a sensitive perception of what he may someday be like himself.

On the other hand, if his mother is flattered by his obvious preference for her, permits an undue amount of snuggling and intimate body contact, and plays along with the child either by rejecting her husband or pretending to, the child also feels guilty. He knows he is not his father or an adult man. Somehow, with the daggerlike penetration of a child he realizes that this is not what a 5-year-old wants. In such a child, the oedipal conflicts are not resolved; they become suppressed and may influence the individual's ability to establish normal heterosexual relationships later in life.

The picture of oedipal love has been painted with the little boy as the central theme. The picture for the little girl is similar. She identifies first with her mother. She dresses up in her mother's clothes, copies her mother's gestures, talks like her, does her best to be as like her mother as possible. Then the notion dawns on her that she would like her mother's prerogatives with respect to her father. She wants only her father to put her to bed. She wants him to stay in her room. She pushes her mother away whenever her father is in the house. The emotional situation with the little girl carries the same ambivalence concerning the pushed-away mother as does the boy's with his father. The little girl needs help in coping with feelings that she does not know how to resolve.

Whatever its basic explanation, the oedipal stage is so frequent an experience in the lives of little children that it is justifiable to consider it a phase in normal maturation. It is a phase, however, that many parents have difficulty in understanding and in coping with in such a way that the child can resolve his conflicts and pass on to later stages, unencumbered with crippling guilts. Goodrich discusses the role of professional help at crucial periods in maturation to aid in establishing mastery experiences rather than disorganizing failures.

SIBLINGS

Another phase of love enters the picture in reference to siblings. When a new child arrives in the family, the displaced baby will find it difficult. This is true regardless of the age of the displaced one, though the problems vary with his age. It is difficult to be an ex. Ex-presidents and ex-wives have trouble accepting the fact that they are no longer what they once were, and an ex-baby is apt to have a hard time of it.

The displaced child is jealous of the attention the new baby receives. He feels he is in competition for his mother's love. If he is very young, under a year and a half, his feeling is an amorphous one of withdrawal from his mother. At this age he may not even be aware that the new baby is the direct cause of what he feels is a change in his mother. He just feels that things are different. If he is in the midst of toilet training, he may give up attempting to control his sphincters, feeling, perhaps, that if he went back a step or two, he might return to the more comfortable conditions of life when mother gave him her full attention. Sometimes he may resort to thumb sucking, either revert to it or increase what he has not yet ceased doing. He seems to have an unfocused feeling that when he sucked, things were better, so he tries to suck his way to satisfaction.

A slightly older child, say between 2 and 3, is quite aware that it is the new baby who is disrupting his life. He is jealous of the baby. He does not want his mother to spend time with the newcomer. He wants to get rid of the baby. If the older child is in the genital phase, he may be aware of the genitals of the baby if they are different from his own. Sometimes this increases a castration fear, if it is already incipient.

If the child is still a little older and in the oedipal stage, the newcomer appears in still a different light. A little boy, wanting the exclusive love of his mother, is violent against this additional rival; the little girl, on the other hand, may leave the squally thing to her mother and turn with renewed enthusiasm to her father. Should he dare to express interest in the baby, she is bitter and resentful.

Awareness on the part of the parents that the older child will react with envy and jealousy can help them ease the burden of displacement and accept the feelings that do emerge. "I know how you feel. It's all right to feel the way you do, but I cannot let you hurt the baby. Mommy loves you very much, but she loves this baby too."

Acceptance of feelings, combined with control of behavior, is the keynote here.

SCHOOLCHILD: BUDDY LOVE—LOVE FOR AN EQUAL

After a few more years have passed, the child's body becomes a more completely accepted phenomenon to him. He has gone beyond the genital phase. He has outgrown his oedipal desires. He has explored his body; he

Girl friends have a deep concern for each other

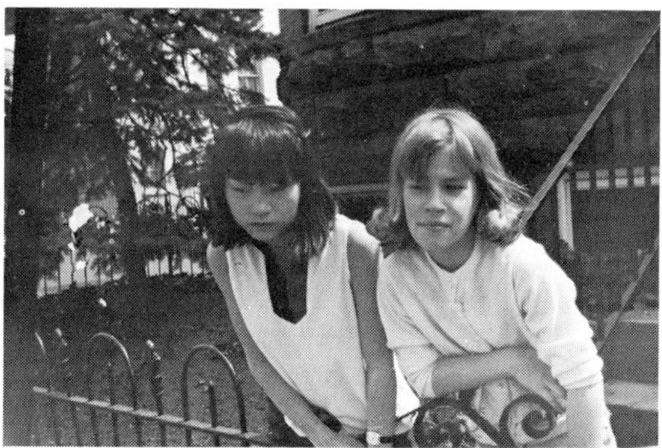

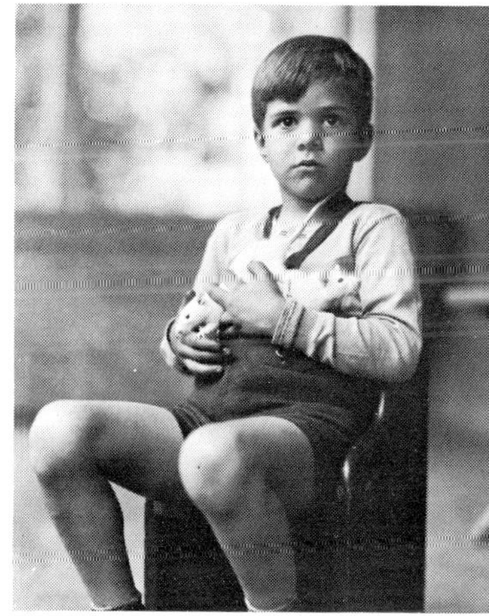

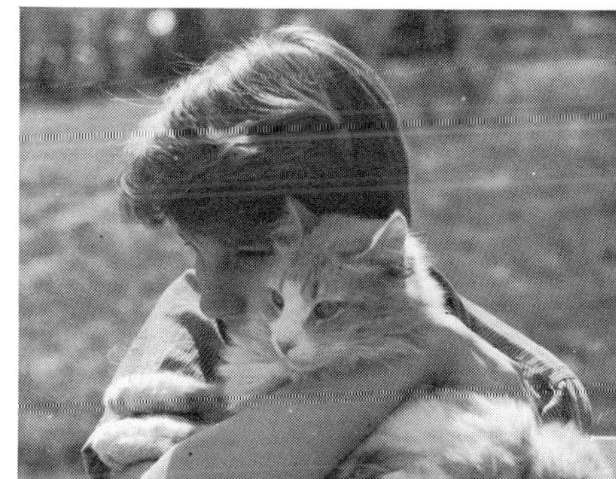

Photograph by Jack James

Preschoolers and school age children learn consideration from pets

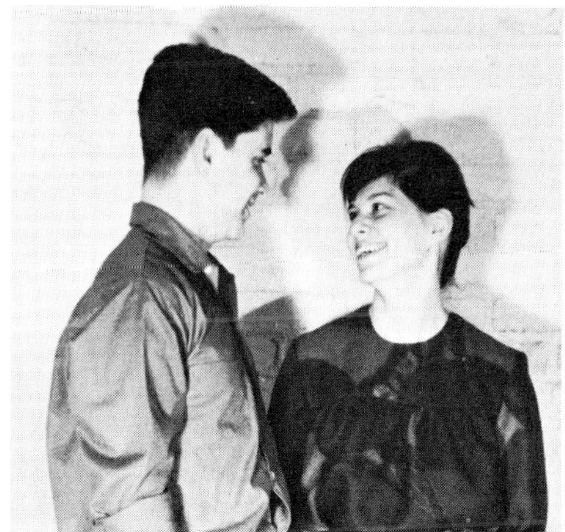

Boy-girl love

Fig. 31-4. As love matures.

knows how it feels, here and there. He still likes it, but it is no longer quite so new and full of surprises. During the in-between years—the elementary school time—the child's main interest is outside his body. This is the so-called "latency period"—latent only with respect to overt sex interests—for the child is far from latent in his explorations of the world about him. He wants to know how things work; he takes part, he builds, he studies, he learns. His curiosity is great. He is forever making new and fascinating discoveries.

He is also relating to people with a new understanding. It is at this time that he discovers his age-mates in a new light—little people like himself in a world of grownups. These children he can comprehend much more completely than he can comprehend adults. He knows about himself, and he discovers that his buddy has needs, desires, joys, sorrows, like his own. A boy's relation with a buddy or a girl's with another girl—an age-mate of the same sex—is an important rung in the ladder of human ability ultimately to relate intimately with a mate (Sullivan, 1953). The love he develops for his friend is the child's first experience with a true mutuality. *I* is becoming *we*. The mutuality in the chumship relation extends to an ability to share gripes, irritations, frustrations. For the first time the child is able critically to evaluate his parents and his home and to discuss and compare the idiosyncrasies of his family with those of his chum.

The mutual love that develops between two children is very different from the love that exists between a child and his parents. From an adult a child expects acceptance and protection. He knows he must learn to deserve some of the acceptance. But for the most part the adult is a "big person" who, in the eyes of the child, can look after himself. The child feels little or no responsibility for the adult. The child may do many things that please his adults and that the adults accept as manifestations of love. Many times these acts are motivated more by the child's desire to exercise mastery over himself than desire to contribute to the well-being of the adult. On the other hand, there are times when a 10-year-old's sincere "Gee, thanks, Mom" expresses a true empathy with a parent.

PUBERTY [1]

As the years go on, the child's body grows, and before long the signs of puberty make their appearance. His reproductive apparatus, in hibernation, as it were, during the years when he is discovering himself in relation to his world of people and things, finally awakens and matures. But it is not only the genitals that mature at this time. Puberty is a time of profound and rapid change, and only part of this is the maturation of the reproductive system. The pubescent child is body-conscious; he is concerned about how big he is, how masculine or how feminine. Although the child in puberty is certainly interested in his changing body, his dominant concern

[1] See p. 573 for definitions of puberty and adolescence.

at this age is now far more apt to be the big questions "Who am I? What am I going to do and be?".

In puberty the child's interest turns back to himself. He is struggling with the last lap in his march to adulthood, and the road suddenly becomes steep. So many changes take place in him so quickly that the job of understanding them and coping with their significance becomes quite difficult. His concern is magnified if he is one of the fringe children not progressing at quite the same rate as his friends (Chap. 12).

But here it is necessary to talk about boys and girls separately. Before puberty, sexual maturation is quite similar in boys and girls, though there are some overtones of difference, as noted above. Children become aware of, and accept, their gender role in early childhood, but the problems in both sexes revolve primarily around the emerging self-awareness and the integrity of the whole self which constitutes *I*.

Puberty in the Girl

While puberty in girls and boys has some features in common, nevertheless it has quite different overtones in the two sexes. The girl is on her way to growing up to be a woman, which obviously is quite different from growing up to be a man.

When puberty begins to make itself evident, the little girl becomes very body-conscious. She is interested in her developing breasts, her change in shape, her feminine curves. These things she sees and enjoys. Her need at this time for good sex education has been stressed by Kestenberg and ideally it should come from her mother. Sex education, of course, begins early in life with honest answers to early questions, in small and simple doses as the child can absorb them, but in early puberty, more information is needed. The little girl needs to know more of what is happening in her body than she can see. She needs to know what is going on in her ovaries and her uterus and that before long she will menstruate. The fact that she will bleed is often distressing to a young girl and may reawaken old fears of castration. The fact that it is a normal phenomenon needs stressing. Even though there is blood, it does not mean an injury. Properly handled, a little girl will look forward to menstruation—a diploma she gets when she graduates from childhood to young womanhood.

The little girl in early puberty, however, wants to know more than the facts of menstruation. She is interested in sexual relations. "What is it like?" "How long does it take?" "Does it hurt?" She needs honest answers. Without them, many a child builds up fantasies of brutality that color her subsequent development. Throughout the girl's development there is the ever-recurring theme of masochism. The frequency with which little girls get the notion that sex is brutal, something to which women must submit, may have deeper origins than the hangover of a Puritan culture.

Little girls are interested in pregnancy and will ask innumerable questions on the subject. How are babies born, and how do they grow inside? Little girls are always interested in the pathologic episodes that have to do with reproduction. "Are babies ever born without heads?" "What makes Siamese twins?" "What is a stillbirth?" Girls' questions are different from those of boys. Girls' sexual interest centers around coitus, pregnancy, delivery, and their aberrations.

The girl also needs to know about sexuality in the opposite sex. She will be in a much better condition to conduct herself if she is aware that the drive for sexual fulfillment in boys is much more direct and more powerful than in girls. This type of education is mandatory in a society in which adolescents are permitted freedom to seek each other's company, without the chaperonage that was such an important part of a bygone era.

The girl in puberty, as the boy, is basically concerned with the big question "Who am I?". The girl's reproductive apparatus contributes only in a vague way to her awareness of her maturity. She may have fleeting tinglings in her genitals, but they are diffuse and not clearly separated from other bodily sensations. Even when the girl has what she recognizes as sexual feelings, they are not a prelude to relief of tension and are not directed toward orgasm as they are in the boy. They are in the nature of a pleasant state to be maintained. The anatomic arrangement in girls is probably a factor in the diffuse character of her sexual awareness, although it is possible that culture also has an influence. While menstruation is genital, it has no erotic element and constitutes no part of the girl's sexual cravings.

The urge to masturbate among girls is not nearly as strong as among boys, and the reasons for the difference are inherent in the physical organism. The term *masturbation* implies the self-stimulation of the genitals to the point of orgasm. Many girls handle their genitals occasionally, especially the clitoris, for the sake of the pleasant feeling they obtain but do not carry the activity to the point of orgasm. Kinsey reports that only 40 per cent of girls have masturbated by the age of 20, although Davis found a higher per cent among college women. (Compare this with boys —see below.)

A teen-age girl is interested in romanticized love, and this interest often transcends her interest in the sexual aspects of her body. As with her sexual cravings, her feelings about love are romantic and diffuse.

Her immaturity is evident in her desire to be loved and sought after. She seeks ways to make her body attractive, techniques by which to snare the males into paying attention to her. She spends long hours, both alone and in the company of other girls, formulating and discussing means of trying out her feminine wiles. In spite of the activity with which she pursues these interests, her attitude is essentially a passive or receptive one. Her success is measured by phone calls, dates, male attention. In the teen-age period the girl begins practicing the art of finding a mate. This stands in marked contrast to the boys, who at this age are interested in sexual gratification and not at all in permanent mate seeking.

Puberty in the Boy

The pubescent boy is faced with a multitude of problems, only one of which is his rapidly maturing physical organism. The sexual aspects of puberty do not make this tempestuous period any easier. The boy's rapidly maturing body poses new problems that add to his basic concern about his identity and purpose in life. As with the girl, he needs a greater intellectual understanding of what is happening in his body than he has already received. The boy should, of course, know about nocturnal emissions before he experiences them, but he will also want to know about sexual relations, about perversion, about homosexuality, about venereal disease. His questions are different from those of a girl. Coitus and perversions dominate his interest. He is only mildly interested in a love relation with a mate, and pregnancy does not concern him at all. The parent who can keep sex a discussable topic can be of inestimable help to a boy.

Additional education for the teen-age boy, as for the girl, is some understanding of what growing up means to the opposite sex. Unless taught otherwise, the boy will assume that the girl feels as he does sexually, and this gross misconception can get the boy into some difficult situations.

While education about his body is very desirable, no amount of intellectual understanding solves a boy's problems. When the reproductive system finally matures, it crowds itself into his awareness. It makes demands. The maturing sperms in his testes create tensions and pressures. The boy's sexual awareness impinges upon his daily life—his contact with girls in school, in social activities, even in a bus, or perhaps through pictures in the newspapers or the reading of a book—all these things make an impression on him. He knows by the tingling in his genitals that he is now a man. Sexual desire in boys is urgent and is directly related to the genitals; its aim is relief of tension by orgasm. In the adolescent boy, sexual cravings are a bodily phenomenon and have little or nothing to do with love. Sexual cravings reach a crescendo in the period immediately after puberty. The peak, according to Kinsey, measured by the frequency with which boys seek orgasm, is reached 1 or 2 years after puberty.

In our culture there is a minimum opportunity for gratification of sexual urges during adolescence. Homosexual activities are condemned by society and usually by the boy himself, though according to Kinsey 37 per cent of adolescent boys have had at least one homosexual experience. Premarital sexual involvements are fraught with many problems. More often than not, the boy's solution is masturbation, which is a very different act from the handling of the genitals in early childhood that is sometimes given this designation. The teen-age boy manipulates his genitals for the purpose of producing an ejaculation which relieves him of built-up pressures in his genital organs.

Almost every boy masturbates. According to various studies by Finger,

Ross, Kinsey, and Giedt, from 90 to 98 per cent of teen-age boys in our culture masturbate with a frequency that varies from once or twice a month to four or five times a week.

Masturbation is not an easy topic to discuss in our society. Judeo-Christian beliefs still dominate the feelings of many people. It is difficult to eradicate the old belief that masturbation is inherently evil. A long list of physical ills has been attributed to the practice; such unrelated conditions as acne, fits, baldness, blindness, impotence, and insanity have been attributed to masturbation (Brady, 1891; Dearborn, 1961). There is not a shred of evidence that masturbation causes any of these symptoms, and yet the persistence of these beliefs has had a devastating effect upon the emotional life of young people in the United States (Dearborn, 1961). Levine states that 75 per cent of the parents of children in a child guidance clinic had threatened their children with some form of physical calamity if they persisted in masturbation (Ford and Beach, 1951).

The evil effects of masturbation lie not in any physical consequences but in the worry concerning possible effects and the guilt in the minds of the young who find themselves unable to control their desire to masturbate. Among some modern counselors of youth who have been convinced that masturbation really has no relation to physical ills there nevertheless remains the feeling that the practice "isn't nice" and should be discouraged, that young people should be encouraged to find "better things to do" and helped to "outgrow the habit." While this attitude is an improvement over threatening a youngster with insanity, it nevertheless represents but a transitional phase on the road to emancipation from the shackles of the past. This attitude too may cause guilt and emotional conflict almost as severe as that of threatening physical calamity.

Some religious leaders, while admitting that masturbation is not related to organic disease, nevertheless insist that the practice should be discouraged. The Roman Catholic Church dogmatically calls masturbation a sin. Some orthodox Jewish and fundamentalist Protestant Churches hold a similar view (Clemens, 1961). However, in spite of the attitude of some churches, there is today a growing opinion, among scientists and people well informed on matters of sex, that masturbation not only is a normal physiologic activity for the release of tension but that it carries positive value (Dearborn, 1961).

The objection has been raised that if a teen-age boy is told that it is all right to masturbate, he will exercise no control and carry the activity to excess. There is, however, no more danger that a normal boy will masturbate excessively than that he will engage in other activities excessively. Life consists of a diversity of pursuits; the normal person divides his time and activities among many interests. The individual who engages in one activity to the exclusion of a repertory is showing signs of abnormality. A disturbed child sucks his thumb to the exclusion of playing; a normal child sucks now and then. The child or adult who eats excessively or talks without letup is using the activity to compensate for failures in other areas. Such an individual needs help—not so much to stop the excessive activity directly as to open up his personality to a fuller life. And so with masturbation, the normal boy who can masturbate moderately and in private finds the activity a useful outlet. On the other hand, the boy who masturbates constantly, often in public, is giving evidence that he is failing to develop a rounded personality. The excessive masturbation is not the cause of his failure but one symptom, probably among others, of a disorganized personality.

A boy who is taught that masturbation is evil, that dire consequences will befall him if he persists, will suffer greatly from guilt, since he will probably masturbate anyway. In the long run, it makes little difference whether the boy fears physical disease or confirmation of his sinful nature. In either case, he feels guilt. His guilt, his feeling of unworthiness, make much more difficult the solution of the most important problem of this age: "What kind of a person am I?" Secretly masturbating, consumed with guilt and feelings of inadequacy, he struggles along trying to keep to himself the knowledge of what a debased person he really is. The boy who feels that there is something evil in his sex organs, who feels that the evil drive is bigger than he is and makes him masturbate even though he tries not to, comes to feel that his body is a threat to him, not an asset. Ultimately, when such a boy seeks a mate, it is difficult for him to share in true mutuality that part of himself which he has not learned to accept as good and valuable. He may never be able to accept his mate as one with whom he can share the best of himself. He remains alone within his own body, using his mate only for biologic needs, but he fails to achieve the pinnacle of human mutuality. His guilt, his debasement of himself, remain in the pattern of his neural and emotional structure. They are such unpleasant and threatening feelings that they are pushed down below the level of his daily thought and conscious feeling, whence they burst to the surface from time to time as neurotic symptoms.

On the other hand, the boy who is told that masturbation is normal will feel free to engage in this practice from time to time. He understands how his body works, he accepts it, it belongs to him, he likes it, he is glad he is growing to adulthood. He is able to incorporate his masculinity into a concept of his self that he respects. When the time comes, he has something he holds in high esteem to share with a mate.

MATURATION OF THE ABILITY TO LOVE

Sexual maturity brings to man and woman alike the full concept of the body. If development has progressed in a reasonably optimal way, the individual not only knows his body but accepts it as part of his total self. He and his body are at peace. With the solid foundation of a good and valuable physical organism whose feelings are integrated into the self, the individual is finally equipped to comprehend the totality of the external world of people and things.

The egocentricity of infancy has matured into a self-respect. Self-respect is the dominant attribute of the mature person's concept of himself. The immature person, on the other hand, has failed to mature beyond the egocentricity of his earlier years. He is the person who grabs for himself; his pleasures are in taking, not in giving. He looks at the world only to see what he can get from it. Instead of a respect for himself, he has contempt and tries to cover up the self inside him for which he has no fondness.

Mature love comes slowly. It does not burst into full flower with the menarche or the first nocturnal emission. The adolescent has to incorporate into his self his new knowledge of his body. He must also resolve his big question, "Who am I?" and he must finally pull away from dependence upon his family. When he has accomplished all this, the adolescent has crossed the threshold into maturity. The chronological age can vary from 16 to 30 depending upon life experiences. Some people never cross the threshold.

Erotic Love—Love for a Mate

Mature, independent, alone—a few people maintain this status for life, but most desire an exclusive intimate relation with some one other human being of the opposite sex, some one person with whom to share the self. From the depth of his own profound self-respect, the mature person is capable of appreciating the basic worth of another. Two such selves can relate in mutuality, because each has an honest realistic appraisal of himself. Each knows and respects what he is and therefore does not attempt to cover it over with false attributes. Love between such people is dominated by tenderness, by concern for the other person's welfare. There is a desire to give, to bring pleasure and happiness to the other. The relation is not dominated by the desire to be loved. This desire has been outgrown. Mature love is a giving rather than a receiving of love. Of course, that which is given must also be received, so there is always an element of accepting in mature love, but it is not dominated by the feeling of "What is in this for me?". The pleasures of receiving in a love relation are a by-product, not the central theme. The mature person's self-respect keeps him on keel; the love he receives is a delightful addition. It is the epitome of Christ's admonition "Love thy neighbor as thyself." To love another person fully, tenderly, it is essential first to love thyself.

Love of mature people is a fusion of their personalities and carries with it the desire for sexual union, which is then a consummation not of animal appetites but of the humanness that has transcended the physical organism. Mature love is forever renewed as the depths of personalities are constantly explored. The selection of a mate with whom to share the deep recesses of the personality is predicated not only on ability to love maturely but also upon compatible interests, intelligence, education, talents.

The desire for sexual union, however, is not necessarily synonymous with love. Sexual desire can be a physiologic appetite for relief of bodily tensions. In our society sexual acts are not infrequently entered into with full knowledge that lust is the motivation. Under such circumstances the individual is aware that love is not his goal, and he is not disappointed when it does not materialize. Sexual desire, however, can also result from many diverse strong emotions. Occasionally the wish to hurt or to be hurt dominates sexual desire. The motive may be that of conquering another for the sake of personal aggrandizement or even social prestige. Loneliness, too, can push an individual into feeling that sexual union will dispel his fear for himself. All these feelings are directed toward the person himself. He desires sexual union in order to benefit himself. These feelings are not love, any more than lust is, and sexual union offers but a momentary relief of physical tensions (sometimes not even that). Under these circumstances sexual union does not create love, as some people are wont to believe. The individual does not gain a tender mutuality with another person; he is still just as alone, as greedy, as in need of status as he was before. He has neither given nor received truly human understanding by means of the sex act. In his disappointment, he may blame his sexual partner and try to seek other relationships which seem to offer new excitement. If the original failure was due to failure in the ability to love, only greater insight into the causes of this deficiency is likely to improve future relationships.

Since the Second World War enormous changes have taken place in American Society, some of which are reflected in radically altered attitudes toward sex. Various studies (Reiss, 1960) have found that approximately half of the high school population has had some sex experience and that three quarters of college students have engaged in premarital or extra marital sex relation. While some (Feucht, 1961) have deplored this situation and urged an enforced return to the traditional attitude that sex is for reproduction only, others (Duvall, 1961; Ditzion, 1961) have taken a more realist view and tried to analyze and understand the forces that have brought about our changed sexual mores. An unusually thoughtful and provocative analysis is that of Kirkendall who feels that the time is upon us when we must truly comprehend the role that man's sexual equipment plays in the human capacity to establish mature interpersonal relations.

Mature Love

Erotic love is exclusive; it is the desire for a relation with one special person. Every individual, however, has relationships with many people. The person who has respect for himself is able to respect other people. He can appreciate the elemental core of humanness in the people with whom he comes in contact. As he grows in knowledge of the world, he becomes able to transcend differences in culture, in intelligence, in education, and in social status, and can relate to most people he knows with an attitude of respect and givingness. A few people are even able to extend this feeling to mankind in general.

In contrast, the individual worried about his own integrity is constantly seeking props to his shaky self and views each human contact with an eye to what benefit he can extract for himself. This is essentially the egocentric attitude of the little child, not left behind, but carried into adult life.

The ability to treat other people with respect for themselves as they are is the pinnacle of human relations, and it is predicated on a reasonably optimal development of love culminating in a sound self-respect. Should the human race ever be able to achieve this goal on a mass level, not only would individual lives be less tension-ridden, but even cold wars might fade from the human scene (Taylor, 1953).

Maternal Love

Human maternal love is a special kind of mature love. Like love for a mate and love for people in general, it rests on the foundation of a true maturing—of the ability to accept the self as a good and valuable possession. There is perhaps no form of love more difficult to achieve in its totality than maternal love—at least in Western culture. The failure of adequate maternal love is disastrous in its consequences, since the child deprived of this essential seldom succeeds in building up his own capacity to love on a mature level.

There are doubtless elements of maternal love that are structured in the organism and come to fruition during the process of childbearing, lactation, and child rearing. These elements may be similar to the instinctive patterns of all mammals and of some species below the mammal who care for their young. They are most obvious in the human during the period soon after childbirth.

In the human maternal love transcends any instinctive patterns. While maternal love is doubtless aided by biologic mechanisms, there are many women who never go through pregnancy who are nevertheless capable of achieving it—witness the many excellent mothers all of whose children are adopted. Some women who never marry or adopt children also achieve a true maternal love. A nurse, a teacher, a social worker, or just a woman is occasionally found who seems to have the innate ability to understand the needs of children and give them the love they need. Nevertheless, the experience of having children, either by natural or legal means, does enhance most women's understanding of children.

Maternal love has a developmental cycle—a cycle which has a reciprocal relation with the child's developing capacity to love. In the beginning a mother's love is unconditional. She loves her child, not because of this or that quality; she loves him simply because he exists. Her desire is to protect and to bring contentment to her child. She asks nothing in return. When the child cries, the mother is uneasy until she can bring peace back to her baby. She has an urge to pick him up, rock him, cuddle him, feed him when he is hungry. She enjoys seeing him asleep. She also enjoys seeing him wake up. She gets pleasure in watching him do whatever he can do. Her manifest pleasure in the infant's activities impart to the infant a satisfaction to his being. When he smiles, the mother is overjoyed at this expression of happiness.

During the early months of life, the mother's care of her child is almost an extension of the complete care she gave him automatically while he was within her uterus. He can, after birth, take care of his own internal biologic mechanisms, but his mother must do everything else for him. She not only protects, warms, rocks, feeds him, but she must even change his position for him. All the baby can do is ask for his mother's care by means of his cry. The baby accepts his mother's ministrations and reacts to them with peace and pleasure. The baby is responding to maternal love with baby love; he is feeling that it is good to be alive.

This is the earliest phase of maternal love, the phase in which the mother is the power that controls the helpless infant's well-being. The infant's manifest need of his mother imparts to her a sense of importance. She enjoys being needed, she gains an added sense of her own value, she knows she is a worthwhile person, but if she is reasonably mature, she is not dependent upon her baby's need to maintain her own integrity. She continues to relate to family and friends, and especially to her mate, on an adult level and fulfills through them her need for adult human relatedness.

A mother who is less mature may discover for the first time in her life a deep sense of her own value as she realizes her infant's need of her. The great majority of women find within themselves the ability to be good mothers during the early infancy of their children. There are, unfortunately, a very few women who, from the beginning, reject their children and never provide them with the unconditional love so needed in the beginning of life.

The next stage of maternal love emerges as the baby's utter dependence gives way to his ability to do some things for himself. His body is coming under his control, he can move it, he can turn over, he can grab with his hands. He can begin to feed himself. He wants to do each thing his developing body makes possible. Ideally, maternal ministrations retreat, the child is encouraged to exercise his emerging powers, and all the while the mother expresses her unconditional approval of everything the baby does and is. She is pleased with his developing independence. The mature mother's competence is not threatened by her baby's powers to do for himself. She does not push him in order to be able to brag about his accomplishments. She permits him to exercise his developing abilities and expresses her satisfaction in each new act he adds to his repertory.

The less mature mother, on the other hand, sees her baby's growing independence as a threat to her. The more he can do for himself, the less important she feels she is. She is reluctant to relinquish the sense of power she felt when her baby needed her to maintain his very existence. She cannot admit that she needs her baby's dependence, so she develops a blindness to his emerging capacities and expresses this by continuing to do for him those things he would prefer to do for himself. The immaturity of her love is manifested by her appreciating in her baby only what he does for her—his bolstering of her self-esteem—rather than what she can do for him by encouraging his independence. Not only in infancy but later on in childhood such a mother is apt to thwart her child's desires for independence and responsibility. She may bathe him when he would rather splash by himself, take him to school instead of letting him go alone, select his clothes, his toys without offering him any choice. Later she may even try to select his ideas and attitudes for him.

The acceptance of the child's independence begins ideally during the first year of life and increases as the child's abilities grow until the child reaches full maturity. It becomes closely intertwined with another aspect of maternal love, the application of discipline.

When the infant matures into a toddler, he must learn to conform. He must act this way, not that way, in order to receive his mother's approval. The mother expresses approval only up to a point; the child is no longer free to do everything he is capable of doing. He cannot destroy the possessions of his parents, he cannot explore the dangerous, he must eliminate his wastes in the bathroom, he must eat his food at prescribed times and in prescribed ways. All these things the child learns through the withholding of maternal approval for nonconforming behavior. The mother is accepting her child's developing independence but guiding it into the culturally accepted patterns. Maternal love can be unconditional only during the early phases of the infant's life. His dawning independence requires that he conform to cultural patterns. Though maternal love now has to be earned, it is nevertheless unselfish (that is, ideally). The mother's interest is the child's well-being, and her satisfaction arises from her child's growing independence from her, and also from his happiness and his ability to conform with a minimum of frustration. The toddler is basically unconcerned about the welfare of his mother, which is quite beyond his comprehension, although he probably does feel some warmth for the person who does things for him.

With respect to all problems of discipline, the immature mother has problems. She has already been threatened by her child's growing independence of her. Try as she will, she cannot keep him dependent upon her by force, so she tries to maintain his dependence by gratitude. She is afraid that if she thwarts him, he will not love her. She does not teach him to conform to the requirements of society. She gives in to him, lets him do almost everything he wants to do, and at the same time, paradoxical as it seems, she overprotects him. This does not produce love for the mother or gratitude toward her. The failure to impose restraints on culturally unacceptable behavior makes the child anxious and fearful. He lacks the security of knowing how to act. He becomes afraid, instead of pleased, with his developing powers.

The spoiled, overprotected child is apt to become rather obnoxious. It is difficult for him to relate to other children and adults, and even his own parents find him unpleasant to live with. Before long he gets jumped on and yelled at, at home as well as abroad. His mother vacillates between babying him and condemning him for failure to conform. Ultimately she becomes bitter and resentful: she has devoted herself to a child who shows neither gratitude nor respect for her.

The oedipal phase poses special problems for all mothers. When a little boy wants the exclusive love of his mother, the mature and informed mother is able to deny her man child his wish to displace his father in her life. She continues to love him unselfishly but insists upon her adult prerogative of loving her mate. Also the mother of a little girl accepts her daughter's jealousy of her during the time the little girl wishes the exclusive love of her father. Again, the ideal mother understands what is going on in the child's feelings, is able to accept the child, feelings and all, and yet maintain her own adult integrity. Her sense of her own value is not even touched by her daughter's temporary rejection of her.

The immature mother, on the other hand, may have a heyday during the oedipal stage of development of her little boy. She is delighted by the child's obvious preference for her. She is glad to conspire with him to eliminate Daddy from the emotional scene. She permits and encourages physical intimacies, lets the child sleep with her, often ousting her husband to the child's bed. Normally the oedipal phase is relatively short-lived, but when no limits are set to behavior or daydreams, it may continue for years with disastrous results to the child's ultimate relations with other people. The same mother may be devastated by the oedipal phase in her little girl and build up a hatred of the child which is resolved, if ever, with difficulty.

Throughout all the years of childhood, ideal maternal love is relatively unselfish. The mother is interested in the well-being of her child. The child's independence is encouraged; his conformity is praised. His feelings are in general accepted without condemnation, whether they are flattering to the mother or grossly condemnatory. His actions are controlled and channeled into socially acceptable behavior. Even those actions during the oedipal phase of the little boy which are profoundly flattering are controlled by the mature mother, because she is not dependent upon her child to maintain her own sense of worth.

With the coming of adolescence, the child establishes the totality of himself. He is struggling to exist on his own; he both wants and does not want protection. Maternal love during adolescence is still concerned with the well-being of the child, but now it is expressed less in protection and more in encouragement of full independence. While independence is encouraged, the adolescent is still in need of some parental controls. The mature mother is able to apply firmly the necessary discipline and to accept the condemnation of the rebellious adolescent without wounds to her self-esteem. The mature mother loosens her reins slowly; she does not suddenly drop them for fear that her almost grown child will turn against her. The years between physical maturity and cultural maturity are marked by the mother's finally passing the reins over to the young adult. He is now on his own. Ideally he is ready to seek a mate and to relate to the rest of the world on a truly mature level. With his maturity there dawns on him an awareness that his mother is a human being like himself. He knows now that she is not the omnipotent person he once thought she was. He sees her as an ordinary person with hopes, dreams, feelings of her own. He finally becomes able to relate to her as a person, not as an authority. A mutuality can build up between an adult son or daughter and a mother provided that the mother has been able to relinquish her protective role and accept her child as a self-directed adult.

The immature mother has many problems during the adolescence of her child. Her almost grownup child rebels violently; often he will have nothing to do with any values held by his mother. He is resentful and determined to break away from all supervision and guidance. Because he has never been allowed to shoulder responsibilities as he became able to, he has not developed self-confidence. To cover up his basic fear of himself, he is often aggressive and domineering. He must constantly prove to the world (though it is really himself he is trying to convince) that he is bold and free and strong.

The mother of such an adolescent is miserable. She feels her child is making many mistakes; she wants to protect him, to guide him, but he will have none of her. The mother is empty and frustrated; she hangs on to her child as tightly as she can—her need of him is desperate. The more she clings, the harder the child fights to be free.

Ultimately the child reaches full physical maturity and leaves home as quickly as he can. His mother is desolate. For years she has had what consolation she could find in life from his dependence. Now he has gone, and the mother has nothing left. She is not capable of a truly mature relationship with her husband, who by this time is quite likely absorbed in his business and perhaps a little bored with his wife. She is a sad wreck of a human being. Though her grownup child is away from home, she may try, when he marries, to wedge herself into the lives of the young couple. She may try to direct, to manage, to advise. If permitted, she may work herself to the bone for them, trying to gain a little gratitude. And the young married person suffering from his lack of adequate maternal care is, like his mother, unable to accept himself as competent and adequate. He continues to be rebellious against his mother. He has not the ability, any more than she, to relate to another person on a mature adult level. So, mother and child continue to quarrel and bicker. They make each other miserable, and the misery is reflected in all the members of the new family.

A few words must be said about the woman who from the beginning rejects her child. She is apt to be the one who, instead of overprotecting her child, is inclined to push him beyond his capacities. In addition, the rejected child may have a succession of caretakers. The rejecting mother finds many reasons for farming her child out to relatives or to nurses. The care the child receives may lack continuity. Discipline is apt to be harsh and severe, even to the point of cruelty. The child is made to conform so rigidly that he is permitted no spontaneity. His failures are met with condemnation, and there are many failures, because he is often required to behave in ways that are impossible for him. Such a child grows to physical maturity with a deep sense of his own failures. He has never felt comfortable with himself. He has been unable to accept the self within him as worthy of his respect. He may turn his feelings inward and become a shy, withdrawn (perhaps schizoid) personality, or he may become excessively aggressive.

Maternal love has been pictured as black or white. In actuality, it is seldom wholly good or wholly bad. No mother is ever an ideal fully mature woman, capable of always giving what her child needs, nor are the childish mothers always on the wrong side of the ledger. The vast majority of mothers love their children and according to their lights do the best possible for them.

Mothers learn with experience. As the eldest in one family put it, "Sure, you are a good mother now, but you learned on me." The adequacy with which a woman carries out her mothering role depends on the degree of maturity she has reached when she begins the job, but it also depends upon her life experiences as her children grow up. Her relations with her husband are of great importance. It is on him that she relies to maintain her self-esteem. A woman's relations with her own mother are also significant, whether that mother is physically present or present only in fantasy. If the young mother identifies with her own mother, she may have absorbed many of the older woman's attitudes; on the other hand, deep rebellion against her own mother may unconsciously make her reject any attitude that identifies her with her mother. The young mother's adequacy depends, too, upon the cultural milieu in which she lives. She can gain support from a society in which she feels comfortable, or she can be undermined, if she feels deeply out of step with her surroundings.

Human motherhood is a big job; its importance for society at large can scarcely be overestimated. It is carried out through acts of choice, not instinctively as in lower species. It requires maturity, intelligence, knowledge, and a favorable milieu. Contrary to a widely held belief, fertility is not its only requirement.

Paternal Love

A human father, unlike a mother, has no instinctive patterns to help him establish a relation with his child. The paternal act of procreation activates no neural pathways in the father. He must build a relation with his infant by acts of will.

Some fathers have little to do with their small infants; others do take part in their care. The mere propinquity of an infant, an awareness of the physical helplessness of the newborn, produces in many fathers the same sort of unselfish and unconditional love that develops in the mother.

The father's love for his newborn infant is compounded of his awareness of the infant's helplessness, his sympathetic relatedness with his wife, and his feeling of responsibility for the welfare of both. When a true mutuality exists between husband and wife, each is alerted to the feelings and needs of the other, and the father absorbs from his wife some of her feelings toward their child. In the United States one of the father's most important roles is the support he gives his wife. The mother is the one who shoulders the major responsibility for child care. The more adequate she feels, the better job she does. Her husband's sympathetic understanding of what she is trying to do, his physical help on occasion, and his moral support at all times help maintain the mother's personal equilibrium. Interest, advice, discussion are all in order, but indifference and nagging criticism can be devastating to the mother's self-confidence and therefore to the adequacy of the care she gives the children.

As the years go on the father relates more and more to his children as people. He establishes a relationship of his own with each of them. Essentially, paternal love is similar to maternal love. It consists of unconditional love and acceptance in early infancy, gradually changing to love that is conditioned on the child's ability to conform to the cultural pattern and always combined with the expression of pleasure as the child slowly takes over his own responsibilities. Finally, there comes the abandonment of all protection and guidance and an establishment of an adult relation built on mutuality.

Fromm feels that maternal and paternal love are essentially different. It is his position that maternal love remains always completely unconditional, that it never has to be earned, that one is loved by one's mother simply because one exists. Unconditional maternal love, according to Fromm, represents one of the deepest longings of every human being all life long. Paternal love, still in Fromm's view, is love that must be deserved. It is the father who imposes discipline, who makes the child conform, teaches him the ways of the world. Paternal love always leaves a doubt that one has not pleased the father and therefore that love could disappear. This picture of the father as a powerful figure of authority was also Freud's position and doubtless represented the family structure of his day. Clarence

Day's portrayal of fatherhood in the United States of the nineteenth century is similar.

In our society, father certainly seldom represents an Olympian figure who metes out punishments, gives commands, and demands immediate obedience. He is far more often a partner in domestic activity who builds his relations with his children not as an assistant mother, as some disgruntled fathers have maintained, but as a masculine figure of strength, albeit he displays consideration and kindness. In our society, both parents contribute to their children what the older psychoanalysts separated into the maternal and paternal poles of love.

BIBLIOGRAPHY

BRADY, E. T.: Masturbation, *Virginia M. Month.*, p. 256, 1891–1892.

CLEMENS, ALPHONSE H.: Catholicism and Sex, in Albert Ellis and Albert Abarbanel (eds.), "The Encyclopedia of Sexual Behavior," p. 288, Hawthorn Books, Prentice-Hall, Inc., Englewood Cliffs, N.J., 1961.

CONN, JACOB H., and LEO KANNER: Children's Awareness of Sex Differences, *J. Child Psychiat.*, 1:3, 1947.

DAVIS, KATHERINE B.: "Factors in the Sex Life of 2200 Women," Harper & Row, Publishers, Incorporated, New York, 1929.

DEARBORN, LESTER W.: Autoeroticism, in Albert Ellis and Albert Abarbanel (eds.), "The Encyclopedia of Sexual Behavior," p. 204, Hawthorn Books, Prentice-Hall, Inc., Englewood Cliffs, N.J., 1961.

DITZION, SIDNEY: Moral Evolution in America, in Albert Ellis and Albert Abarbanal (eds.), "The Encyclopedia of Sexual Behavior," p. 82, Hawthorn Books, Prentice-Hall, Inc., Englewood Cliffs, N.J., 1961.

DEUTSCH, HELENE: "The Psychology of Women," Grune & Stratton, Inc., New York, 1944.

DUVALL, EVELYN M., and SYLVANUS DUVALL (eds.): "Sex Ways in Fact and Faith," Association Press, New York, 1961.

ERIKSON, ERIK H.: Childhood and Society, 2d ed., W. W. Norton & Company, Inc., New York, 1963.

FEUCHT, OSCAR E.: "Sex and the Church," Concordia Publishing House, St. Louis, 1961.

FINGER, FRANK W.: Sex Beliefs and Practices among Male College Students, *J. Abnorm. & Social Psychol.*, **42**:57, 1947.

FORD, CELLAN S., and FRANK A. BEACH: "Patterns of Sexual Behavior," Harper & Row, Publishers, Incorporated, New York, 1951.

FREUD, S.: "Basic Writings of Sigmund Freud," Vintage Books, Random House, Inc., New York, 1938.

FROMM, ERICH: "The Art of Loving," Harper & Row, Publishers, Inc., New York, 1956.

GIEDT, F. HAROLD: Changes in Sexual Behavior and Attitudes Following Class Study of the Kinsey Report, *J. Social Psychol.*, **33**:131, 1951.

GOODRICH, D. WELLS: Possibilities for Preventive Intervention During Initial Personality Formation, in Gerald Caplan (ed.), "Prevention of Mental Disorders in Children," p. 249, Basic Books, Inc., Publishers, New York, 1961.

HARLOW, HARRY F.: The Nature of Love, *Am. Psychologist,* **13**:673, 1958.
HATTENDORF, KATHERINE WOOD: A Study of the Questions of Young Children Concerning Sex, *J. Social Psychol.,* **3**:37, 1932.
KANNER, LEO: "Child Psychiatry," 3d ed., Charles C Thomas, Publisher, Springfield, Ill., 1957.
KESTENBERG, JUDITH S.: Menarche, in Lorand Sander and Henry I. Schneer (eds.), "Adolescents: Psychoanalytic Approach to Problems and Therapy," p. 19, Paul B. Hoeber, Inc., New York, 1961.
KINSEY, A. C.: "Sexual Behavior in the Human Female," W. B. Saunders Company, Philadelphia, 1953.
———: "Sexual Behavior in the Human Male," W. B. Saunders Company, Philadelphia, 1948.
KIRKENDALL, LESTER A.: Sex and Social Policy, *Clin. Pediat.,* **3**:236, 1964.
LEVINE, MAURICE: "Psychotherapy in Medical Practice," The Macmillan Company, New York, 1942.
REEVY, WILLIAM R.: Child Sexuality, in Albert Ellis and Albert Abarbanel (eds.), "The Encyclopedia of Sexual Behavior," p. 258, Hawthorn Books, Prentice-Hall, Inc., Englewood Cliffs, N.J., 1961.
REISS, IRA: "Premarital Sex Standards in America," The Free Press, Glencoe, Ill., 1960.
ROSS, ROBERT T.: Measures of the Sex Behavior of College Males, Compared with Kinsey's Results, *J. Abnorm. & Social Psychol.,* **45**:753, 1950.
SULLIVAN, HARRY S.: "The Interpersonal Theory of Psychiatry," W. W. Norton & Company, Inc., New York, 1953.
TAYLOR, G. RATTRAY: "Sex in History," Thames and Hudson, London, 1953.

32

Communication and Language

THE NATURE OF COMMUNICATION

Communication consists of imparting something to someone else. Two quite different kinds of things can be communicated: one is an emotion; the other is an idea—a thought, a warning, a command. There is a significant difference between these two types of communication.

An emotion can be expressed in a variety of ways. It *can* be communicated with words; it can be expressed also, not so much by the actual words as by the tone of voice, the pitch, the stress, the pauses employed. Grunts, growls, groans, squeals, yelps are effective means of expressing feelings. Feelings can be communicated with muscular activity (kinesthetically), entirely without vocalization, by gesture, facial expression, or posture. Autonomous reactions can convey emotion—the red face of anger, the blushing face of embarrassment, the blanched face of fear, the tense muscles of agitation. The individual communicating his emotions may intend to tell another person how he feels; on the other hand his performance may be without awareness that he is communicating his feelings. Emotional messages are sometimes understood through the eyes, sometimes through the ears, and sometimes through body contact.

An idea can be communicated only by the use of symbolic language, usually words, although occasionally gestures have symbolic significance. The communication is always intentional.

Only human beings learn to use symbolic language (leaving out for the present the possibility of "dolphinese," to be discussed below). This late phylogenetic achievement is also late in the development of the individual. Babies do not talk, but babies communicate their feelings by the primitive tools of their bodily organism. Throughout all of life much is communicated by these same primitive tools. Communication other than by symbolic language is phatic—the transmission of emotion.

Phatic[1] Communication

The "language" of animals is entirely phatic, again with the possible exception of "dolphinese." Lorenz discovered that the jackdaw is capable

[1] La Barre, from whom the present author has borrowed the word *phatic,* credits Malinowski with its prior use. The word is not in the dictionary but comes from the Greek *phasis,* meaning "to show."

of making four or five different sounds which it uses when it is dominated by certain emotions. Hearing one jackdaw emit the fear sound, other jackdaws become aware that danger is imminent and act accordingly. The jackdaw and many other birds are vocal animals. Vocal animals use sounds to express the state of their feelings; many vocal animals, notably parrots, are able to imitate sounds they hear and can be taught to make sounds that resemble human speech. But such sounds are not speech. If they express anything, it is but the state of the bird's feelings.

A dog is much less vocal than most birds, but he "tells" his master many things, some with his voice—a bark of joy, a yelp of pain, a growl of anger. He also communicates his feelings with his whole body. Who can doubt how a dog feels when he slinks to his master with his tail between his legs?

The "language" of the primate has been extensively studied. Yerkes was able to distinguish some fourteen different sounds made by gibbons and used by these animals to proclaim their feelings. Yerkes could differentiate sounds of anger, contentment, sexual excitement, and fear. The Kelloggs, who brought up a young ape, Gua, with their own child, were never able to teach her any real words. Nevertheless, Gua expressed enthusiastic approval, fear, contentment with distinct vocal expression. The primates do not confine their expressions of emotion to vocalization. An angry gorilla adds to his growls by beating on his chest or thumping on the ground—gestures as expressive of the state of his feelings as the sounds he makes (Yerkes, 1945).

Phatic expressions are the direct result of feelings. They occur only when the emotion is present. To paraphrase Langer, they cannot be used between outbursts to discuss the nature of the enemy or to plan a campaign for his extermination. At the moment of the expression, however, both the sounds and the gestures are extremely revealing to others of how the animal feels.

A human baby communicates his feelings by these same techniques. When he is distressed, he cries (vocal expression), he thrashes his arms and legs, he tenses all the muscles of his body (kinesthetic expression). When he is content, he relaxes, he coos, he gurgles. The baby is not consciously trying to tell his adults anything. He is reacting to stimuli, but the way he acts conveys meaning. When a neonate roots around with head motions and mouth seeking, it would be an imperceptive adult who did not grasp the fact that the infant was hungry.

All through life the human "says" much with his body and with his voice, much of which is unintentional communication. Postures convey fatigue, alertness, boredom, depression, excitement. The sound of her husband's footsteps as he comes into the house in the evening tells a sensitive wife what kind of day he had at the office. Tone of voice, regardless of the words said, displays the emotional state. All human beings communicate with each other in these ways. The more intimately two people know each other and are sensitive to each other's feelings, the more is told without words. Much of what is called *intuition* is the receiving and understanding of phatic communication.

The motivational advertising of Madison Avenue, insofar as it induces emotional states in would-be buyers, is phatic communication. Adults share phatic communication with animals and with babies. It is primitive and powerful and constitutes an important part of all our interpersonal relations.

When a hungry man smelling good food dilates his nostrils rubs his abdomen, and says "yum-yum," no one doubts that he is expressing delight at the prospect of gustatory pleasures to come. He is responding much as the Kelloggs' little ape Gua responded to the same kind of stimulus. When two youngsters pass on the street and yell out, "Hi," they are but expressing pleasure in the sight of a familiar person. Much of trivial conversation does no more than express the attitude of the participants. In some adolescent gatherings the laughter, the nudgings communicate just as much as, perhaps more than, the words used. Even among adults there are times when not much is communicated but feelings—pleasure, hostility, suspicion—regardless of the words tossed around, and often in spite of the words.

A mother who talks and croons to her baby is aware that he does not understand her words. The baby understands her mood. This is an ability he does not have to learn. He is born with it fully developed. He senses by the tone of her voice, by her gestures, by the tension of her muscles whether she is warm and loving toward him or whether she is indifferent or even hostile. It is next to impossible to fool a baby.

In addition, the sensitive mother also knows how her baby feels. Her receptors pick up his phatic signals. She knows when his cry means hunger or fatigue or illness. Her knowledge is not based on the acoustic quality of the sound alone but on her total awareness of his needs. Sherman demonstrated that medical students, nurses, and even mothers could not distinguish the cause of an infant's crying when they could not see the infant. This, however, does not negate the mother's ability to absorb phatic communication when she has access to all the cues given by the infant.

All through the growing years children are extremely sensitive to phatic communication. They cut through the words used and understand the primitive message. Not infrequently they understand more than the sophisticated adult is conscious that he is communicating. Phatic communication comes from the deep and real feelings, little influenced by the superficial overlay of conventional society, and children seem to understand this. Later the armor of self-protection may dull these sensitive perceptions, and phatic communication may be less well understood.

"Sit down and eat your dinner" may convey to a little child nothing at all about the pleasures of eating. It may convey anger. If so, he will respond far more to the emotion than to the words. On the other hand, "You stupid little dumbbell" may mean "I love you dearly just the way you are." With varying inflections, with gestures of body and face, words can convey something entirely different from their literal meanings.

True Speech

True speech is different from phatic communication. Language depends upon the ability to comprehend a symbol.

A symbol is something which stands for something else. The sound of the word *table,* that combination of air waves that reaches the ear, stands for the article of furniture. The sound is not the table, but every time that particular sound is heard, it creates the mental picture of *table.* There is no need to see *table;* the sound is sufficient. This ability to comprehend a relation between two completely different things—a sound and a table—is a supreme evolutionary achievement. It comes about because of the unique function of a special area in the cortex, the speech center.

Human language has made use of man's capacity to make sounds. Man hit upon sound as the tool of his symbolization, but it is the capacity to comprehend symbols that is the great human achievement rather than the capacity to make sounds. It is possible to build up a true language by using gestures in place of sounds, as has been done in some deaf-mute languages and as was done for intertribal communication among some of the American Indians (Langer, 1942). Those unfortunate human beings who have suffered loss to the speech area and "forget" how to speak are as unable to use gestures as they are to use sounds for semantic communication.

While our true language is built on the use of sounds to symbolize reality, nevertheless we do use both kinesthetic and visual clues as symbols. The flexion of the forefinger in the semantic gesture *Come here* is as much a word as the sounds *Come here,* and the two can be used interchangeably. The nonverbal highway signs designating curves, winding roads, sharp turns, etc., are "words" in the same fashion, and can serve as international communication.

The bulk of our language depends upon sounds as symbols. Langer has a theory that man developed an auditory, rather than a kinesthetic, language because in his infancy he is a babbling creature, in contrast to the primates, who are relatively silent in infancy. The human infant appears to have an instinctive drive to use his vocal apparatus early in life to make a great variety of sounds. Therefore once the human brain achieved through evolution the special area in the cortex capable of conceiving symbols, man used his repertory of sounds as the tool with which to develop symbolization. Langer points out that the primate shows the rudiments of the capacity for symbolization, but it uses gestures, not sound, as the tool. Yerkes commented that vision seems to be more important than hearing among apes for their mutual understanding. The Kelloggs found that Gua was capable of using some gestures in a truly symbolic way, though she was able to use sound only phatically.

In some completely unexplained way human beings made a sharp break with the primates when babbling during infancy developed. The change from the primate to man in the speech areas of the cortex is quantitative rather than qualitative, even though the amount of change is great.

While sound is the basis of human symbolic language, sound has other uses both in man and animals. Sound is used for the expression of emotion, as stated above. Sound is a background sense and is used for orientation in space (p. 507). Man is not as adept as some animals in this use of sound; sight is his chief method of getting about. Deprived of sight a blind man listens to the tap of his cane.

Some species have elaborate techniques for appraisal of their environment by sound. Bats have evolved a technique called *echolocation.* These night-flying creatures emit a blast of sound too high-pitched to be audible to the human ear. As these sound waves impinge upon objects, they send back echoes which the bat is able to interpret and by means of which he can control his flight so that he avoids obstacles and simultaneously locates the insects he needs for food (Griffin, 1958). Echolocation is so highly developed in bats that these animals can fly through a dark, enclosed space successfully avoiding a multitude of fine wires stretched across it.

Dolphins have evolved a similar system, which is called *sonar.* The word is a contraction of so(und) n(avigation) a(nd) r(anging)—a technique man has attempted to develop for navigation beneath the surfaces of the ocean without the use of vision. Dolphins have a repertory of sounds they emit under water which are returned to them as echoes. The dolphins' ability to interpret these sounds far exceeds not only the human biologic capacity but also any machines man has so far been able to construct.

The dolphin possesses a brain larger in proportion to his body size than that of any other creature except man (p. 140). Examination of this brain indicates that auditory mechanisms are more fully developed than in any other species. The eighth nerve is very large, and what is interpreted to be the auditory cortex is also large and densely packed with nuclei. The dolphin apparently is much more capable than man of interpreting auditory sensation. Lilly makes a comparison with man's visual capacity. Man is capable of distinguishing a spectrum of colors in white light. Lilly suggests that the dolphin is capable of breaking down "white sound" into a spectrum. The dolphin can apparently distinguish an echo reflected from a piece of wood from one coming from a piece of metal or from a fish with the same ease with which man can distinguish red from yellow.

Echolocation in bats and sonar in dolphins, though auditory, are not languages, nor are they a means of communication with others. These are techniques used by these animals for orientation in space and water and are similar to sight and smell when used to avoid the dangerous and locate the desirable.

Since dolphins have a highly developed brain, it is within the realm of possibility that in addition to the use of sound as sonar they are capable of some symbolic use of sound. Lilly, who has done extensive work with dolphins, is convinced that these animals have a means of communication with each other. He is doing his best to devise experiments by means of which he can demonstrate "dolphinese," and he even hopes to understand it some day.

For speech to develop in a human child he must have (1) an oral mechanism that can make sounds, (2) an ear that can hear these sounds, and (3) a speech area in his brain that can conceive of these sounds not just in their phatic quality but as symbols that refer to objects or events in the world of reality. Among all the creatures on this planet only man and possibly the dolphin possess all three mechanisms.

Speech has developed in all races of mankind. However, the nature of the symbolism involved is a long way from being universal, in marked contrast to the vocalization of most animals. Lorenz, for instance, found that jackdaws in Northern Russia made exactly the same sounds to warn of danger as did his jackdaws in the United States. Man, on the other hand, confronted with more or less the same external world, finds astonishingly different ways with which to refer to it.

Components of Language

According to La Barre, language consists of three things: (1) sense—vocabulary, (2) sound—phonetics, and (3) structure—grammar.

Sense—Vocabulary

Given the human being capable of understanding symbols and given the world of nature which is roughly the same over the entire planet, one might assume that all languages would come up with about the same interpretation of reality. This is far from the case. In different parts of the world different languages have evolved by means of which people communicate with each other, and in each of these languages the external world is carved up differently. Not only are the words different, but the little pieces of reality they denote may have different boundaries. Once an individual learns his native tongue, the symbols of that language are firmly fixed in him. He comes to feel there can be no other expression of reality. His ability to communicate becomes crystallized in his own language; he is unable to communicate with people of other cultures. Many objects of language are untranslatable, because the basic symbol is different.

A symbol exists only in the human brain. It is not a unit of nature; it only stands for that piece of reality which the user of the symbol chooses to select. He is at liberty to select aspects of reality that seem significant to him and equally at liberty to ignore others (Whorf, 1956).

La Barre has described this phenomenon in relation to the word *snow.*

The word brings up a definite picture. Actually snow consists of an infinite number of crystalline forms; in fact each snowflake is uniquely different from every other one. These differences are ignored in English; all kinds of snow are lumped together; a common property is abstracted; the totality adds up to *snow.*

In the Eskimo language there is no word translatable as snow. The Eskimo is not interested in individual snowflakes, either, but he is concerned with what snow can do to him. He has a word for *hard-driving-snow-in-the-air,* another word for *snow-packed-hard-like-ice-on-the-ground,* still another word for *soft-snow-on-the-ground.* In English these differences are ignored and snow is *snow.*

In translating from English to Eskimo, the Eskimo might quite understandably feel that he was being deliberately misled if *snow* were translated as *snow-packed-hard-like-ice-on-the-ground* when as a matter of fact it was *hard-driving-snow-in-the-air.* In the first case the Eskimo could safely build an igloo; in the second, he could not. Both the Eskimo and the English-speaking American assume that with his word he is dealing with a basic reality of the universe. Neither has the words to do otherwise, for, as La Barre says, as soon as the human infant learns to speak any language at all, he has a "hardening of the categories."

Our own language family—the Indo-European—originated from a common ancestral language. There is therefore much in common among all the languages of the Western world. Nevertheless each of these languages has evolved in sufficient isolation to be now not only quite mutually unintelligible but often quite untranslatable. The French *tu* does not have the same connotation as the German *du,* and neither means the same as the English *thou.* The French *monsieur,* the German *Herr,* and the English *mister* have shades of meaning that we often have to ignore in translation, to the detriment of our ability to communicate nuances to our language cousins.

There is a theory that misinterpretation of one word in a Japanese reply to the Potsdam surrender demand subsequently resulted in the needless dropping of the atomic bomb on Hiroshima. The word was translated as "ignore," rather than as "withholding comment pending discussion." (Coughlin, 1953).

Sound—Phonetics

The physical quality of sound is universal, but sound patterns vary enormously from language to language. Sound in the physical sense consists of (1) duration—the length of time a sound is heard, (2) amplitude—the volume or loudness of the sound, (3) frequency or pitch—the number of vibrations produced in the air, and (4) timbre—the number of overtones in addition to the basic sound. These qualities of sound *are* universal. An Eskimo, a Hopi, a Chinese, or a Russian can recognize a musical note and distinguish the four qualities of its sound. Any one of them can tell an A from a C. Anyone will know, or can easily learn, to distinguish the sound of a flute from an oboe or from a piano, and it does not matter whether he hears it in New York, Moscow, or Timbuktu. But speech is a different matter, because different cultures give different meaning to the four qualities of sound.

Duration of a sound has no meaning difference in English. Southerners drawl out some words, but the duration of the sound does not change its meaning. In some American Indian and African languages, duration of the sound of a vowel has as much difference in meaning as a *b* and a *p* in English.

Amplitude, or volume, of a sound is used in English for stress or accent. It has no symbol value. It can, however, express changes in the meaning of a sentence. "*Tom* acted like a dog." (The last person in the world you would expect to act this way.) "Tom *acted* like a dog." (Tom might be like a dog, but you did not expect him to show it.) "Tom acted like a *dog.*" (You knew Tom was peculiar, but not in this way.) The Chinese coolie, again according to La Barre, uses stress only when angry; therefore he might get quite the wrong impression when he heard any of the above sentences.

Pitch is combined with volume in English to give melody, grace, and expression to conversation, without changing the symbol structure. In French, as in English, stress and pitch have no symbol meaning. They are used as a sentencewise phenomenon, rather than as a syllablewise one. There is no accent in the French word, but there is inflection in an entire sentence which is quite different from even melodious English. In all the Indo-European languages pitch and volume are used as expressive modulations of the voice, as punctuation, as sentence melody.

Some languages do not use volume or stress at all.

In Chinese, differences in pitch distinguish different words (symbols). A single word in Chinese may mean a completely different object, depending upon whether it is spoken with a high-rising or low-falling pitch.

With his many languages man utilizes duration, volume, and pitch of speech to reflect quantitative differences in sound. He uses timbre to represent qualitative differences.

Most languages use vowels and consonants as their basic sounds, but Hottentots add clicks. We use a click when we talk to a horse, but we do not very often click at each other, and we do not put clicks in our dictionary. The basic sounds of languages consist of vowels and consonants in various combinations. A vowel is a sound made with the mouth open. It comes more or less unmodified from the vocal cords. A consonant is a sound modified by lips, tongue, palate.

A group of enthusiastic linguists attempted some years ago to construct an international phonetic alphabet. Their aim was to construct an alphabet in which each distinct sound in every human language was given a specific symbol. Their goal proved unattainable, because the number of physically distinct sounds, even in one language, was enormous. The linguists were surprised at this finding. They had thought that the number of vowels and consonants was not great, maybe not more than about thirty or so in any one language, and perhaps not more than a hundred in all languages (Lado, 1957). When they carefully analyzed, acoustically, each "single" vowel or consonant, they found not a single unvarying sound for each vowel and consonant but a whole group of sounds for each.

In any one language, the speakers of that language learn to be unmindful of many variations in sound. In English the *p* in *puff*, in *lip*, in *poor* are all called *p* and yet, in actuality, each of these *p*s is a different phonetic unit.

Phonemics is based on the concept of phonemes which grew out of the awareness of the almost infinite number of phonetic sounds used by human beings. A phoneme is a unit of sound, used in any one language, as an entity. It is sometimes, but not always, represented by a letter of the alphabet. The *p*s listed above, though phonetically different, can be represented as single English phonemes, usually written /p/. People who speak English are unaware of the differences and quite willing to call them all *p* and represent them by that letter in the alphabet. In English the problem is further complicated by the fact that there are *p*s in the language which are readily recognized as not being represented by the phoneme /p/. What better illustration than the words *phonetics* and *phoneme?* There are also *p*s which are completely ignored in pronunciation, as in *psychiatry*.

The phoneme is a unit only within one language. Some phonemes are similar in many languages. On the other hand, the variations in sounds grouped as a phoneme in one language may be grouped differently in another language.

For example, one of the Canadian Indian languages, cited by La Barre, does not distinguish between our phonemes /p/ and /b/. They combine these two sounds into an intermediate *b*. Thus the speaker of this language would fail to distinguish between an English pat and bat (linguistically)!

The Chinese language has no phoneme like either *v* or *r* in English. Since the ear of a Chinese is not attuned to these sounds, he has difficulty in distinguishing them in English. In trying to say *very*, an adult Chinese is apt to come out with *belly*, the nearest sounds in his language.

In learning a foreign language, phonemes which are radically different from those of the mother tongue are more easily learned than those in which the variation is so slight as to be unheard by the ear accustomed to his own language. The American has considerable difficulty in pronouncing correctly the French *u* in *tu*, and the German has trouble in changing his rolling *r* to an English *r* as in *drive*.

Sounds found in human language seem to have no rhyme or reason. According to Brown, linguists have tried hard to relate sound to basic meaning, to relate the sound to the symbol for which it stands, to try to find some universal reason why one sound, rather than another, has been picked to stand for some reality.

There are some onomatopoeic words in all languages like *bang* or *splash* —words which sound like the object described, but except for these relatively few correlations between word sound and reality sound, there is no consistent relation between phonemes and meanings.

Structure—Grammar

In the structure of language there is the same kind of disparity as that found in meaning and sound. Language has not been put together in the same ways by the human brains who created and are creating it throughout the world.

In the Indo-European languages there are parts of speech: words are specialized into nouns, pronouns, verbs, adjectives, adverbs, conjunctions, prepositions, and interjections. English-speaking people seem to assume that it is not possible to talk unless there are different kinds of words to string together in a sentence. Yet the Chinese manage to do a good bit of talking and communicating among themselves without a single part of speech in their language. Chinese have what are called *full words,* which are hitched together in sentences by means of *empty words.* The full words have meaning—are symbols of reality; the empty words relate the words to each other. Neither change their form; there are no declensions, no conjugations; there are no changes in prefixes or suffixes to designate gender, number, or tense.

In contrast to a language like Chinese or Turkish, there are the highly inflected languages in which a root word is added to, fore and aft, to indicate gender, number, subject, object, possessor, or past, present, or future conditions. Finnish has eight declensional forms of its nouns and six conjugations of its verbs.

HUMAN SPEECH

This glimpse into comparative linguistics gives us insight into what is going to happen to an American baby lying in his crib, playing with his toes and hands and voice. He is going to restrict his amorphous human babble into the language of his parents. He is going to mimic them, not only in the actual sounds he makes, but in the quality, pitch, frequency, and amplitude of his oral expression. Other sounds he makes in his infancy will slip away from him as his utterances crystallize into those acceptable to his parents. He will likewise come to copy the semantic gestures of his parents.

But more than this—much more—he is going to accept the symbolism of his parents and his culture. His world will soon be bounded by the rigidities of his ability to communicate with the tools of the language he will be learning. Without language our baby could achieve nothing truly human, but with language he will live and have his being understanding reality as his culture understands it.

There have been in ages past some rather naïve concepts of how speech was learned. Ross and McLaughlin quote an experiment carried out in the thirteenth century: Frederick II wanted to find out what language children would speak if they heard or spoke to no one in early childhood. He thought they might speak Hebrew, which was the oldest language known to him, or Greek or Latin or Arabic, or perhaps the language of their parents. He instructed foster mothers to feed and care for a group of children but not to fondle them or talk to them or croon to them. His experiment met with failure, because the children all died before any language developed. They were unable to survive without affection and human warmth.

A somewhat similar experiment, also quoted by Ross and McLaughlin, was set up in which infants were cared for by nurses who were deaf-mutes. These nurses, however, were given no special instructions, so they fondled and loved the children and communicated with them as they did with each other, through gestures. The youngsters grew up without oral language but used gestures for semantic communication.

Man has evolved the capacity for speech. Nevertheless, speech has to be learned. There have been two cases reported in modern time (Davis, 1947) of children deprived of contact with speech. These cases bear remarkable similarity to the experiments just discussed. The first is a child, Anna, discovered in 1937 tied to a chair in a second floor attic room. She was the illegitimate child of a woman with an IQ of 50 and had been hidden away to avoid the anger of her grandfather. She had received the barest minimum of physical care. When discovered, she was about 6 years old and could not walk or talk or care for herself. She was severely malnourished. She was removed to a home for retarded children. She lived for only 4 more years; she learned to walk, to dress herself, and to say a few words. The opinion of the school was that Anna was feebleminded, which, considering her mother's mental capacity, was not surprising. Up to the age of 6 she had learned no speech, and in her additional 4 years of life she never learned really to use language, but whether this was due to innate lack of capacity or to her extreme isolation is indeterminable.

Another child, Isabelle, found at about the same time as Anna, presented a different picture. Isabelle was the child of a deaf-mute. Mother and child had been kept for 6½ years in a darkened room, completely isolated and away from the rest of the family. Isabelle had had human contact but had never heard speech. When found she used no verbal speech; she communicated with her mother by gesture. She was removed and given expert care by doctors and psychologists. Her language development went through the developmental pattern of a normal child, but at a greatly increased pace. In 2 years she went through the language development that usually takes

6 years. At 8½ Isabelle was not easily distinguishable from normal children her age. Isabelle's ability to learn speech considerably after the usual age would suggest that at 6½ years of age she had not yet passed beyond the critical time when this learning was possible.

Isabelle and Anna were different in two important aspects: although neither had heard speech, Isabelle had had plenty of human contact of which Anna had been deprived. Isabelle was normal intellectually, and probably Anna was not, although Anna's retardation was doubtless accentuated by her lack of human contact.

How mankind first achieved language is shrouded in mystery, though there have been many ingenious theories as to how it came about. Regardless of the origin of the ability to talk—hence to think—the human child does not repeat in his lifetime the ancestral pattern of the race. The child does not create his own language. Unless a child hears the spoken word, he will grow up without the ability to use speech.

DEVELOPMENT OF SPEECH IN THE CHILD

Developmental Stages

Speech is the latest of the evolutionary accomplishments. It is late phylogenetically, and it is late to develop in the individual. However, while true speech does not occur before the second year, the infant begins making sounds and using gestures, the preludes of symbolic communication, from the time of birth.

Unlike many other functions, sounds are not practiced in utero. The fetus is silent (as far as is known). He has developed vocal cords, uvula, pharynx, tongue, cheeks, lips—the organs he will someday use to talk, but he has not given them a trial run.

The Birth Cry

An infant becomes vocal within moments after birth. He clears his air passageways and emits the long wail of the birth cry, his first sounds. This is a purely reflex action, and even though it is called a *cry,* a word which signifies distress, there is probably no emotional content to this sound. It is vocal only because the infant is equipped with vocal cords so designed that they vibrate when air rushes past them. That the birth cry signifies wrath or anger or frustration, as postulated by Rank, seems rather adultomorphic.

Crying

The newborn soon ceases to cry as he gets his breathing apparatus under reasonable control. He subsides into regular breathing and sinks into sleep. Ultimately he awakens from this sleep, aroused by physiologic discomforts. His cry then is a true distress signal. He cries because this is his

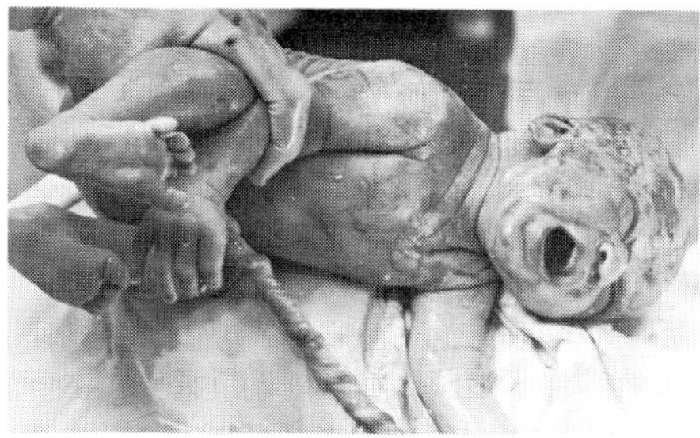

Vocalization begins with the birth cry

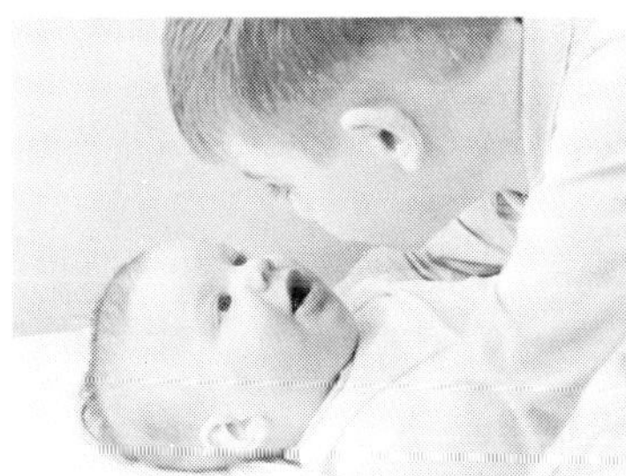

The infants early "talk" is met with a responsive audience

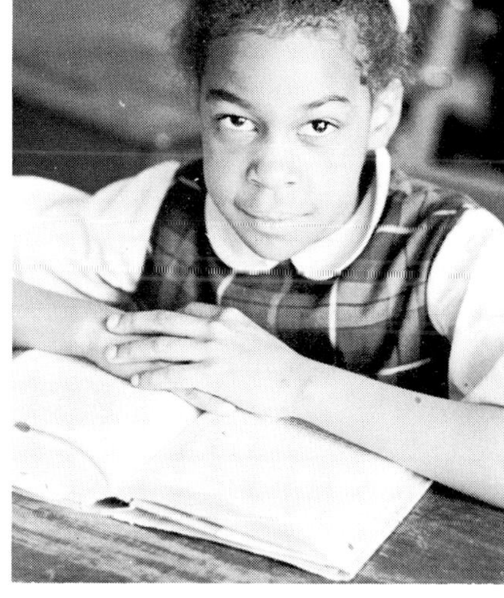

Much pleasure lies between the covers of a book

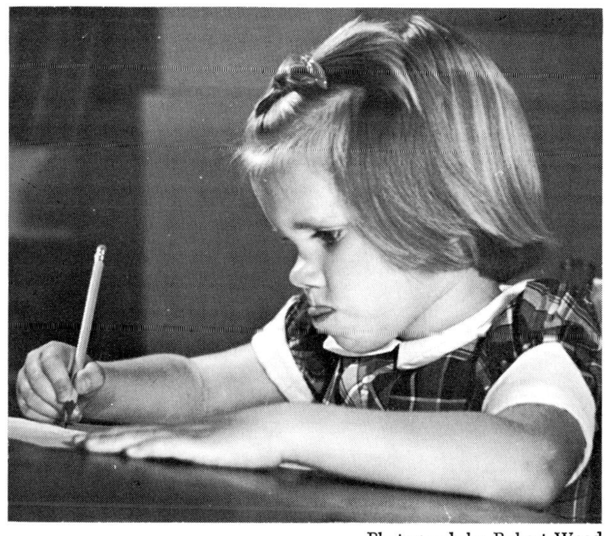

The urge to be literate

Photograph by Robert Wood

Fig. 32-1. Communication skills.

instinctive response to a need (p. 390). As soon as his needs are satisfied, he stops crying. The pattern is discomfort—crying—gratification—silence. A newborn infant is not really silent even when his needs have been attended to. His respiration is noisy, he often emits a grunt or sigh, he coughs and sneezes and hiccups after he expels air from his stomach, but these noises are mere by-products of his respiratory activity.

Karelitz found that the cry changes as age advances. The cry of the very young infant is short, staccato, and repetitive. As the infant grows, there is a lengthening of the duration of each individual cry, and more than one syllable becomes audible. The pitch becomes more varied and inflections more meaningful. When cooing and gurgling (see below) make their appearance, these sounds become part of the cry. Later, babbling can be heard in the cry. As speech development progresses, imitations of words appear in the cry, and finally real words and simple phrases can be detected. In his study of the cry Karelitz discovered that the cry of a normal child could be distinguished from that of a brain-damaged child. Not only was the tempo of progression slower in the defective child, but the quality of the sounds was sufficiently distinctive for Karelitz to use the cry as an early diagnostic sign of a child whose speech development would be impaired.

In the early months it is through his mouth that important activities take place. The infant uses his mouth to express his distress by crying. The mouth is an important part of rooting behavior which alerts the mother to his need for food (Spitz, 1957). It is through the mouth that gratification comes when he finally gets the nipple. The infant uses the sensitive tactile receptors in his mouth to feel and taste his world, and it is also through the mouth that his vocal expression will come. Ultimately the child develops additional means of maintaining contact with his environment, but throughout life the mouth remains, through language and through dining, a permanent and mature organ of human communication.

Comfort Sounds

For the first month of life crying is the chief vocalization of the infant, and the sound is elicited by discomfort, but even during this first month the infant adds a new type of sound. He begins to gurgle as he sucks, and watching an infant one has the distinct impression that this gurgle is a sound of satisfaction in contrast to the cry of distress. By the end of the first month the infant stays awake for appreciable times after his needs are met, and during these contented wakeful periods he begins to coo, another comfort or pleasurable sound.

His sounds express the way he feels, and he communicates his feelings to his associates. Soon after a baby learns to smile, at about 1 month of age, he adds a laugh, a rollicking chuckle, to his repertory that leaves no doubt that he feels pleased with the world.

Babbling

As the months go by and the infant begins to gain more control over his body, he plays. He plays with his hands and toes, and he plays with his vocal apparatus. He makes all sorts of sounds. He makes a single sound with his lips open, he runs through all the vowels, he experiments with opening and closing his pharynx and combining this with the motion of his lips and tongue to produce consonants and diphthongs. He combines his vowels and consonants and produces syllables: "agoo," "tahu." This is the babbling stage. It is a form of play. He makes many, many sounds at random. By the time he is half a year old the human infant has produced and reproduced just about all the sounds found in any language and many, many more than are present in any one language.

A baby babbles because of an urge within him to do so. The baby is not yet imitating anything he hears (except perhaps himself). He babbles when he is content with the world, when his body feels pleasant and good and he feels safe and secure. A happy baby babbles much more than an unhappy one. Failure to babble is an ominous sign.

Jargon

At about 6 months of age the babbling baby adds a new accomplishment: he begins to imitate sounds. For this step in development he must be able to hear. Deaf children cry, gurgle, and babble, but a deaf child can go no further. The normal child begins to listen to himself, to sounds from his environment, and he comes out with syllables that he repeats over and over. When imitation enters the picture, the baby's sounds are called *jargon.*

His ear is not too accurate as yet, nor is his control of his vocal apparatus. At random he is capable of a great variety of sounds, but when he tries to make a particular sound in imitation of what he hears, it is apt to come out only vaguely resembling the original. He keeps on trying, hour after hour. The more he is talked to—the more he has to imitate—the greater will be the variety of the sounds he makes. Also, the happier he is, the more he will engage in this kind of play. The baby needs his mouth for babbling. Excessive use of a pacifier (p. 370) may slow down his vocal experimentation.

During the babbling and jargon stages a baby picks up much of the quality of the voices he hears. His jargon will have the tone, the pitch, the amplitude of his mother's voice. He listens and imitates her voice qualities long before he uses real words. He will string his sounds together into "sentences" as she does; he will stress syllables or leave them unstressed as she does; he will inflect his whole sentence or paragraph according to what he hears. There will not be a single word that is recognizable, but in his jargon the comma, the periods, and the paragraph marks are recognizable.

In this jargon inflection and voice quality are so accurately picked up by the child that it is possible to recognize what language he has lived with, even though not a single sound is identifiable as a word. Long before the baby can use his language as a tool of communication, long before he has the cerebral capacity to understand a symbol, he has learned the melody of his native language.

Occasionally in a child's jargon it is possible to hear sounds other than human speech, sounds which the baby paid attention to. He may tick like the clock, bark like his dog, baa like a sheep, or make sounds like rain on the window pane. Any sounds he hears he tries to copy. He will imitate angry yells and screams with the same devotion to repetition that he uses to imitate more agreeable voices.

Irwin and Chen studied babbling by recording the sounds on a chimograph. They found that in the early months most of the sounds of adult speech were quite lacking in the infant's babble, but as the months passed, the infant made more and more sounds similar to adult speech; that is, there was a phonetic drift in the direction of the speech of the infant's culture. Babbling and jargon have been formally studied only in the English, French, and German languages. It does not seem too far a flight of fancy to assume that the early babbling of all human infants, the world over, has much in common and that a phonetic drift toward the language heard by the infant occurs in all cultures. While the human baby is imitating the sounds he hears, he is also imitating the gestures and motor actions of his adults as rapidly as his increasing autonomy makes possible. He shakes his head, wags his finger, waves bye-bye, plays pat-a-cake in imitation of action he sees. These early gestures as yet have no symbolic significance. As the sounds are preliminary stages of auditory language, so the gestures are preliminary stages of kinesthetic communication.

Babbling, listening, imitating are essential for later speech, but they are not speech. Motor control and imitative gesture are essential for ultimate symbolic gesture, but they appear before the capacity for symbolization matures. A vocal apparatus is essential for babbling, a functioning ear is essential for the imitative babbling called jargon, and a functioning area in the speech center of the brain is essential for the next stage: the awareness that a sound or a gesture can be a symbol that refers to something outside the child's own body.

From Sounds to Symbols

Before the infant says any real words, what Myklebust calls an *inner language* develops. He recognizes the familiar objects in his environment. At this stage when the infant sees his bottle in his mother's hands, he knows what it is and will reach up for it. A little more maturity brings the next stage, when the infant comprehends simple auditory expressions; he will then look around and prepare himself when he hears his mother say "Bottle." Recognition that a sound (a word) stands for an object

Myklebust calls *auditory receptive language.* Both the inner language and the auditory receptive language are taking-in processes. The infant must incorporate these concepts into his developing ego before he is ready for the next and final step in learning to talk. This last step is the giving forth of meaningful words. The infant says the words he has already come to understand. This is *auditory expressive language.* In order to bring forth a word, the infant must first take in the concept of the symbol. This is the progression of events in the normal child. The deaf child is able to comprehend the look of *bottle,* but he fails to learn the sound *bottle.* He must be taught symbolization through the other sensory receptors (sight or touch), since a receptive language must precede an expressive language (p. 517).

A child's first real spoken words are usually names of concrete objects—nouns. He has heard these words over and over and has come to understand what they mean; then one fine day he says "Bot," and he really means *bottle,* or he says "Dog," and really means the furry quadruped. He then will expand his vocal expressions and learn more and more words.

The child will use a noun in place of a whole sentence or several sentences: "Mi'k" means "I am hungry, give me some milk," or "Baa" may mean "I want my teddy bear," or a shake of the head may mean "No more banana, thank you." Frequently a child uses words which, to the adult, are two- or three-word combinations but which serve him as a single word. Such expressions as "All gone" or "Go bye-bye" are in the class of word combinations copied as a unit from what he hears.

Sentences

A child can be considered to be using a true sentence when he combines his own words in a meaningful way. The first sentences are usually a combination of two nouns: "Da-da home" may mean the baby heard the front door open and close, or it may express a wish to see his daddy, or it may be a greeting as his father walks into the room. Similarly "Da-da car" may be said as the baby watches his daddy drive away or come up to the house, or as a question when neither Daddy nor car are within visual range.

Verbs usually enter a child's vocabulary soon after he has become aware that words mean things. Like the nouns, verbs are often used as single- or as double-word sentences. "Mama come" or "Eat" are all expressive of his desires or demands. Verbs, however, unlike the nouns, are not naming what he sees. They represent an abstraction. Words—sounds—can now mean action as well as concrete objects.

Negation—the First Abstractions

At the time in his life that sounds are acquiring symbol value, the child is becoming more mobile, first by crawling and soon by walking. His increased mobility brings him inevitable prohibitions. He is forever hearing "No, no"; he sees the wagging finger and the head-shaking gestures of his mother. Both the sounds and the gestures convey to the child the meaning of prohibitions. An enormous number of activities of the little child end in this frustrating experience. Spitz has pointed out that the frustration prevents the child's "discharge of tension," which must then seek another outlet. It is apt to become a desire for identification with his mother, and when it does, the child finally is able to handle his frustration by incorporating into his self as much of his mother's behavior as he can. He copies her gestures and words. He tells himself "No, no," and he tells his mother "No, no." Before long it dawns on the child that these experiences have a common property—the quality of negation. With this concept comes the child's first understanding of an abstraction. He can now shake his head, wag his finger, or say "No, no" when he wishes to express negation. Spitz points out that the symbolic value of the word and the gesture mature simultaneously and doubtless have to do with the maturing speech area in the cortex.

The child has diverted some of his frustration at prohibitions into identification with his mother (and/or other adults) and through this mechanism has been able to internalize the adult's symbols and use them for his own ends. Abstract negation is an enormous step not only in symbolic communication but also in the growth of the self. The child's use of "No" signifies a growing comprehension of the difference between the *I* who is refusing and the *mother* to whom he is communicating this idea. He is now able to use "No" *against* his mother. Prior to the child's concept of the abstract quality of negation he had expressed refusal by motor activity, by pushing away an unwanted object or by running away himself. In these acts he was concerned only with his own rejection—he was not trying to communicate negation to anyone. The negation was directed toward himself, not against his mother. Now with his newfound ability to use a word or a gesture symbolically, the child has a more efficient tool at his disposal. As with other newly acquired abilities the little child practices his new power incessantly. He says "No" and shakes his head on appropriate and also on most inappropriate occasions. To the adult this is the period of stubbornness when "No" is the answer to almost everything. It is, however, for the child, a time of great triumph. It is almost as though he sensed the significance of this step in development.

Once the first abstraction is comprehended, the baby begins to apply his new-found insight to the things he has already named. Previously *bot* meant his special bottle filled with milk; *dog* meant Corky. Now he is on the brink of being able to define a category of similar objects. He catches on that *dog* can mean his own black cocker spaniel and can also mean the big collie he sees through the window. Mother keeps saying "Dog" when she pats the family pet and also when she and the baby look at other dogs. The concept dawns on the baby that *dog* is a class of objects, not just one. The child still has to sharpen up and limit his categories. He calls a cat "Dog," and mother says, "No, that's a cat." By constant repetition, by persistent trying out of his ability to name things, the child absorbs the knowledge of the limits and the extensions of the categories of words used in his immediate environment.

Language is developing into a useful tool. By it a child can make his wants known, but more than this he uses language to orient himself into his world. By naming objects and events he is beginning to classify them in the same way his parents do.

Prepositions come into the child's vocabulary and with them his first orientation into space and time. *Up* and *down* begin to have meaning. He wants to be picked up, and the combination of the gesture of the outstretched arms with the word *up* conveys more, not only to his mother, but to the baby himself. Before long *on* and *under* mean places, and so the child's world is dividing itself up into *where.*

Time is more difficult. The word is *now* for the baby, and this is apt to be his first word in relation to time. If only a matter of moments, *soon* can be distinguished from *now,* but *later* is no different from *never.*

Modifying words come quickly into a child's understanding. Big Daddy, a big bang, fast train, hot cereal. He is grasping the fact that there are qualities to the objects he names. It takes quite a bit of abstraction to apply the word *big* to Daddy and to a noise, yet our human child can do this almost as soon as he can use the word at all.

Pronouns are a difficult concept. A little child calls himself by his own name: "Tommy wants milk" or "Tommy's wagon." Sometimes he will call himself "You." Mother calls him "You," so Tommy calls himself "Tommy" and sometimes "You." Sometimes he will carry this further and refer to his mother as "I." With the understanding of the words *me, mine,* and *I* one more step is mastered: "I am me," but Mother is "me" too, to herself. That everyone possesses a *me* is a profound idea. Little children do learn this concept, however, and they learn it long before they can engage in philosophical discourses on the entity of the self. Language is certainly a help in the development of awareness of self.

After the concept of *I* and *you* is established, the little child learns the difference between *he* and *she,* and sometime during the end of his second year, he learns the categories *boy* and *girl.*

Understanding of grammatical construction comes along toward the end of the second year. If he says, "Corky runned out the door," he has made a mistake in grammar, but a great deal of abstract understanding has gone into that construction. He has never heard anyone say "runned," but he has learned how to alter a verb to indicate that the act is over and done with.

Once this concept of grammatical construction is grasped, the child is well on his way to use his language proficiently. He will learn new words—new categories of things, new qualities, greater precision in place and time. All these refinements will come with the years, but the fundamentals of communication with others is firmly established.

It is through language and its symbolism that the child will be able to have ideas, to think, and to communicate more than his feelings to his fellow man. Without some kind of symbolism, abstract thought is impossible. It must not be forgotten, however, that the symbolism of any language is never identical with external reality, nor is the symbolism of any two languages the same. Any set of symbols limits comprehension of all aspects of reality, but without some symbolic system there is no abstract comprehension.

The Tempo of Language Learning

As with most kinds of development the rate of acquisition of speech varies greatly from child to child. On the whole, girls learn to talk at an earlier age than boys, but there is much individual difference even between members of the same sex. Regardless of the tempo, the progression is roughly similar in all normal children learning English as their basic language.

In recapitulation the sequence is about as follows:

First year:

- Prelanguage vocalization.
  - Crying.
  - Comfort sounds.
  - Babbling.
  - Jargon.
- Prelanguage gestures.
  - Rooting.
  - Head shaking.
  - Bye-bye.
  - Pat-a-cake.
- Comprehension.
  - First stage: recognition of objects, inner language.
  - Second stage: recognition of spoken word, auditory receptive language.

Second and third years:

- Single words, usually nouns: *bot* (bottle), *car*. Expressions such as *all gone, bye-bye* used in direct imitation are in the class of single words.
- Sentences: combinations of words which the child himself puts together —*Mama come.*
- First abstraction: *no* as a word and negation as head shaking.
- Further abstractions: *dog* as a category instead of a particular dog. *Daddy* is different from all other men.
- Adjectives and adverbs: quality is being discovered—*big Daddy, hot cereal.* This is another type of abstraction, in which a quality can be abstracted from the thing.
- Prepositions: concept of time and space is being grasped.
- Pronouns: *me* as a person and different from the *me* that is in *you.*

Gender role: comprehension of *he* and *she*.

Third and fourth years:

Sentences: grammatical structure. Parts of speech are now put together into full meaningful sentences.

It is far more important that the child progress from one stage to the next than that he accomplish a given degree of proficiency at any specific age.

Some children (as some adults) are more verbal than others. The verbal youngsters learn to talk earlier than the less verbal ones. Only within very wide limits is this correlated with intelligence. Some very bright people have been late talkers. Early talking (and/or much talking) is probably a genetic factor inherent in the child from conception. But genetics is not the only factor that influences the speed with which children learn to talk.

Talking is accomplished with the mouth and the oral structures. It begins in the prelanguage phase at the time when the mouth is the child's most important organ of contact with his environment. Language is the means of moving on from the interpersonal dependency of the sucking infant to the more mature interpersonal relation of the talking child. The contented child is eager to push ahead in development.

While speech progresses along a fairly well-determined pathway, it may speed up or slow down depending upon what else is going on in the child's life. A child often concentrates on one phase of learning at a time. When a child is first learning to walk, he puts all his energy and interest into perfecting that skill. He forgets about his toys for a time, and he may slow up in his acquisition of new language skills. Once his walking is perfected to his own satisfaction, he will return to his interrupted interests in other spheres. The same thing can happen over weaning or toilet training. These are the normal and expected changes in pace.

Disturbances in the child's life may also slow the pace of language as well as of other development. Minor and temporary episodes, a disrupting trip, a visit from an undesired guest can slow up speech for the duration of the experience, but once life calms down, development picks up and goes on. Constant emotional deprivation may slow the full flow of the developmental river to a trickle.

Language—the Child's Tool

By the time a child is about 3 years of age, he has the fundamental concepts of his culture at his disposal. An American 3-year-old can talk in full sentences and use the grammar of the English language, but in spite of his technical linguistic competence the little child's use of language is far from mature. Language reflects personality, and the 3-year-old has as yet amorphous concepts of himself and of the world of people and things about him.

A normal toddler talks as he plays. He is not talking *to* anyone; he is just talking. He verbalizes what he is doing, what is going on in his mind. He is quite incapable of keeping ideas to himself. As Piaget says, he has "verbal incontinence."

A little girl playing with soap bubbles sings to herself: "Bubbles, bubbles, bubbles, big shiny bubbles, whoops, bubble broke, broke, broke, all gone bubble." She may go on and play with the words: "Bubble, jubble, wubble" and then laugh at her nonsense syllables.

At other times the little child will verbalize what goes on in his memory. As he lies in his crib, the day's events run through his mind, not silently, but audibly, sometimes to the consternation of an eavesdropping parent: "Daddy talk big to Mommy," says the 3-year-old as he snuggles down for his nap. "Mommy spill coffee, drip on floor." Then, after a pause, "Bad Daddy."

The little child uses words as a part of play rather than a means of communication with others. Words, or sometimes just sounds, extend the imagery of the object with which he is playing. As he pushes a toy car up an incline, he announces what he is doing. "The car is going up the hill. Grrr, change gears! Chug, chug." Words extend reality. They are part of romancing and inventing. They are a kind of magic which can endow physical objects with desired abilities (see Imaginative Make-believe, Chap. 33).

Word play of the young child is different from the phatic sounds made by infants or by animals (p. 451). The child says real words which are correctly used as symbols of the world of reality; nevertheless he is not using them to communicate anything to others.

Even when little children play in groups, much of their talk is this same kind of individual play accompaniment. A child will comment on what he is doing. He may be aware of the audience of the other children, but he is not really talking *to* them. He neither gets nor expects an answer. He is talking aloud to himself in the presence of others. His talk accompanies and extends his activities, but the child is unconcerned with communicating his ideas to others.

Piaget calls this type of talk *egocentric language;* it bubbles up from within the child and has little relation to the people in his environment. It helps to create a world of imagination; it is related to feelings, not to facts in the world of reality. It occupies a large percentage of the verbalization of young children. Little by little the egocentric talk fades as more mature talk takes its place. When the child comes to have an increased understanding of the identity of himself as a unique being, he has a greater desire to communicate *his* ideas to other people. This is what Piaget calls *intelligent talk* in contrast to the earlier egocentric talk.

Though egocentric talk fades, the egocentric thought that lies behind the talk never completely disappears. Throughout life, flashes of imagination come to mind and images are conceived not as step-by-step logical processes but as whole concepts, seen and perceived in their totality. It may be that the sympathetic understanding of the child's early flights of fancy helps to maintain and to nurture the ability of the older individual to create ideas, insights, and feelings about the world.

There is a great temptation on the part of many adults to attribute to the remarks of children the same significance that similar remarks would have if uttered by an adult. This adultomorphic attitude can cause much misunderstanding of a child. A 3- or 4-year-old frequently does not distinguish between what goes on in his mind and what goes on in the world about him; he talks about both, often indiscriminately. He may relate a purely imaginary event as though it were an external fact. To the child it is important that "it" happened. That the happening takes place in his imagination is of little significance to him. He tells about the fire engine he saw (which he really did see) and the exciting ride he had on it (which is purely imaginary) as all part of the same event. The adult may call this a lie and condemn the child for it, without realizing that not only is he demanding of the child concepts that are far beyond the maturity level of the youngster, but also he is denying to the child the significance of his flights of imagination.

Children pick up what they hear. Many a mother is horrified to hear her sweet, innocent young son come out with a most expressive "God dammit." It is to be expected that the child repeats bad language as he repeats good talk. If some of his words are met with a charged emotional reaction, he soon discovers that these words have special attention-getting value, and he will use them to achieve this purpose. The child, like the adult, can get a good bit of pent-up aggression out with a vehement verbal explosion.

Bathroom language makes its appearance in almost all children. Bathroom activities are important and interesting to the toddler, and he likes to talk about them, but, as with his curse words, if he discovers that these words get a special reaction from his parents, the words take on an added importance to him, and he may continue to use them.

Little children ask questions. Piaget analyzed the questions of a group of children and found that in the 3-year-old many questions were not truly questions seeking an answer but were mere statements of observation put in this form. If unanswered, the child would supply his own response: "Is the paint wet?" Then, after a pause: "Paint is wet." Questions concerned with human action need an answer. They are egocentric and are concerned only with their effect on the child: "Why do you go away?"

When the child reaches the school years, his language reflects his greater maturity. School-age children are interested in words as symbols; they have outgrown their earlier interest in the mere sound of words. They now love puns and an infinite variety of jokes and "little moron" stories. The egocentricity of the early years has given way to a world-centered interest. The child begins to ask questions concerning the world about him. He wants to know "What is it?" "How does it work?" "Why is it so?" He is developing curiosity about things and people apart from what they do to him. This is a big step in maturity. It is the beginning of intellectual and logical thought and comes with the personality development of the middle years. These questions need carefully considered answers, answers that not only supply the needed information but that enhance the child's awakening interest in abstract thought. The child who matures with the feeling that to know is good is forever pushing on to know more and more.

Crystallization of Culture Concepts through Language

Our children learn to see and know the world as we know it and as we talk about it. This is inevitable. We have words that stand for the concepts we accept. All our "of courses" we teach our children.

Time is important, of course. We do things on schedule. Meals are on time, we keep appointments. We must go to bed *now* because it is bedtime. We can't play *now* because it's time for school. This is our cultural heritage and eventually most of our children accept it, although many a youngster does a good bit of rebelling before he settles down into our concept of time and speed and tempo. In other cultures time is handled differently. People from the United States in many Latin American countries are hopelessly frustrated by the Latin lack of concern about time schedules. The Latin American keeps an appointment if and when he feels like it. The culture itself—hence the person—attributes no importance to being on time. This cultural difference is absorbed in childhood, not entirely, but largely, through language.

We also teach, through language, our special feelings, our beliefs and prejudices. In some families the word *Negro* means a human being whose skin is dark in color. In other families the same word means a human being of a lower order whom one does not associate with as an equal. These definitions set up emotional tones as the child learns the word.

There are basic overall cultural categories which almost everyone in the society accepts; then there are categories within a given family. The child learns to see the world through the same spectacles as his parents. He comes into awareness of the world with many definitions and concepts firmly established. He "knows" Jews are aggressive, he "knows" Negroes are inferior, he "knows" women are stupid, just the way he "knows" rocks are hard and water is wet. Sometimes in the same learning fashion he comes to "know" that no one is to be trusted, that old people are a nuisance, that it is smart to grab what you can for yourself. Or maybe he learns that honesty is a value worth cultivating. Although it is not entirely through language that children learn these and many more concepts from their parents, language is one of the most dominant ways in which learning takes place.

Learning a Second Language

The adult who tries to learn a second language usually never succeeds in speaking that language without an accent, and yet a child can pick up another language and speak like a native. For this reason parents often want to teach a child two or even more languages as soon as the child begins to use speech.

Language is more than sound. Each language has its own categories of meaning. Each language interprets the world in a different way. Not only is the vocabulary different, but grammatical structure, syntax, and reality concepts are different.

The amount of learning involved in speaking any language is enormous. The more difficult the task, the slower is the learning progress, and if it is too difficult for any given child, he may be seriously delayed in the whole matter of communication on a verbal level. In all aspects of growth there is a critical time for learning the basic human skills. If at the crucial time of relating sounds to symbols and meaning the child is confronted not just with one way of getting his meaning across but with two, he may be sufficiently confused not to make the necessary effort. Thus it may be that his ability to communicate verbally is slowed down to a degree that is never quite made up for later.

The general consensus is that a child does better to learn to communicate in one language until he gets the feel of his ability to use sound meaningfully. The age at which this happens varies, of course, from child to child. Usually a youngster at 5 can talk quite freely. Very verbal youngsters may accomplish this by 3, and others may be 6 or even 7 before they are easy with language.

Once a child can talk freely, he can be introduced to a second language without disturbing his understanding of the meaning and desirability of communication. Almost any time under the age of 10 a child can pick up a foreign language by ear and use it as well as those from whom he learns it. He will pronounce correctly, his intonation will be accurate, his grammar will be correct, and he will learn to distinguish the shades of meaning of the new set of categories.

Many children do learn two languages from the beginning—children who grow up in bilingual families. Some of these children do very well; whether or not they would have done better had they learned one language first is impossible to say.

There is, however, considerable argument for beginning a second language in the primary grades rather than waiting for the high school years.

READING AND WRITING

Reading and writing can be considered rungs in the developmental ladder of communication. By the time the normal child is about 6 years old, he has acquired the use of some ten thousand words in his spoken vocabulary (Smith, 1941), and he is ready to learn how these words can be understood through the eyes as well as through the ears.

Children are *able* to learn to read because they are human; they *do* learn because they are taught. A human being can grow up without the ability to talk if he is never taught speech, and he can certainly grow to physical maturity without reading and writing if he is not taught these skills.

The Alphabet

Man probably learned to speak before he learned to write. The early attempts to write probably began with pictures which in the course of time became more or less stylized representations (Bodmer, 1944). In these early writings, the written symbol represented the thing, not the word. The character may represent *dog*, but it has no connection with the sound of the word *dog*. Seeing this symbol on the printed page, one could learn to say "dog," "chien," "hunt," "perro." The symbol gives no clue to its pronunciation. In certain languages in the world today, notably Chinese and Japanese, pictographs are used as the written symbols.

Human beings in some cultures hit upon the idea of a phonetic alphabet (Ogg, 1948). Instead of making a written symbol to represent the *thing*, they made the symbol represent the *sound* of the word; thus the alphabets came into existence. Basically an alphabet is a list of written symbols which represent each of the sounds used in the spoken language.

Theoretically, learning to read phonetically could be accomplished by memorizing the alphabet and learning what sound goes with each written symbol. Once this is accomplished, a child should be able to spell all the words he can say and recognize these words on the printed page. Learning to read and write in English would be this simple if our language were really a phonetic system. Unfortunately English is far from a truly phonetic system. While there are phonetic rules in English, there are so many exceptions that a list of simple rules of pronouncing the written symbols does not provide the tools needed for reading and writing.

Take the letter *A*. This letter is named *ay*, and in a few words that sound is actually used, as in *ate* and *able*. But the letter is pronounced differently in *and, as, ask*, and quite differently still in *boat* and *beauty*. Again, compare the way the letter *B* is pronounced in *but* and *bill* with the way *B* is written but completely silent in *doubt* and *debt*. The letter *H* we call *aitch* but this is a sound not at all like H in *he* or *here*. Likewise the letter *W*, called *double you*, has a sound quite unrelated to its name.

Phonetic Teaching

As a phonetic system, English leaves much to be desired. For many generations children have been taught to read and write English as though it were a phonetic system. Such teaching begins by teaching the child the alphabet and the sounds of the various letters. The number of exceptions to the rules which the child must learn is so enormous that progress in reading skill is slow and it is possible that some children never become as proficient as they might be in both reading skill and in spelling.

Look-and-say Teaching

About thirty years ago in the United States an effort among educators to find a better method of teaching reading and writing resulted in the "look-and-say" system (Brown, 1958). By this method children are taught to recognize whole words rather than to build up words from individual letters. Teaching begins with short common words with which the child is familiar in his spoken vocabulary. The word is printed in large letters on cards, with a picture of the object beneath it. The teacher flashes the card before the child, says the word, and points to the object. Ultimately the child learns to recognize the printed word without the picture.

This method of teaching ignores the phonetic value of the letters. Children are taught to read as though each word were a picture. The printed word—the visual image—is related to the thing, not to the spoken word. A child learns to recognize the word *dog* and knows what it means when he sees it printed on a page, but he is not aware that the three letters have special sound values. He learns the printed word *dog* just as he might learn as a symbol meaning the spoken word *dog*.

The look-and-say method of teaching children to read English is based on a great deal of research (Brown, 1958). It has been found that competent adult readers recognize a number of word shapes at a single glance; they do not read each letter separately. The eye goes across a line of print in jumps and pauses; the pauses are the time it takes to recognize a series of words. The advocates of the look-and-say method thought it desirable to begin children with the reading technique they would ultimately come to use rather than drill them with less valuable and often boring phonetic symbolism.

Children *do* learn to read by the look-and-say method. They also learn to read when taught by a strictly phonetic system. The big controversy in educational circles, recently publicized by Flesch in *Why Johnny Cannot Read,* is over which method is better. Unfortunately there is no clear answer, since reading involves many skills. The look-and-say method seems to be somewhat superior for learning to read quickly and with comprehension. The phonetic system is superior in teaching the ability to tackle the unfamiliar words and in learning to spell (Agnew, 1939; Russell, 1943; McDowell, 1953).

A child taught by the look-and-say method has to learn each word individually. Once learned as a whole word, it is quickly grasped when seen again. However, when he comes across a word entirely unfamiliar to him, he has no clue to its meaning except by the context of the sentence. The phonetically trained child, on the other hand, can attempt to sound out the letters. If the word is familiar to him in his spoken vocabulary, he may well be able to hit upon it through vocalizing its sounds. He has a tool, even though imperfect, at his disposal, which the look-and-say–trained child does not have.

There are advantages in both methods of teaching. Good teaching at the present time is a combination of phonetics and of look-and-say, and it includes the good points of each method (Agneu, 1939).

Regardless of the method used, normal children learn to read before they learn to write. As with learning to speak, the taking-in phenomenon precedes the giving forth. According to Myklebust the stages in communication skills are:

1. Inner language—recognition of objects
2. Auditory receptive language—understanding spoken words (taking in)
3. Auditory expressive language—talking (giving forth)
4. Visual receptive language—reading (taking in)
5. Visual expressive language—writing (giving forth)

Reading Readiness

Custom and the law in the United States say that children enter first grade at the age of 6. Many school systems are very rigid concerning the child's chronological age at school entry. If the child's sixth birthday comes before October 1, November 15, December 1, or some other specified time, he may enter first grade in September. If he fails to meet the deadline, even by a week, he must wait another year before he can attend first grade. This rigidity creates problems for some children, because there is, at best, only a rough correlation between the number of years a child has lived and the amount of maturing he has done in that space of time.

Reading is universally taught in first grade. Some 6-year-olds, probably the majority, are mature enough to learn this skill. Some, however, are by no means ready; it may well be another year before they have the level of maturity required for this complicated skill. A few children, on the other hand, are fully ready to acquire reading skills at the age of 5, though there is a difference of opinion as to whether even these early-maturing children might not be better off if their learning to read were postponed.

It is very desirable to be able to distinguish between those ready and those not ready to begin reading instruction. Tests for reading readiness and for general maturity, rather than the mere accident of the birth date, are more and more being used as criteria for entering first grade. This subject is further discussed below under Reading Failures.

Optimal Development of Language Skills

A child absorbs his language from his family. The more he is talked to, and with, the better he learns to talk, to use language for all the subtle meanings that constitute human intercourse. Language, of course, is not a thing apart from the rest of development; it is just one aspect of the child's emerging awareness of himself in a world of people. The more smoothly his general development goes, the more easily he will absorb the ability to use talking, reading, and writing. Some family practices, however, are more conducive to language development than others.

In the early months, singing has special value. The baby who hears his mother's voice associates its soft sound with his own comfort and pleasure. When he begins to imitate, his jargon is met with interest, his mother talks back to him, he has more and more to imitate. Finally when words and sentences come, again he has a receptive and appreciative audience.

As soon as the child can understand, he loves stories. Stories that are told to him, stories that are read to him from books. Little children like the same story over and over again. Repetition and practice is the pattern of toddlerhood. A favorite story is like a familiar person: the child knows what is coming; he can count on an ordered world. In fact, if the teller of the tale or the reader of a story deviates by a single word, the child is apt to correct the mistake. The child knows what is right, and he wants it that way.

Stories, stories, stories—the little child is insatiable. He loves books with pictures, and long before he can comprehend the printed word, he enjoys turning the pages and "reading" the story from the pictures.

Early association with books prepares the child for later pleasure when he grows up enough to learn to read. During the school years, in a family whose members read and discuss what is read the youngster is stimulated to partake of the pleasure to be found in books. Interest and participation breed reading skills.

In Larry's family both his parents told him stories as well as read them. Larry knew what stories were Daddy's and which were Mommy's. Stories were told at bedtime and whenever there was a lull in the day's activities. The magic words "Once upon a time . . ." were enough for Larry to be all attention. He developed an extraordinarily rich vocabulary.

Larry was the youngest of several children, and the family played many word games, trying to adapt them to the capacities of the various ages. One of their favorites was the old game: "I'm thinking of a color that begins with *R*." To Larry someone would say: "That's *rrr*," sounding the letter. Larry played this game with his family long before he entered first grade.

Another word game that the family loved to play was called adverbs. One person left the room. The rest picked out an adverb such as *politely*.

Then the guesser had to determine from the way everyone acted and responded to his questions what the word was. Larry played along with everyone else. He especially liked to act out *gruffly, loudly.* When it came to *badly,* there was a big discussion as to what the word really did mean. Did it mean "naughty" or did it mean "poorly"? Or could it mean both?

Games and stories were part of life in Larry's family, and language skills grew rapidly. One time Larry was sick and had to stay in bed. He was sitting up "reading" his books. He told his mother he wished he could "read" the story about the olden days when Mother was a little girl. Well, why not? Mother got a notebook and began writing the story down, a few words to a page and little stick figures for illustrations.

Larry finally got to first grade and began to learn formally to read. He learned quickly. He was ready and eager. He already knew a lot about words and their meaning, and he knew that fun and pleasure lay between the covers of a book. Larry was taught the look-and-say method, but phonetics were also used. Larry was so eager to read that it would have been difficult to prevent him.

Once Larry learned to read, learned that those little marks on the page meant things he could understand, he had an inner excitement of great discovery. As Larry grew older, the family added other games to its repertory. They read plays out loud together, each person reading and acting out parts.

DANGER SIGNALS IN COMMUNICATION SKILLS

While it is impossible to set up a definite time schedule for a child's language accomplishments, nevertheless, there are signs of trouble to be watched for.

In the first year there must be babbling and then a progression from babbling to inflected jargon. If babbling does not appear or if it does not progress, trouble may be in the offing. By the age of 1 year, the normal child is paying attention to what he hears. This awareness is reflected in his vocalizations and in his obvious understanding of simple things said to him. Some children will have 15 to 20 single words at 1 year, but other perfectly normal (contented and intelligent) children may not have a single word before the age of 2. This is nothing to worry about provided the child is reasonably happy, babbles a lot of sound in which inflections can be detected, and responds to the speech of others.

Once speech has been established, the normal child talks more and more and passes through the stages described above. Failure to progress constitutes a danger signal. The child who stops talking or talks very little, the child who remains in an immature phase as his chronological years pass, is obviously not developing normally.

Attempts have been made to standardize the speech of children and thus come by some objective measure of their speech maturity. Kirk and

McCarthy have published a test for psycholinguistic abilities in which the length and grammatical complexity of the child's utterances are recorded and analyzed.

The Child Who Does Not Talk

If a child has no recognizable words by the age of 2 years, one *should* be concerned. Failure to talk can be due to one of several factors, or to a combination of factors (Bangs, 1961):

1. Mental retardation—a generally slow process of development, only one aspect of which is speech (p. 148)
2. Deafness—sensory impairment due to damage or defect in the external, middle, or inner ear [for tests to determine deafness, see p. 269; for discussion of the effects of this sensory impairment, see p. 517 (Ewing, 1954)]
3. Aphasia—defect or damage in the central nervous system involving the auditory apparatus (Morley, 1955)
4. Autism—failure of ego development resulting in lack of desire to communicate.

These are serious reasons for lack of speech. None of these conditions appears suddenly, and it is often possible to suspect trouble early in the life of the child. It is not always easy, however, to make an accurate differential diagnosis. Occasionally a child may have multiple defects which affect speech. Deafness and aphasia may coexist. Any child who fails to learn to talk for any reason has difficulty in establishing and maintaining normal interpersonal relations and may therefore add symptoms of autism to his functional disorder (Eisenson, 1963).

Deafness, aphasia, autism do not disappear with normal growth. A child with any of these conditions needs special treatment, and the earlier in life it can begin, the better is his prognosis.

The Child with a Speech Defect

A defect in speech is a defect in sound quality. It has to do with the ways a child uses his voice, the way he combines sounds into words and words into sentences. A speech defect does not involve the child's ability to understand speech.

Maturing of Speech

In the early years *all* children have speech defects. They mispronounce words; they repeat sounds, syllables, or whole words; they use inaccurate inflections, they use pitch and quality and timbre of voice which is neither pleasing nor socially acceptable.

Almost all children outgrow these mistakes just by living and hearing good speech. But occasionally a child does not outgrow these normal growing pains of speech and needs help. Some guides are needed as to when to accept and when to ignore and wait, when and how to treat. These are important decisions, because considerable harm can be done to a child by nagging him to a perfection he is not mature enough to achieve. On the other hand a great disservice can be done him by letting him grow to maturity with speech that will forever handicap him in all his social relations.

It is reasonable to expect that a child will speak as well as his parents. It can hardly be demanded that he improve upon them, even though this might be desirable. A child picks up the intonations he hears, and he may keep these voice qualities all his life. Often it is impossible later in life to distinguish between the voices of mother and daughter on the telephone.

Sometimes a child's strident voice may be an expression of the mother's tensions which she expresses sometimes vocally and sometimes in gestures but which the child picks up vocally.

Speech defects due to the mispronunciation of words are not usually so much the direct copying of adult speech as they are signs of immaturity in the child (Burgi and Matthews, 1963). A common defect is the substitution of one sound for another. All children do this when they begin to talk, but some are quicker to grasp correct articulation than others, and, of course, the more a child is talked to *correctly*, the sooner he picks up the mature way of speaking. If his baby mistakes are repeated back to him, he will make little effort to change them, especially if they are considered cute and appealing. A 2-year-old "frows his ball to his muvver," but by 5 he should be "throwing" and he should have a "mother." At 5 he should "ride," not "wide," in the family car, and he should go to "sleep," not "seep."

If progress seems slow but there *is* progress, patience is the guiding principle of treatment. The child needs to be talked with, sung to, read to. He needs to hear good speech and lots of it, and he needs *not* to be nagged. Records and songs are particularly good, and so are games. Little children like to play with words and sounds. A child will say a word and then try other sounds like it "Ride, row, run," then just "r-r-r," or "Mumble, jumble, wumble." The more he can be encouraged to use his vocal apparatus in these vocal feats, the better, especially when Mother or Father can play along with him. Always, the more relaxed he is, the more spontaneous experimenting he will do. The child who is nagged and corrected every time he opens his mouth becomes discouraged. He stops trying, because he cannot ever seem to get it right. Progress stops short when a youngster no longer tries.

Some children lisp. Lisping is a special problem of the sound of S. There are several varieties of lisping, but none are pleasant to hear. The child may say "loth" when he means "loss" or "thing" when he means "sing." As with other faulty articulation, patience, talk, singing games, and lack of tension are the best remedies during the early years.

But if at the age of 4 or 5 a child is still not speaking clearly and not improving, it is time to see a speech therapist, who must exercise great care in coming to the correct diagnosis of the trouble. If a child's speech is poor because his life is upset, because he is tense and afraid, exercises in better pronunciation may make him more tense and give him an even stronger sense of failure. A child's speech may be poor because he is shy and afraid to make verbal contact with people or because he would rather not have much to do with them. On the other hand, maybe he is just sloppy about his speech—it has always got him what he wanted, so why bother to improve it? A skillful speech therapist can often help in coming to an accurate diagnosis of a particular child's problem. Treatment must be tailored to the underlying cause. Sometimes treatment will include speech therapy sessions for the child, but quite often such sessions do more harm than good.

Stuttering

Stuttering is a special kind of speech defect in which the child repeats sounds, syllables, or sometimes whole words and cannot seem to get on to the next word. The defect is in the rhythm of speech.

Under the age of 5, hesitation in speech and disturbance in the rhythm of talk are common—almost universal. The more completely they can be ignored, the better. Wendell Johnson is of the firm belief that labeling a child a stutterer in the early years is a big factor in actually helping him keep the pattern rather than outgrow it.

Some children, however, do keep this pattern into later years. Stuttering in children over the age of 6 or 7 almost always revolves around hostility, a battle between child and parent for control. The stuttering is apt to occur at moments of repressed anger or fear. Why some children should respond to tension by stuttering and others by wetting the bed or sucking the thumb or having tantrums is a difficult question to answer. It may be that the stutterer has a more labile speech mechanism than the nonstutterer. It is as though speech were his weak point, and when life goes sour with him, his feelings and tensions show up in his speech. Other children can undergo what seems to be very nearly the same upset and yet never develop disturbances in speech, though they may have other symptoms.

There is some evidence that stuttering runs in families. This does not mean there is a gene for stuttering. If it should be true that some people have a more labile speech mechanism, it is possible, though surely not proved, that such mechanisms are gene-determined. It is also true that a family plagued by the presence of a stutterer is more actively aware of the problem than a family who has no such member. Awareness of the problem doubtless alerts parents to the hesitation in a child's speech.

Stuttering is no mere mechanical speech defect; it is an emotional problem. It is a serious handicap and in children over 5 surely needs treatment, but treatment must be directed toward the elimination of the tensions that produce the writhings of voice and body. Seldom is speech therapy, as such, called for.

Stephanie began to stutter at the age of 6¾. There were no stutterers in her family. She was a small, average little girl whose birthday made it impossible for her to enter first grade in the public school when she was almost 6. Her parents sent her to a small private school where she was placed in first grade. She did very well, and at the end of the year the private school recommended her for second grade. In September she entered the second grade of the large local public school. She was one of a class of 40 children. She was small, immature, and frightened. By the middle of October she began to stutter, and the stuttering rapidly became worse. At first she stuttered only in the classroom, but before long she stuttered at home too. When she was called upon in school, her whole little body went through contortions, and the words just would not come out. The school sent her to their speech therapist, but fortunately for Stephanie, before speech lessons were begun, her parents consulted their pediatrician, who had known the child since her birth. The diagnosis was not difficult. The child was being pushed far beyond her capacity. She could not cope with the confusion of the big classroom, and the schoolwork was considerably beyond her. She was frightened—of herself and of her inability to do what was expected of her. She was also angry with her parents for expecting her to do what she knew she could not do. To have given that little girl lessons in better speech would only have accentuated her problems. She was put back into the first grade, which fortunately was a smaller class, and given a great deal of reassurance but no speech training, and in another month she was talking quite smoothly again.

Faulty Structure

There are two conditions present at birth which interfere with the ability to control the vocal apparatus: cleft lip and palate, and cerebral palsy.

Cleft lip, with or without cleft palate, is a defect due to failure of normal fusion of these parts during intrauterine life. Modern surgical procedures can do wonders for this condition. Some children born with such a defect can have it so repaired that there is no interference whatever with the development of speech. However, in the more extreme cases, where the defect, especially in the palate, is large, surgical treatment may not completely restore normal function during infancy. A hole in the palate means that air goes up through the nose and it is therefore difficult for the child to produce acceptable speech sounds. Such a child needs help, and he needs it early. Toward the end of the first year exercises in the form of games can help such a child acquire reasonably good articulation. Sucking and blowing games are especially useful. A child with a cleft palate needs to be under the guidance of a skilled speech therapist beginning in the latter part of his first year.

Cerebral palsy is usually caused by a birth injury with damage to the central nervous system. There can be all degrees of damage done, from very minor and insignificant injury to almost total paralysis. The paralysis is of the spastic variety, since it is the upper motor neuron which is damaged. If the nerves to the lips, cheeks, palate, and tongue are involved, the child will have difficulty in articulating. In extreme cases speech never becomes possible, but where the damage is less severe, the child can be helped by exercises to use what control he has. A child with cerebral palsy needs a team of specialists, one of whom should be a speech therapist.

Reading Failure

Inability to read at a level that can reasonably be expected, taking into account the child's intellectual endowment and his educational opportunities, is called *dyslexia*. It is a complicated problem. It may be related to aphasia and be part of a general language disability; it may be the outcome of trying to learn to read at a time when the child's maturity level was incapable of this accomplishment. Dyslexia is sometimes due to visual or auditory impairment, to illness necessitating absence from school during crucial learning periods. Failure to learn may stem from an emotional problem; it may be the means of expressing hostility toward parents who put undue pressure on the child (Critchley, 1964).

Once inability to read as well as his peers has been established, regardless of its original cause, secondary problems almost always arise. The child feels incompetent and worthless; he ceases to try. He may become aggressive, in an effort to overcome his fear of his own inadequacy, or he may withdraw from normal contacts with other children or adults. The secondary emotional problems compound the child's handicap. The longer the reading failure continues, the harder it is to institute remedial measures. Seldom will a child outgrow his early failures. Unless he is helped, he will grow up unable to function adequately in a literate society.

Dyslexia is a common problem. Betts has estimated that from 5 to 20 per cent of school children have some degree of dyslexia. Boys are more prone to this disability than girls. About 4 out of 5 poor readers are boys. The problem has been extensively studied in the last 50 years, and the literature is voluminous. Orton and Blau each feel that dyslexia is related to cerebral dominance, though they have different theories to account for reading failure in the presence of weak left or right dominance. Gallagher is convinced dyslexia is a disturbance in neurologic function in a specific area of the cortex. He thinks the disorder is hereditary and can involve all areas of language skills—talking, spelling, reading, penmanship, or expressing oneself in writing or speech, and can exist in all degrees of severity, from the very mild to the extremely severe. However, unlike almost all other forms of neurologic disorders, dyslexia is amenable to treatment.

It is impossible to review here the extensive literature on the causes of dyslexia. The condition, however, should be suspected in any child who fails first or second grade. Concept of numbers (Guttelius and Layman, 1960) appears different from that of ordinary reading skills, and often the child who has trouble reading is nevertheless quite competent in arithmetic in the early grades. Later, when mathematics involves word problems, he begins to fail in this subject too. Spelling is notably poor, as is penmanship (Money, 1962).

Prevention of dyslexia seems possible in many cases. If children who are likely to have reading difficulties can be detected before they have experienced failure, given special training, and not pushed ahead more rapidly than they are able to proceed, they can quite often acquire normal reading ability.

Children whose speech development has been slow, who come from families where dyslexia has been known to be a problem, or whose general ego development seems to lag need special consideration. Reading readiness tests (Castner, 1935) can help select the child who needs special help. Remedial reading classes in the school or a special tutor for a year or so can save some children many of the secondary problems bound to eventuate from failure in first grade. Many school systems are well prepared to cope with this frequent and now well-recognized problem, and the special classes are part of the school regime. Where such classes do not exist, parents need to be alerted to the need for an individual tutor early in the child's school life.

Older children who have already experienced the secondary problems resulting from their failures may need psychotherapy before remedial reading can be effective. The causes of dyslexia are so numerous that each case must be handled on an individual basis. However, the sooner a child can be helped, the more adequate will be his future development. If he has been a poor reader in the early grades, he is not likely suddenly to overcome this handicap, nor will mere repetition of a grade solve his problem.

BIBLIOGRAPHY

ABRAHAM, KARL: "Selected Papers," Chaps. 12 and 24, The Hogarth Press, Ltd., London, 1927.

AGNEW, D. C.: The Effect of Varied Amount of Phonetic Training on Primary Reading, The Duke University Press, Durham, N.C., 1939.

BANGS, TINA: Evaluating Children with Language Delay, *J. Speech & Hearing Disorders*, **26**:6, 1961.

BENDER, L.: Psychiatric Aspects, in Spencer L. Brown (ed.), "American Speech and Hearing Symposium," Washington, D.C., 1958.

BETTS, E. A.: "Foundation of Reading Instruction," American Book Company, New York, 1940.

BLAU, ABRAM: The Master Hand: A Study of the Origin and Meaning of Right- and Left-sidedness and Its Relation to Personality and Language, Research Monograph 5, American Orthopsychiatric Assn., Inc., 1946.

BODMER, FREDERICK: "The Loom of Language," W. W. Norton & Company, Inc., New York, 1944.

BROWN, ROGER: "Words and Things," The Free Press, Glencoe, Ill., 1958.

BURGI, ERNEST J., and JACK MATTHEWS: Disorders of Speech, *J. Pediat.*, **62**:15, 1963.

CASTNER, B. M.: Prediction of Reading Disabilities Prior to First Grade Entrance, *Am. J. Orthopsychiat.*, **5**:375, 1935.

COUGHLIN, WILLIAM J.: The Great Mokusatsu Mistake, *Harpers Magazine*, 206 (March), 1953, p. 31.

CRITCHLEY, MACDONALD: "Developmental Dyslexia," William Heinemann Medical Books Ltd., London, 1964.

DAVIS, KINGSLEY: Extreme Social Isolation of a Child, *Am. J. Sociol.*, **45**:554, 1940, and **52**:432, 1947.

EISENSON, JON: Disorders of Language in Children, *J. Pediat.*, **62**:20, 1963.

EWING, I. R., and A. W. G. EWING: "Speech and the Deaf Child," Volta Bureau, Washington, D.C., 1954.

FLAVELL, JOHN H.: "The Developmental Psychology of Jean Piaget," D. Van Nostrand Company, Inc., Princeton, N.J., 1963.

FLESCH, R.: "Why Johnny Cannot Read," Harper & Row, Publishers, Incorporated, New York, 1955.

GALLACHER, J. ROSWELL: Specific Language Disability, Dyslexia, *Clin. Proc. Child. Hosp.*, **16**:3, 1960.

GRIFFIN, D. R., and A. D. GRINNELL: Ability of Bats to Discriminate Echoes from Louder Noises, *Science*, **128**:145, 1958.

GUTTELIUS, MARGARET F., and EMMA M. LAYMAN: Reading Disability, or Developmental Dyslexia, *Clin. Proc. Child. Hosp.*, **16**:15, 1960.

IRWIN, ORWIN C., and H. P. CHEN: Infant Speech, *J. Speech & Hearing Disorders*, **13**:31, 123, 1948.

———: Infant Speech, *J. Speech &Hearing Disorders*, **12**:397, 402, 1947.

———: Phonetic Speech Development in Cerebral Palsied Children, *Am. J. Phys. Med.*, **34**:325, 1955.

JOHNSON, WENDELL: Perceptual and Evaluational Factors in Stuttering, *Folia Phoniatr.*, **8**:211, 1956.

KANNER, LEO: "Child Psychiatry," 3d ed., Charles C Thomas, Publisher, Springfield, Ill., 1957.

KARELITZ, SAMUEL, RUTH F. KARELITZ, and LAURA S. ROSENFELD: Infants' Vocalizations and Their Significance," in P. W. Bowan and Hans V. Mautner (eds.), "Mental Retardation," Proceedings of the First International Conference, Grune & Stratton, Inc., New York, 1960, p. 439.

KELLOGG, WINTHROP N., and LOUISE A. KELLOGG: "The Ape and the Child," McGraw-Hill Book Company, New York, 1933.

———: "Porpoises and Sonar," The University of Chicago Press, Chicago, 1961.

KIRK, SAMUEL A., and JAMES J. MCCARTHY: The Illinois Test of Psycholinguistic

Abilities: An Approach to Differential Diagnosis, *J. Ment. Deficiency,* **66:**399, 1961.

La Barre, Weston: "The Human Animal," The University of Chicago Press, Chicago, 1954.

Lado, Robert: "Linguistics Across Cultures," The University of Michigan Press, Ann Arbor, Mich., 1957.

Langer, Susanne K.: "Philosophy in a New Key," Mentor Books, The New American Library of World Literature, Inc., New York, 1959.

Lilly, John C.: "Man and Dolphin," Doubleday & Company, Inc., Garden City, N.Y., 1961.

Lorenz, K.: "King Solomon's Ring," Thomas Y. Crowell Company, New York, 1952.

McDowell, J.: A Report on the Phonetic Method of Teaching Children to Read, *Catholic Educ. Rev.,* **15:**506, 1953.

Money, John (ed.): Reading Disability: Progress and Research Needs in Dyslexia, The Johns Hopkins University Press, Baltimore, 1962.

Morley, Muriel, Donald Court, and Henry Miller: Delayed Speech and Developmental Aphasia, *Brit. M. J.,* **2:**463, 1955.

Myklebust, Helmer R.: Aphasia in Children: Language Development and Language Pathology, in L. E. Travis (ed.), "Handbook of Speech Pathology," p. 503, Appleton-Century-Crofts, Inc., New York, 1957.

Ogg, Oscar: "The 26 Letters," Thomas Y. Crowell Company, New York, 1961.

Orton, S. T.: "Reading, Writing and Speech Problems in Children," W. W. Norton & Company, Inc., New York, 1937.

Pearson, Gerald H. J.: A Survey of Learning Difficulties in Children, *Psychoanalyt. Study Child,* **7:**322, 1952.

Penfield, Wilder, and Lamar Roberts: "Speech and Brain Mechanisms," The Princeton University Press, Princeton, N.J., 1959.

Piaget, Jean: "Play, Dreams and Imitation in Childhood," translated by G. Gattegno and F. M. Hodgson, W. W. Norton & Company, Inc., New York, 1951.

———: "The Language and Thought of the Child," translated by Marjorie Gabain, Routledge and Kegan Paul, Ltd., London, 1924. (See Flavell above)

Rank, Otto: "The Trauma of Birth," Robert Brunner, 1952.

Ross, J. B. and M. M. McLaughlin (eds.): "A Portable Medieval Reader," The Viking Press, Inc., New York, 1947.

Russell, D. H.: A Diagnostic Study of Spelling Readiness, *J. Educ. Res.,* **37:**276, 1943.

Sherman, M.: The Differentiation of Emotional Responses in Infants, *J. Comp. Psychol.,* **7:**335, 1927.

Smith, Mary K.: Measurement of the Size of General English Vocabulary through Elementary Grades and High School, *Genet. Psychol. Monog.,* **24:**311, 1941.

Spitz, René A.: "No and Yes, On the Genesis of Human Communication," International Universities Press, Inc., New York, 1957.

Whorf, Benjamin Lee: Four Articles on Metalinguistics, U.S. Department of State, Foreign Service Institute, Washington, D.C., 1949.

———: "Language, Thought and Reality," Cambridge Technical Press, Cambridge, Mass., 1956.

Yerkes, Robert M., and Ada W. Yerkes: "The Great Apes," Yale University Press, New Haven, Conn., 1929.

33

Play and Discipline

THEORIES OF PLAY

All children in all cultures play, and children have undoubtedly played since before the dawn of recorded history. It is only within comparatively recent times that serious thought has been given to the meaning and significance of children's play. Even now many adults think of play as amusement, as leisure time activity, as a pleasant but unnecessary frill to life. Work is considered the serious business of life; play, in contrast, a luxury. Play has even been considered by some people to be harmful in that it wastes time and interferes with useful occupations.

Some of the earlier theories of play reflect this attitude of the nonessential character of play. Herbert Spencer felt that a child's play served merely to drain off his surplus energy. He did not conceive of play as a constructive force. Why a child was endowed with so much energy, why he continued to play even when exhausted Spencer did not elucidate. Karl Gross suggested that play was a preexercise activity and prepared the child for the serious work of later life. It was his feeling that the more play could be directed into the channels that would some day become serious work, the more useful to the child would be his years of childish play. Unlike Spencer, Gross thought play could be useful to the child, but only insofar as it had a specific content. He did not think of play as a constructive end in itself. Stanley Hall looked upon play as a recapitulation of the activities of primitive ancestors. As the physical organism repeats in embryonic development the evolutionary adaptations of the past, Hall, who was called "the Darwin of the mind," felt that activity in the form of play also retraced the evolutionary pattern.

It is certainly true that the play of very young children has elements in common with the play of the higher mammals. Puppies, kittens, young foxes, young monkeys engage in the same sort of sensorimotor play as do human children. Both children and the young of higher mammals learn their way around their worlds through the same basic technique of sensory exploration and inherent discipline. As with so many aspects of human development, the early stages repeat phylogeny. But the human soon leaves behind his evolutionary ancestors and plays in ways that bring to him his human concept of the cosmos. Sensorimotor play, which is the totality of animal play, in the human is only the prelude to the full orchestration of variations on the play-discipline theme.

It is only within the twentieth century that the idea has arisen that play is an essential medium through which children acquire a knowledge of themselves and of the world about them. Quite contrary to an old view that saw play as a means primarily of getting children out from underfoot, modern concepts consider play as essential (Harlow and Harlow, 1962). Children *must* play to achieve their human potential. In addition, it is through play that discipline is first achieved. And discipline, as well as play, is necessary for optimal development in every human cultural milieu.

Play is a spontaneous pleasurable activity which begins in infancy and progresses through a series of overlapping developmental stages. While there are many forms of play, there is a unifying quality to all play. Piaget sees in play the activity by means of which the child comes to understand the attributes of the world about him.

SENSORIMOTOR PLAY AND THE BEGINNINGS OF DISCIPLINE

The newborn does not play. He is an extraordinarily serious little piece of humanity struggling to satisfy his basic needs for survival. It is not until his cortex begins to establish its connections with muscles and with sensory nerve endings that the infant begins to experience the pleasures his body can give him. He then begins to play. The infant is concerned in the beginning only with the way objects affect him. He enjoys the variety of sensations he can produce in himself by looking at, listening to, tasting, smelling, squeezing, shaking, or throwing whatever comes his way. Everything is full of surprises and interest. He has no taboos; he reaches out with eagerness to experience as much as he can from the world. The baby is interested only in how he feels. He has no concern, as yet, with the objects and the people which give him the various feelings.

However, within the first half year of life, it begins to dawn on the baby that objects in the external world have qualities that he must adapt to, if he is to receive the sensations he enjoys. If he throws or drops a rattle, he can no longer shake it. It is gone, and so is the enjoyable feeling he was receiving from it. If he squeezes a scratchy substance, it hurts him; it is not like his soft toy. This adaptation to the realities of objects outside the baby himself is the beginning of discipline. The child learns that he must alter his behavior to adjust to the qualities in objects outside himself. Thus there begins in the baby the dim perception that things "out there" have an entity in and of themselves and apart from the sensations "in here."

People too, and of course Mother above all others, give the baby pleasurable sensations, but he must adapt his behavior and play in certain ways to gain those pleasures. The infant's total egocentricity is lessening as he appreciates that things and people have qualities he must take into consideration. The baby uses his powers of doing and feeling to gain for himself the maximum in satisfaction. Through his manipulation of in relation to the objects in his environment, his dim awareness gro there is an *I* in himself that feels and acts, and that there are obj people outside himself that are different from his *I*. Play is the taking-in phenomenon; discipline is the adaptation necessary to obtain the pleasant sensations of play. Piaget calls the former assimilation, the latter adaptation, and defines play as the activity dominated by assimilation.

Toward the middle of the first year, as the infant is learning about the attributes of things outside himself, the pure joy of doing and feeling evolves into a desire to accomplish specific purposes. The undirected sensorimotor play of the baby merges into practice play. The older infant begins to do *things*, instead of just doing. The initiative for the early practice play comes from within the child. He does, because he discovers he can; he repeats, because he enjoys the familiar sensation and also because he is becoming goal-directed. Ultimately he learns to sit up, to manipulate his toys, to get around his crib, later to crawl and to walk (p. 399). Each new accomplishment spurs him on to even greater effort.

As practice play advances, imitation makes its appearance. The child watches and listens and tries to copy what goes on about him. One of the earliest forms of imitation is with voice play (p. 465). Imitation and repetition remain a part of play throughout life.

The child learns what he must do and how he must act to obtain the joy his sensory apparatus is capable of giving him. Early discipline is inherent in the nature of the objects; it is consistent, it can be understood, it produces no anxiety. It is there and must be coped with. The infant and young child absorbs a sense of his own power in his growing ability to deal with externals.

The discipline which comes not from objects but from people introduces other aspects of control. The child's relation to his mother involves his need of her acceptance of him. If the mother's discipline is gentle and above all reasonably consistent, the baby can accept it as he accepts the inherent attributes of inanimate objects. He *wants* to learn how to control his body so that life is pleasant.

For a mother to be able to apply discipline in these ideal ways she must meet certain requirements. The first requirement is knowledge of what to expect from her baby. She needs to know something about developmental trends and drives so that she does not push the child and demand behavior beyond his capacity, and at the same time her knowledge should be sufficient so that she does not hold him back and thwart the powerful drives within the child that are directing his maturing. For example, she needs to know and accept the fact that a yearling handles and mouths whatever comes his way and cannot be expected to distinguish a toy from a cloisonné vase. Second, the mother, again ideally, should be a mature woman capable of genuine maternal love. She should be able to give unselfishly and unstintingly to her child—to give without asking anything in return (see Maternal Love in Chap. 31). These are not easy requirements to fulfill. The first is a matter of education. The second involves the whole life history of the mother.

The ideal mother attends to her baby's needs as they arise and builds up in him a basic trust (p. 356). She encourages his explorations and at the same time sets limits for his behavior. The mother who sometimes permits the child to do things and at other times thwarts him with angry words, irritable gestures, or physical hurt confuses the child and makes him anxious and fearful. Sometimes he is allowed to squeeze his cereal in his hand and enjoy the warm, wet, slippery sensation, but sometimes his mother's response to the same act produces in him a fear that she is denying him her love. His pleasure in the play is destroyed by his panic at the feeling that he is losing his mother and does not know why.

The child messing with his cereal is not naughty. He is not even trying to annoy his mother. He is only trying out an agreeable sensation. A baby *is* messy; he has to mess to learn what it is like. If his behavior can be accepted, he will add valuable knowledge to his fast-increasing store and in time will outgrow his messiness. When he becomes too enthusiastic in behavior that the mother cannot accept, he can and should be stopped, gently, consistently, and without anger. He is quite capable of learning that cereal is to eat, not to play with, and he can learn it without being hurt or made angry and fearful. It is because he is so inexperienced and because everything in him requires his mother's love that he reacts to every episode totally. It will take a lot of living, loving, and maturing before his self is organized enough to withstand the jars of harsh adult inconsistencies.

Once the little child learns to walk, his desire to play with everything he can get hold of inevitably runs into more and more mother-applied discipline. Ideally, if these disciplines can take into account his developmental stage and be absolutely consistent and free from anger, the child will accept them with a growing sense of his own competence. He knows how to control his body so that through play he can obtain the pleasurable sensations he so much desires. Discipline under such circumstances becomes a constructive force that helps the child gain mastery over himself and his immediate world. At this stage the little child is also learning to talk, and speech becomes incorporated into his concept of discipline. Spitz has pointed out that the child first hurdles the semantic concept of an abstraction by means of negation (p. 467). The child's first use of verbal symbols is to designate a specific item. Before he understands that *dog* can mean a whole category of objects, instead of just Corky, he has already understood that the word *no* or the semantic head-shaking *no* gesture can mean many different prohibitions (see Language—the Child's Tool, in Chap. 32).

Sensory pleasures of play and consistent discipline condition the child to full appreciation of the joys and learning to be had through his senses.

The toddler limits his bouncing, swinging, shouting, tasting to the permitted expressions, and within these clearly defined limits he gets joy and understanding free from anxiety. The school child and the adolescent still enjoy the sensations his senses bring him, but within the limits of his culture (that is, ideally). It is a utopian dream to think that any child could grow up without encountering fear and anxiety in relation to his sensory pleasures. If these emotions are not too severe, the child can cope with them without destroying his eagerness to continue exploring the world. The human child develops techniques for coping with moderate degrees of anxiety (see Symbolic Dramatic Play, below). However, the constant repetition of fear-laden experience can so overwhelm the child that his desire to reach out to the world is curtailed. He then grows to physical adulthood without the urge to experience ever more of the world.

Thus the sensory pleasures to be had from the world begin in early infancy and in modified and sophisticated forms continue through life. In mature adult life the joys of the senses can be part of the good life. In adult life, it is apt to be called *aesthetic pleasure* instead of play. The adult who can enjoy with his whole being the sound and sensation of a symphony or a beautiful landscape or a good meal is appreciating the world with the same elemental pleasures as the baby who squeezes and listens to his squeaky toy or the child who flies skyward in his swing.

IMAGINATIVE MAKE–BELIEVE–UNDERSTANDING THE WORLD

While sensory play and its concomitant discipline begin early and continue through life, other forms of play make their appearance as the child matures. Once the child has the concept that objects and people have an existence quite apart from his own being, he tries to understand these objects. His first understanding is his acceptance of their qualities—what has been called discipline. But this is not adequate in and of itself. He wants to know more about the qualities of these objects, what they are like quite apart from himself. The child's technique is to act as though he were the object. By this time his language development has progressed to the point where he can understand and use many symbols and abstractions.

He now enters the realm of imaginative make-believe. The child tries out by identification what it feels like to be other people and things. He chugs like a train, he flops his arms like a bird, he crawls around on the floor like his kitten, he calls his father on the phone as does mother. To understand more completely what an airplane is, he must *be* an airplane. When he is an airplane, he is not a little boy. The airplane exists quite apart from him, and he exists quite apart from it—a profound realization. The little child may also pretend to be a dog, a lion, maybe an earthworm. He acts out not only the living things he knows but also the inanimate ones' and frequently he acts several roles at the same time. He can be a

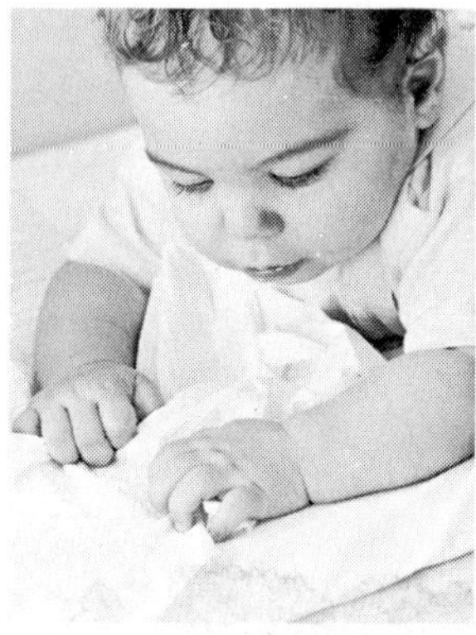

The first play is a sensori-motor pleasure

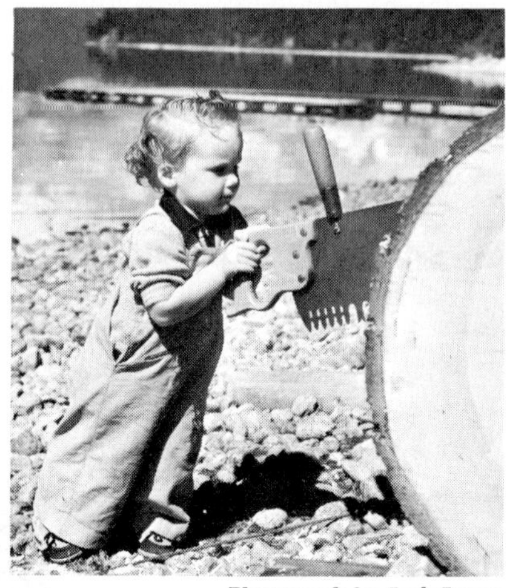

Imitation enters into many play activities

Photograph by Jack James

Dramatic Play

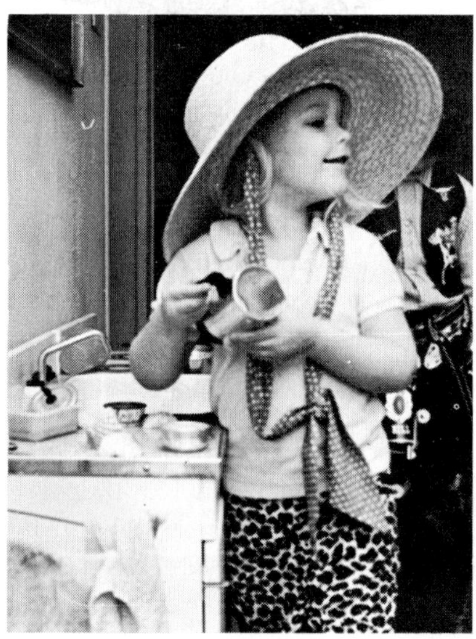

She identifies with mother

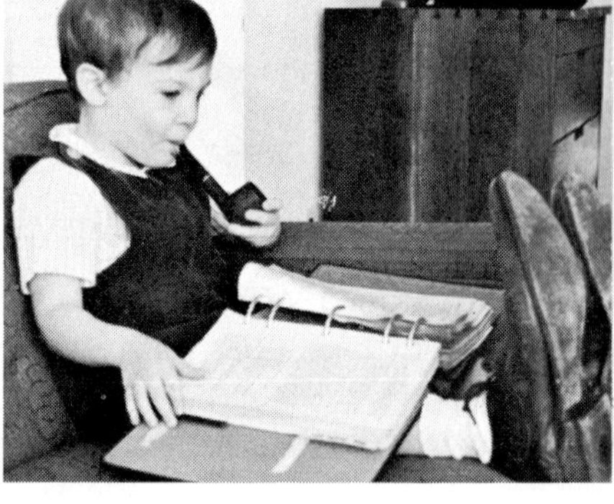

He identifies with Daddy

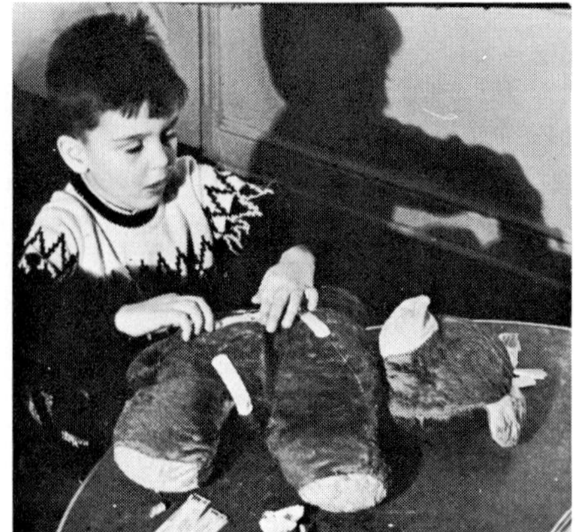

Symbolic play frustrations are being worked out

Fig. 33-1. Play in the early years.

tree and at the same time a squirrel running up the trunk; he can be a steam shovel and its operator. He superimposes one role on another. Time and space are no problems to him. In his play he is feeling the way he conceives that these objects feel, and it is quite logical to him that a tree and a squirrel have feelings at the same time.

During the years of toddlerhood and preschool life, children dress up in adult clothes and play at being mother, father, baby, teacher, garbage man, postman, doctor. In this way the child begins to grasp the fact that there are many adult roles and many kinds of adults. He will pretend to be a nasty neighbor or an admired parent with equal devotion to detail.

Imaginative play is the dominant activity of the little child. He uses all his play material to pretend. Blocks, sand, dolls, paints, dress-up garments—all serve the purpose of helping the child live out the experiences of his daily life. Sensory pleasures in the materials are still much in evidence, but more and more materials are being put into the service of the imagination. A toddler may taste his paint or wiggle his toes in the sand for pure sensory delight, but he will also build structures with his blocks, people the buildings with other blocks, and carry out a drama of domestic play. In the early years, the child's attention flits from one thing to another in rapid succession. Each thing he spies suggests a use, so that play jumps from theme to theme, but in spite of the distractibility of the little child, the imaginative play which occupies such a large part of his waking life serves the purpose of giving him an understanding of the world of things and people about him.

As with sensory play, imaginative play continues in modified form throughout life. To be able to feel as another feels is called sensitivity later in life, and it finds expression in art, in music, in literature. It is also an essential ingredient in the relationships of truly mature adults.

SYMBOLIC DRAMATIC PLAY—FRUSTRATION AND CONTROLS

The active, distractible toddler is forever barging into everything. He has learned some self-discipline by this time, but much more is ahead of him. The insatiable curiosity of the exploring child is often frustrated by adult-imposed rules. He cannot be permitted to injure himself or hurt another person. He cannot destroy the precious possessions of his parents or of anyone else. The toddler years are necessarily full of discipline. Again, discipline which is consistent, firm, and friendly and which does not ask the impossible is better accepted by the child than unpredictable outbursts of angry, threatening, love-withholding adult behavior.

No matter how well a mother manages, frustrations of the child are inevitable. He will become angry and resentful at the necessary restrictions put upon his free behavior. It is normal for a child to feel anger at frustration. He has no control over his feelings. These feelings just come to him. Sometimes he will express this anger directly in words and actions.

"I hate you." "I wish you were dead." The words, to the child, do not have the same meaning they have for the adult. To the child "I wish you were dead" is likely to mean "I don't want to be interfered with." Not for a single instant does the child really want to get rid of his parent. Such expressions need to be accepted by the parent at the child's level and with an understanding that the vehemence with which the words are uttered also serves as an outlet for frustrations. With parent understanding and acceptance, the child is helped to vent his pent-up emotions without the fear of losing love. The child discovers that it is all right to have feelings—even bad feelings; mother loves him, bad feelings and all. The firm conviction in the child of mother's love strengthens the child's confidence that the self he is discovering is a good self, and this conviction takes the edge off his anger, because there is no fear to compound his anger. If the child can accept and express his own bad feelings, there is no need for him to repress them and try to pretend they do not exist. Expressed feelings are over and done with; repressed feelings fester in the unconscious, a potential source of future trouble.

However, when the child tries to use kicks along with his verbal expressions, these must be stopped as part of adequate discipline, but always with the understanding that the emotion behind the action is acceptable to the mother. "I know it makes you angry when I won't let you do so-and-so. It's all right to be angry, but you cannot kick me." The child's feelings, which he *cannot* control, are accepted as they are; his actions, which he *can* control, are channeled into acceptable behavior. Thus the child learns how to behave at the same time that he is discovering the range of his feelings.

In addition to his overt manifestation of frustration, the child uses play as a means of coping with his anger. Imaginative play merges into symbolic play, in which the child acts out, not the feelings of the object being dramatized, but his own feelings. A child playing a family scene may push a father figure off the roof or hold a baby under the water of a bathtub, or cover a mother with Band-aids. The child is acting out his desires to be free from the restraints or interference imposed on him. In the fantasy of play, he does the things he does not dare to do in real life. Sometimes the acting out gives him a considerable sense of power within himself and of relief of pent-up emotions. There is one essential difference between this kind of emotion-laden dramatic play and the previously described imaginative play. In imaginative play, the child knows he is pretending. He acts like a lion, but he knows quite well he is a little boy pretending to be a lion. In much of symbolic play the child is not aware of what he is acting out. He does not realize that his own resentments are being expressed. If he did, he could not express them.

In the play life of children, these two elements are often simultaneously present; nevertheless they serve quite different purposes. In the one, the child is trying to assimilate the qualities of people and things. In the other, he is using play as catharsis to rid himself of tensions. Symbolic play is the child's way of incorporating the necessary discipline into the structure of his personality. Viewed in this way, symbolic play, like other forms of play, is a taking-in phenomenon, as pointed out by Piaget. Later in life, sophistication makes this direct use of symbols impossible for most adults, and symbolic acting is confined for the most part to dreams and the fantasy of daydreams. (In primitive societies, the burning of an enemy in effigy is an example of symbolic play carried into adult life.)

WHEN DISCIPLINE GETS OUT OF HAND

It would certainly make life simpler for all adults who live with children, especially mothers, if the child's own play technique of dealing with the frustrations of discipline were adequate to take care of all disciplinary problems. Such is far from the case. There are bound to be difficulties in persuading children to conform in ways which adults consider essential.

It is well to bear in mind that basically children *want* to conform. A child must have love. The love the child wants is a one-way phenomenon—he wants *to be loved*. To the little child being loved means approval and acceptance of himself as he is, the bad parts of him as well as the good. It means encouragement to be his real self. It is expressed by words, looks, actions, physical contact. Often the giving of expensive material goods is part of love shown the child, but no amount of things can replace the feeling of love (Baruch, 1949).

The reasonably well-behaved child, one who is usually a pleasant person to have around, may have a bad day or a bad afternoon. He may on occasion refuse to follow directions, eat little, and find everyone else in the wrong. Such a moment in his total life span may be nothing more than passing growing pains, or a brief relaxation from living up to his idea of his self, or a mustering of courage to discuss a worry with a parent. This child's behavior is of no great concern. Next day he will probably be his usual cheerful self. All his annoying behavior needs is a little parental patience and forbearance.

It is the youngster who chronically misbehaves who is in real trouble. He feels deeply deprived of his mother's love, and he will use every means at his disposal to get for himself the love he craves. The means he uses are not likely to make him lovable from the adult point of view. He may whine, he may run away, he may deliberately do things which he knows are forbidden. Behavior of this sort is bound to get his mother's attention. The child seems to get some satisfaction from being the center of the stage. What he wants most of all is love, acceptance, and approval, but in the absence of these he will accept any kind of notice and even punishment as a substitute.

Since "bad behavior" seldom or never brings the child the love he craves, it does not solve his problems. He is apt to go from one type of unacceptable behavior to another. He may turn to his own body for comfort and indulge in excessive thumb sucking or bed rocking, or may handle his genitals more than usual. Another child may show fits of rage—tantrums. He may be cruel and aggressive to playmates or pets. There are a thousand ways in which a child may act unacceptably. The technique he uses may be related to specific trauma he has sustained and to his own particular nature. Regardless of the form his behavior takes, the child is saying that he has needs which are not being fulfilled. A child does not behave badly because of any innate instinct for aggressiveness or because he is willful. His bad temper is not inherited from Aunt Alice, nor his tendency to steal from Uncle Henry.

It is unfortunate that nature has not endowed the child with more successful techniques for rectifying the inadequacies of his environment. A month-old baby is endowed with the ability to enchant his mother with his toothless grin. The irresistible quality of his smile helps to ensure the continuance of the love he needs. The older child needs love, too, and while he can be lovable, he also has a genius for devising ways that can try the patience of the most saintly mother.

The "bad" child is in some way a deprived child. He is acting the way he does because he is struggling desperately to squeeze from his life those things his very being demands as essential for his development. His technique often produces irritation and annoyance in adults and is apt to result in the age-old methods of disciplining a misbehaving child—spankings and deprivations. These methods provide the adult with a means of relieving his own anger but are not likely to convince the child he is loved. They do not remove the cause of the misbehavior any more than bribes and rewards do. If the punishment is severe, the child may not commit that particular misdemeanor again, but some other equally undesirable acts are apt to recur if the basic condition is unchanged. Repeated punishments not only do not help a child become responsible for anything but the concealment of his bad behavior, but they also stimulate distrust of adults.

Parental intelligence must take over and find ways to convince the child that he is loved. It is up to the adult, first, to make an accurate diagnosis of why the child feels unloved and, second, to alter what needs altering.

Occasionally a parent who does genuinely love a child is so absorbed in the mechanics of providing for the child that there is no time for her to express the feeling of her love. The child is utterly unconcerned with laundry and cleaning and cooking; he is only interested in his mother's attitude toward his own little person. When such a mother comes to understand what her child's bad behavior means, she is usually able to find ways of rectifying the situation.

A mother who truly resents the child, who feels abused and restricted by the necessity of providing care, cannot conceal her feelings from her child. The child feels unloved because he *is* unloved. Treatment of misbehavior in this situation involves treatment of the mother's total personality.

The fundamental way of handling children's misbehavior is to try to look at life through the child's eyes, an adult exercise in the use of sensitivity. If a child is given a chance, he will often tell us what is worrying him.

Kathy, age 4, was jumping around the floor, pretending to be a dog. She barked and yelped and began pulling the tablecloth off the table with her mouth. Disaster was imminent. Her mother scolded: "Stop that, Kathy! What are you up to anyway?" To which Kathy replied: "I'm a dog and I want you to do what you're supposed to do to a dog."

"You want a whipping?" asked her mother, quite ready to give it.

"No, pat me," said Kathy.

Oftentimes it is not that easy, but neither is it so impossible as many parents think. Once the parent has an inkling of how the child feels, it helps the child to be accepted as he is, without condemnation. Sometimes to put into words how the adult imagines the child feels—"You're angry because I went away" helps the child accept his feelings without the dread of losing love.

The cues in handling misbehavior can be outlined as follows:

1. Misbehavior is a symptom that the child's needs are not being adequately met. Look for the cause and try to rectify it.

   a. Is the child being pushed beyond his capacity? Are demands made on him which he is quite incapable of fulfilling? If so, his inevitable sense of failure destroys his feeling of self-competence.

   b. Is the child being held back and not permitted to do what he is capable of doing? Is he not being allowed to shoulder those responsibilities he can easily handle? Or is he being asked to make decisions that are beyond his degree of maturity? While a little child should be permitted to make decisions within the range of his competency (will he wear blue socks or brown socks today?), he should not be permitted to make decisions that are the prerogative of his parents (will he go to nursery school today or stay home?). His self-confidence grows as he is able to manage himself successfully.

2. Try to look at life through the child's eyes, and find out how he feels.

3. Accept his feelings, even the bad ones. He cannot help feeling. He needs to know that his mother understands how he feels and that she loves him and accepts him, bad feelings and all. He then does not have to cover up and try to deny his feelings in order to have her love. If his bad feelings can be accepted by his parents, he too can accept them and will feel that the self he is discovering is all right (Baruch, 1949).

4. Bad behavior must be stopped. While the child's bad feelings need to be accepted, overt acts of aggression do not help the child cope with him-

self; they only make him feel guilty and remorseful afterward. He needs to be protected from himself.

5. Parents often need help to understand the meaning of the misbehavior of their children. They need encouragement to seek this help from physicians, teachers, or a social agency, without embarrassment or shame.

These are the basic principles in helping children grow up in a complicated society. For adequate execution, they require love, understanding, sensitivity, patience, and time, from a reasonably mature adult. The adult is rewarded not only by a pleasant life during the child's growing years but by the satisfaction of helping the children reach full human maturity.

While disciplinary problems have been discussed more or less in relation to the young child, the basic principles are similar through all the years of childhood. Manifestations of bad behavior vary, of course, with the age of the child, but the drives that make children act in unacceptable ways are similar at all ages and need the same sort of sympathetic understanding in their management.

GAMES AND RITUALISTIC PLAY

As children pass on into the school years, they enter a new phase of development which is reflected in their type of play. School-age children form gangs and cliques. To belong to some group is of vital importance. Belonging means abiding by the rules, which may be not only bizarre but extraordinarily rigid.

In play, this need for conformity is manifest in all sorts of ways, and especially in the games that are such a big part of the life of the schoolchild. The child has played many games in his earlier years, but games that he himself invented or that he and a friend (even an adult) evolved, with rules that just grew as the game grew. Now games have fixed and unvarying rules. Much of the fun of a game is knowing the rules, and knowing means belonging. The child who does not conform is ostracized; individuality is not tolerated.

While the rules are essential, children acquire many skills during these years in the practice of their games. A child will practice and practice to attain a skill which is considered worthwhile in his group. His ability gives him pleasure in bodily accomplishment, and his performance gives him stature with his peers. Both feelings add to his self-confidence.

Conformity and ritual are the keynotes of school-age play. They are present not only in the games but also in much of the ritualistic language. Childhood is full of chants and taunts: "Eeny, meeny, miney, mo," "Susie's mad and I'm glad," and "Last one is a rotten egg." Children get an enormous amount of pleasure from these and other age-old sayings, often embellished with particular variations of their special group. The undeviating ritual often is endowed with some magic quality and helps the child gain a sense of power over the unconquerable world about him. Clubs

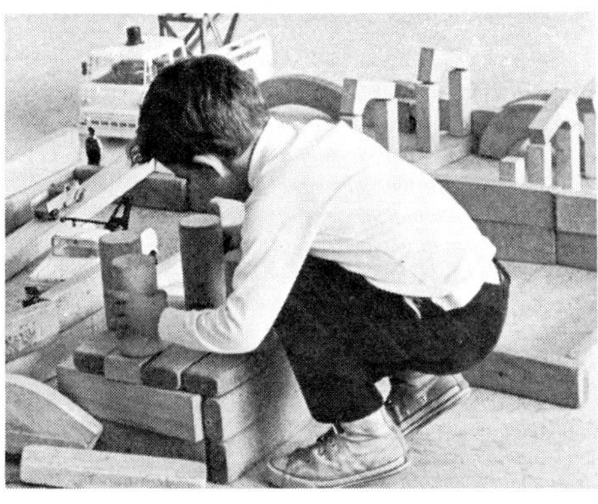

Creative imaginative play

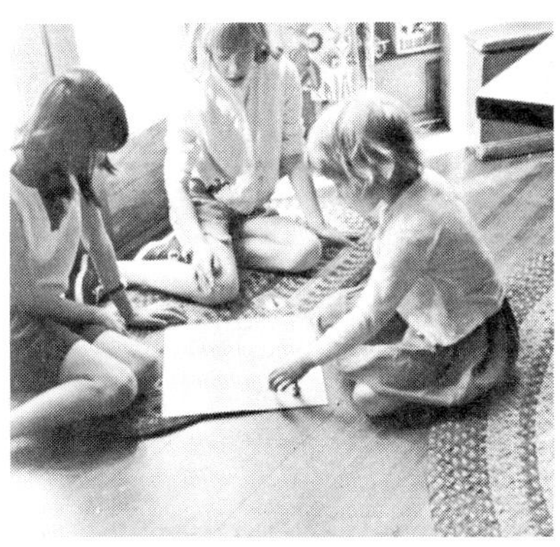

Games - knowing the rules is part of the fun

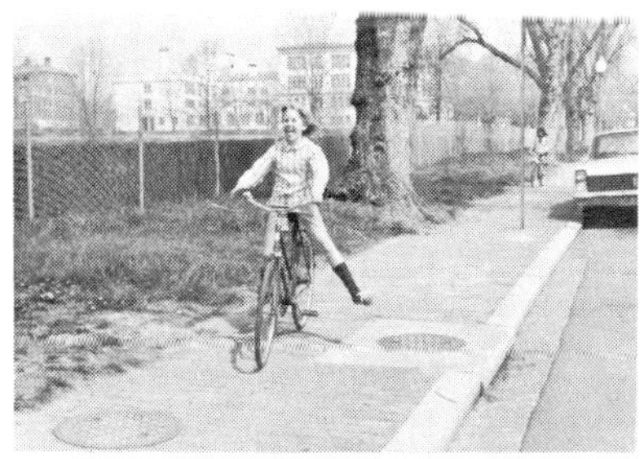

Skills learned during the school years provide pleasures throughout life

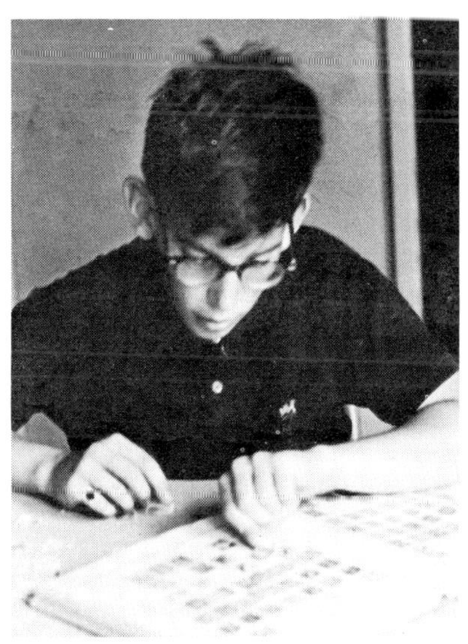

Collections: Learning to manipulate material possessions.

Fig. 33-2. Play in the school years.

and secret societies make their appearance. To be accepted in the inner circle, the child must conform to an arbitrary set of rules which are often bizarre in the extreme. He may have to learn to write his name in mirror writing or master a secret language or always wear a red shirt on Thursdays. The club members meet and giggle and eat and give each other support. An excluded child may have a hard time.

During the middle years children may be as conforming about ideas as about behavior. They accept as right the values of their group concerning morals or aesthetics just as rigidly as they accept the idea of what is funny or what clothes to wear.

This is also the age of collections—another ritual. In the early school years, collections consist of the oddest assortment of objects; drawers or pockets full of colored stones, matchbook covers, bus transfers, playing cards. At first these are messy, disorganized piles—but extraordinarily precious. Later in the school years, collections tend to become somewhat more orderly and more organized. Stamps are pasted neatly in an album, horses are arranged on a shelf, movie stars' pictures are hung on the wall.

All ritualistic play of the school years serves the same basic function as the earlier play. It helps the child understand and cope with the world as he finds it. The child's developing skills give him assurance of his own competence and his ability to compete with others, his collections represent fragments of the big external world, reduced to a level he can control and manage. His clubs, his secret societies—in short, his oneness with his peer group—help him establish himself as a person independent of his family. He must cut his family ties before he can become self-reliant. It is too terrifying to take this step in one leap. The technique of the child is to move from family to peer group.

As with earlier forms of play, the ritualism and conformity of the middle years, while outgrown in its rigidity, nevertheless pave the way for many adolescent and adult pleasures.

Athletic skills learned in childhood are enjoyed for many years—swimming, skating, hiking, dancing. Such activities give sensory and bodily delight but are no longer needed to prove status. Gliding across a frozen river on a clear, cold winter day, swimming in a beautiful lake, or almost flying on water skis—such are the mature dividends of childhood skills.

Other types of skills learned as play in childhood serve different purposes in adult life—sewing, cooking, music, painting, carpentry, and many others. Some can eventually have vocational value; others serve as tools for creative expression. New skills are, of course, learned in later years, but often the ones that have some tie with childhood are those that are most enjoyed in later life.

The collections that mean so much to the child of the middle years may also evolve into adult collections of books, records, pictures, antiques which are a means of expanding horizons of knowledge rather than mere aggregations of things.

While the play of the middle years leaves a rich residue for later life, its major value is its contribution to personality structure. Failure to leave behind childhood rituals is all too often seen in many adults who have not achieved full maturity. Rigid social conformity, conversation splattered with clichés, displays of material goods are all mementos of a childhood not left fully behind.

RECREATION VERSUS PLAY IN THE MATURE YEARS

Once maturity is reached, play in the sense used here fades from the picture for many people. The adult has learned his way around, he uses what he has learned for the serious business of life. Sometimes, but all too infrequently, there is a true play element in an adult's experimenting with a new medium; he explores it, tests it out, looks at it from many aspects, and takes it in as does a child. When an adult does this, he brings the imaginative zeal of childhood to bear on his adult occupation. An artist, a poet, a scientist, or just an ordinary being who can play in this sense has been able to distill from childhood the essence of human creativity.

This kind of play is very different from the leisure time activities of adults more properly called *recreation.* Recreation is a lull in the usual activities of life, used, as the word implies, to renew vitality and provide a change in pace. Failure to distinguish play from recreation is doubtless the reason it has taken man so long to realize the essential nature of the play of childhood. When the two were equated, especially in cultures which looked aghast at any form of pleasure, it is understandable that many people thought play was a waste of time, interfering with the serious business of life.

BIBLIOGRAPHY

BARUCH, DOROTHY WALTER: "New Ways in Discipline," McGraw-Hill Book Company, New York, 1949.

GROSS, KARL: "The Play of Man," Appleton-Century-Crofts, Inc., New York, 1901.

HALL, G. STANLEY: "Youth," Appleton-Century-Crofts, Inc., New York, 1920.

———: "Life and Confessions of a Psychologist," Appleton-Century-Crofts, Inc., New York, 1923.

HARLOW, HARRY F., and MARGARET K. HARLOW: Social Deprivation in Monkeys, *Scientific American,* Nov., 1962.

———, and ROBERT R. ZIMMERMAN: Affectional Responses in the Infant Monkey, *Science,* **130**:421, 1959.

PIAGET, JEAN: "Play, Dreams and Imitation in Childhood," translated by C. Gattegno and F. M. Hodgson, W. W. Norton & Company, Inc., New York, 1951.

SPENCER, HERBERT: "The Principles of Psychology," Appleton-Century-Crofts, Inc., New York, 1873.

SPITZ, RENÉ A.: "No and Yes, On the Genesis of Human Communication," International Universities Press, Inc., New York, 1957.

34

Sensation, Learning, Cognition[1]

The development of the organs by means of which the human receives stimuli from his environment has been discussed in Chap. 23. The present chapter is devoted to the nature of the sensations received, the meaning of these sensations to the child, and their contribution to his developing personality. Learning and cognition are largely dependent upon stimuli received through the sense organs.

Since sensation enters into almost every aspect of human behavior, some of the topics in this chapter have been mentioned elsewhere. However, at the risk of burdensome repetition, an attempt will be made here to bring together some aspects of the significance of the human capacity to receive and react to afferent stimuli.

THE NATURE OF SENSORY EXPERIENCE IN MAN

In the mature human being, sensation provides contact with the environment—contact with the physical aspects of the surroundings and contact with fellow human beings. Sensation functions at several levels: (1) a primitive biologic awareness, (2) an inwardly directed, egocentric sensation, and (3) an outwardly directed, world-centered perception.

The Primitive Level of Awareness

The recent work on sensory deprivation has pointed up the importance of a constant barrage of afferent stimuli. When adult human beings are deprived of such stimuli, they develop a multitude of bizarre symptoms. Experiments, varying somewhat in detail, have been done in which young men were placed in small rooms, in dead silence, with an opaque or translucent mask over the eyes. Heron had his subjects lie on a comfortable bed, Wexler et al. used a respirator (with vents open), and Lilly immersed his subjects in a bath. Heron permitted his subjects to get up for meals and

[1] Sensation, perception, learning, and cognition are subjects wihch have interested philosophers, neurologists, and psychologists for centuries. The literature is enormous. All that can be presented here is a brief and cursory discussion of some aspects of developmental trends.

to go to the toilet; Wexler provided bedpans and arranged a tube from which his subjects could drink a rich eggnog as desired.

In all these experiments, exteroceptive sensations were reduced almost to the zero point, and proprioceptive sensations were severely diminished. The only sensations left at a more or less usual level were the enteroceptive ones, those emanating from the viscera.

As the experimental conditions varied in detail, so, too, did the results show minor variations. Nevertheless, there was a fundamental concordance in the findings. All the subjects showed abnormal behavior. Hallucinations were universal; there was confusion about space and time; simple problems were solved poorly if at all. Some subjects showed anxiety, and a few had such severe panic reactions that the experiment had to be discontinued.

There has been much speculation concerning the physiologic and psychologic mechanisms responsible for the results obtained. Electroencephalographic studies in various animals (Lindsley et al., 1950) suggested that brain changes accompany cessation of normal afferent stimuli. Reison, working with chimpanzees, found that visual deprivation altered the structure of the visual system and that the age at which the deprivation took place was a critical factor in the development of vision. Hebb and others have suggested that the nervous system functions like the cybernetic systems described by Norbert Wiener, that is, that a constant feedback mechanism is at work. Afferent stimuli enter the CNS and activate efferent responses, some of which result in appropriate action and some of which return to the CNS and keep the total system in something like a state of tone. In the absence of afferent stimuli, the feedback fails to function, and the CNS is unable to maintain homeostasis. This is a new concept of the CNS and stands in contrast to the older view (Sherrington) in which the CNS was seen as a sort of switchboard which merely directed afferent and efferent impulses.

The work on sensory deprivation demonstrates beyond a question of a doubt the essential nature of afferent stimuli. Though the physiologic mechanism is not well understood, it is postulated that an awareness of what is outside the body enables the individual to define the limits of his body and so maintain a concept of his own bodily integrity, to know the difference between *I* and *non-I*.

Egocentric Sensation

Mature man, in normal contact with his environment on a visceral level (if one may use such a term), receives in addition sensations which have an emotional tone. Some of these sensations he likes and seeks to prolong or repeat; others cause him displeasure, and he tries either to terminate or avoid them. Sensation which has its focus on how *I* feel about what *I* sense can be termed *egocentric;* it gives little information about the object sensed except its ability to affect the individual. Much of man's egocentric sensation is on a simple everyday basis; man uses sight to avoid bumping into things, sound to attract to the desirable or warn of the dangerous, smell and taste to be aware of food.

Man's capacity to obtain feelings from his senses has transcended the purely useful. Man can obtain pleasure from the look of a sunset, the sound of a symphony, the feel of a delicate shell, the smell of a field of new-mown hay, the taste of a vintage wine. However, even these "higher" pleasures from the senses are the result of how *I* feel. Egocentric sensation reinforces visceral sensation; the latter defines the limits of the physical being, the former gives quality to that being. The ego becomes more satisfactory as the individual is able to bring to himself desirable sensations.

World-centered Perception

In addition to sensation directed toward the individual doing the sensing, man has acquired a further ability to use his senses. Man can interpret what he senses; he can combine different sensations, make use of past experience, and recognize the inherent traits in the object sensed. Instead of being directed toward how *I* feel, this type of sensation is directed toward what *it* is. It can be termed *world-centered* perception. Man can look, listen, and feel an object, not only to find out what it can do to him, but also to find out what the object is, what it is made of, how it works. Man takes apart and puts together to comprehend qualities that have no immediate bearing on him.

Egocentric sensation as described above arises from the feeling tones of pleasure or displeasure received through the senses. Between the pleasurable and displeasurable sensations lies a whole realm of sensation that is neutral, or indifferent, with respect to its effect on feelings. Egocentrically these sensations are ignored, but from the point of view of world-centered perception, this neutral zone comprises the bulk of sensations available for exploring the nature of reality. Man listens to speech not to obtain pleasure from the sound but to understand what is said; he reads the printed page with the same objective. He handles objects to find out what they are. There is, of course, much overlapping: a voice can be melodious, pleasing, comforting, or it can be raucous or threatening. In spite of these egocentric qualities, speech is listened to primarily for its content, and books are read to understand what the author has to say.

Egocentric sensation carries the connotation "What can this object do to me?" and stands in contrast to world-centered perception, which carries the connotation "What is the nature of this object?" World-centered perception is late phylogenetically and late ontogenetically. While in all adult human beings some measure of world-centered perception develops, the ratio between the deep-seated primitive egocentric sensation and the superimposed world-centered perception varies greatly from person to person. Fear and anxiety can so keep the focus on the self that every new encounter is viewed as "What is in this for me?" Such an attitude tends to dampen the desire to explore and keeps the individual encased in his own emotions.

One of the objects of nurture is to strike a balance between the powerful and primitive egocentric view of the world and the human capacity to appreciate and understand that which bears no relevance to the individual. World-centered perception constitutes the human dimension of sensation.

These, then, are the uses to which adult man puts his sensory apparatus:

1. Primitive sensory contact with the physical environment, which, in ways not well understood, maintains the integrity of the neural mechanisms and keeps the limits of *I* in focus.

2. Egocentric sensations which produce feeling tones of pleasure or displeasure and give quality to the *I*.

3. World-centered perception which is directed away from the *I* and makes possible an understanding of the inherent attributes of people and things that may not have any relation to the individual doing the sensing.

SENSATION FROM THE VARIOUS SENSORY RECEPTORS

Man uses all five exteroceptive sense organs at all the levels at which he receives sensation. However, each sense modality has unique contributions to make. The distance senses, hearing and vision, are what Myklebust calls "lead senses." Hearing is present all the time, even during sleep, and provides constant contact with the environment (Ramsdell, 1947). Sounds come from all directions and constitute a permanent background awareness. Such phrases as "dead silence," "silent as the tomb" convey the idea that life cannot be separated from sound. Familiar and understood sounds keep the individual oriented; he knows where he is, and he knows who he is. An unusual sound causes an alert; it rises from the background, is consciously listened to, then is either relegated to the background or investigated with other senses. The individual feels confident he will be alerted by sound, so in the absence of an alert, he feels safe within a known milieu. Sound operates 24 hours a day for the duration of life.

Sound is capable of producing egocentric sensation. Soft melodious sound is pleasing, and music is one of the joys of life. In contrast, noise can be most annoying (Church, 1961).

Sound at the human level has acquired a special world-centered significance. Man has endowed sound with symbolic value and therefore has been able to build up language. By means of language man is able to conceptualize the reality about him and thus to develop cognitive thought. Through speech man communicates with other human beings and maintains contact at the human level. Speech constitutes the human dimension of the sensory ability to hear sound.

Vision is neither as constant nor as all-pervading as sound. Vision is a foreground sense in contrast to the background quality of hearing. The individual looks only at the area immediately in front of him; he has no eyes in the back of his head. Vision can be blotted out by the simple device of closing the eyes (there is no means of closing the ears). In general, hearing is the sense that alerts to a change; vision, the sense used to explore the nature of the change.

Hearing and vision, though for the most part background and foreground senses respectively, can reverse their roles (Cobb, 1958). Either one can become the lead sense. Hearing can become the foreground, when one listens intently—to speech, for example—while vision does the background scanning and keeps the individual in comfortable and safe contact with his surroundings.

Hearing is a temporal sense. A sound is heard and then gone; it cannot be held in time. Even when a sound is recorded and played back, it is again heard only momentarily. Vision, on the other hand, is a spatial sense. One can take his time in examining an object visually; the image remains in space; it does not disappear as does a sound.

Vision, like hearing, is capable of producing egocentric sensation. Much of what is looked at is appreciated with a feeling tone. All the visual arts create egocentric sensation; much of daily living includes visually stimulated feelings of pleasure or displeasure.

Again like hearing, vision at the human level has acquired the ability to be used symbolically. Reading the printed page is man's supreme achievement with respect to vision. It is world-centered perception in one of its most important forms. World-centered vision, however, is used by mature man in ways other than reading. Once can look at an object from many perspectives to discover its inherent traits.

Taste and smell, proximity senses, do not serve mature man as lead senses. They are not used to scan the environment, to provide the constant background awareness that hearing and vision supply. In some species, such as the dog, smell *is* a lead sense and provides constant environmental awareness. In man smell can cause an alert, but it is of minor importance compared with the pervasiveness of sound (Pratt, 1954).

For most people, most of the time smell and taste remain for life sources of either pleasure or displeasure and are therefore egocentric sensations. Neither of these senses has any cerebral component capable of translating a sense perception into a symbol. It is impossible to conceive of a language built up on the basis of odors or tastes. There is almost no world-centered quality in these sensations.

The tactile organs provide mature man with two basically different senses, total body tactation and touch in the hand. The former, combined with the proprioceptive sense, provides a background orientation in space. It contributes to the knowledge of where I am and who I am. It can be an alerting sense, as when an unusual touch impinges on the body. Body touch is an egocentric sensation and has virtually no world-centered possibility. The leg is scratched by a chair; to learn what qualities in the chair are capable of scratching, the chair is examined with eyes and hands, not with the leg.

Touch in the hand is almost never a background sense. In general the hands are idle when not actively engaged in investigation. When man "handles" an object, he usually does so to find out something about the object itself. Man is able to touch, feel, explore with his hands and discover something of the inherent qualities of the object. He can find out whether the object is heavy, light, hard, soft, rough, smooth, wet, dry. These attributes belong to the object and constitute world-centered perceptions. Sensation in the hand may, of course, produce feeling tones in the toucher, and therefore the hand is an organ of egocentric sensation as well as of world-centered perception.

Like vision and hearing, touch in the hand can be used symbolically. It is possible for man to "read" with his fingers, as the blind read braille.

SENSATION PRIOR TO BIRTH

The proximity sense organs and the organs for receiving sensations of hearing and equilibrium mature before birth. While the capacity to see as a human being is not mature until much later, nevertheless the receptor organs which have the capacity of distinguishing light from dark are mature quite some time before birth. The opportunity for stimulation of any of these receptors is minimal in the confines of the uterus. Temperature is maintained at a constant level; the amniotic fluid cushions and dampens tactile and auditory sensation. What sensations of taste and smell there are come from the relatively unvarying amniotic fluid. Sight is not stimulated at all in the dark confines of the uterus. Therefore the majority of the sensations received by the fetus are due to equilibrium changes in the mother's body and those tactile sensations resulting from her movements, which pass in waves through the amniotic fluid. These sensations serve no useful purpose to the fetus, as far as can be detected. They do not help him adjust to the uterus; they only disturb him. The human being seems not to need his sense organs until he has emerged from the uterus.

Avery has recently published a provocative comparison of the "sensory deprived" fetus in utero with man in outer space. She comments that further study of the mechanisms whereby the neonate (full-term or premature) adapts to the rich sensory extrauterine existence may shed light on the reverse process of how adult man can adapt to a space capsule.

SENSATION IN INFANCY

The newborn can receive sensory stimulation. He is equipped at birth with mature sensory receptor organs (except for vision) which function as capably in the neonate as at any time of life (p. 263).

Sensory impulses come to the neonate through his peripheral receptors, proceed to the primary sensory ganglia and ascend to the specific nuclei in thalamus or midbrain (depending upon the nature of the stimuli), but the further neural pathways to the cortex, being unmyelinated in the neonate, carry impulses somewhat haphazardly.

The neonate feels warmth, cold, pain; he hears sounds, appreciates equilibrium changes, smells, tastes; and is aware of light and darkness. His felt sensations from any of his receptor organs are diffuse, poorly localized, and poorly differentiated. In fact, Werner suggests that stimulation of one receptor organ may be experienced by the infant in more than one sense modality; that is, a soft light may convey not only a color but a sense of warmth or even a tone. This primitive synesthesia is probably more prevalent in early infancy than later in life, although it is never completely lost. Most adults feel that some colors are warm and others cold, and many children attribute colors to numbers.

All sensation in infancy, both that experienced synesthesically and that experienced in a single sense modality, conveys to the infant a feeling tone. Even though his felt sensations are diffuse, the infant is aware of whether the experience is pleasant or unpleasant.

The infant's reaction to all sensation is global. If the sensation conveys displeasure, the infant cries and thrashes his arms and legs about; if the sensation conveys pleasure, the infant relaxes and may attempt to prolong the pleasurable feeling.

The infant gains no awareness of objects in the external world from his sensations. At this time of life there is no distinction between "in here" and "out there." The infant has no awareness of himself as an entity in a world of objects.

The human infant can do little to bring pleasant sensations to himself nor to get rid of unpleasant ones. He can, however, express his feelings and thereby let his mother know how he feels.

Newborns not only wish to be relieved of unpleasant sensations; they want pleasant ones. It was Freud's view that pleasure for the neonate consisted only in the removal of displeasure and that once this was accomplished, the infant would return to a state of quietude resembling that of the womb. In recent years evidence seems to point to the fact that even very young infants appear to turn toward pleasurable sensations and attempt to prolong them (Schachtel, 1959). An infant snuggles his body next to his mother, obviously enjoying the tactile sensation; if rocking or singing cease, he wiggles and whimpers, asking, with the only techniques available to him, to have these sensations continued.

Sensation in the mouth is particularly acute in early infancy (Spitz, 1945). It is not only the organ for taking in food, but it is the area wherein lie sensitive tactile and gustatory receptors, stimulation of which appears to give the infant much contentment.

All of the young infant's sensation is directed toward how he feels and is therefore egocentric. However, this term is really a misnomer when applied to a neonate who has no conception of his own unique identity. He and his world are to him one amorphous gob of sensation, some good, which he would like to hang on to, some bad, which he would like to get rid of.

As maturity advances a step or two, the infant becomes able to appreciate the differences in quality of sensation. He can distinguish between smooth and rough, between soft and hard (he could feel these textures earlier, but their only impact on him was whether or not he liked the sensation). At this stage in maturation, motor control has advanced to the point where the infant has some voluntary ability. He uses his muscles to bring as much pleasant sensory stimulation as possible within reach of his receptors. As soon as his hands become manageable, he uses them to gain sensations. He also uses his hands to put objects into his mouth, where he can make use of his sensitive oral receptors. In early infancy the mouth seems to convey as much as the hand. An infant mouths as well as handles. In fact the infant uses all the equipment he can possibly bring to bear. He uses his hand to scratch the starched sheet on which he lies, listening to the sound, feeling the substance under his finger. He strokes the satin binding on his blanket, squeezes his rubber toy. He not only uses his hands, but he examines with his eyes, listens to whatever makes a sound, explores with his mouth, tastes and smells everything he can bring within his reach. This is sensorimotor play (p. 490).

Toward the end of the first year of life, the infant begins to grasp the concept that objects can exist even when he cannot see them. It is then that he will peer over the edge of his crib to look for a dropped toy. At this age, the pleasure he received earlier from all-over body feelings is beginning to wane. He wants now to explore with eyes and ears and with the tactile receptors in his hands and in his mouth. As he experiences a greater and greater variety of sensations, he sharpens up his focus on "in here" and "out there." By the end of infancy, the child is fairly clear about where *he* ends and *it* begins. Sensation is now unequivocally egocentric, since now he is beginning to have an *I*. Sensorimotor play and its inherent discipline (p. 490) becomes what Piaget calls "sensorimotor intelligence" and what Myklebust calls an "inner language." It precedes vocal language, and enables the infant to establish himself among the objects about him. Objects have become detached from the infant's own actions and have begun to exist for him as elements of his environment—an environment in which he too is an object. Thus the infant has learned that his body is an object among many others, all of which have some permanence. He knows that things do not cease to exist just because he cannot see them. He can now include mother in the permanent objects of his universe, provided his sense of basic trust is maturing with reasonable competence. This is a big step from the neonate's vague amorphous awareness created solely by his own sensory impressions.

SENSATION AND AUTONOMY

Once the baby begins to accept the fact that there is an *I* within him, he begins to try to establish mastery over that *I*. He enters the ego stage of autonomy (p. 356). Much is made of his need to control his body at this stage, to make it do what he wants it to do. But it must not be forgotten that to feel is as important as to do. The toddler uses his muscular powers not only to perform physical feats but also to bring into his range ever new sensory feelings.

As the toddler grows into a preschooler, his egocentricity begins to merge into a greater degree of world-centered sensation. Speech is becoming more mature. The child talks less to himself now. He begins to listen with greater understanding to what is said to him. Eventually he comprehends that there are not only *things* in the world with which he must cope but there are also *thoughts* of other people which produce feelings in himself. With the concept that thoughts (which one cannot sense with any sense organ) exist in others dawns the notion that he too has thoughts that can give him feelings. He is entering the realm of imagination (p. 493). He is beginning to get beyond the immediate physical experiences to the world where ideas as well as objects and sensations are important. This is what Piaget calls the stage of "egocentric thought."

Throughout the toddler and the preschool years, children thrive in an environment which supplies rich opportunity for sensory experience combined with warm adult interest in their activities. Toys that give scope to the imagination, books and people to read them aloud, trips about the community, contact with people outside the family—all contribute to the richness of sensory perceptions.

WORLD-CENTERED PERCEPTION DURING THE SCHOOL YEARS

When the school years are reached, the child, who has succeeded so far in establishing a reasonably competent ego turns his full attention to the world outside himself. He now wants to know about everything. It is at this age that he begins to learn to read, at least in our culture. The ability to read opens wide the door of learning. The discovery that all those little marks on a printed page can convey ideas and stories can fill a child with

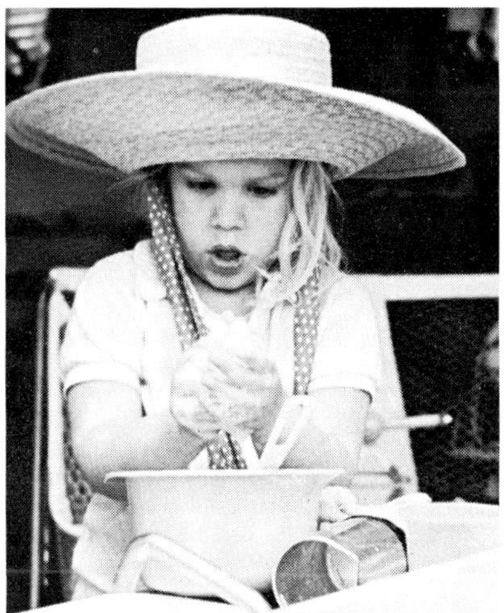

The feel of soap

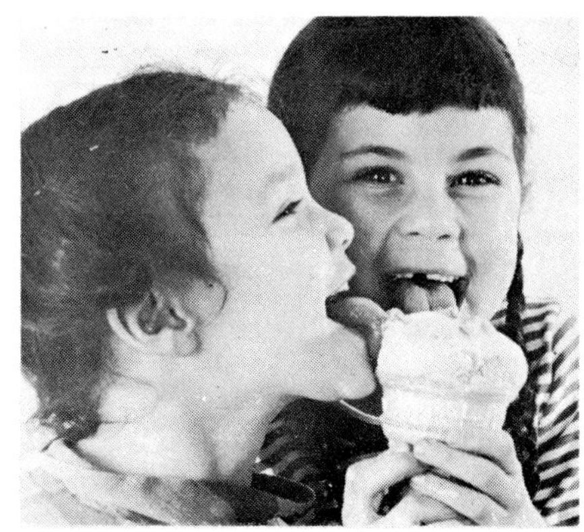

Taste is a special pleasure

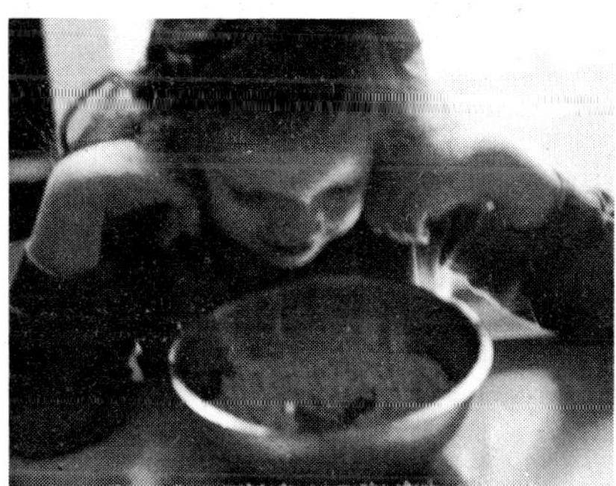

The smell of things to come

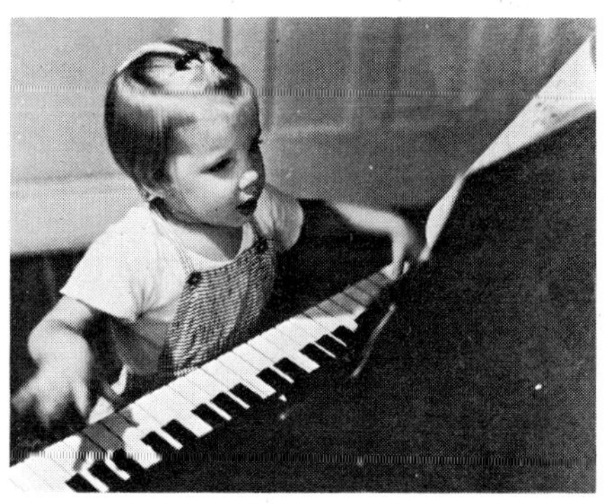

Photograph by Robert Wood

Absorption in sound

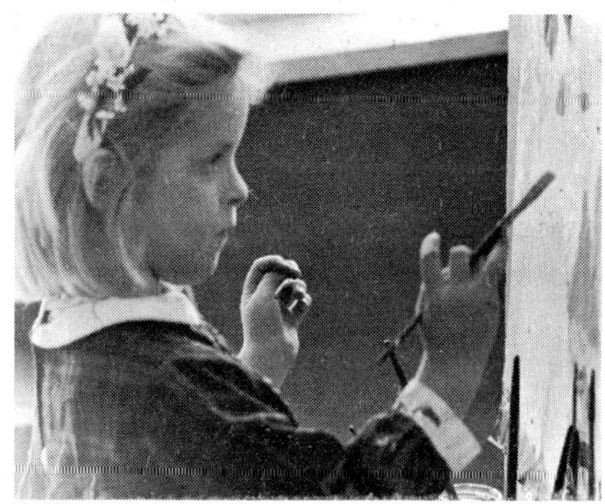

The look of paint

Fig. 34-1. Experiencing the senses.

the excitement of discovery. Now he wants to know for the pleasure of knowing, not for the pleasure of a sensory experience. With the ability to read, world-centered sensation crescendos. There have been many preliminaries in the earlier years, but now the child's enthusiasm is as unbounded as was his enthusiasm to feel a few years back. He wants to know, not only through the printed page and through talk, but also with his hands. This is the age when children want not only to take things apart but also to put them together. Earlier, taking apart was destructive; now, the taking apart is to learn how a thing works, the putting together to try out his skills.

Early in the school years, children come to grips with the problem of relativity. What is an object? Is it what he sees, feels, hears, when he stands in the middle of a room? Is it what he senses when he looks down on it from the top of the stairs? Is it the desirable object of play, or the dirty nuisance his mother calls it? The realization that it is all these things and perhaps many more all at the same time is an amazing idea. When a youngster can grasp this idea, he has progressed a long way from his infantile notion that an object ceased to exist when he could not see it. He now conceives of an object as having permanence, a permanence that is the same even though it looks different when seen from different perspectives and even when seen by different people.

When a child can conceive of this sort of relativity, he is capable of understanding logical relations between objects and even between people. His thought can now be world-centered as well as egocentric.

With the acquisition of the capacity to understand logical relations combined with the ability to read, the child has the tools at his disposal for exploring his world. He wants to talk, to read, to experiment, which adds up to the fact that he wants to learn.

Throughout child development, the emotional climate in which the child lives can either foster or thwart the march of events. The youngster who in the earliest years was able to establish a reasonable trust in his world is sufficiently free from anxiety to have time and energy to explore his sensory powers; later, if he is convinced of his own basic worth, his desire to know is not consumed in fruitless efforts to prove that he is what he is not, and he can use all his drive to find out what is to be known in the world about him. The more the excitement of his discoveries is met with interest and tolerance from his significant adults, the more his drive to continue his education is enhanced.

THE SENSORY–DEPRIVED CHILD

A child (or an adult) deprived of any or all contact with the environment has problems. These problems are enormous if the deprivation occurs in infancy before ego functions necessary to evaluate the world have been formed. Emotional problems arise at any time of life that sensory stimulation is reduced. Needless to say, the greater the loss, whether it be in a single receptor or in several, the greater the problems.

In infancy, sensory deprivation is basically of two kinds: One is due to organic failure of sensory receptors—as in the deaf, the blind, the amputated. In the other, deprivation is based not on organic sensory defect but on failure of the environment to supply the needed stimulation. This latter type of deprivation is spoken of as *maternal deprivation*.

Maternal Deprivation

Sensation in the neonate is closely associated with the care the infant receives from his mother. He is unable to eliminate unpleasurable sensations or prolong desirable ones by his own efforts. He can obtain an abundance of desirable experiences only by being exposed to them by his mother's ministrations. The newborn is endowed with instinctive techniques (Bowlby, 1958) with which he reaches out toward his environment. The earliest of these techniques is the cry. If no one picks up the crying infant, cuddles him, rocks him, sings to him, the infant fails to receive these pleasurable sensations. He lives in a world where what felt sensations he does receive he experiences as unpleasant. His world becomes a threatening place; to reduce its terrifying quality, the deprived infant withdraws from it as much as possible; he ceases even to reach out with his cry. When he is old enough to smile, he finds out that this technique is no more useful than his cry (Spitz and Wolf, 1946); he may try it a few times, but if it does not bring him pleasant sensations, he abandons it. As he gets a little older, he is able to bring voluntary muscular activity into operation, but, again, if his outward thrusts toward his environment are not met with maternal warmth, he does not find them satisfying and soon ceases to use them. Such an infant does not reach out with eyes and ears and hands to bring to himself what he can; rather he becomes apathetic, he lies still, he moves sluggishly when he must move, he does not smile and laugh and babble, he does not even cry; he has little urge to use his emerging powers to move out toward his environment. In the absence of use, development proceeds at a sluggish pace.

Spitz has shown that sensory-deprived institutionalized infants fail to progress at the usual tempo; they do not sit up, crawl, babble, play, or walk as do normal infants. Such children have failed so utterly in the first phase of ego development that they have established no basic trust. In addition failure to use sensory and motor powers may have caused structural and functional deterioration in the nervous system. Such deprived infants are not only unprepared for subsequent stages of ego development but may have suffered irremedial organic damage. Extreme maternal deprivation in the first year of life produces irreversible growth failure.

Hebb, working with animals, demonstrated that an impoverished sensory environment during very early life resulted in adult animals with reduced abilities to discriminate, with less taste for exploration, with decreased ability to learn from experience. Hebb also found there were critical periods for learning. Unless a puppy had adequate opportunity to obtain sensory stimulation before a certain age, irreversible changes took place. Harlow's work with monkeys has also demonstrated the essential quality of early sensory stimulation.

In the early months of life, sensory deprivation results from lack of adequate care from any competent person. The syndrome in its severe form is seldom seen except in some institutionalized infants; less extreme forms are occasionally seen in infants whose mothers (or mother substitutes) are cold, rejecting women.

Toward the end of the first year, when the infant is old enough to distinguish mother from everyone else, and up until the age of about 3 years, sensory deprivation can result if the child is separated from his mother or from some equally familiar substitute. Bowlby describes this phenomenon as one of grief. The child is so panic-stricken at the loss of his love object that he withdraws from contact and, if the separation is long, sinks into a state of apathy and may even regress and act like a child younger than his chronological age.

Separation anxiety may cause varying degrees of damage, depending upon the duration of the separation and the previous ego development of the child. The possibility that severe separation anxiety may cause permanent damage to personality is suggested by Bowlby, Spitz, and others.

Hospitalization can be a very traumatic experience for a young child if his mother is not permitted to accompany him. A child confined to a respirator or an oxygen tent needs special consideration to maintain adequate contact with his familiar world.

Sensory Deprivation from Organic Impairment

Organic sensory impairment present from birth or acquired in the first 2 years of life interferes profoundly with the development of the ego. Impairment later in life has its effects upon personality. It is, however, less difficult to maintain ego identity once it has been established than it is to develop it without adequate sensory stimulation. The great problem in the deprived infant is helping him establish and maintain a satisfactory identity. He must be provided with means of obtaining sensations with which he can define himself, with which he can communicate with other human beings, and with which he can obtain perceptions that adequately convey appreciation of the world in which he lives.

In very early life, the proximity senses dominate the infant's sensations. Organic malfunction of total body touch, of taste, and of smell is extremely rare, so that even deaf or blind children are able to manage fairly well. They can respond to cuddling, to rocking, to body warmth as normal infants can. But the time soon comes when the child who is unable to see or unable to hear or who cannot feel with his hands shows evidence of handicap. An accurate appraisal of his handicap by 6 months of age is of great help in planning for his future care. Blindness is usually suspected by the appearance of the infant—his vacant stare, his obvious failure to look. Deafness is not so easily suspected. The deaf infant's ears look like those of a hearing child. Suspicion of deafness must be aroused by the infant's behavior (p. 267). Loss of hands with which to feel is, of course, obvious.

Sensory impairment is sometimes so profound that the child has no residual function. Sometimes, however, the impairment is only partial, and efforts can be made to use what limited powers the child has—with hearing aids, with glasses, with prosthesis. Each child must be evaluated individually, but, in general, the earlier in life his limited sensory powers can be augmented, the better chance he has for normal development.

The Deaf Child

Congenital deafness is more often than not due to impairment in the inner ear, and acquired deafness is generally, though of course not always, due to impairment in the middle ear. Hearing aids are most useful when disease of the middle ear is the cause of hearing loss. Hearing aids, however, should be tried in any deaf child, since it may be possible to raise the hearing threshold to the point where speech can be understood. However, it must not be forgotten that raising the hearing threshold from say 90 to 80 db may result only in permitting the child to hear the human voice raised in angry shouts.

Deafness so profound as to interfere with hearing the human voice prevents the infant from learning to talk. Deafness produces many other disabilities. Hearing, as stated above, is a background sense constantly alerting the individual to environmental changes. Vision for the deaf child must serve the dual service of background scanning and foreground attention. The deaf child cannot concentrate for long on a visual image but must frequently look away from it and scan his surroundings to detect any changes. It is quite likely that he will discover, by frightening experiences, that his world changes suddenly. Since he cannot hear voices or approaching footsteps, he is startled by sudden appearances. The more frequently and severely he is frightened by unexpected sights, the more he concentrates his visual powers on the landscape. The deaf child becomes adept at recognizing minor visual cues at a distance; he sees changes in shadows, small movements, differences in brightness. However, so much of his normal attention is consumed in scanning his environment that he is less able than the hearing child to devote vision to exploring visual-tactile-motor experiences. Motor coordination develops more slowly in the deaf child. The deaf infant needs an abundance of whole body tactile contact to compensate for his inability to make auditory contact with his adults.

Deaf children must be taught language through vision, tactation, or kinesthetics. The sign language of the deaf permits communication of a somewhat limited extent among those who know the technique. The sign language has a more serious drawback: it is not the kind of introduction to language which will permit the learning of reading and writing. These skills are predicated on the ability to use the symbols of the spoken language. The sign language cannot be translated to the printed page. The deaf child must learn the symbols of auditory language before he can comprehend these symbols translated to a visual image. The deaf child must learn "auditory" language through his eyes and fingers. The technique found most useful for this purpose is what is called speech reading. It needs to be started by the time a child is 16 months to 2 years of age. Under favorable conditions the child gains considerable proficiency in about a year's time, and from then on he increases his vocabulary and his understanding of language as does the hearing child. Speech reading is mandatory for the deaf child, and it is often helpful for the hard-of-hearing child.

Once a deaf child has learned to understand ordinary speech and learned to talk, he is on his way toward normal development. He will, of course, have greater difficulties than the hearing child.

The importance of recognizing deafness very early in life can hardly be overemphasized (p. 269). The child who gets to school age without the ability to use language is severely and perhaps permanently damaged in his intellectual development, since he is unable to conceptualize or use symbols and has passed the critical age when these skills should have matured.

Most cities have speech and hearing clinics associated either with a children's hospital or with a general hospital with a pediatric department.[2] In such a clinic a child's hearing can be tested to determine whether or not a hearing aid will benefit him.

The Blind Child

A child totally blind from birth develops no visual imagery. He does not live in total darkness, because darkness itself is a visual quality with which he has no experience. (Lowenfeld, 1950). It is impossible for the seeing person to imagine the world of the congenitally blind person. The seeing person can shut his eyes, but he does not shut out all past experience with vision. An individual who becomes blind later in life retains a visual frame of reference; he can feel an object and immediately form a visual image of it, but the child who has never seen can have no concept of the *look* of an object. His understanding of the world must come from other forms of sensation.

The basic limitations of the blind child are in relation to his range of experiences. This poses problems in his ability to comprehend himself in a

[2] The John Tracy Clinic, 806 West Adams Boulevard, Los Angeles, California, has compiled a correspondence course for parents of deafened preschool children.

world of objects, in his ability to comprehend these objects, and in his ability to exercise control over himself, things, and people.

The blind child must rely on hearing and tactation, but there is much that these sensations cannot convey. A sound cannot give any conception of shape and size and physical characteristics. A blind child can hear a cat meow, and if he can feel the cat, he can obtain some conception of what a cat is, but he cannot feel a bird when he hears him sing, and he cannot feel the branches of a tree crackling in the wind. Many visual experiences are utterly closed to the blind child. He can have no comprehension of clouds in the sky, of buildings down the street, of mountains in the distance. He cannot conceive of perspective or of reflection. Not only objects in the distance but many of the little things close at hand are out of the experience of the blind child. He may experience the sting of a mosquito bite, but he cannot get much impression of a mosquito by touching it.

Blind children can learn to talk and to understand speech. In the beginning of speech, the blind child learns word symbols for those objects he comprehends through sound, smell, taste and tactation. These words have meaning for him, but what can *butterfly, cloud, mountain* mean to a blind child? How can he comprehend *blue, yellow, green?* Many words are meaningless symbols to a child deprived of visual imagery.

The blind child is restricted in his mental orientation to the world about him. He is also restricted in his ability to move about. In a familiar setting, the blind child learns many cues of avoiding obstacles, but he is at a great disadvantage in an unfamiliar environment. He remains more dependent than the seeing child, a dependence which may extend beyond mere locomotion. The blind child is in need of considerable encouragement to take over as much responsibility as possible.

Like the deaf child, the blind child may have many frightening experiences as he discovers that hearing is not adequate to monitor his environment. Since he cannot see approaching objects, he may be hit or injured without warning. The more he is frightened by such experiences, the more he is likely to develop timidity and fail to reach out to explore what he can of his environment.

The blind infant does not have the same incentive as the seeing child to reach out to his environment. Sounds and smells are a poor substitute for vision. Since he cannot copy the actions of others, he is apt to be slow in acquiring behavior patterns. Some retardation is to be expected in posture control, in crawling, in walking, in the manipulation of objects in play. While the blind child does learn to talk, he does not use gestures or facial expressions.

Infants blind from birth are of course not immediately aware of their handicap, but that they are different becomes borne in upon them. A blind child, who knows well his mother's voice, hears her, from across the room, make some comment about what he is doing, most frequently a "No, no." Slowly it dawns on the child that mother has a mysterious power over him, a power which he does not have over her. He becomes conscious of being observed. This is probably his first awareness that he is different, and it happens long before he can verbalize that he is blind. Different children react differently to being observed, but in general this phenomenon detracts from the integrity of self; it is as though the edges of the blind child were fuzzy to himself—others seem to know more about him than he knows himself.

The blind child, however, reacts emotionally as does the seeing child. A frightened child, a frustrated child (whether blind or seeing) reacts in just about the same ways. The blind child has more such experiences to cope with. In any child such experiences interfere with ego development. The blind child, therefore, has more difficulty than the seeing child in establishing trust in his world, in accomplishing mastery over himself and his environment, and much more difficulty in achieving independence (Fraiberg and Freedman, 1964).

Burlingham discussed the role of hearing in the blind child and comments on the apparent passivity of the blind child toward auditory stimuli, which she feels may represent active listening rather than indifference. The mother of a blind child needs understanding of the responses of her infant lest she misinterpret his apparent lack of response to her overtures and build up a feeling of rejection toward him.

Knowledge of how to educate the blind has increased enormously in the past couple of decades. This education, however, needs to begin before the end of the first year of life. It is not a blind child but a *whole child* who is to be educated, and that education begins when the youngster first begins to reach out toward his environment. This early education is best done in the home. It is the parents of a blind child who must learn how to interpret the world to their handicapped child (Meyer, 1950).

Parents can be aided by the resources of the community which are of course much better in some areas than in others. The National Society for the Prevention of Blindness in New York City can supply information on local facilities.

The Partially Sighted Child

Children whose vision in the better eye, after correction, is between 20/70 and 20/200 are classified as partially seeing. While such children need help to learn academic skills, their problems are quite different from those of the blind child. Partially sighted children are able to form visual imagery and therefore do not have the fundamental difficulty in conceptualizing the world that the blind child does.

Partially sighted children usually manage fairly well in a good home environment until they reach school age. Then they need special instruction, since they are unable to see adequately the materials used to teach reading to normal children. Many cities provide special classes in the regular school program. In these classes the partially sighted child learns the close skills and is able to participate with normal children in other activities. Writing is usually taught with the use of a typewriter.

Colorblindness and Tone-deafness

These are often considered minor handicaps, and obviously they do not compare in degree of seriousness with blindness and deafness. Nevertheless these qualitative sensory deficiencies can cause a child considerable emotional trauma when he realizes that he is less well endowed than his peers.

Neither of these conditions is amenable to treatment; they must be accepted for life with as much equanimity as possible. In adult life they restrict vocational choice. A colorblind person will not be a success in any of the visual arts, and a tone-deaf person makes a poor musician. The handicaps, however, are more all-pervading than choice of a vocation, since colors and tones enter into much of daily life. Awareness of the problems in early life, compensatory activities and interests, and above all protection from ridicule can help a child accept himself as he is.

The Child without Hands

Tactation in the hands is an important part of man's armamentarium for discovering and comprehending the world. Man fingers and handles, as well as looks and listens, to understand.

Several cities in the United States provide services for child amputees. The Michigan Child Amputee Service is the oldest, having started its clinic in 1946 (Aitken and Frantz, 1960). They have devised means of fitting prosthesis to children as young as 5 months, and Lund comments on the desirability of early use of these devices. The first prosthesis has a passive terminal device (pylon) with which the child can push. If fitted early, the child becomes acclimatized to his artificial hands and uses them during his early kinesthetic development. By 17 months of age, this passive device can be changed to an active pincer hook, which the child operates himself and with which he learns to pick up objects. Children develop amazing skills with these cleverly devised prostheses, especially when their parents can come to accept the appearance of a hook instead of a hand.

The normal infant uses his hands almost every waking moment. He pushes, pulls, bangs, shakes whatever is within reach. He uses his outstretched index finger to discover the third dimension, as Gesell puts it. He picks up big things and, later, minute ones. He discovers the feel of his surroundings; he learns about texture and form and shape; he finds out what his fingers feel like in his mouth. Later those same hands are essential in the manipulation of objects. An enormous number of skills are manual.

However, no device, no matter how adequate its mechanical action, can be endowed with sensory receptors. No hook can convey a sense of roughness or softness, and a hook in the mouth must feel and taste quite different from a thumb. Mechanical hands certainly aid in motor manipulation and give the child amputee the opportunity for near-normal ability to manipulate; nevertheless, many sensory experiences must be unattainable for the child without hands.

Aitken, who has had a great deal of experience with child amputees, made the following statement in a personal communication:

> We do not know at the present time what is the result of a child's inability to explore the "third dimension" as the result of congenital amputations. I feel quite certain, however, that there is not a complete absence of exploration of the "third dimension." My reason for saving this is that in the unilateral amputee the contralateral extremity is used as the mechanism of exploration. In the bilateral upper extremity amelia, the feet are used as hands. This is not something that we have to teach these children—it is something that develops in a nearly identical manner and phasing as would upper extremity function. Whether or not the sensory perception of objects by feet and the development of prehension faculties with feet alters the cerebral perception of this I do not know. In such cases it is reasonable, I believe (this cannot be documented) that the homunculus would probably be of a different shape than the one which we customarily believe is a standard pattern for normal people. Whether or not tactation of the feet in these cases is a reasonable substitution for that same function of normal hands, I do not know either. I do know, though, that bilateral upper extremity amelias become so adept with their feet that they can pick up coins, brush their teeth, take the tops off tubes of toothpaste and replace them, feed themselves, shuffle and deal cards and write.

The Children's Bureau in the U.S. Department of Health, Education, and Welfare, through its Crippled Children's Services, is aiding the states in establishing amputee clinics in various cities and can furnish information concerning facilities now in existence.

BIBLIOGRAPHY

Aitken, George T., and Charles H. Frantz: Management of the Child Amputee, *American Academy of Orthopedic Surgeons Instructional Course Lecture,* **17**:246, 1960.

Avery, M. E.: Altered Environments: Space Medicine and Adaptation at Birth, *Pediatrics,* **35**:345, 1965.

Bowlby, John: The Nature of the Child's Tie to His Mother, *Internat. J. Psychoanalysis,* **39**:350, 1958.

———: Grief and Mourning in Infancy and Childhood, *Psychoanalyt. Study Child,* **15**:9, 1960.

Burlingham, Dorothy: Hearing and Its Role in the Development of the Blind, *Psychoanalyt. Study Child,* **19**:95, 1964.

Church, Joseph: "Language and the Discovery of Reality," Random House, Inc., New York, 1961.

COBB, STANLEY: "Foundation of Neuropsychiatry," The Williams & Wilkins Company, Baltimore, 1958.

FRAIBERG, SELMA, and DAVID A. FREEDMAN: Studies in the Ego Development of the Congenitally Blind Child, *Psychoanalyt. Study Child*, **19**:113, 1964.

FRANTZ, CHARLES H.: Child Amputees Can Be Rehabilitated, *Children*, **3**:61, 1956.

HARLOW, HARRY, and MARGARET K. HARLOW: The Effect of Rearing Conditions on Behavior, *Bull. Menninger Clin.*, **26**:213, 1962.

HEBB, D. O.: "The Organization of Behavior," John Wiley & Sons, Inc., New York, 1949.

———: Drives and the CNS (Conceptual Nervous System), *Psychol. Rev.*, **62**: 243, 1955.

———: The Mammal and His Environment, *Am. J. Psychiat.*, **111**:826, 1955.

HERON, WOODBURN: Cognitive and Physiological Effects of Perceptual Isolation, in "Sensory Deprivation," Harvard University Press, Cambridge, Mass., 1961.

LILLY, JOHN C.: Mental Effects of Reduction of Ordinary Levels of Physical Stimuli on Intact, Healthy Persons, *Psychiatric Res. Rep.*, **5**:1, 1956.

LINDSLEY, D. B., L. H. SCHREINER, W. B. KNOWLES, and H. W. MAGOUN: Behavioral and EEG Changes Following Chronic Brain Stem Lesions in the Cat, *Electroencephalog. & Clin. Neurophysiol.*, **2**:483, 1950.

LORENZ, KONRAD, and NICHOLS TIMBERGEN: Taxes and Instinct, in Claire Schiller (ed.), "Instinctive Behavior," International Universities Press, Inc., New York, 1957.

LOWENFELD, BERTHOLD: Psychological Foundation of Special Methods in Teaching Blind Children, in Paul A. Zahl (ed.), "Blindness," p. 39, Princeton University Press, Princeton, N.J., 1950.

MEYER, GEORGE F.: Education of Blind Children in Public School, in Paul A. Zahl (ed.), "Blindness," p. 109, Princeton University Press, Princeton, N.J., 1950.

MYKLEBUST, HELMER R.: "The Psychology of Deafness, Sensory Deprivation, Learning and Adjustment," Grune & Stratton, Inc., New York, 1960.

PIAGET, JEAN: "The Origins of Intelligence in Children," translated by Margaret Cook, International Universities Press, Inc., New York, 1952.

PRATT, KARL C.: The Neonate, in Leonard Carmichael, "Manual of Child Psychology," 2d ed., John Wiley & Sons, Inc., New York, 1954, p. 190.

RAMSDELL, DONALD A.: The Psychology of the Hard of Hearing and Deafened Adult, in H. Davis (ed.), "Hearing and Deafness," p. 459, Holt, Rinehart and Winston, Inc., New York, 1960.

REISON, A. H., K. L. CHOW, J. SEMMES, and H. W. NISSEN: Chimpanzee Vision after Four Conditions of Light Deprivation, *Am. Psychologist*, **6**:282, 1951.

SCHACHTEL, ERNEST G.: "Metamorphosis," Basic Books, Inc., Publishers, New York, 1959.

SPITZ, RENÉ A.: Hospitalism, An Inquiry into the Genesis of Psychiatric Conditions in Early Infancy, *Psychoanalyt. Study Child*, **1**:53, 1945.

———, and K. M. WOLF: The Smiling Response, A Contribution to the Ontogenesis of Social Relations, *Genetic Psychology Monograph*, **34**, 1946.

———: The Primal Cavity, *Psychoanalyt. Study Child*, **10**:215, 1955.

SULLIVAN, HARRY STACK: "The Interpersonal Theory of Psychiatry," W. W. Norton & Company, Inc., New York, 1953.

WERNER, HEINZ: "Comparative Psychology of Mental Development," translated by E. B. Garsiae, Harper & Row, Publishers, Incorporated, New York, 1960.

WEXLER, DONALD, JACK MENDELSON, P. HERBERT LEIDERMAN, and PHILIP SOLOMON: Sensory Deprivation, A Technique for Studying Psychiatric Aspects of Stress, *A.M.A. Arch. Neurol. Psychiat.*, **79**:225, 1958.

WIENER, NORBERT: "Cybernetics," Houghton Mifflin Company, Boston, 1948.

Section VII

HORIZONTAL PICTURES

INTRODUCTION

Human development is a drama with many actors; sometimes one, sometimes another player has the center of the stage, but in this drama no one player is ever on stage alone. The preceding sections of this book give the script of some of the players. In the present section scenes from the whole drama will be presented.

Children vary so much in so many ways that it is manifestly impossible to describe a child at a specific age and make the description applicable to all children at that age. All children, however, do pass through similar phases of development, even though each child progresses at his own tempo and with his own uniqueness. There is a recognizable quality of being a newborn, of being a 3-year-old, or of being a 10- or 20-year-old. An attempt will be made, in the descriptions to follow, to capture this quality of ageness.

Parents, too, go through stages as their children grow up. The mother of a newborn reacts to life differently from the mother of a toddler or the mother of an adolescent, and the mother of several children lives in a different environment from the mother of an only child. Since so much about a child depends upon the attitude of his parents, no picture of a child is complete without a consideration of the ways of his parents.

35

The Premature and Low-birth-weight Infant

DEFINITIONS

The normal period of gestation is approximately 40 weeks; an infant born before the thirty-seventh week is considered premature. However, since gestational age is often difficult to determine, birth weight has, for many years, been used as a criterion of prematurity. The First World Health Assembly in 1948 established an international definition of prematurity based on a birth weight of 2,500 Gm or less (5½ lbs). The arbitrary selection of weight as evidence of prematurity produces some distortions. An infant, especially if born to small parents, may be genetically a small individual and even at 5½ lb birth weight may be as mature as a term infant; contrariwise, an infant whose birth weight is over 5½ lbs, if genetically a large individual, may not have reached the maturity of a term infant. In addition infants who have been carried in utero a full 40 weeks but who have suffered growth retardation from any cause are classified as premature when weight is the criterion. Twins and other multiple-birth infants are not infrequently lighter in weight than single infants of the same gestational age.

The inadequacy of weight as a measure of prematurity has prompted the Expert Committee on Maternal and Child Health of the World Health Organization (WHO) to use the designation *low birth weight* for all infants of 2,500 Gm or less and reserve the term *premature* for infants born before the thirty-seventh week from the onset of the last menstrual period. Using gestational age as the criterion of prematurity makes a sizable number of infants fall in the *unknown* category, with respect to gestational age. As Silverman (1963) points out, the change in nomenclature does not *create* unknowns but merely gives them recognition. A clear distinction between size and age in classifying newborns has many advantages in properly assessing the newly born. The Committee on the Fetus and the Newborn of the American Academy of Pediatrics has adopted the WHO classification.

MORTALITY

Low birth weight is correlated with death during the first year of life in the United States. Infants who weigh 2,500 Gm or less at birth account for about one-third of all deaths in the first year of life (p. 20).

A great many deaths attributed to prematurity occur in the neonatal period; about one-half of such deaths take place within the first 24 hours of life and four-fifths within the first week (p. 25). The survival of a premature (given optimal care) depends upon his degree of maturity and his freedom from abnormality. While these are different factors, nevertheless, survival is closely correlated with birth weight. Holt and McIntosh give the following figures for survival of low-birth-weight infants given optimal care:

Birth weight, Gm	Survival, per cent
2,001–2,500	90
1,501–2,000	80
1,001–1,500	50
Less than 1,000	10

Births before the end of the normal period of gestation or birth of an unusually small infant are sometimes due to a pathologic condition in the mother and sometimes to aberrations in development of the fetus; not infrequently both factors contribute to early termination of pregnancy.

Among maternal factors may be mentioned disorders of the genital tract (placenta previa, premature separation of the placenta, pelvic deformities); disorders related to the state of pregnancy (the toxemias); chronic illness in the mother (chronic nephritis, heart disease, tuberculosis, syphilis, malnutrition); some acute illnesses in the mother (German measles, possibly other viral infections); drugs taken by the mother. Some of these maternal conditions may interfere with placental circulation; others may permit the transfer of noxious agents to the fetus (p. 64).

Among fetal factors contributing to prematurity or low birth weight are congenital abnormalities, some of which may be due to defective genes, some to defective intrauterine conditions, some to other events.

If adverse conditions have caused aberrations in development of the fetus, it is possible that his body has been put together in such a way that independent existence is impossible. His failure to survive is basically due to pathologic development, and such an infant might not survive even if carried to term. On the other hand, some prematures have developed normally during their brief intrauterine stay; they suffer from immaturity, not from abnormality. For survival to be possible the fetus must possess the structures and have reached a degree of maturity such that he can carry on his own vital life processes. Before the sixth month of gestation this is almost never possible, but after the sixth month, when the fetus weighs about 1½ lb, survival is possible for some infants.

NEONATAL CARE

Care of the mother during labor is a factor in the ability of an immature infant to survive. Since anesthetic and analgesic drugs tend to suppress the infant's immature respiratory system, these drugs should be given the mother only in minimal doses.

Immediately after the birth of a premature, if the cord is left unclamped until it stops pulsating, the infant receives the advantage of the blood contained in the placenta (p. 177).

Resuscitation of a small infant who does not breathe immediately is similar to that used for the larger infant. Excessive care must be exercised not to injure the delicate respiratory apparatus (p. 77).

Once respiration has been established, the immediate care of the low-birth-weight infant is characterized by conservatism. He is placed in a heated crib and handled as little as possible. The initial examination must be gentle but thorough enough to detect gross abnormality, cyanosis, jaundice, or edema. It should be as rapid as possible in order to reduce the chilling effect of exposure to a room temperature considerably below that of the uterus (Parmelee, 1959).

Temperature and humidity of the incubator are adjusted to help the infant maintain his body temperature with a minimal tax upon his metabolic processes (Adams et al., 1964). The immature infant is under a double handicap with respect to thermoregulation: (1) he is unable to increase his heat production by shivering when his body temperature falls, and (2) he is unable to sweat to increase his heat loss when his body temperature rises.

Thermoregulation in the newborn is maintained largely by chemical means (Day, 1963). The metabolic rate increases when additional heat is needed (Bruck, 1961). Such a waste of energy for thermogenesis may put an undue strain upon the immature mechanisms of very small infants and may be responsible for the higher mortality of chilled premature infants (Silverman, 1958).

Silverman's (1964) recent work suggests that 89°F is the optimal incubator temperature for small infants, rather than the 80 to 84°F previously recommended. The same investigator (Silverman, 1964) found that high humidity in the incubator had little beneficial effect other than that of maintaining body temperature. High humidity carries the added hazard of infection through contamination of the water used to produce the water vapor. Agate, Silverman, and Parmelee have devised a method of supplying a low-energy infrared radiation to an infant in a conventional incubator. By the use of this apparatus the infant is placed in a neutral thermal environment in which body temperature is maintained at a normal level with a minimal metabolic effort and an untaxed circulatory effort.

Oxygen is not infrequently needed for the small infant. The smallest amount of oxygen necessary to maintain normal color is the goal sought. This frequently requires constant regulation of the oxygen flow, especially in infants whose cyanosis is due to central nervous system conditions causing periodic apnea.

Oxygen in excess may cause changes in the retina leading to retrolental fibroplasia. Smith (1964) suggests that excess oxygen may cause other pathologic changes in premature infants which have not as yet been identified.

The most common signs of inadequate development within the first 24 hours of life are cyanosis, respiratory distress, jaundice, edema, and convulsions. Some pathologic conditions in the premature infant can be treated adequately; it is not to be expected that all such conditions can be remedied.

The first 24 hours of postnatal life are crucial to the young premature. During this time he must stabilize his physiologic processes. He can be helped if he is kept in an environment that does not tax his metabolic processes. He needs to be disturbed as little as possible. He needs neither food nor water. At the end of this crucial day, if the infant is breathing fairly regularly and his color is good, he has made his first big hurdle and demonstrated that he may possess a degree of maturity and sufficient freedom from abnormality to be able to maintain independent life.

The American Academy of Pediatrics has prepared a manual on the care of both full-term and premature infants, the contents of which have been endorsed by all the major organizations in this country interested in the care of the newborn. Anyone responsible for infants will find this manual an invaluable source of information.

THE PREMATURE OF 28 WEEKS' GESTATION

An infant born at about the sixth month of gestation offers a marvelous opportunity to understand what happens in the final refinements of preparation for extrauterine life.

Such an infant is small indeed. He can be held in one hand, and his forearm is no larger in diameter than the adult's thumb against which it rests. His head seems abnormally large. The infant feels loose; his head, his arms and legs flop unless held up for him. His muscle tone is poor. He is thin to the point of scrawniness; there is no subcutaneous fat over his body. The skin over his face is wrinkled and gives the look of extreme age, because of the absence of layers of fat. The skin over the abdomen may be so thin that peristalsis is visible. Lanugo hair may be present over much of the body. In the male the testes may not have descended into the scrotum; in the female the labia minora are large and thick and may protrude beyond the labia majora (Kagan, 1962).

This tiny creature will move, sometimes by himself, sometimes in response to stimulation, but the movements are sporadic, without seeming purpose, and not well sustained. The arm may start a movement, but it may stop before it gets anywhere and remain for a time in a sort of catatonic pose. Myoclonic twitchings of the muscles are frequently seen.

The young premature slips into a torpor rather than a true sleep. It is hard to distinguish between the sleeping and the waking state; he never seems to be fully awake or fully asleep (Gesell, 1945). Sometimes his cry is soundless, and sometimes a high-pitched wail comes from his vocal cords, but crying, like other activities, is not sustained for long. It seems to fade out rather than stop. His eyes move both vertically and horizontally but they do not move coordinately. He will blink if a bright light shines upon him. Similarly he will show distaste for a loud noise by a wincing of his face. He does not show a true Moro reflex (p. 387).

His breathing is often shallow and irregular with periods of rapid breathing followed by periods of apnea. The lungs of small prematures may contain areas that are incapable of expansion because of lack of development of the alveolar buds and poor muscle tone. In addition pulmonary function may be interfered with because of inadequate development of capillaries around the alveoli.

Capillary inadequacy may exist in other parts of the premature, as well. The respiratory center may have a poor supply of blood and therefore be sluggish in responding to changes in oxygen level. Immature capillaries in the liver and kidney or throughout the whole organism may contribute to failure of function. Not only is the vascular network immature quantitatively, but the vessel walls are so thin and fragile that hemorrhage takes place easily. Intracranial hemorrhages are frequently found at the postmortem table in prematures who fail to survive. An additional factor predisposing to serious hemorrhage in prematures is the low level of prothrombin in the blood, which means that blood clots slowly and tiny breaks in the capillary walls permit the blood to seep into adjacent tissue. The vascular tree completes its development late in pregnancy, and therefore it is not infrequently too immature to permit adequate function in prematurely born infants.

The heart, on the other hand, is formed early in prenatal life, and unless its basic development is abnormal, it seldom creates problems due to immaturity.

The kidney matures early in prenatal life; it is usually reasonably competent in the premature. It is, however, unable to stand stress. The immature kidney has scant power to concentrate urine and therefore is unable to conserve water in time of dehydration. It cannot handle electrolytes in concentrations much removed from physiologic balance. For these reasons diarrhea is catastrophic in the premature.

The small premature is unable to suck, partly because he lacks the fat pads in his cheeks that facilitate sucking but more importantly because the reflex neural pathways upon which sucking depend have not matured. Even swallowing may be imperfectly developed; he may be able to swallow liquid if it is dropped into his mouth, but he seems quite indifferent about it, and his swallowing cannot be relied upon as a feeding method. He is not much interested in eating; he does not wake up and cry vigorously for food; he does not seem to be bothered internally by hunger pains. He must be fed by gavage. He is slightly aroused when so fed but may doze off in his characteristic torpor in the middle of a feeding.

At the end of his first crucial 24 hours he can be given small amounts of water or 5 per cent glucose by a polyethylene catheter passed through one nostril into the lower esophagus. This catheter can be left in place for several days and the infant fed through it at intervals without disturbing him or removing him from his incubator.

The gastrointestinal tract of the premature exhibits its immaturity by its inability to handle some dietary ingredients and by the speed with which food is propelled from mouth to anus (p. 188). The premature tends to react to many kinds of stress by developing diarrhea, which further complicates his fragile equilibrium. In the first week of postnatal life the young premature's requirement for food is low, his metabolic rate is low, his muscle tone is poor, he does not move very much. However, once his vital organs are stabilized, he begins to grow, and then his need for food becomes large (p. 340).

He grows at the rate he would have maintained had he remained in utero; this is a rate faster than that of the normal full-term infant (p. 108). To maintain this rapid growth the premature needs more calories per pound of body weight than the full-term infant; however, the premature has a smaller gastric capacity than does the full-term infant; therefore he must have a more concentrated food. For these reasons unmodified breast milk is not the best food for the premature. He can handle protein and mono- and disaccharides fairly well, but fats, especially saturated fats, are poorly used, and polysaccharides are not adequately digested. The most satisfactory food for the premature consists of a milk mixture fortified by the addition of extra protein and the substitution of unsaturated fats for saturated fats. Several such products are available (p. 340).

If the young premature has sufficient maturity to maintain his breathing and is free from developmental aberrations, he may survive and complete his development in his incubator as satisfactorily as though he remained in his mother's uterus. He does not need handling and fondling; he does much better if left alone as much as possible, left alone to mature as he was doing when interrupted by being born. He has not yet matured to the point where he can respond to social contacts. If he survives—and the limiting factor is usually his respiration—in a month's time he will have made considerable strides in maturation.

THE PREMATURE OF 32 WEEKS' GESTATION

A 32-week-old fetus presents about the same picture whether he is just born or has already been breathing air for a month. The month's difference in maturity has produced much change. This premature is about twice as big as he was a month earlier. He weighs about 3½ to 4 lb, no mean achievement in a month's time. He has more subcutaneous fat, though not yet as much as the full-term infant. He looks thin rather than scrawny.

He has developed the fat pads in his cheeks and can suck with considerable vigor. When food is offered, he will suck with interest but may tire before his nutritional needs are met. The balance of the food may have to be given by gavage.

He is more interested in the world. His muscle tone is better developed; he moves as though he means it, though he still cannot sustain much movement. When stimulated by a blow on the mattress near where he is lying, he now responds with a full-bloom Moro reflex (p. 387). He can cry when disturbed and will thus announce that he is hungry. His cry is apt to be thin and not long continued. Unlike the very early premature this child probably has a few satisfactions such as food satiety, warmth, perhaps stretching. He may suffer frustration and annoyance if these satisfactions are not forthcoming, but he does not show any need for social contact.

This premature is remarkably more alert than he was a month earlier, but compared with what he will be a month hence, he seems an unfinished, drowsy, distant little creature. As soon as he is able to maintain his body temperature fairly well, he can graduate first to a heated crib and finally to a regular crib. He is usually ready for home care when he reaches 5½ lbs. This is, however, an arbitrary figure, and under favorable conditions some infants can be sent home at lower body weights.

THE PARENTS OF THE PREMATURE

No human baby, not even a premature, lives in a social vacuum. All human babies have parents. The premature, however, needs his physical organism cared for by trained and skillful professionals with the aid of good modern equipment. Until he is mature enough for home care, he has no need for his parents and is quite oblivious of their existence. But the premature's parents cannot spend the incubator weeks in emotional hibernation. The mother of a premature feels anxious, sometimes guilty. She may blame herself for his early birth, or sometimes her husband may blame her. They want to know: Will he live? Will he be all right? What can they do for him now? How must he be cared for later?

The mother, and her husband too, need sympathy and understanding explanations. There is always doubt whether or not a tiny premature will survive, and dishonest optimism does not allay anxiety or remove guilt. Fear is real and must be faced squarely. But the parents can be brought in on the team, told just as much as they are able to understand. When they can be made to feel that they are sharing the responsibilities, some of their anxiety can be channeled toward a positive interest in each new development, instead of an amorphous dread of each new moment.

When the mother goes home from the hospital, a daily phone call can do wonders for her, combined with a firm promise to call immediately regardless of the hour of day or night if any untoward development takes place. She is still on the team and, if things are going well, it is hoped that she is beginning to lose her anxiety.

Eventually, when the baby finally reaches a degree of maturity such that home care is suitable for him, this mother needs to be able to take over the care of her baby as a normal mother free from fear, free from anxiety. He needs to be treated as the normal baby he is, not overprotected and unduly swamped with agitation and anxiety. The baby's chance for ultimate happiness will be greatly improved if there can be as much success in bringing the parents through the incubator stage as in bringing the baby through.

BIBLIOGRAPHY

ADAMS, FORREST N., TETSURO FUJIWARA, ROBERT SPEARS, and JOAN HODGMAN: Gaseous Metabolism in Premature Infants at 32–34°C Temperature, *Pediatrics,* **33**:75, 1964.

AGATE, FREDERIC J., JR., and WILLIAM A. SILVERMAN: The Control of Body Temperature in the Small Newborn Infant by Low Energy Infra-red Radiation, *Pediatrics,* **31**:725, 1963.

BRUCK, KURT: Temperature Regulation in the Newborn Infant, *Biol. Neonatorum,* **3**:65, 1961.

DAY, RICHARD L.: Maintenance of Body Temperature of Premature Infants, *Pediatrics,* **31**:717, 1963.

GESELL, ARNOLD: "The Embryology of Behavior," The Beginnings of the Human Mind, Harper & Row, Publishers, Incorporated, New York, 1945.

HOLT, L. EMMETT, and RUSTIN McINTOSH: "Pediatrics," Appleton-Century-Crofts, Inc., New York, 1953.

KAGAN, B. M.: The Premature Infant, in Joseph Brennemann (ed.), "Practice of Pediatrics," vol. 1, 1962, p.43.

PARMELEE, ARTHUR HAWLEY: "Management of the Newborn," 2d ed., The Year Book Medical Publishers, Inc., Chicago, 1959.

SILVERMAN, WILLIAM A.: "Dunham's Premature Infants," 3d ed., Paul B. Hoeber, Inc., New York, 1961.

———, JOHN W. FERTIG, and AGNES P. BERGER: The Influence of the Thermal Environment upon Survival of Newly Born Premature Infants, *Pediatrics,* **22**:876, 1958.

———, FREDERIC J. AGATE, JR., and JOHN W. FERTIG: A Sequential Trial of the Nonthermal Effects of Atmospheric Humidity on Survival of Newborn Infants of Low Birth Weight, *Pediatrics,* **31**:719, 1963.

———: Use and Misuse of Temperature and Humidity in Care of the Newborn Infant, *Pediatrics,* **33**:276, 1964.

———: Low Birth Weight, *Pediatrics,* **32**:791, 1963.

SMITH, CLEMENT A.: Use and Misuse of Oxygen in Treatment of Prematures, *Pediatrics,* **33**:111, 1964.

"Standards and Recommendations for Hospital Care of Newborn Infants, Full Term and Premature," American Academy of Pediatrics, 1964.

36

The Infant

THE FULL–TERM INFANT

The full-term infant presents quite a different picture from the little creature who has been pushed out into the world only partly equipped to cope with the problems of independent existence. The last months of gestation do much to prepare an infant for the hazards of living outside the uterus.

The Newborn

The full-term baby is chubby. In the last month of gestation large amounts of adipose tissue have been laid down under his skin and around his internal organs, and he will keep on gaining fat in the next few months. The fat pads in his cheeks are well developed. They are larger and firmer now than they were a month ago, although they do not seem as prominent, because now there is subcutaneous fat all over his face. His arms are rounded, there is fat over his abdomen, his rump is plump, and even his legs have their quota of fat below the skin. He may even show creases in his buttocks and legs from the accumulation of fat. In girls there is a fat pad over the pubis.

Immediately after birth the newborn is covered with the vernix caseosa, which dries in an hour or so and leaves a chalky velvety covering over the entire skin. This material has some bactericidal qualities, and no attempt should be made to remove it. After a few days the vernix wears off.

The skin is thin and translucent. The reddish color of the newborn is due to the glow from blood coursing through superficial capillaries. Flat irregular hemangioma are frequently observed over the eyes, across the bridge of the nose, and in the occipital region. They disappear within a month or so.

In the lumbosacral region there are often irregular areas of bluish or brownish pigmentation, which disappears in later infancy. Occasionally these pigmented areas are found over the scrotum, on the buttocks, or on the thighs. They are more frequent in the Oriental race than in the Caucasian.

Many but not all newborns have a considerable amount of dark coarse hair on the scalp and also elsewhere on the body, especially in the lumbar regions of the back. Most of the coarse hair is lost, and there may be a period of baldness on the scalp before the true hair comes in.

The genitals of the newborn appear large. In males the testes are usually in the scrotum. Hydrocele is frequent, and unless there is so much fluid that it might cause pressure on the testicle, it can be ignored. It will disappear in a week or so. Phimosis is almost universal in the newborn male.

In girls there is frequently a thin white discharge from the vagina. Occasionally the discharge is blood-tinged. The breasts of either male or female may enlarge within the first few days of life and may actually secrete a milklike substance (p. 205).

The eyes may show a mild conjunctivitis due to the instillation of silver nitrate at the time of delivery. The eye muscles are not coordinated, but the pupils react to light.

Temperature regulation is considerably advanced over that of the premature although it is not yet fully mature. The full-term baby is not able to shiver or sweat (Day, 1964). Recent work suggests that the newborn has some ability to maintain thermogenesis by changes in metabolic rate (Oliver, 1964).

As soon as the infant draws his first breath, the circulation through the umbilical cord slows down and stops within a few minutes. Respiration is shallow and rapid (30 to 50 breaths per minute). It may be irregular but within a day or so establishes a regular rhythm. The oxygen level of the blood rises to about 90 per cent of normal within 3 hours. Blood pressure does not become stabilized until about 10 days of age. The heart rate of the newborn is about 150 beats per minute and usually shows considerable sinus arrhythmia, a characteristic evident through most of childhood.

In palpation of the abdomen of the newborn both liver and spleen are usually felt, and often the lower edge of the kidney, as well. Marked distention of the abdomen is suggestive of congenital obstruction of the gastrointestinal tract.

The secretions of the gastrointestinal tract, saliva and gastric, biliary, and intestinal secretions, are functioning and are adequate for the digestion of milk. Peristalsis is under fairly good control, although far from completely mature. Most of the food consumed is pushed in the right direction from mouth to anus, but not infrequently peristaltic waves go in the opposite direction, and some regurgitation takes place.

The intestinal tract contains meconium, a stringy dark-colored substance, the accumulation of "practice" efforts of the digestive glands prior to birth. It is passed by rectum during the first day or two of life and usually before the infant has started digesting food.

The full-term baby's periods of sleep and wakefulness are much more definite than those of the premature. He now definitely goes to sleep and stays asleep until some urge makes him wake up. Then he stays awake for a time.

Muscle tone is now quite well developed. The full-term baby can move his body and hold his movements; they do not fade out in midair as do those of the premature. He moves his arms and legs with vigor; he raises his head when lying on his abdomen, though he cannot balance his head on his shoulders when held erect. While his muscular activity shows much more maturity than that of the premature, nevertheless his movements are spasmodic and purposeless. He thrashes his extremities; he does not *do* anything with them. When quiet, he does not appear relaxed. His arms and legs are flexed against his body, his hands are held tightfisted. He will respond to stimulation with characteristic reflex motor patterns (p. 387).

The legs are normally bowed at birth. Asymmetry of the gluteal folds suggests dislocation of the hip. Limitation of abduction of the hip when the thighs are flexed on the abdomen also suggests dislocation of the hip. The feet of the newborn show a low arch, but the normal foot does not show valgus.

The neonate can *receive* and *feel* sensory stimuli, but his felt sensations are diffuse, poorly localized, and poorly differentiated. He is but dimly able to distinguish one type of sensation from another. He is, however, quite aware of whether a sensation is pleasant or unpleasant (p. 510). His reaction to any sensation is global. He demonstrates distress vocally and kinesthetically, and he relaxes when pleasant sensation comes to him.

While hunger is the most obvious of the unpleasant sensations with which the infant must cope, he will demonstrate his global displeasure in response to other stimuli. He does not like loud noises, bright lights, bitter tastes; he does not like to be cold or to have a pain; and, above all, he does not like a tense, nervous person.

There is a quality of being newborn which stamps a long list of characteristics on all these little people; nonetheless each of them has, in addition to the universal traits of his age, his own special unique qualities. When an adult who has had little experience with babies comes in contact for the first time with a number of newborns, he is apt to be struck by their common characteristics. After a little familiarity with babies it is not difficult to see their individuality.

Some newborns are dynamos right from the beginning. They go at life hard. Their muscles are strong and tense. Asleep, they look as though they were curled up and ready to jump. When they are hungry, their reaction is violent; they thrash around with strength and vigor, and their cry is a loud demand for immediate attention. When the nipple is forthcoming, they grab it and suck for dear life, and when they have had enough, they are through; there is no coaxing another swallow. They go to sleep with the same vigor with which they demanded food.

At the other extreme are the gentle, passive babies. Their muscles are more relaxed; they feel almost limp when picked up; and while they too cry for food, they can wait a minute. It is almost as though they said: "If you please, and when you can get around to it, I'd like some milk."

Between these extremes there are all sorts of gradations. No single description fits all newborns, any more than a single picture can be drawn of all 20-year-olds.

Babies and mothers begin reacting to each other from the first time they meet. If a dynamo of a baby has a gentle, passive mother, quite a different situation develops from that in which the qualities are reversed.

The Parents of the Newborn

Giving birth to a baby is a profound emotional experience as well as a physical ordeal. Women react to this experience in a thousand different ways. Some are euphoric, some sentimental, some depressed, some vindictive, but there is hardly a woman whose emotional equilibrium is "as usual" in the days following childbirth. It is in this charged emotional climate that a mother first meets her child. The more she understands prior to actual delivery that her emotions are apt to work overtime, the better able she is to cope with herself.

No matter how well-prepared she is (and some mothers are not prepared at all), she will have many questions about her infant and about her care of him. Awareness of her emotional instability and a sensitivity to the direction her wayward emotions are taking are essential for anyone who would guide her.

The father of a newborn is often in need of understanding. He may have been catapulted into an emotional whirlwind that leaves him anything but enthusiastic about the joys of parenthood. The girl he married may seem to have vanished, and in her place he may find a weepy, volatile creature who seems to have forgotten that he is anything more than the payer of bills and the doer of chores.

In the hospital there are nurses and doctors to help both parents, but once at home the full responsibility of the baby inevitably falls on the parents, who may feel overwhelmed by their lack of knowledge. It is to be hoped that this transitional period will not be too long and that ultimately life will calm down as the mother begins to get the feel of her new job. The adjustment will be speeded along if the young mother has confidence in some strong kindly person who will answer her questions, guide her, and simultaneously build up her confidence in herself.

In the early weeks of life the infant begins to tackle the task of developing his ego. The more he can be immersed in an environment which is free from tension and in which his call for care brings reasonably prompt and adequate attention, the more he absorbs the conception that the world about him is a good place to be.

ONE MONTH

The first month of extrauterine life is characterized by stabilization of physiologic processes. Respiration is now regular and slightly slower than at birth (p. 154). Cardiac rate is strong and slightly slower (p. 166). Kidney function is adequate; urination is involuntary and frequent. The blood count has dropped almost to the level that will be maintained through infancy (p. 179). Temperature regulation is more stable than at birth, although neither sweating nor shivering have developed. The baby looks chubbier than he did at birth because of the rapid deposition of subcutaneous fat.

The month-old baby is competent at sucking. The stomach has increased in size, so that larger volumes of milk can be taken at a time. Therefore feedings are less frequent than soon after birth; however, few month-old infants can go the night through without food. Schedules are somewhat more regular than soon after birth but far from predictable, and demand schedules are still indicated. Digestion of breast milk is adequate. There is still no starch-splitting enzyme in saliva or pancreatic secretion, so polysaccharides cannot be handled. Saturated fats are poorly digested. If breast milk is not available, cow's milk still needs modification (p. 339). Peristalsis continues to be rapid, and food is pushed quickly from mouth to anus. Stools are soft and moist, and while the frequency of defecation has decreased slightly since birth, stools are more frequent than they will be later. Peristalsis remains unstable and may reverse direction occasionally, causing vomiting.

Tears have made their appearance. Persistent tearing of one eye suggests an occlusion of the tear duct.

In the examination of a 1-month-old baby, attention needs to be paid to the growth of the head and its size compared to that of the chest. The feet and hips need special watching. Muscle tone is firmer than at birth; the infant will tighten his muscles when picked up. He still lies curled up with the head held to one side. When lying on his abdomen he can raise his head a little, but he cannot hold his head steady on his shoulders when held or propped up. All the reflexes present at birth are still in evidence.

The cortex is just beginning to come into function; voluntary behavior, while rudimentary, is becoming evident. Structures at the head end are getting their cerebral connections, and the cephalocaudal law is becoming evident.

During the infant's brief waking periods (longer now than at birth) he begins to perceive his world through his sensory apparatus. His proximity senses of touch, taste, and smell give him sensations of apparent pleasure which he gives evidence of wishing to prolong. Although his visual sense is rudimentary, he can now move his eyes coordinately and will follow a bright moving object with his eyes; however, he will not turn his head to watch it (p. 282). Hearing is better developed than sight, and the month-old baby will pay attention to sound. He will stop crying to listen to a soft sound and cry out at a loud noise. He also is sensitive to equilibrium changes and will fuss when rocking ceases, only to quiet down again when it is resumed.

When uncomfortable for any reason, his cry is violent and is accompanied by thrashing of arms and legs. His distress is still global. Even if it is due to hunger, the most frequent causes, and evidenced by rooting movements, he will quiet down momentarily when picked up and soothed. He grabs violently for the nipple with his mouth, and sucks vigorously. He demonstrates an intensity of global satisfaction as great as his global distress of a few moments before. His sucking is accompanied by throaty sounds of apparent pleasure.

Adequate weight gain is the best criterion that the infant is progressing satisfactorily. However, adequacy of weight gain has to be determined clinically; figures are as yet of little use, unless the weight is ½ lb or less above birth weight, in which case the infant is definitely undernourished. Even greater poundage may not be adequate for a specific baby. Adequate weight gains can be judged by the feel of the baby. Color should also be good. Some infants who are underfed cry a great deal, but this is not an infallible sign. Sometimes a severely undernourished infant is apathetic, and the mother reports that he is a "good" baby.

In the absence of a detectable abnormality the most frequent cause of malnutrition at 1 month of age is inadequate food. If the infant is breast-fed, a supplemental bottle is indicated; if bottle-fed, the formula recalculated and strengthened.

Excessive crying at 1 month, or earlier, may be due to a slightly inadequate food intake or to indigestion. Indigestion is rarely due to the milk fed in these days of an abundance of good milks for infants. However, occasionally an infant is intolerant of cow's milk and straightens out miraculously on one of the soybean preparations. A history of allergies in the family background suggests that allergy may be a factor.

Colic and irritable crying in spite of adequate food and a good weight gain may be due to organic immaturity (p. 193) but also are frequently related to emotional stress.

The month-old baby, like the newborn, will accept care from any comfortable arms and voice. He is quite indifferent concerning the person who cares for him, but he is extraordinarily sensitive to the quality of the care he receives. Tension or nervousness in the adult who ministers to him is perceived by the infant and so distresses him that he cannot quiet down. He may refuse to suck even if hungry.

If the baby cries a great deal, inquiry into the mother's way of life is in order. How does she feel about this baby? What is her relation with her husband? What is the state of her health? Are there financial worries or problems with in-laws? Many of these problems are difficult to solve, but helping the mother realize where her trouble lies helps her face them more constructively. Sometimes the judicious use of a little sedation to both mother and child can tide her over until the infant's physiology is more stabilized and better able to cope with moderate stress. Reassurance that the baby will not be spoiled by being rocked, if it comforts him, is often helpful. Some babies *do* cry more than others even under the best of circumstances.

Very rarely an infant at 1 month is malnourished and apathetic because of severe maternal rejection. The care the child receives is so lacking in warmth that he has already discovered that crying is of no value. He lies listlessly in his crib; he does not bother to eat enough for his physiologic needs. This state of affairs will be recognized by both the condition of the baby and the attitude of the mother. It is serious. Unless the atmosphere warms up, the prognosis for both physical and emotional health is bad. A consultation with the father is in order. It is possible that the detachment of the mother is a lifelong attitude; on the other hand, it is also possible that it is part of a temporary postpartum depression.

The human infant is endowed with innate mechanisms for survival and techniques for obtaining from his environment what he cannot obtain for himself. If his mother responds to his demands and attends to his needs as they arise, he is not subjected to long periods of panic. Before long he begins to build up a basic trust in the goodness of his world (p. 356).

TWO MONTHS

Weight gain and thereby general health still are judged clinically for the most part. A growth chart can be started, but it is too early to get an impression of a given baby's growth tempo.

A 2-month-old baby still needs holding and cuddling while he takes his milk—automatic with breast feeding but sometimes a point that needs emphasizing if the baby is bottle-fed.

A large or rapid-growing baby may need pureed food added to his diet; however, if he is content on milk alone, he needs no additions. If crying has been a problem, it begins to subside at 2 months, though it will not have disappeared.

The baby can be pushed a little into a schedule more convenient for the mother.

Most babies are smiling by 2 months, many at 1 month.

THREE MONTHS

This is the smiling age. The smile develops at about 6 weeks. In some babies it appears at a month (p. 392) of age and in a few even a little earlier, but by 3 months all babies are enchanting every passerby with a grin; many have already added a chuckle. The smile is the baby's first real social contact. He is making his way with the people who care for him. He needs love, and he is making himself lovable. He can do many other things at this age, but his smile is his 3-month tool par excellence.

By 3 months the baby and his mother have had time to adjust to each other. If the mother's care has imparted to her child warmth, love, security, the baby will be responding to her with basic trust. When he calls to her, he knows from experience that he will be made comfortable. When he hears her on the way, he can wait a minute. Such a baby is comfortable with what he is finding out. He expresses comfort by smiling and responding pleasantly to overtures made to him.

The baby who does not smile at 3 months of age has learned that fear and the anxiety it engenders come frequently. Perhaps he did smile a few times when the neuromuscular pathways matured, but he did not find it a useful activity and soon ceased doing it. At this very early age he has already begun to turn away from the world, or perhaps it would be more accurate to say he is failing to turn toward the world. It is quite likely that his gain in weight is skimpy. At 3 months this is an ominous sign (p. 394).

At 3 months eating patterns have stabilized. The baby wants his food at regular times and is capable of waiting a moment or two if his mother calls out to him that she is coming. Meals now include pureed food from a spoon as well as milk to suck (p. 371). Some 3-month babies sleep through a 12-hour night, though many need one milk feeding between supper and breakfast. The 3-month-old is awake more in the daytime and is frequently content to lie in his crib or, better, in his playpen, watching the world go by, without crying.

His motor development now permits fairly competent use of his head. When he is lying on his back, his head is usually held in the midline; it only occasionally flops to the side. He struggles to raise his head when he is on his back but is not very successful; however, when on his abdomen, he can raise his head about 90°, supporting his weight on his arms from elbow to wrist. When supported in sitting or upright position, his head is steady on his shoulders (p. 398).

When lying on his bed, the infant will clasp and unclasp his hands and spend long periods of time examining them. This is the rudiment of sensorimotor play (p. 490). Some 3-month-olds will grab for a toy, but most will not attempt this for another month or even two. The reflex grasp is now fading from the picture (p. 386), and when grabbing for an object does occur, it is a voluntary act. When the infant is able to grab, he lets go involuntarily—his hand just relaxes and the object falls. Releasing is a later accomplishment. Any object in the hand or the hand alone goes frequently to the mouth, where lips and tongue aid fingers and eyes in getting what sensations are to be had.

The eyes are better coordinated, and the infant looks at things, focusing sometimes on far objects, sometimes on near ones. At 3 months of age, neither fovea nor cone cells are developed in the retina, so sharp outlines and color probably play little part in the baby's visual awareness. The baby will follow a moving object with his eyes and turn his head to keep it in view. However, once it is out of visual range, he will make no effort to go after it with his eyes. He seems unaware that it could be found by looking over an edge or under a slight barrier. Out of sight seems to be out of existence for the 3-month-old. Hearing, however, is more mature: the baby at 3 months will turn his head in the direction of a sound.

Language development has progressed. During play the baby makes many sounds, usually guttural ones from the pharynx. The tongue and lips as yet take little part in his vocalizations.

He cries much less than previously, but he has not forgotten how and will bellow if anything is wrong.

Clinical judgment is still important in evaluation of overall progress. Figures for weight gain are beginning to be of use but are still tricky.

The 3-month-old baby is a friendly little person, ready and willing to get along with everyone. He has begun to take part in the life around him.

SEVEN MONTHS

Anxiety in strange situations is beginning to enter the picture. Up to this time the infant has responded to any reasonably comfortable and friendly person. He would quiet down on any shoulder, accept food from a variety of persons, and play with whoever came along. He has discriminated only against tense, nervous people, whom he has firmly rejected. Beginning at about 6 months and continuing well beyond the first year, the baby reacts adversely to strangers and to new situations. When confronted with the unfamiliar, the baby shows anxiety and wants to clutch his mother; hanging on to her, he seems more able to withstand the vicissitudes of life. He now knows his mother as different from everyone else, and he feels most comfortable with her. This fear of the strange and desire to cling are not a regression (as many parents seem to think). They represent a step forward in the baby's ability to distinguish mother from everyone else, and the familiar from the strange. This is a phase of development and as such must be taken seriously and coped with.

When clinging enters the picture (between 6 and 9 months), separation from mother, or from an equally familiar person, needs to be handled with great care. Separation should be brief—a matter of hours—and the substitute person should be someone with whom the baby is familiar, not someone brought in as the mother is leaving the house. A baby will often accept, reasonably well, an adult whom he sees quite often—his father, a grandmother, a baby sitter. He will prefer mother above all others, but another familiar adult will do for a time. However, the baby becomes uneasy if mother does not come back before long. A long separation from mother, especially in strange surroundings, can be devastating for a baby over 6 months of age. If a baby should need hospitalization, his mother should accompany him. When a baby is sick or hurt, he needs the comfort of his mother even more than when he is well.

When in familiar surroundings, the 7-month-old is a happy, friendly little person. He has developed many new skills. He is struggling to sit up but

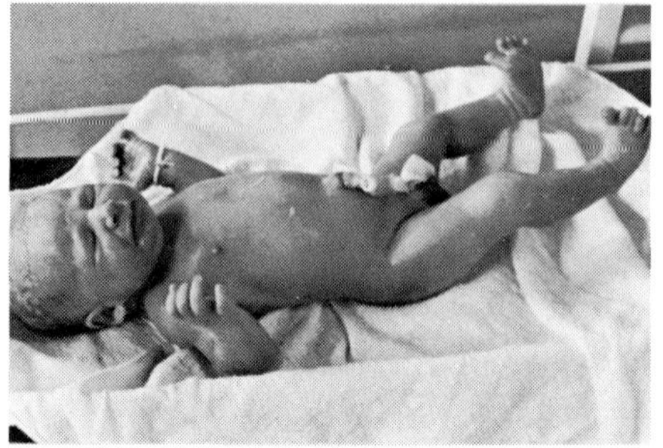

Neonate
A bundle of drives with a
will for fulfillment

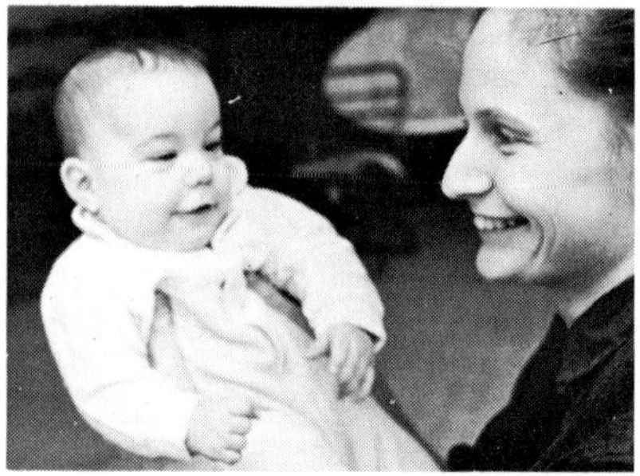

The first quarter year
smiling acceptance

Middle infancy-
everything is
inspected with
eyes and hands
and mouth

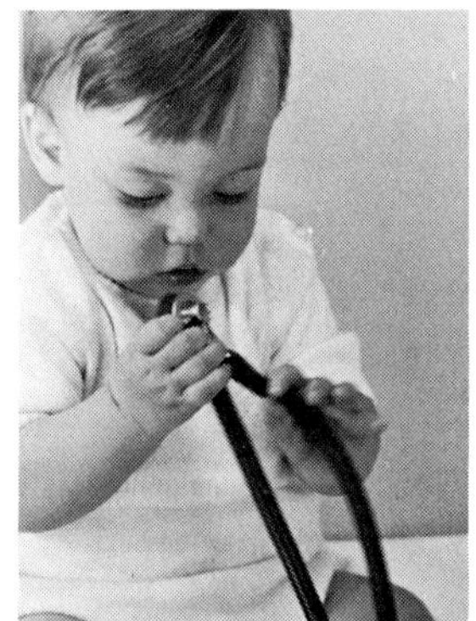

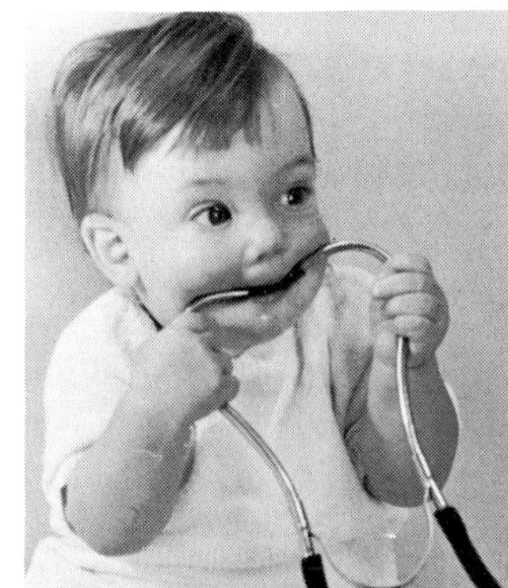

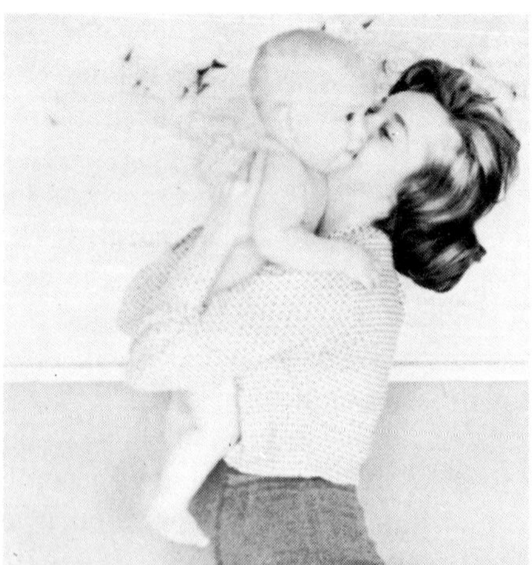

Late infancy age of anxiety

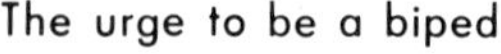

The urge to be a biped

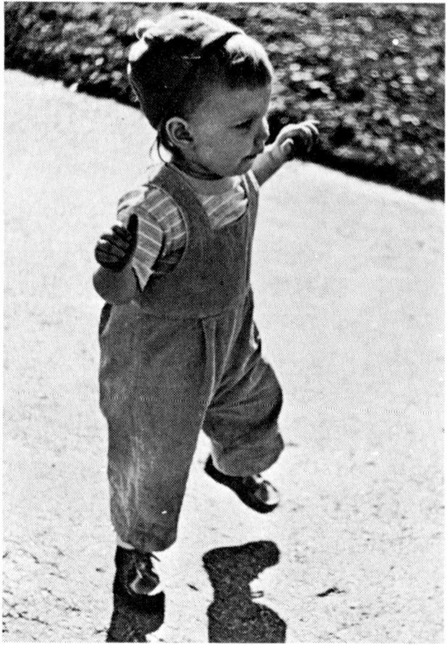

Photograph by Robert Wood

Fig. 36-1. The first year.

usually cannot quite manage it. If supported, he loves to bounce and will laugh and chortle with glee. He grabs a toy with both hands but cannot as yet put it down on purpose. He can shake a rattle; he can bang. He can transfer a toy from one hand to the other, but if an object drops out of sight, he still does not look for it. He often discovers his toes at about this age and will give them a chew now and then. He puts most things into his mouth. He is now more apt to chew them than just feel them with his mouth.

His teeth are beginning to erupt. The irritation they produce in the gums stimulates an excessive flow of saliva. When the baby is awake, this overabundant saliva drools out of his mouth. The 7-month-old is apt to be damp around the mouth and chin most of the time. When he sleeps, especially if on his back, the saliva may trickle down into his trachea and cause him to cough occasionally.

The erupting teeth stimulate the baby to bite on whatever he gets into his mouth. If he is breast-fed, he may experiment with biting his mother's nipple (p. 373). Since the infant is biting and chewing on everything, this is the appropriate time for the introduction of foods to chew (p. 372).

The 7-month-old may want to help feed himself. He is not very expert, but he is extraordinarily eager to use what skills he can muster. He cannot yet oppose thumb and forefinger. He picks up objects with a palmar grasp, so that small objects are elusive. He can grab a bone and gnaw on it. He can almost hold his own bottle if it is not too heavy. Some 7-month-olds like a few sips of water or juice from a cup, but most of them are not yet interested in cups.

Physical well-being is reflected in weight gain, and figures for weight gain are now useful. If the infant's weight is plotted on a curve, it is easy to see at a glance if he is more or less in his expected channel of growth. The mother will be interested in the chart, and it will reassure her that all is well, especially if her child is appreciably larger or smaller than the average child (p. 113).

Hearing and sight are important aspects of the 7-month-old's orientation. A hearing loss should be suspected if the baby does not respond to a loud noise either by turning his head or by crying. He should also respond to his mother's conversation and show enjoyment of singing.

Sight is easier to test than hearing. A 7-month-old baby should follow a light with his eyes and try to keep it in view by turning his head. He should reach for a toy and respond to his mother's gestures.

Vocalizations have increased in both quantity and variety. The lips and tongue are now used as well as the throat and pharynx. The infant can run through all the vowels and most of the consonants.

NINE MONTHS

Fear and anxiety in strange situations and with strange people and clinging to mother under these circumstances are more than ever in evidence. It is important for the baby's sense of self-competency that he not be subjected to long periods of panic because the familiarity of his world has disappeared. Some adult with whom the baby is familiar is a godsend to any mother. Such a person permits her a little time off, of which she is usually in considerable need.

In motor development the baby is now competent at sitting unsupported. He is able to crawl expeditiously and can get himself across a room in record time. He will object to long periods in his playpen once he has discovered the joys of free navigation. With his enlarged domain come inevitable frustrations, both from objects he bumps into and from parents who set limits on his explorations. Discipline is entering the picture (p. 490). He may be able to pull himself up to a standing position at the side of his playpen or crib.

The hands have become useful tools. The child reaches with one hand instead of both hands. He no longer uses his hand as a rake but can accurately oppose thumb and forefinger and pick up tiny articles, most of which go immediately to his mouth. He is more interested now in small objects than in large ones, and can release voluntarily. His first approach to an object is usually with outstretched index finger. He is reaching out to explore his world, through play, and he needs the opportunity to feel, touch, taste, bang, shake, pound. Eternal vigilance against the dangerous is called for.

At 9 months the baby enjoys games of give and take with an adult. The baby's enjoyment of the simple game can far outlast most adults' enthusiasm.

A 9-month-old baby will object if something is taken away from him. This is quite a step in development; he is beginning to realize that objects exist when he cannot see them. His awareness that "out there" contains real objects with an existence of their own is developing. He will now not only look over an edge for a lost article but will seek for it under a blanket or a box.

Vocalization also shows progress. The baby not only makes his own sounds, but he also is beginning to imitate sounds he hears. He plays a great deal with his voice, both by himself and when in company with a familiar adult. From time to time it is possible to distinguish what it is he is imitating. At this age his imitations are, for the most part, single syllables, or possibly two syllables strung together. They are sounds only to the baby, not words as yet. Imitation, however, is evidence that the baby hears.

It is at about 9 months that the baby will be fascinated with his own stool, should he come across it in his constant manual explorations (p. 408). It is also the time when he is likely to discover his genitals and the pleasant feeling to be obtained when he handles them. Many children of his age grab for their genitals when their diaper is being changed (p. 420).

The 9-month-old baby is ready to take an active part in feeding himself, although he is far from expert. He can pick up some articles of food in his fingers and get them fairly accurately to his mouth, but spoons and forks are difficult. Fingers are far handier tools than spoons. With ingenuity, a wide variety of foods can be so arranged that the child can pick them up and get them to his own mouth. Cereals and soft pureed foods cannot be eaten in the fingers, and this degree of messiness need not be tolerated (see Chap. 33 for discussion of discipline). He can probably hold his own bottle and may prefer to lie down by himself instead of being held in his mother's arms. He is probably interested in drinking some water or juice from the cup, but most 9-month-olds will have nothing to do with milk from a cup.

Weight gain is a fairly reliable guide to physical health, and the weight chart is a useful tool both in evaluating his progress and interpreting it to the mother. He is not gaining as rapidly now as in early infancy, and occasionally this normal phenomenon needs to be explained to a mother, lest she struggle to get more food into the child than his body needs.

THE YEARLING

Walking dominates the scene at about the first birthday. Some children have already accomplished this feat; however, most children are just on the verge. They can cruise around hanging on to an adult's finger or a piece of furniture. The desire to walk is insatiable. Nothing seems to be as important as to master the skill of being a biped. For a time all other interests are secondary, and the child frequently prostrates with fatigue and boredom the adult whose finger he wants to clutch while he walks. He is no longer pleased with his playpen except for brief periods. His new horizons bring him frustration as he learns the inevitable lessons of discipline.

When he is not practicing his pedestrian skills, he plays with small objects. He can build a tower of two blocks. He can put small things into a container and dump them out; often he prefers the dumping operation. He still explores with outstretched index finger.

Language has made real strides. He imitates much that he hears and runs his sounds together into full paragraphs, not one syllable of which is a real word. He has picked up the melody of the language he hears. He may have a few real words in addition to his jargon. Sounds that he makes mean objects that he knows. His words at this age mean specific things: "mi'k" means his bottle filled with warm milk. It has nothing to do with milk in a glass or milk spilled on the table. He is not yet capable of any verbal abstractions (p. 467).

The yearling usually likes to sit at a table for meals and take an active part in feeding himself. He is still messy but somewhat better coordinated than a month or so before. He prefers his fingers to spoons and chews small lumps in his food. He probably drinks water or juice quite competently from a cup and may even take sips of milk in this way. He probably wishes to finish his milk from a bottle and usually wants to hold it himself.

The weight at a year is roughly three times the birth weight but should be close to the child's own channel of growth.

FIFTEEN MONTHS

At about this age the thrust in development is in language. The child has already conceived the rudimentary concept of verbal symbols and is able to name a few specific objects. Now he grasps the concept of abstraction. This is an enormous hurdle in intellectual development. In our culture, his first abstraction is very apt to be "No," both the spoken word and the head-shaking semantic gesture (p. 467). Instead of using his whole body to express refusal—pushing away, kicking—he can now *say* "No." He is so fascinated with the amazing power of this word that he uses it to excess, just as a few months ago he wanted to walk to excess. This ushers in the stubborn period when the child's response to almost everything is "No." In many situations "No" is just a nice word to use, and the child will proceed to do what is expected to the tune of a repeated "No." While he has hurdled the human ability to comprehend an abstraction, he has to refine his understanding and limit the categories to which "no" applies.

The 15-month-old has progressed with motor development. He is now mobile on his own two legs, though clumsy. His hands are efficient tools; he can reach and grab. He gets into everything and is ceaselessly active. Discipline is entering with a vengeance (p. 490).

In eating, the child is taking the big hurdle of graduating away from sucking milk to drinking from the cup. Some children give up the bottle for good at or before 15 months, but many are anxious to hang on to the comforting sucking, especially at bedtime, for some time to come (p. 374).

The 15-month-old is verging on toddlerhood, and many of the phenomena discussed under that heading are beginning to apply.

RECAPITULATION OF THE PERIOD OF INFANCY

At the end of infancy the criteria for general well-being are:

1. Physical growth within the channel characteristic of the individual child.

2. Freedom from signs of chronic disease, though there may have been episodes of acute infections of the respiratory tract, of the gastrointestinal tract, perhaps skin infections.

3. Motor activity. The normal child is busy every waking moment. He walks, runs, skips, and jumps, though he may be clumsy and falls frequently. He uses his hands with a prehensile grip and is eager to handle and mouth everything within reach. His attention span is short, and he flits from one thing to another.

4. He has begun to use the language of his parents.

5. He is cheerful, laughs, smiles, jabbers constantly, cries relatively little.

The following are danger signals at the end of infancy:

1. Inadequate growth, poor muscle tone, droopy posture, poor color, fatigue, listlessness, and irritability. All these are indications that there is some interference with the physical organism.

2. Apathy. A child who lies still or sits without doing anything, who smiles relatively little, who does not jabber, who is unresponsive to familiar people needs a careful investigation into both his physical well-being and the emotional climate in which he lives.

3. Excessive thumb sucking, handling of genitals, head banging, crib rocking. Most children engage in one or more of these activities occasionally, especially if fatigued, temporarily frightened, or just bored. These activities become pathologic if engaged in so constantly that they interfere with normal play.

BIBLIOGRAPHY

Day, Richard L.. Thermoregulation of the Newly Born, in S. G. Thompson (ed.), Supplement 2 to Reports of Ross Conference on Pediatric Research, Ross Laboratories, Columbus, 1964.

Oliver, Thomas K., Jr.: Thermoregulation of the Newly Born, in S. G. Thompson (ed.), Supplement 2 to Reports of Ross Conference on Pediatric Research, Ross Laboratories, Columbus, 1964.

37

The Toddler

The time between 18 months and about 3 years constitutes the period of toddlerhood.

PHYSICAL HEALTH

Weight gain is slow but steady. Growth levels off during this period, and food consumption is correspondingly small. This is the age when parents are apt to complain that the child has a "picky" appetite.

Physiologic processes have achieved considerable stability. The child can withstand minor stress without becoming physically ill. His gastrointestinal tract is reasonably mature. He can digest adequately almost everything normally consumed by adults. He is not too competent in managing reflex control of swallowing and breathing, so that hard substances, such as nuts, may be aspirated instead of swallowed. He may also aspirate nonfood items he puts into his mouth, such as small toys, coins, beads, stones. Eternal vigilance to keep such items, as well as medications, away from him is mandatory for his safety. Stools have decreased to once or twice a day, and he is not as vulnerable to diarrhea as he once was. He is able to concentrate his urine, and therefore dehydration is no longer the ever-present danger it once was.

Infections are frequently a problem, especially infections of the respiratory tract. The child has built up but little immunity and succumbs to many pathogenic agents. It is a mistake to oversterilize his environment, to try too hard to isolate him. The contact with other children does him more good than the occasional cold does him harm. On the other hand, moderation in this respect is valuable. Crowded stores (especially at Christmas time) and movies are places where children pick up many infections, some of which may be serious.

GENERAL BEHAVIOR

Toddlerhood is the period of "Me do it," or the period of autonomy. The child is becoming aware of himself as an independent person, but he is a long way from having a concept of self as such-and-such a sort of person with known limitations and abilities. His self becomes real to him only as he tests out his powers. If he has developed a fair degree of basic trust, he wants to explore his own capacities. He wants to act *his* way, he objects to being told this is right and that is wrong. He wants to find out for and by himself. While the toddler appears to feel omnipotent, he nevertheless becomes aware of the many things he cannot do. He tries the impossible, becomes angry, and may burst out in a temper tantrum, or he may revert to babyhood and suck his thumb or want to be cuddled or carried. Once reassured of his safe place in the world, he is off again on his explorations. Not only does the toddler want to act, but also he wants to feel—to test out his capacities in this area as in all others. He seeks the good feelings—competence, triumph, pleasure—but he also seems to seek bad feelings—anger, hate, hostility. Sometimes feelings are mere by-products of his attempts at the impossible, but there seem to be times when they are actually ends in themselves.

He needs latitude to explore, to make mistakes, to find out for himself, within the framework of adult love and acceptance and of prohibition, as well. It is only as the child can accept both the good and the bad in his self that his respect for, and love of, this self matures. There will be angry outbursts of temper, occasional regressions—these are part of learning one's way around. They will be incorporated into the total worthwhile self if the general attitude is loving and accepting and gently firm. It is only constant criticism and reproach which dampens the child's enthusiasm and instills a feeling of worthlessness.

MOTOR ACTIVITY

The toddler not only has mastered walking, but he can run and jump, sidle backward, hop. However, he is often clumsy and unsure of himself; he falls easily and frequently. His legs are short; in early toddlerhood, he is often encumbered with bulky diapers. In spite of his limitations, he trots around incessantly, pulling, hauling, shoving. He lugs chairs, tables, toys, big blocks or boards, everything he can lay his hands on that is not nailed down, not to get them anywhere but just for the joy of doing. He may gravely carry a spoon to his Daddy tucked between upper arm and chest as though it weighed many pounds. He loves to pull things around on a string and may become furious when they get caught. Everything the toddler spies suggests a use to him, and there is no delay in acting on the impulse. Out on a walk, a low wall must be clambered onto and walked along, a big piece of pipe must be crawled through; at home, an open door must be closed, a closed one opened. The toddler is very distractable. He flits from one thing to another. If he bumps into a hammer lying on the floor, he is quite likely to stop, pick it up, and hammer on anything handy before he goes on.

PLAY

While almost everything the toddler does is a form of play—a finding out about the world and about himself, these are the years when imaginative make-believe occupies a large part of his waking life. He is forever copying what he sees, acting and feeling as he imagines other things and people feel (p. 493). Toddlers do not play much with other children, even though they enjoy being in company with their age-mates.

LANGUAGE

In the beginning of toddlerhood language is just becoming a useful tool. The child has the concept that sounds have symbol value, he has grasped the idea of abstraction. He can talk instead of expressing his feelings and notions with motor activity. He still does use his body to let the world and himself know how he feels, but he is becoming more and more adept at putting ideas and feelings into words. He still uses "No" to excess. "No" is a powerful and often emotionally charged word, the cause of much conflict with parents (p. 467). While the toddler can talk in whole sentences and use the syntax of his native language, nevertheless, his use of language reflects his immaturity. He talks to conceptualize the world to himself, and he is often quite indifferent about his audience. As toddlerhood advances, he begins, more and more, to use language maturely and to communicate his ideas to other people (p. 471).

EATING

The toddler's desire for "Me do it" is nowhere more evident than at mealtimes. When he comes to the family table, he must begin to conform to family patterns both in relation to the foods eaten and with respect to table manners. Failure to appreciate the toddler's total needs in relation to eating is the cause of ever-recurring problems in our society (p. 375).

TOILET TRAINING

Often one of the real problems of this age is persuading the child that the bathroom is the place to deposit his urine and stools (Chap. 30). In Freudian literature the central theme of this age is considered to revolve around the child's need for autonomy with respect to the holding on and letting go of his feces. It is therefore often spoken of as the anal stage of development. While the establishment of culturally acceptable toilet habits is certainly an essential part of the toddler's need to understand and control his body, it is certainly not the only way (perhaps not even the most important way) his dominant interest in autonomy manifests itself.

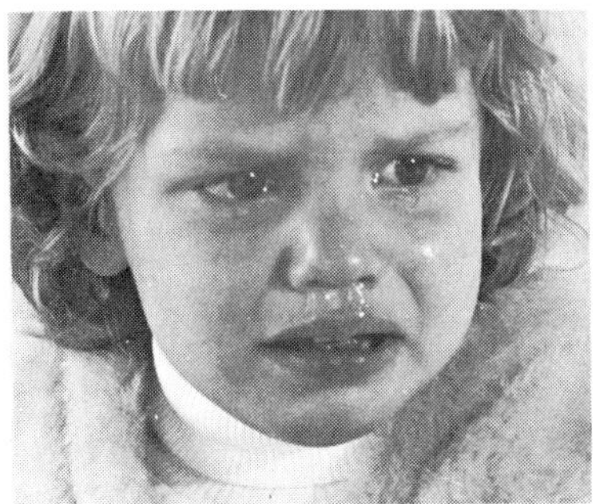

Respiratory infections are at an all time high

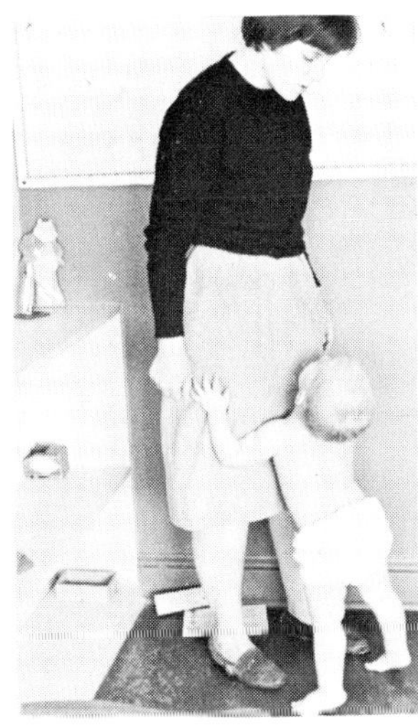

Constantly underfoot

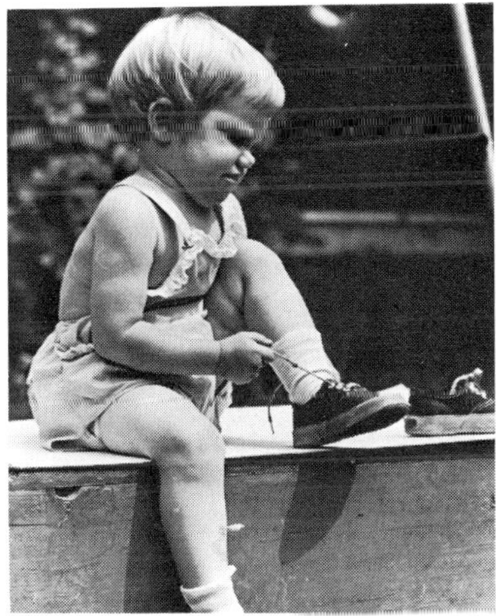

Photograph by Robert Wood

"Me do it by myself"

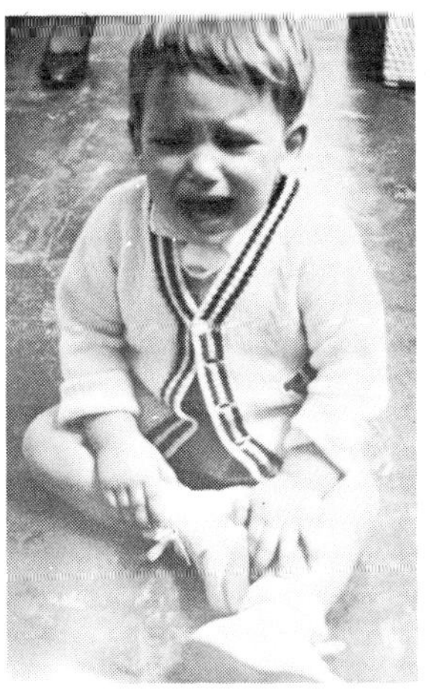

Age of tantrums

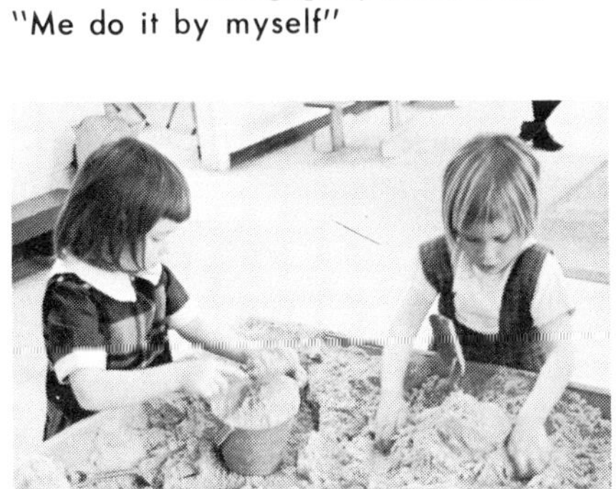

Parallel play
Toddlers enjoy playing near but not with each other

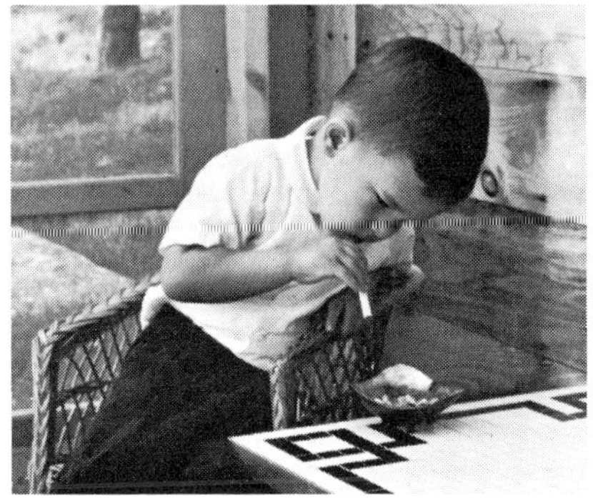

Play imitates any activity

Fig. 37-1. The toddler.

THE HANDLING OF THE TODDLER

The toddler's judgment is inadequate; he cannot distinguish the safe from the dangerous, and he has no concept of the values of material goods. He may have little concept of the feelings of others and may hurt pets or other children as well as adults, not because he is naturally sadistic, but simply because he is not yet aware that other people feel as he does. His ceaseless activity and genius for discovering new uses for the most unlikely articles mean that he must be under supervision at all times.

A constant succession of "No," "Don't, "Stop" is not the answer. There are a few basic principles in dealing with a toddler, some of which have been mentioned elsewhere (p. 495) but which may be reiterated. An awareness of what to expect in developmental trends is essential so that a child is not jumped on for behavior which is normal and expected or held up to standards of performance which for him are quite impossible—table manners, sitting politely still when there is company. He needs freedom to act as a normal toddler acts. Insofar as possible prohibited acts should be made impossible. The objective is not so much restraint of the child's activity as channeling it into acceptable ways. For a few years the first editions, the valuable bric-a-brac need to be out of reach so that prohibitions can be reduced to a minimum. Some prohibitions are essential, but a child can accept some if not every move is met with an angry reprimand. Ideal discipline is consistent and free from anger (p. 497). A toddler is not mature enough to understand all the reasons why he cannot do such-and-such. It is a waste of time to try to explain why an electric outlet is dangerous or why the dials of the hi-fi cannot be monkeyed with. "You cannot do it because I say so" is adequate. Too many explanations give a little child a handle for delaying necessary conformity. "Why can't I?" or just "Why?" become burdensome and useless.

Transitions from one activity to another are best made gradually to give the child time to get used to what is to come next. "When you finish that picture, it will be time for lunch" rather than an abrupt "Come to lunch."

The mother of a toddler needs a mature self-confidence to enable her to carry through what she started and not give in because the child puts up a fuss. Toddlers often want the impossible, and it must be denied them, even when the denial makes them angry.

There are times when a screaming, kicking child just has to be carried where he must go. If the parent can carry through these inevitable turmoils of toddlerhood without becoming angry, she is likely to have fewer of them to cope with than if she resorts to childish behavior herself.

Toddlerhood is full of prohibitions. It is impossible for a child to live through these years without frequent frustrations. Hopefully he can be taught that some things are forbidden, but it is too much to ask that he will not get angry at the limitations put on his free behavior. The mother must learn to accept the child's angry outbursts without being herself hurt (physically or emotionally). The child needs to know that he is loved in spite of his bad feelings.

SEPARATION ANXIETY

As long as the toddler is in a familiar and comfortable environment and mother is nearby, he is full of curiosity and trots around in ceaseless activity, but the toddler has not developed enough self-confidence to depend upon himself alone except for brief periods. He frequently must reassure himself that mother's all-pervading protection is ever-present. The more firmly he has established basic trust during infancy, the longer he can permit his mother out of sight and still be confident that she will return. It is a devastating experience for a child in early toddlerhood or even in late infancy to be playing contentedly with his back to his mother and suddenly find that she has slipped away when he was not looking. When he turns and discovers his aloneness, which he was not prepared for, his confidence is shattered. He comes to feel he must keep his eyes on his mother constantly or she will disappear. On the other hand, if he is told she is leaving the room but will be back soon, the toddler with reasonable trust can accept her temporary absence, knowing full well that she can be counted on to return.

Even the most secure of toddlers needs to "Go see Mommy" frequently. The more secure his basic trust, the longer he can manage by himself. However, if the toddler finds himself in a strange situation, especially if he sees in it something threatening, he not only needs to "see Mommy," but he also needs to clutch whatever part of her he can reach. He will move right along with her if she tries to walk away. This is the following pattern described by Bowlby (p. 396). It is a slightly more mature version of the clinging pattern seen in late infancy. Like the clinging pattern, the following pattern needs to be accepted. Without his mother's protection the child is unable to establish confidence in himself, but with it he ultimately becomes so convinced that he is protected and secure that he can withstand longer and longer periods of dependence on himself alone.

An interesting corollary of the following pattern, as pointed out by Bowlby, is the child's ability to find a substitute for the security of his mother in some article he totes around with him. The toddler may be devoted to the same old dirty blanket he loved as an infant, or he may pick a new object, a teddy bear, or a pillow. Such a cherished object is enormously important to the child; its familiarity gives him comfort that his world has constancy. This is a security he needs when frustrated, especially if it is his mother who has imposed some discipline. At the moment he may feel too hostile toward his mother to get satisfaction by clutching her. He may find his totem comforting at bedtime, when by the dictates of our culture he is supposed to sleep in his own bed alone.

Separation from Mother during toddlerhood, as in late infancy, needs to be handled with care. A substitute for the mother needs to be a person with whom the child is familiar. A toddler left suddenly with strange people for any appreciable length of time suffers first anxiety, then grief, and finally apathy. This does not mean that parents of a toddler can never go away on a trip without the child, but it does mean that a toddler cannot be dumped suddenly on relatives without serious repercussions to his security. For a hospital stay it is most desirable that the mother be with her child.

THE MOTHER OF THE TODDLER

Toddlerhood is a difficult time for the mother. The child is at home all day—he is too young for nursery school. Every waking minute he must be under supervision. He is so distractible that it is not safe to assume he will stay at any one activity more than a moment or two. His mood swings are rapid and as unpredictable as his behavior. He is very dependent upon his mother. Many, many times a day he has to "Go see Mommy." His insistent demands for "Me do it" make routine procedures, like dressing, bathing, eating, interminably slow. The young mother has her housework to do; perhaps she has other children who also need her care. It is quite understandable that she should become fatigued, irritated, and desperately in need of some adult company now and then. Her fatigue and irritability are often reflected in her child by emotional outbursts on his part, which only add to her state of despair.

Sympathetic understanding of her predicament can, at times, give her a great moral boost. Toddlerhood does not last forever. The suggestion that a little money spent on a familiar baby sitter so that she can get away from the child for short periods may be so welcome that she can do it without feeling guilty about using limited family resources just for herself.

DANGER SIGNALS IN TODDLERHOOD

The normal toddler is an active, distractible, busy little person, cheerful, talkative, affectionate, constantly under foot, and in need of 24-hour vigilant care. Some tantrums, some thumb sucking, some generally bad behavior are normal and expected.

A serious sign of trouble in a toddler is being "too good." A child who sits quietly for long periods doing nothing or engaged in some ritualist motor behavior, such as stirring a bucket of sand or pounding with hand or toy, is not acting like a normal toddler. He may stand at the edge of a group of children, with thumb in mouth or hand on genitals, but neither plays by himself nor enters the group's activities. Such a child moves sluggishly; his voice is flat and toneless. His speech may show the same ritualist repetition as his motor behavior. He seldom smiles at people, though he may smile occasionally at things. He is not affectionate, and in fact appears to withdraw from contact with people. While such a child is relatively little trouble to care for, his development is not progressing normally. These are danger signals of early childhood schizophrenia and need expert care quickly.

Occasionally a toddler who has not progressed as well as he might is overactive. He acts as though he were constantly on a hot griddle. His voice is loud and shrill. His movements are jerky; he is overly aggressive. His hits, bangs, kicks to an excessive degree. He may have night terrors (p. 317), and he probably has an excessive number of tantrums when thwarted. He too needs expert care as soon as possible.

38

The Preschool Child

The preschool years begin roughly at age 3 and end when the child is ready for first grade, usually at about 6.

PHYSICAL HEALTH

Gain in weight and height continue to be slow but steady. A child whose growth continues to follow his individual pattern meets the first prerequisite of physical well-being (p. 110). Failure of expected growth calls for investigation. The failure may be due to chronic physical illness or too long-standing emotional problems. Acute illness may cause temporary cessation of normal growth, but once health is restored, growth jumps back on its normal course.

Total well-being includes good posture (p. 236), adequate muscle strength, good color, and good nourishment, all of which are usually, but not always, reflected in total growth. Hearing (p. 269) and vision (p. 282) must be adequate for the child to pass muster as a healthy physical specimen.

The body of the child changes shape as he enters the preschool years (p. 120). He loses much of his baby fat, his legs lengthen, he grows taller and appears more slender than the toddler. His earlier clumsiness disappears, and he becomes a lithe, graceful little child who no longer views the world from the bottom side of things. He can go up and down stairs by alternating feet, instead of by the one-foot performance of the toddler. He can hold his spoon instead of clutching it. All his motor skills have increased; he is more dexterous with his whole body.

The main health problem in the preschool years is infection. This is the age of maximum susceptibility. It may be that the toddler is even more susceptible, but his environment is usually more home-bound, so he does not come in contact with quite so many pathologic agents as does the slightly older preschooler, who ventures forth into the neighborhood and may go to nursery school. At all events the preschool years are the time infections are at their peak, especially infections of the respiratory tract (p. 11). If each respiratory infection is treated seriously and the child given optimal care, he will live through this period without developing the serious complications that all too frequently follow in the wake of a neglected minor cold.

GENERAL BEHAVIOR

Many of the problems of toddlerhood fade away during the next 3 years. The child's body is better organized, he is less distractible, he is less mother-bound, and his mood swings are not so sudden or so violent. His activities have gained a greater purposefulness. Instead of just lugging things around, the preschool child begins to build with his blocks. He no longer picks up a hammer just to pound; he hammers a nail into a piece of wood and later will nail pieces of wood together with an eye to the finished product. He makes castles in the sand instead of just digging and sifting sand. His scrawls and scribbles are beginning to take on form and color.

The preschool child is becoming much more adept with people. He is learning that mother and the members of his immediate family are not the only trustworthy members of the race. He can form a relation with a teacher or with a neighbor and feel secure and comfortable without mother or some well-known person. The following pattern is subsiding. He is also relating to children in a new way. As a toddler, he enjoyed the company of his age-mates, although paradoxically he ignored them for the most part. Parallel play is now giving way to cooperative play. Groups of children work together on a single project. Imaginative make believe and now symbolic play (p. 495) occupy a large share of the preschool child's time.

Language is becoming a more useful tool. Instead of banging another child over the head when he gets in the way, verbal abuse is coming to the fore. Language is used as an accompaniment to play, and while the preschool child is more capable than the toddler of keeping some thoughts to himself, nevertheless he verbalizes much of what goes on in his head. His flights of fancy are often confused with reality. Imagination and dreams seem as real to him as the things he can touch. A 5-year-old may object to sleeping in his bed where the bad dream is. These are the years of imaginary companions who become so real to the child that such a "friend" must have a chair at the dinner table, must be greeted and patted and lived with by the whole family. Such a companion has a name and personality. Though usually a child, the companion may be an animal or even an adult. Imaginary companions are usually pleasant people to have around, but occasionally they are quite the reverse and scold and terrify their creator.

GENITAL INTEREST

During the preschool years children become interested in their genitals (p. 427), and their talk about their bodies and bathroom activities is woven

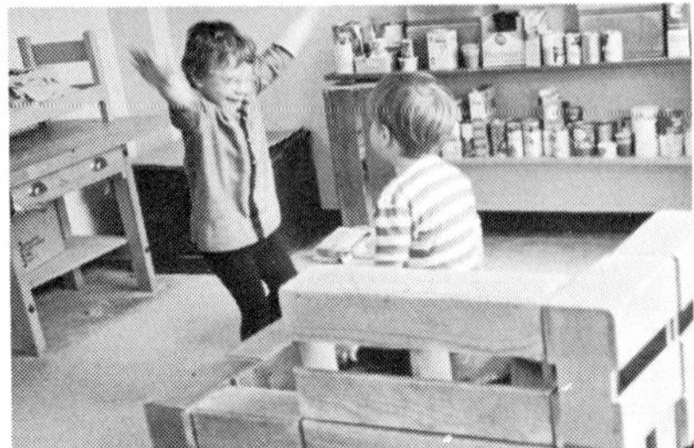

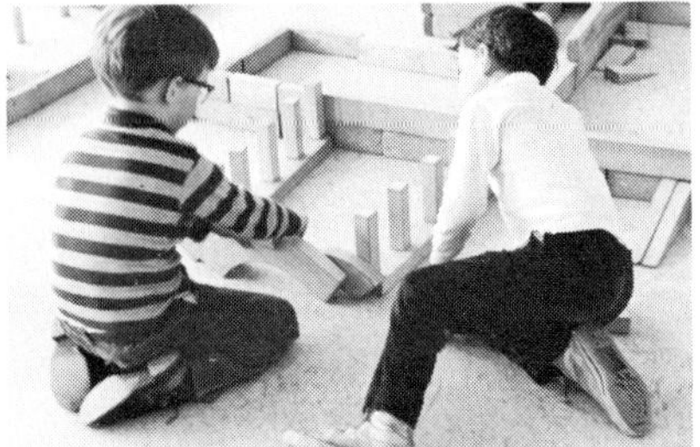

Cooperative Play
In this age group children work out elaborate projects together

Preschoolers understand adult roles by being and feeling like their model

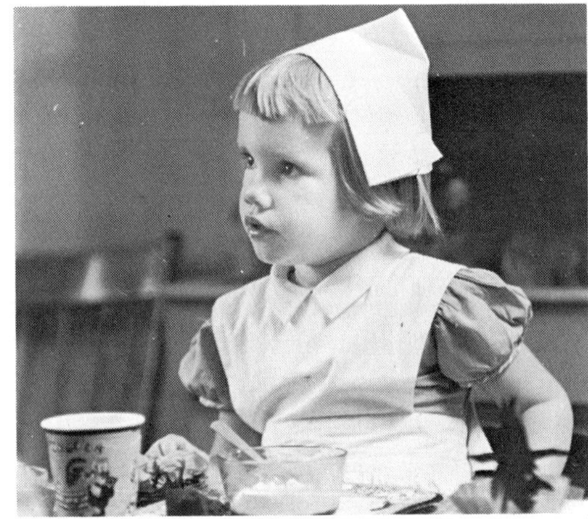

Photograph by Robert Wood

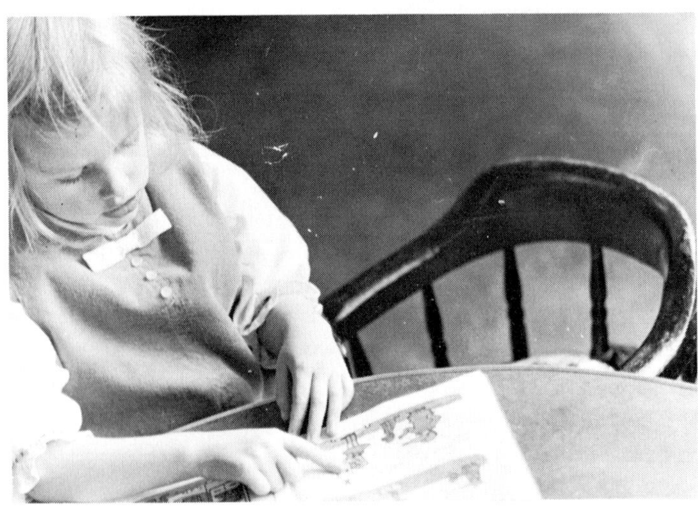

An imaginery companion

Fig. 38-1. The preschooler.

into much of their play. This is the age when castration fears develop in some children. Occasionally excessive belligerence, especially in boys, may be a castration fear (p. 428).

Although in Freudian literature this age is spoken of as the genital stage and interest in the genitals is assumed to dominate the development of the preschooler, in our present culture this is debatable. The little child is busy sharpening his concept of what kind of person he is. His gender is important, but so too are his muscular skills, his language, his ability to exercise his independence.

Toward the middle of the preschool years many children become involved in the oedipal situation, in which they desire the exclusive love of some one person (p. 429).

THE FIRST TENTATIVE BREAK FROM HOME

During the preschool years the child begins to experiment with separation from his mother and the home circle. Play in a friend's house or perhaps a meal in someone else's house without mother give him the feeling that he can be safe on his own. Longer visits to familiar grandparents or old friends aid in a slow but progressive accustoming of the little child to separation from home and family.

The break from home must be in easy stages. A preschooler suddenly dumped into an unfamiliar situation, especially with people he does not know, is apt to be deeply disturbed. A preschooler who needs hospitalization should be accompanied by his mother.

NURSERY SCHOOL

A good nursery school can be of great benefit to a little child, especially if he has already experimented with brief sojourns away from home. The regularity of leaving home every morning, of developing friends and interests outside the family circle and away from his mother helps him establish confidence in himself.

A good nursery school, however, is not a parking place for children where they are kept safe and busy and out of their mothers' hair. A nursery school is an educational institution—as much so, in the fundamental sense, as a university. It is tailored to the growth and educational needs of its students. A good school provides creative toys and encourages imaginative exploration. The children are taken on short trips in the neighborhood where they see and experience the broader life of the community. They have the opportunity to relate to age-mates and to teachers. The nursery school teacher is trained in the ways of children. She spends her full time during school hours with the children (unlike their mothers, who have but half an ear and eye on them as they try to carry on their household activities).

Nursery school experience, short trips away from home, with or without the family, help prepare the child for the school years ahead. The child who has spent all his preschool years within the close confines of home may undergo much emotional turmoil when he suddenly has to enter first grade.

39

The School-age Child

The school age is the period of elementary school life, roughly from 6 to 12 years of age. Physiologically, it begins with the shedding of the deciduous teeth and ends with the growth spurt of early puberty.

PHYSICAL HEALTH

During the middle years, growth in weight and height is slower than in the earlier years and slower than it will be in the years immediately ahead. Between the ages of 6 and 12 children gain between 1 and 2 ft in height and roughly double their weight. The type of body build is now fairly clear, and height/weight figures can be compared with standards (p. 110). Physical growth is a useful guide in estimating health. A child whose growth pattern is going along more or less in its expected channel usually has a body that is functioning adequately. Deviations from expected growth may be the first indication that something is amiss. Growth failure calls for a complete appraisal of the child. Organic disease can be of infinite variety and should be searched for assiduously. Occasionally organic malfunction is due to inadequate nutrition, lack of sleep, or inadequate physical exercise. It can be due to emotional stress.

Height, weight, and bone age can be used also to predict, with reasonable accuracy, the time of appearance of puberty and the ultimate height that will be attained (p. 112). This information is often useful in helping both parents and child accept the child's own pattern of growth. It is especially valuable for fringe children (p. 128) to understand why they are different from their peers.

Physical health is usually good during the school years. Infections decrease in frequency as greater immunity develops. Specific problems arise with certain children, but there are no overall health problems during these years.

Vision and hearing need to be checked periodically. Impairments in these sensory functions can affect the child's personality development and can be the cause of school problems.

PERSONALITY DEVELOPMENT

The thrust in personality development that takes place during the middle years has two aspects: one is directed toward attaining some independence from parental protection, and the other is directed toward intellectual growth. They are simultaneous, and each affects the other.

At the onset of the school years the child has lived through the first three phases of ego development (p. 355), during which time egocentricity has dominated the picture. The little child has been concerned almost entirely with his own feelings; he has defined the world only in its relation to himself. By so doing, he has achieved, by the time he enters the school years, confidence in his own basic worth. He has a concept of who and what he is and is ready to turn his attention outside himself. The egocentricity of the early years slowly fades, though never completely, and makes way for the development of world-centered interests (p. 506). Secure with his own solid little self the child ventures forth into a larger world, establishes an image of himself distinct from that of his home identity, and at the same time turns his attention toward things outside himself. It is important to understand that it is not the chronological age of 6, the loss of the front teeth, or the entrance into first grade that truly usher in the developmental phase of the middle years. It is rather a degree of maturity such that the child is able to get his mind off himself and put it to use absorbing human culture. The stage of development can be characterized by the ability of the child to pass from "how *I* feel" to "what *it* is."

At the beginning of the school years the child's independence is tentative, his knowledge meager. He has roughly 6 years to organize his human qualities before he will be in the turmoil of puberty and the problems of full maturity.

The human child has several techniques at his disposal for the personality development scheduled during the middle years. His motor development helps him acquire skills which give him a feeling of competence (p. 402). His sexual development contributes to his relations with people and especially to a buddy of his own age and sex (p. 433). His play gives him security and knowledge and helps him acquire cultural values. His sensory development permits speech and reading and the acquisition of further knowledge (p. 475). All these lines of development weave themselves together and make possible the solution of the tasks of this age period. Throughout the school years the attitude of the home can be of enormous assistance in helping the child achieve his goal.

Independence

While traveling the path of human development, the child is pushed from within to be independent. Even if he is well prepared for this phase,

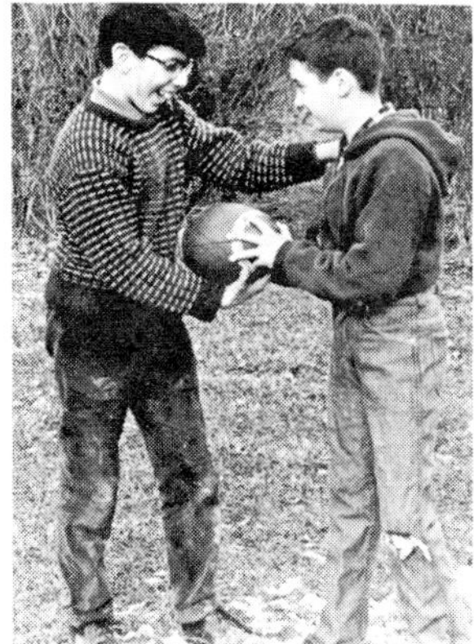

Buddies
Dirty, dishelved
and inseperable

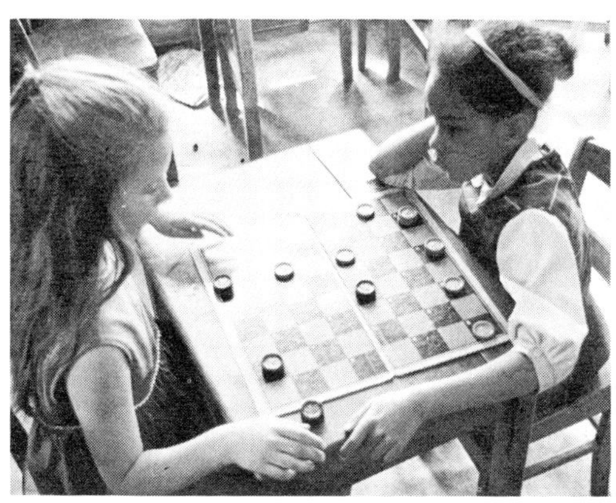

Girl friends-devoted to each other

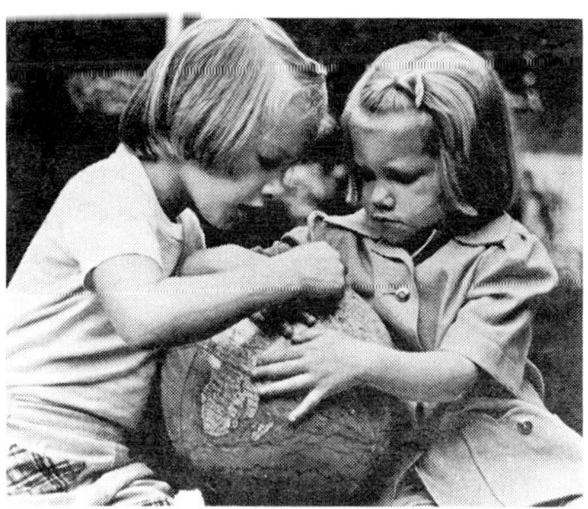

Photograph by Robert Wood
The urge to know

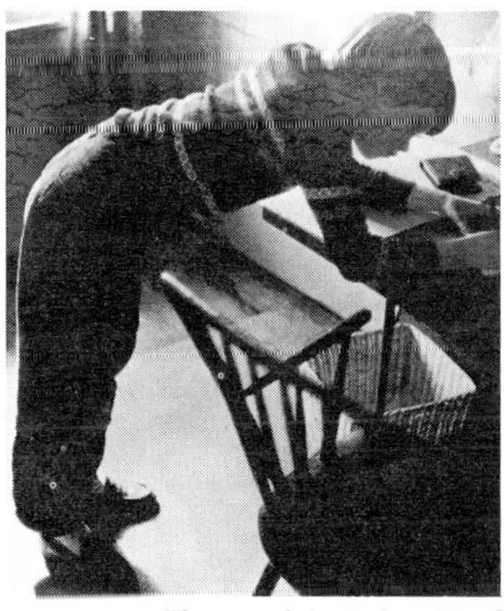

Photograph by Robert Wood
Secret societies flourish

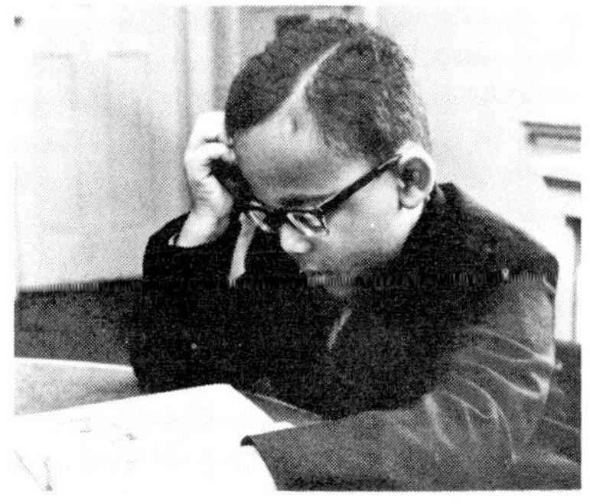

Reading is a big part
of the school years

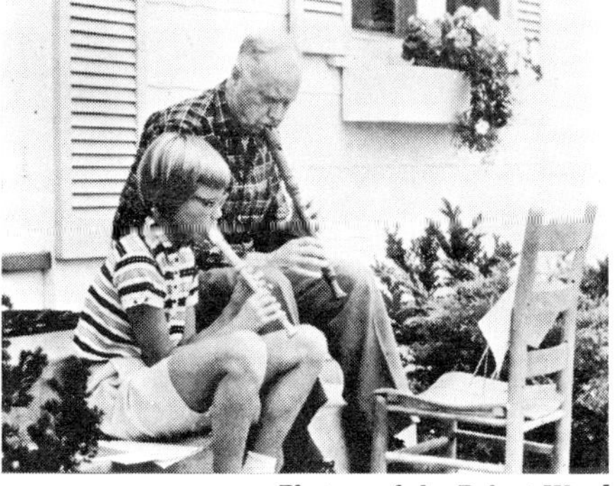

Photograph by Robert Wood
A bond that spans the years

Fig. 39-1. The school-age child.

independence is apt to bring apprehension. Within the confines of home the youngster has felt quite secure; however, venturing away from home, in the beginning of the next phase, is another story. It is inevitable that he find new and strange situations, some of which create fear. He does not yet know how to cope with the whole world. The jump from home to outside society is an enormous one. Yet he *must* take this leap.

The child finds the solution to this dilemma through association with his age-mates. When he can establish a bond with another child of his own sex and age, he gains confidence to make the tentative break with home. Not only does the child find one friend with whom he establishes a close bond, but he immerses himself in the group of his peers. The school years are the period of gangs.

The transition is gradual. The 6- or 7-year-old hangs around on the outskirts of the gang, watching, listening, practicing his skills, taking part as often as the older children will permit him to. After a year or two on the fringes of the gang, especially if he can be in company with a buddy, the youngster will move into real participation with his peers.

Now he feels he belongs. The school-age child achieves independence from home by merging his identity with that of his peers. His own shaky little self is held up by the support it receives from other equally shaky little selves.

The outstanding characteristic of the gangs of the school child are the rigid rules they impose on each other. Conformity is the keynote of this age. To belong to the gang the child must behave exactly as the others behave. The rules relieve the child of the necessity of making decisions; he is freed from the fear of mistakes. Belonging gives him a secure niche in society. He has traded conformity to a family pattern for conformity to a peer group pattern. His comfortable niche with his peers, outside his home, gives him confidence and courage to seek further independence.

For the child to step from family to peer group he needs the sympathetic encouragement of his family. It takes parental understanding and tolerance to cope with some of the behavior, ridiculous in the extreme from the adult perspective. As the child stands solidly with his group, he may appear to turn his back on his parents. He seems to have become quite a different person from the cooperative, parent-oriented preschooler of a few years back. The school-age child may become sloppy in appearance and violently resist the least contact with soap and water. He is intolerant of the ways of his parents when they deviate from those of his gang. He may be rude and indifferent to their feelings at the same time that he is acutely sensitive to the feelings of a buddy and concerned over his welfare. The school-age child may seem anxious to get away from the house as often as possible and join his friends.

While independence is a goal to be striven for, nevertheless the child is not yet ready to abandon parental control. It is essential that there be restrictions to his behavior. He may complain about restrictions which interfere with his wishes of the moment. However, in spite of his complaints, he really wants to be prevented from the necessity of coping with the whole world. He feels more secure when he knows his behavior is controlled by authority greater than his own wishes; he also senses parental love that expresses itself in concern for his welfare.

The child has respect for adults who consistently prevent him from acting on every urge that bubbles up within him. He may try his best to break down restrictions imposed by his adults, but he is uneasy if he succeeds. He wants reasonable, firm, and consistent barriers to his behavior. One 10-year-old, after a storm in which she had tried her best to be allowed to do something rather unreasonable, announced some time later: "Well, Mother, if you had allowed me to go out last night, I would have been ashamed of you."

The child in the middle years needs his parents, as adults. It is a sad sight to see a parent, deeply hurt at the child's turning away from him, try to maintain love and gratitude by attempting to be a pal to the child. Children have little respect for an adult who tries to act like a child. The child is acutely aware of what is a child and what is an adult. He can relate to either, but not to someone whose identity is jellylike. The child can treat his true pal as an equal; he wants to treat his adults as beings with strength and maturity. He needs their strength when he is in trouble. He needs a haven when in the vicissitudes of child life he is temporarily at odds with his friends. He needs it acutely if family moves disrupt his life and separate him from the security of his friends. Parents can be the secure anchor which steadies the youngster through periods of failure or lonesomeness or illness. Even when life is going smoothly for the child, at times he wants parental companionship and interest.

The school-age child is full of many paradoxes. He may hotly argue against a parent's point of view and yet the next day expound this same philosophy as though it were his very own. While he may express contempt at home for his parents' ways, he is quick to come to their defense if any outsider should criticize them.

As the school-age child rejects his parents, he often rejects his brothers and sisters, and for some of the same reasons. They represent the family tie he is trying to break. In the case of siblings other factors enter, such as jealousy, the feeling that he is less favored than a brother or sister. Most children do a good bit of bantering, teasing, and open battling in the confines of home. Nevertheless, as with parents, there is a loyalty to brothers and sisters outside the home that is sometimes remarkable. And as there are times when the school-age child wants and enjoys his parents, so, too, there are times when he appreciates his brothers and sisters and takes part with enthusiasm in family enterprises.

Adults need to let the child know the solid base on which they themselves stand. To a child it is important to have come from a family he respects. As he establishes himself free from them, he tests his new values against theirs, and while he may reject them temporarily (or seem to), he will ultimately incorporate into his own value system that which he found good in his parents' values. The more solidly the child can accept himself in his tentative breaking with his family, the greater strength he has to move on to greater maturity in the years immediately ahead when he will be able to break loose from the security of the gang and truly stand independently.

Intellectual Growth

Secure with his buddy, his peer group, and his family, the school-age child turns his attentions toward the world in which he lives. Early in the school years the child learns to read. He has known about books before, but always some grownup had to "make the book talk"; now he finds that books will talk to him when he is all by himself. The sensitive adult can sometimes feel this excitement as he watches the expression on a child's face as he stands before his bookshelf deciding which book to take down.

The child's desire to know is as insatiable as was his desire to walk when he was a yearling. He will find out as much as he can by his own efforts. He uses every power within him to understand. He looks (reading is a vital part of looking), he listens (speech is the human way of listening), he manipulates with his hands.

Children talk among themselves; they observe and experiment. But in their quest for knowledge, they turn to adults. They want to learn skills and welcome adult help in sports, in mechanical and domestic pursuits. They ask questions—an infinite number of questions: Why are trees green? What is God really like? Why is Mrs. Jones so mean? What is it like on the moon? Why can't a fish live out of water? The response of the child's adults to his intellectual explorations determines in large measure how far he carries his interests. School and home can foster or thwart his development.

If a child's questions are met with interest, if conversations follow in which child and adult pursue a subject, the child comes to realize that knowing leads to more knowing and even greater interest. Talk, books, trips, experiments, keep the intellectual fires burning (Cutts and Mosley, 1957).

Formal learning goes on in school. Good schools kindle interest. Much learning goes on away from school. Children like to talk about what interests them. A good lesson at school, a movie, a TV show, a book, an article in the newspaper, an event during the day—the interests of the child cover the whole gamut of his life (Coleman et al., 1959).

A good parent keeps abreast of the child's interests and is prepared to converse on the child's level. Such a parent knows what is going on in school, reads some of the child's school books, sees some of the TV shows, occasionally goes to a movie either with the child or independently, and so is able to encourage with interest and enrich with added knowledge.

During the school years children come to realize that grownups—parents and teachers—are not the paragons of knowledge they once thought them. This is an essential bit of understanding. No one knows everything a child wants to know, but an inquiring attitude toward the unknown is more important than a pretense of omniscience. The parent who is always willing to admit his ignorance, who knows how to find some answers in books, can fire the child's desire to know even more. Indifference squelches the child. It is no fun to ask questions if they are met with ridicule, or even if they are just put off.

From his grownups a child not only absorbs an attitude toward learning, but he also absorbs moral values. If he lives in a household where courtesy, consideration, honesty, integrity are part of daily living, he incorporates these values into himself. He may ask a lot of questions, he may test out the values his parents live by, but in the long run, what gets across to the child is the integrity of his parents or their lack of it.

The child who frequently hears a parent brag about a sharp deal or describe ways of getting even with a competitor even though he gives lip service to the principles of honesty is apt to pay more heed to the values lived by than to those merely talked about. In similar fashion the child accepts his parents' prejudices at face value and comes to "know" that foreign accents are a sign of stupidity or that a mink coat clothes a person whose friendship should be sought.

The school-age child is open to learning, and he learns what is available. He can grow up with his childish zeal to know undimmed and become a person who continues to cherish learning his whole life long, or he can discover that learning carries little pleasure.

DANGER SIGNS DURING THE SCHOOL YEARS

Many things can go wrong during the school years. Some are transient problems which can be overcome if the child is given a little special help. Others are more serious and may need long-continued psychotherapy.

The half decade of middle childhood is a vital period in personality development. As the uniquely human capacity of world-centered perception emerges, with it comes the concept of individual identity different from that of his protecting parents. Interwoven with these attributes is that of responsibility for himself and ability to relate to others. The school-age child's empathy is confined for the most part to human beings like himself. Relatedness to people different from himself is a task of later periods of development, but it is predicated on the accomplishments of the middle years (Korsch et al., 1961).

Without reasonably successful accomplishment of the tasks of the middle years full human maturity is impossible. Signs of inadequate development during the middle years make themselves manifest in many ways.

School-age children are apt to be troublesome to parents. The child *must* break some of his home ties, if he is ever to establish full maturity in the years ahead, and his techniques do not always endear him to his parents.

The child who is too good is a cause for worry. The youngster who is unable to establish bonds with his age-mates may turn toward adults. He becomes teacher's pet, Mommy's boy, a goody-goody. His behavior may cause little disruption, but it means he is failing to establish his necessary separateness. He needs a buddy to help him into the world away from adult protection. Why he has been unable to accomplish this for himself needs investigating. It may be lack of propinquity with others, frequent family moves, or inadequacies in earlier stages of development. In any case the child needs help to move adequately toward solution of the developmental tasks of the middle years.

School Problems

More obvious signs of trouble center around school problems. If the child is not doing well in school, the reasons for his failures need to be sought. Is his physical health good? Chronic illness, a low hemoglobin level, poor nutrition may be sapping his energies. Are his hearing and vision adequate? Occasionally a pair of glasses or a tonsillectomy will solve the problem. Failure to learn to read at the usual time influences all subsequent schoolwork (p. 485). Is he being pushed beyond his capacity? His intellectual endowment may not be adequate for the load he is asked to carry. A battery of tests should provide the answer. Going back a grade or transfer to a special school may be what he needs. Changes of this sort need to be made in such a way that stigma of failure does not compound the child's troubles. Here, the parents' ability to accept their child as he is, instead of as they hoped and dreamed, can spell the difference between good and poor progress (Glaser, 1965).

If the child's poor schoolwork cannot be attributed to organic or intellectual inadequacies, one must look for explanations of his inadequate motivation to learn. Sometimes the fault lies in the school, sometimes in the home, sometimes in the child himself. School inadequacies stem from crowded classrooms, poor teachers, overrigid or overlax discipline, and dull lessons. Home inadequacies are related to indifference on the part of the parents, to tensions, to rigid discipline, to sibling rivalry, to lack of real love for the child as he is. Inadequacies in the child himself may be related to his failure to establish comfortable relations with his age-mates. The child who is not comfortable with himself has little incentive to learn.

None of these problems is easy to solve, but exploration of the possible sources of trouble, with the cooperation of concerned parents, not infrequently brings to the surface attitudes that can be altered (Holt, 1964).

Neurotic Symptoms

Some children protect themselves by developing symptoms that keep them away from the situation that distresses them. The symptoms can involve any part of the body. Vomiting, abdominal pain, pains in the legs, wheezing and asthma, dizziness, and faintness are frequent but by no means exhaust the list of possible complaints.

Such symptoms can be transient and attributable to a specific cause such as an examination, a feared teacher or child. If the child can be made to understand the nature of his fear and helped to cope with it, the symptoms disappear.

On the other hand, neurotic symptoms may have more deeply lying causes and represent an overall fear of coping with life outside the safe confines of home. Regardless of the chronological age, a child with deep-seated and constant neurotic complaints has not matured to the point where he is ready for the break from home necessitated by school. Time alone will not accomplish this for him; he needs psychotherapy to help him accomplish the maturation steps he should have accomplished during his earlier years.

Neurotic symptoms most often stem from failures in the ego stage of the preschool years when the child was struggling to establish his concept of what kind of person he is. Failure at this stage leaves a large residue of guilt and sense of lack of inner worth. The child suffers greatly from his low opinion of himself; he suffers, too, from his psychosomatic symptoms, but this suffering is less devastating to him than having his inner emptiness paraded before the world. Neurotic symptoms are often amenable to verbal psychotherapy, although adequate treatment may be long drawn out.

Antisocial Behavior

Unlike the neurotic child, who develops symptoms that keep him away from that which he cannot handle, the antisocial child makes no effort at all to handle difficult situations. He simply does what he wants to do regardless of normal social demands. He takes no responsibility and feels no guilt over his inadequacies. He grabs what he can for himself regardless of consequences. He steals or lies if the occasion warrants it. He does not go to school if he does not want to. He is aggressive with adults and children alike. This is predelinquent behavior. It is the most serious of all types of school-age problems. The failure in ego development from which it stems began in infancy. Basic trust was never established; the child has neither respect for himself nor confidence in the world. Since the psychic trauma dates back to preverbal experiences, it is not amenable to treatment through the spoken word. Even so, treatment of the school-age child with this syndrome has a better chance of success than that of the same child once he has become a true delinquent a few years hence.

BIBLIOGRAPHY

COLEMAN, J. M., IRA ISCOE, and MARVIN BRODSKY: The "Draw-A-Man" Test as a Predictor of School Readiness and As an Index of Emotional and Physical Maturity, *Pediatrics,* **24**:275, 1959.

CUTTS, N., and N. MOSELY: "Teaching the Bright and Gifted," Prentice-Hall, Inc., Englewood Cliffs, N.J., 1957.

GLASER, KURT, and RAYMOND L. CLEMMENS: School Failure, *Pediatrics,* **35**:128, 1965.

HOLT, JOHN: "How Children Fail," Pitman Publishing Company, New York, 1964.

KORSCH, BARBARA, KATHERINE COBB, and BARBARA ASHE: Pediatricians' Appraisals of Patients' Intelligence, *Pediatrics,* **27**:990, 1961.

40

The Adolescent

DEFINITIONS OF PUBERTY AND ADOLESCENCE

Puberty is physiologic maturing; adolescence is cultural maturing. Puberty and adolescence are closely related; yet a delineation between them sharpens the focus of each.

Puberty, being a biologic process, is essentially similar in all races of man and in all cultures. It begins at the end of the long, slow growing period of middle childhood, with a rapid spurt in growth and maturation of the sexual apparatus. Puberty ends in the girl soon after the menarche, with the establishment of regular ovulation, and in the boy soon after the first nocturnal emission, when spermogenesis is established.

Adolescence is not as sharply fixed a period as puberty. It begins simultaneously with puberty, as the child gets his first glimmering comprehension that he himself is really going to become an adult. Adolescence does not end abruptly but slowly merges into adulthood as the young individual ultimately takes over responsibility for himself. Acceptance of his adult role is the major concern of the adolescent.

In a loose metaphor puberty and adolescence can be compared with hunger and appetite (p. 367). Both puberty and hunger are biologic phenomena. Adolescence and appetite are human—both make significant contributions to personality formation and therefore have human dimensions of function.

ADOLESCENCE IN VARIOUS CULTURES

Adolescence, unlike puberty, varies greatly in different cultures. There is a correlation between the complexity of the civilization and the length of time it takes for the youth to attain adult status.

In some primitive societies (Mead, 1939) full cultural adulthood is recognized soon after puberty or even simultaneously with it. The event is solemnized by some form of puberty rite, after which the young adolescent assumes all the rights, privileges, and responsibilities of full maturity. The child in such societies knows from early life what it will be like to be an adult. He sees his grownup self mirrored in the life about him. Throughout childhood he prepares for a known adulthood by increasingly participating in adult activities. There is no ambiguity in his future; he slips easily into adulthood when the time comes and is accepted in his foreordained role by his parents, his society, and himself. Adolescence in such societies is brief and relatively tranquil. What is thought of in our society as the inherent turmoil of adolescence hardly exists. In some primitive societies puberty rites are painful and fearsome. Doubtless such practices cause anxiety in those who must endure them.

In much of man's history, the transition from child to adult has been relatively brief. It comes as a shock to most twentieth century Americans to realize that Shakespeare's Juliet, with all her mature emotions, was but 14. In the United States today adolescence is prolonged probably longer than in any previous culture, though even here there is a class difference. In the economically less privileged, full adult roles are assumed at an earlier age than in the middle and well-to-do classes. College and even graduate school training are considered mandatory as preparation for the assumption of adult roles in the higher echelons of our complicated society. Youth in the United States, though physically mature, remain economically and often psychologically dependent, sometimes for as long as a decade.

Not only is the period of transition long, but there is no sharp cutoff point recognized by the youth himself or by his society which announces full cultural maturity. Is he adult when he leaves home to go to college? When he gets a job? When he is financially independent? When he marries?

The Christian confirmation and the Jewish Bar Mitzvah, residuals of old puberty rites which once signified the attainment of adulthood, are nowadays but social events. The 13-year-old has a good time at the ceremonies but after they are over he is as much a child as ever. There is no ceremony which signifies the end of adolescence. In fact, society reflects the vagueness of the transition into adulthood. A boy can be drafted at 18, a girl can marry in most states without a parent's consent at 18, but neither can vote until 21. Either boy or girl is legally permitted to drive a car as young as 14 in some states and not until as late as 18 in other states, but automobile insurance companies will not grant the boy adult premium rates until he is 25. The ambiguity of society and of parents adds to the young person's own ambiguity about himself. During much of this transitional time he is unsettled. He is neither child nor adult.

Not only is the apprenticeship long in our culture, but the issues are magnified by the fact that the ultimate adult goal is by no means clear. In early life the child has no clear vision of what it will be like to be an adult, as has the child in simpler societies. The child in the United States does not identify with a set pattern, nor is he apprenticed in adult activities. His future is fluid. He is going to school and preparing, but for what? He does not know. He is getting a general cultural background, which, if he thinks about it at all, he hopes will help him live an enriched life in modern society, but his future is amorphous. The youth *can* follow in his father's footsteps, or a girl in her mother's, but neither has to do so. Each is free to choose not only a very different occupation but also moral values and political and social ideals at variance with those of the parents. Adolescence is the time when these momentous choices must be made. While many an adolescent seems, at times, in a rush to grow up, he nevertheless resists pressures put upon him to decide on a vocation. So many possibilities open up before him that he wants time to make up his mind. He craves adult privileges but is often reluctant to assume the corresponding responsibilities. It is not surprising that adolescence is a time of turmoil.

ADOLESCENT PROBLEMS IN OUR SOCIETY

In puberty the child is primarily concerned with the changes taking place in his body—its size, its shape, its appearance, and its new feel. After puberty the body is more or less accepted, and the young person's attention is focused upon emancipation from the ties of his family, upon making a heterosexual adjustment, upon establishing himself vocationally, economically, and ideologically. Throughout adolescence, but with increasing concentration after puberty, the young person is absorbed with answers to the questions "Who am I?" "What am I going to do?" "What sort of a person am I?" "Where can I fit into the world?".

The young individual has a host of problems with which he must cope. There are two facets to the working out of these problems, one internal, the other external. The internal forces are the qualities within himself—his own personality. The external forces are the experiences he meets—with his family, with his peers, and in society at large as he struggles to become adult (Williams, 1959).

Internal Forces

The personality of the child as he enters puberty is a distillate of his whole past life. He has already built up an internal environment which exercises a controlling influence over his responses to new events in his external environment. To a large extent his personality determines how he will feel and therefore how he will act.

Ideally he established a basic trust in his world during infancy (p. 356). This trust was internalized into a feeling of self-competency during toddlerhood as self-awareness developed and he discovered his powers of making his body do what he wanted it to do (p. 356). In his preschool years he consolidated his feelings about his gender role and experienced the world of fantasy (p. 357). In the middle years his now competent little self experimented with a tentative independence as he made his way with his age-mates without the constant protection of his family (p. 358). As he enters puberty, the child, ideally, has achieved a feeling of his own inner worth, some ability to appreciate the feelings of other people, and the beginnings of understanding of the moral values of society (p. 359). With this preparation he is ready for the next step in maturation. The thrust toward independence is universal in adolescents. It bears no relation to whether or not the young person is prepared to cope successfully with what independence means.

Throughout all the growing years the physical organism is pushed ahead relentlessly by the compelling forces of development. This process begins far back during uterine existence. If an untoward event slows development of one part, the faulty structure has to make out as best it can; nature provides no mechanism for repeating a grade. As soon as a structure is formed, whether optimally or not, the organism puts it to use. The embryo pumps its own blood just as soon as it creates its heart. The fetus twitches his muscles and practices sucking as quickly as he has the necessary structures. The infant manipulates his hands to explore as soon as his neuromuscular system permits such activities. The yearling is possessed with the desire to walk, the toddler with the desire to control his body. The school-age child is absorbed with learning about things and about people. Whether a structure is well made or poorly constructed, the organism has an insatiable demand to use what it has. This is as true of physical structure, which permits action, as it is of mental and emotional equipment, which permits thoughts and feelings.

The adolescent's urge for independence is as great as was his urge to become a biped when he was a yearling. The child with a congenital dislocation of the hip is not inhibited in his desire to walk. He does not walk as well as the normal child; nevertheless, he waddles about with the same enthusiasm as his better-made contemporaries. And so at puberty the child whose personality has not matured adequately has the same urge toward independence as the child who is better equipped for this step in maturation.

Many of the problems of adolescence are the result of early trauma which has not permitted adequate preparation for independence. Like the child with a congenitally dislocated hip, the adolescent with inadequate personality structure waddles with eagerness toward independence, often oblivious of his own inadequacies.

External Forces

Not all adolescent problems, however, are due to inadequacies within the individual. Even the well-prepared young adolescent has needs to meet. He is still immature and he still needs help to accomplish the tasks ahead, just as he needed help to accomplish all the preceding steps. The attitude of his family and of the larger society in which he lives can help or hinder his ultimate maturation.

The child whose personality development has been traumatized will have greater difficulty during adolescence, the amount of difficulty depending upon the severity of the early trauma. He too can be helped or hindered by his experiences during the crucial years of adolescence. In puberty, that is, in the very beginning of adolescence, the child must cope with the problems of his changing body; later he must cope with his cultural identity.

BODY CHANGES IN BOTH SEXES DURING PUBERTY

Puberty comes earlier in girls than in boys. On the average girls reach the menarche at 13 and boys do not reach maturity until about 15. This places the beginning of puberty in girls at about 11 and in boys not until 13. There are, of course, wide individual variations, which, if too far from the mean, create additional problems for fringe children (Chap. 12).

The tradition of grouping children in school according to chronological age throws together youngsters in widely different stages of development. Some girls enter puberty as early as 9, some boys not until as late as 16. This 7-year spread in the onset of puberty covers the entire period of junior and senior high school and for some of the early-maturing girls dips down into the elementary school years. As a result there are youngsters in all stages of maturation participating in common activities. Rather suddenly the child discovers that his chronological age-mates, with whom he has always compared himself, are no longer his peers. He has to establish new bases of comparison, and most children need adult help to comprehend the normality of these differences.

In both sexes the first evidence of puberty is usually an increase in appetite, as the slow growth of the middle years gives way to the rapid spurt which precedes puberty (p. 381). The picky eater suddenly begins finishing his meals and asking for seconds. The child who has always eaten fairly well suddenly becomes ravenous and is constantly raiding the refrigerator. Girls have good appetites during early puberty, but boys' appetites are prodigious. This, of course, reflects the fact that boys actually gain more pounds during this growth spurt than do girls. It is difficult to predict the age at which puberty will occur in any particular child unless his growth has been followed with bone age studies (p. 116), but increased food consumption is a readily observable sign that foreshadows puberty.

Concomitantly with the growth spurt, secondary sexual characteristics begin to make their appearance—the girl's breasts bud; the boy's genitalia increase in size. With the development of the sexual apparatus, strange new feelings begin to stir within the youngster. His interests, which during the middle years were focused on outside events and on his age-mates, suddenly are turned inward. He becomes interested and concerned about what is happening to himself.

The jump in appetite offers an excellent opportunity for conversation about bodily changes in the offing. With their increased concern about their bodies boys and girls in early puberty are anxious to know what is happening to them. They want to grow big, and if approached with sympathetic understanding of their feelings, they are amenable to learning some facts about nutrition (Chap. 26) and sleep (Chap. 25) and are apt then to cooperate in programs for their physical well-being. Ideally this education should come from the home in small doses as specific situations arise. Some schools have instituted educational programs for adolescents on nutrition with gratifying results (Whitehead, 1960; Roth, 1960). Where neither parents nor school undertake this responsibility, the physician can assist. If instead of being educated the adolescent is nagged, forbidden gustatory pleasures, made to go to bed early, without reasons which seem adequate to him, the stage is being set for rebellion in the years immediately ahead.

The increase in size and also in shape is so rapid that the child has trouble in adjusting to his new body image. He reaches out his hand, and it goes farther than he expected, so he knocks over his glass of milk. He tries to sit in the small child's chair he has always used in front of the fireplace, and his rear gets stuck in it. The boy's voice plays tricks on him; he suddenly squeaks in the middle of a sentence. Size often outstrips strength as well as coordination. The youth may fatigue more easily than he did as a child, and since he looks so big, he may be pushed into activities that leave him exhausted (p. 157). Fatigue, exhaustion, lack of coordination all pile up to make him feel inadequate, embarrassed, and self-conscious. Accusations of clumsiness, laziness, stupidity do not help him adjust to his new body and his new self.

Some embarrassment is inevitable during these years, but good-natured amusement from his family over his silly predicaments, combined with genuine pleasure in his maturing, can be of real help. He needs the sympathetic understanding of a perceptive adult who can discuss with him the physiology of puberty, point out what is happening to him, why he seems awkward, why he is so hungry and so sleepy, and help him appreciate the fact that this is a transient stage. His present inadequacies will soon pass; they are not indications of lifetime patterns. An awareness of the universality of these problems and an understanding of their temporary nature help the youngster accept his changing body without destroying his feeling of self-competency.

Since the body is of such concern to the pubescent youngster, any blemish is apt to be magnified into a major catastrophe. Unfortunately this is the time of life when glands hypertrophy, and in some youngsters acne becomes a real problem, though an insignificant pimple is not infrequently viewed by the young teen-ager as though it were a monumental disfigurement. The physiology of skin metabolism and the need for more than usual cleanliness can be explained (p. 251). The control of severe acne is not too successful at the present time, and therefore the unfortunate youngster plagued with the disease may need help to accept himself as adequate.

Minor deviations in development can also disturb the youngster. The girl who grows excessive hair on her face or extremities (p. 254), the boy with gynecomastia (p. 206) are embarrassed, and their capacity to adapt is under increased strain. These problems are hard to deal with, since there is usually little that can be done for the troublesome symptom. Sympathetic understanding, an assurance that these symptoms, while annoying, in no way mean a failure of femininity or masculinity can frequently help the youngster live with them.

The appearance of sexual characteristics and the need for adequate sex education have been discussed elsewhere (p. 436).

Physical changes are so obvious that the child constantly compares himself with his peers. This is more apt to increase rather than decrease his worry over his own normality, since puberty comes at such different ages in perfectly normal individuals. The teen-ager is most comfortable when he is just like his friends. He is worried lest there be something wrong with him, if he deviates from the group norm. Once again, assurance of his normality and explanations about tempo of growth can help restore his confidence in himself and his own rate of maturation. If bone age studies are done, some youngsters take an enormous interest in this scientific approach to growing up (p. 116).

During puberty the thrust in physical growth is accompanied by a thrust in psychic growth. The child abandons the fantasy life of the middle years, develops a better orientation to reality, and begins to reach out for a tentative independence. The psychic growth in puberty has different overtones for boys and girls.

PSYCHIC DEVELOPMENT IN THE GIRL DURING PUBERTY

During the middle years the little girl has identified with her mother. In our society the girl's identification with the mother is apt to be a good deal stronger than the boy's with the father. As she grew up, the little girl felt that some day she would be just like her mother; then in her teens comes the realization that her mother does not represent all the good of womanhood. The child looks about her and sees many versions of the feminine role. Mother is one kind of woman; maybe the child still admires her, but she feels that to establish her own identity she cannot be a carbon copy. The only way she knows to establish her own identity is to be different from her mother. If the mother has truly encouraged independence, the child's break will be gradual; it may involve an enormous amount of conversation in which the young girl questions her mother's values, criticizes her mother's behavior. To the mother this may seem a sudden change in character. Previously mother and daughter had gotten along well together; then all of a sudden, everything the mother

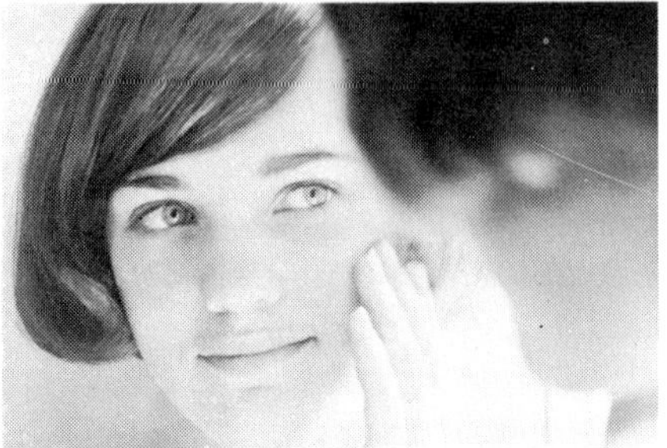

Appearance is of vital importance

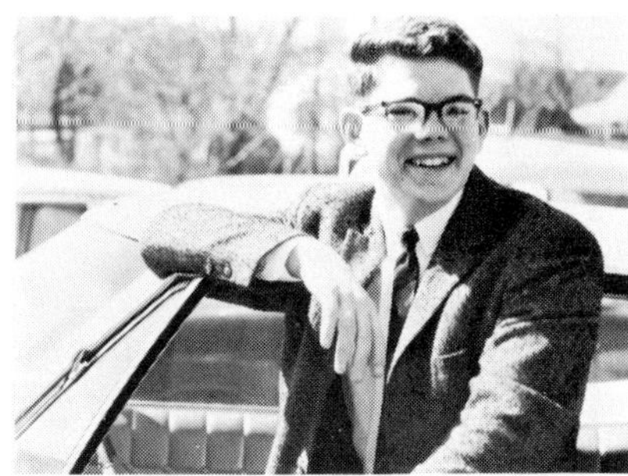

Desire for adult prerogatives

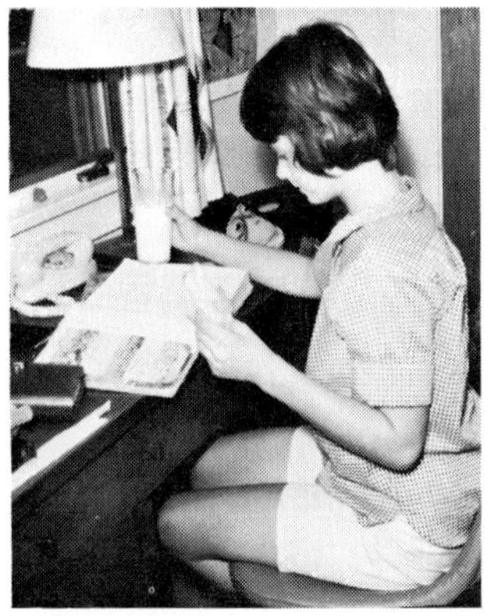

Constantly hungry

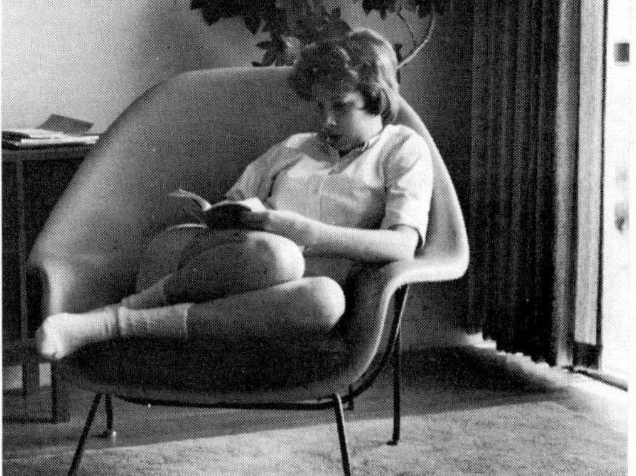

Photograph by Robert Wood

Moody

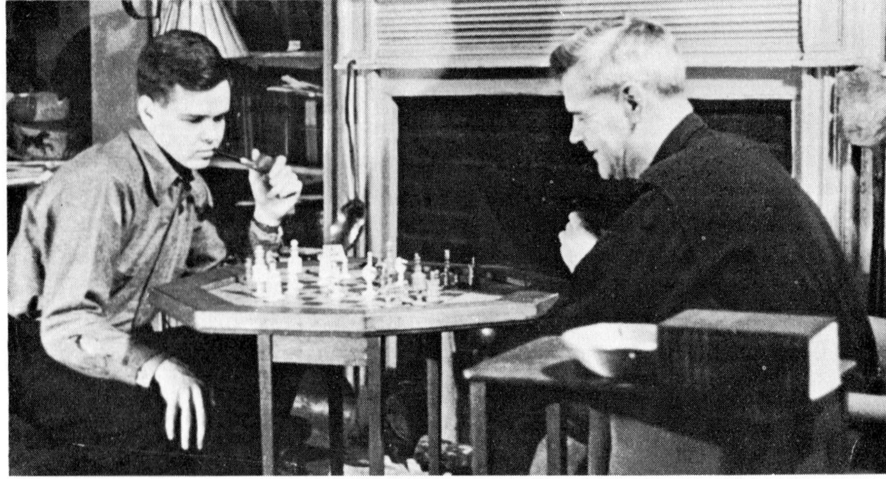

Photograph by Robert Wood

Parent and adolescent share an interest

Fig. 40-1. The adolescent.

does is wrong in daughter's eyes. This can be very disconcerting for a well-intentioned mother and is apt to add numerous tensions, unless the mother is very wise about the feelings and actions of a maturing girl.

The girl may develop a crush on some other woman, often a teacher. By such a friendship the child is replacing dependence upon her mother with dependence on an outside person. At home she extols the virtues of her new-found friend, to the detriment of her mother. However, at school she may sing quite a different tune, glorifying her mother and her whole family in quite extravagant terms. Thus she dispels the guilt she feels at rejecting her mother. Instead of selecting some flesh-and-blood woman she knows, the little girl occasionally identifies with an ideal image—a movie star, a character in a book, a public person.

Turning away from the mother is a forward step for the child. She must relinquish her childhood dependence to achieve maturity. The person with whom she identifies plays a significant role in her life. If it is a mature woman with some understanding of the psychology of little girls, she can be of great help. On the other hand, a less desirable character, flattered by the child's devotion, can tempt the child into relations and escapades for which she is not ready and which do her considerable harm.

In addition to adult ideal images the girl in puberty is likely to have one close and intimate girl friend. The two girls support each other, and each gains strength to take steps forward toward independence. They make a twosome against the fearful adulthood ahead of them. The intensity of this friendship can be very great. The two girls have a need for each other; it is almost as though neither girl feels complete alone. Forced separations due to family moves can be sufficiently traumatic to lead to symptoms of depression. While a bosom friend serves a useful purpose in the period of puberty, the very intensity of the relation can lead to trouble. So long as the two girls are more or less equal in strength of character, they support each other and all is well. However, if one is much more dominant than the other, the submissive one may regress, and the independence she is struggling to achieve may not take place. Under normal and usual circumstances this friendship consists of hours spent together talking and giggling, playacting, and sharing secrets. Seldom is there physical intimacy, and overt homosexuality or mutual masturbation is very infrequent. Much of the private talk is about romantic love and about sexual matters (Fraiberg, 1961).

The renewed interest in the genital organs distinguishes puberty from the preceding phase of childhood, during which genital interest is at a low ebb (p. 359). The two girl friends are vitally interested in pregnancy and may stuff pillows under their dresses and play at being pregnant—a delightful combination of early childhood play and more grownup interests. They are also interested in their own changing shapes and want to wear brassieres, which they puff out with wads of cotton. Good sex education at this stage is mandatory (p. 436).

In spite of the little-girl talk with her bosom companion about love and sex, a girl at this age is not interested in boys in a dating sense. Some girls are not interested in boys at all; others enjoy active sports with boy companions and often develop tomboyish qualities, which fade away when the menarche is reached (Deutch, 1944).

In her attempt to establish herself as different from her mother, the girl does a lot of playacting, sometimes alone, sometimes in company with her girl friend. She imagines herself a great actress, spends hours before her mirror, falls for every cosmetic advertised, reorders her life to fit an image, then in a few weeks alters the image and her behavior. Her various images may at times include what she feels the family of such a great person should be, and she will attempt to alter the family pattern.

The attitude of her family and especially her mother is a potent factor in the girl's maturation. She needs tolerance and love to help her structure her experiences and avoid an exacerbation of masochism. And yet there are times when a young pubescent girl is a great trial to her family. She is vague and diffuse, talkative but not very communicative. She is often belligerent toward her mother and disorderly around the house. Sometimes her schoolwork falls off. Her appearance may become sloppy and dirty, or she may be excessively concerned with her outward appearance and yet utterly unconcerned about the condition of her underwear.

Both parents need to be willing to loosen the reins of early childhood, but nevertheless they must have the strength to hold firm on the discipline which they feel is really necessary. The father of a young girl needs to take a new look at his budding daughter. A few words now and then in appreciation of her developing femininity can do wonders for a child shaky in her new role.

The arrival of the menarche alters the girl's outlook on life (Kestenberg, 1961). Fantasies are now replaced by realities. Even if the girl was well prepared intellectually for the coming event, nevertheless her anticipations had a dreamlike quality. Now she knows "what it is like with me." The definite experience, its sharpness, the mechanics of taking care of herself all give her a sense of relief. Even discomfort sharpens the experience. Frequently the vague diffuse qualities of early puberty fade away as the girl accepts her femininity.

Throughout feminine development there is a masochistic element, first evident in the genital phase of early childhood, when the little girl has to accept the fact that she has no penis (p. 428) (Deutch, 1944). At the time of the menarche feminine masochism is much in evidence. It can be a constructive force that helps the girl define her body to herself. She must incorporate an invisible part into her total self image. Sensations, even unpleasant ones, help in this integration.

Feminine identity, however, does not happen overnight with the menarche. It takes time for a young girl to make the necessary integration. Some girls accomplish the feat more easily than others. Acceptance of gender role in early childhood and identification with the mother begin the process. Later, accurate sexual information combined with a sense of deep love from her parents for herself as she is help the little girl accept, with satisfaction, the fact that she is feminine.

Tomboyishness in puberty is a detour for many girls and to some extent indicates an unresolved envy of boys. Usually it fades as the child gains the definiteness of her femininity evidenced by menstruation. Sometimes it takes time, and for a year or so the pubescent girl tries to deny her femininity by flattening her breasts and pursuing active sports in a masculine fashion.

Soon after the menarche puberty comes to an end, though adolescence continues for some years. The intimate relation with the bosom friend often fades as the girl, sure of herself now, seeks other friendships and pushes forward to free herself from all dependence on her family as she establishes herself as an adult.

PSYCHIC DEVELOPMENT IN THE BOY DURING PUBERTY

Along with the physical thrust in growth at the onset of puberty, the boy also experiences a thrust in psychic growth. In boys this forward thrust is much more direct than in girls. The diffuseness of the pubescent girl is lacking in the boy, possibly because in the boy the genital organs can be seen and felt (Blos, 1941). Unlike the girl, whose reproductive organs are unseen and therefore have an indefinable quality, the boy knows in an objective, concrete fashion that his masculine character is definite. He is apt to be aggressive rather than vague. The boy goes after independence in a straight line, as it were, not in circles and by detours. True, he has ambivalence about growing up and is apt to go forward three steps and back two as he vacillates between wanting independence and being afraid of it.

As puberty advances, the boy spends less and less time at home. His interests are with other boys of his age, and, like the girl, he may have one close buddy. His friends may be the same old gang he played with as a younger child, or because of his greater mobility now he may select other friends farther away from home base. In puberty the boy "clams up" at home, unlike the girl who is often very talkative. Only with one or two intimate friends does the adolescent boy confide his feelings. The boys talk together about many things, but sex and their body changes are always part of their intimate mutual revelations. They are concerned about their new feelings; masturbation is a universal problem (p. 437). The boy is less apt than the girl to bring his sexual worries to the attention of parents; nevertheless, he needs adult guidance. It takes a perceptive adult to pick the right time to raise the question of sexual maturation, its meaning, its significance, its normality. The boy in puberty needs good sex education; without it he may be deeply disturbed about feelings which, though new to him, are quite normal and usual in the human race (p. 437).

The high school population of both boys and girls breaks up into cliques, sharply drawn on sex lines. Each little group is exclusive; usually there is a drawing interest, such as fraternities or sports among the boys and sororities or social activities among the girls. Sometimes the groups divide academically, those planning to go to college forming a nucleus quite different from those waiting for the day they can leave school and get a job. Popularity is vital to both boys and girls and is based on being accepted by the right group. The boy or girl who does not make the group he feels gives him status may have a hard time.

BREAKING THE TIE WITH THE FAMILY

In puberty adjustment to body changes dominates the scene in both boys and girls. There is a tentative effort to break away from the family at this stage, but it is not until after puberty, when the new body has been more or less accepted, that the young person turns his full attention to the job of establishing himself on his own two feet. To accomplish this he must free himself from protection from his family. Under ideal conditions the family, in a reciprocal thrust forward at this time, breaks its habit of exercising authority over the maturing youngster (Stone and Church, 1957).

There is almost always, in our culture, an ambivalence on the part of the young adolescent as he views the vista of full independence ahead of him. He wants to grow up and be free from all parental restraints, and yet even the well-prepared, relatively competent youngster has moments of fear and even panic as he comprehends the responsibilities that are part and parcel of independence. As a result, he vacillates between a maturity that amazes his parents and an equally amazing regression to childishness.

There is also an ambivalence on the part of the parents, even parents who are genuinely dedicated to the idea that independence of their fledgling is the desired goal. Parents take pride in the growing maturity and competence of their adolescent; they may also look forward to freedom from their responsibilities for his care. At the same time, there is often a reluctance to relinquish their own importance in his life. Parents, as well as adolescents, vacillate, and unfortunately the vacillations of the two are apt to pull in opposite directions. At one time parents tend to encourage, and even demand, independence and responsibility, and all too often these are the very moments when the adolescent is fearful of his future and wants to sink back into their protecting arms. At other times the adolescent wants to barge ahead. He demands privileges at a time when his parents feel he is ill-equipped to assume the necessary responsibilities. Parents tend to hold back lest the fledgling injure himself with his untried wings. Conflicts arise over different feelings about the tempo of gaining independence (Salinger, 1951).

These swings up and down, back and forth, are almost inevitable. Under the best of circumstances, adolescence is seldom without its upheavals. But the family which has genuinely encouraged independence during all the child's growing years may surmount the problems concerning tempo and may weather adolescence with bearable friction. In such a family the delights of adolescence may outweigh the inevitable moments of tension. In adolescence intellectual maturity makes its appearance. Parents and child can now read the same books, enjoy the same plays, read the same newspapers, and at times engage in conversation on an adult level. A mutuality of intellectual interests can spring into being with a true exchange of opinions.

While concern about the intellectual and esthetic problems of his society develops in the adolescent, he may well not share his parents' opinions. As his parents can accept with respect his ideas and values, regardless of how much at variance they may be with their own, the adolescent learns what it feels like to be respected as an adult. To feel like an adult is a milestone on the road to acting like one. Discussions of world affairs, of philosophy, of literature, of art, conducted in an atmosphere of mutual respect, encourage independence of thought—a vital need for the adolescent.

Adolescents who have grown up in a family with strong family ties and with considerable self-sufficiency within the family group may find it difficult to wean themselves from this dependency. This is especially true if the parents are strong, competent people. The very force of their personalities increases the adolescent's problems in establishing himself as different from them. If he feels overwhelmed by his parents' competence, he will be reluctant to discuss his ideas at home—he is not sure he can stand up against parental values. His reticence, his apparent rejection of his parents may cause considerable estrangement, especially in a family that has always prided itself on its warmth of mutual understanding. The adolescent is torn between his desire for adult status and his feeling of disloyalty to parents, especially when he has a genuine love for them.

The parents too may be in a quandary. They see the youngster's struggles, feel his rejection; if they withdraw and make no demands, the youngster accuses them of lack of interest, lack of love; if they attempt to influence or control him, he accuses them of holding him back and of refusing him adult prerogatives.

A further difficulty of parents in our tumultuous world is confusion about their own values, especially when challenged by youth. What was acceptable to the parents in their own youth as a code to live by no longer seems adequate. Business ethics, sex morality, religion, political beliefs which once seemed so clear cannot stand up under the penetrating questions of an adolescent torn between what he has been taught and what he finds exists in the outside world. In his effort to carve out a niche for himself in the big world away from home the adolescent may identify himself with some cause—and the more dramatically opposed it is to home values, the greater seems his dedication to it. He may try to establish his own identity through a religious or political or esthetic movement.

These are growing pains of adolescence—painful but essential. The youth must find some way of being himself. Once he can accomplish some self-identity, he can take a more mature view of parental values. It is possible that he may then find some of them good and worth returning to, not because they represent his family, but because he can incorporate these values into his concept of his own world without feeling like a carbon copy of his parents.

These are the conflicts that develop under the best of conditions. When conditions are not optimal, problems mount and are often expressed in antisocial behavior. The major conflicts arise with parents who never truly solved the earlier conflicts of emerging self-awareness and self-dependence. The parents who have only given lip-service, if even that, to their child's self-competency will be met in adolescence with outright rebellion. No matter how ill-prepared the child may be for independence, he is nevertheless possessed with the demands from his genes to be free from restraints. Hemmed in by parental authority, the only way he can achieve freedom is to fight for it. Parents of such a child lose real contact with him during adolescence. To avoid overt war, the adolescent pulls away. He has little to say to his parents; he uses his home as a hotel where he sleeps and eats and drops his clothes for someone else to pick up and launder. When he does become ensnared with his parents, it is usually over their disapproval of some behavior of his. The parents are irritated and attempt to use authoritarian measures to demand conformity, against which the adolescent blurts out vindictives and escapes as quickly as possible. Guidance during adolescence can be accomplished only with a loose rein; a tight bridle is apt to snap, after which there is no guidance.

VENTURING OUT INTO THE WIDER WORLD

Not only must the adolescent break his bond of dependence on his family, but he must establish himself in the outside world. The two processes, of course, go on simultaneously.

The outside world in our society is not very helpful to the adolescent. Independence and adequacy, at least in boys, is measured to a considerable extent by the ability to hold a job, the ability to earn money. The boy yearns for a paid job which to him is the symbol of adulthood and by means of which he identifies with men and establishes a sense of his own worth in society.

High school and college boys, and girls too to a lesser extent, want jobs during school vacations; some want to drop out of school and enter the labor market on a permanent basis. But jobs are hard to get. Teen-age youngsters are not wanted in industry. In many places there are laws against the hiring of anyone under 18. Young people have higher accident rates than more mature workers, and now that employers must assume responsibility for the safety of employees, many companies have fixed policies against employment of young people.

Some boys succeed in getting jobs in gas stations, in grocery stores, but, more and more, even these jobs are denied them, as each small store loses its independent status, becomes a link in a big chain, and must relie on a central employment policy.

High school boys all too often are reduced to jobs with friends and neighbors. They can cut lawns, clean cellars, maybe even scrub floors. Sometimes a boy's family is very incensed that their son refuses to cut the home lawn though he grabs at a job cutting the lawn down the street. The family seems unaware of the fact that cutting Mr. Jones's lawn for pay gives the boy a status impossible to attain by the same amount of exertion on the home lawn even if his father pays him for the job. Adolescent girls have the advantage over boys in that baby-sitting jobs are usually readily available.

In his first tentative attempt to assume an adult role in the community the youth is met with what he interprets as rejection. He feels he is unwanted and denied status and the opportunity to compete. The rejection can have a far-reaching effect on his concept of his competence. Once again a perceptive adult can be of some assistance. Some conversation about the evolution of the present laws against employing young people can help a little. A description of the exploitation of children in sweat shops, of accidents in unprotected factories can perhaps convince the youth that he is not being personally discriminated against. Society has corrected an old abuse and has not yet been awakened to new needs—decent jobs for young people—not mollycoddling jobs where the youth is treated like a child, but real jobs where he must make good or face being fired. Understanding the social forces does not get the youth a job, but it may make him feel less rejected, may even help him identify with constructive social forces.

While a job is important for status, the high school boy (or girl) is interested in thinking about his ultimate career, though he will resist being pushed. He needs information on what sort of work will provide him satisfaction in life. He needs vocational guidance. Some schools have competent people to help him, but many do not. The *Occupational Outlook Handbook* published annually by the U.S. Department of Labor lists every type of occupation in the United States with some comments on education needed and prospects for employment advances in the decades ahead. A boy or girl perusing this book and given an opportunity to decide what appeals to him can be helped to make constructive plans for his future. If those plans include college, the next questions are what college, how to get in, how to finance it.

Getting into college, however, poses another problem. With the increasing number of young people wanting a college education, it is more and more difficult for an individual boy or girl to be accepted in the college of his choice. Failure to get into the chosen college is again often interpreted as further rejection at the hands of society.

DELINQUENCY

In the last 20 years the juvenile delinquency rate has trebled. What is wrong with our society that we cannot provide a climate in which the young can grow to acceptable maturity? There is a huge literature on the subject. As a society we are certainly concerned.

Delinquency is antisocial behavior in an adolescent. The same acts in an adult are called criminal, which indicates that delinquency is recognized as a developmental phenomenon. Some adolescents who engage in delinquent acts progress in the same pattern and become adult criminals, but certainly not all do (Noshpitz, 1960).

During adolescence a huge number of young people have delinquent fantasies. In the turmoil of solving his personal adjustment the young person has periods of vindictiveness when he wants to get back at the world that thwarts him. A great many act out some of their fantasies. An honest recall of the adolescence of most of us would include an occasional episode we would just as soon forget, yet since these acts were not brought before the court, we were not labeled delinquent, nor did we become delinquents.

In the relatively normal adolescent these antisocial acts are infrequent. There is, however, a qualitative difference as well as a quantitative one between the growing pains of a normal adolescent and true delinquent behavior. The normal youth "knows" better; he feels guilty after he has acted badly. The true delinquent does not distinguish between his fantasies and reality. He has no inhibitions against his acts, and he feels no guilt after the act.

Blos describes three classes of delinquents:

1. Functional delinquency. This, he feels, is a means of discharging inevitable tensions. It occurs in many normal youths and is fairly soon outgrown. It is important that the label of delinquency not be pinned on normal youngsters whose behavior has slipped occasionally from acceptable norms.

2. Facultative delinquency. This sort of antisocial behavior largely depends upon the environment of the adolescent. If he happens to get in with a gang planning a window-smashing expedition, he goes along. He is not mature enough to hold out against the gang, but neither is he pushed from within to behave in an antisocial way. There is no substratum of delinquency. If he can be protected from undesirable influences, he will behave acceptably, and he will probably mature normally even though there may be unpleasant episodes during his adolescence.

3. Pathologic delinquency. These are the serious cases and represent a

failure of normal development. This sort of delinquency does not appear suddenly in adolescence. The trauma of development occurs early and is evident as latent delinquency in the middle childhood years. If the condition is diagnosed then, treatment has more opportunity for success than it does later, when the ill-prepared personality is further traumatized by the failures of adolescence (Deisher, 1960). In adolescence the latent failure in maturation bursts forth into overt acts precipitated by the inevitable problems at this age. These can be either inner turmoil in the youth as his urge for independence is thwarted or hyperstimulation from a gang of aggressive youths or adults. Probably both inner and outer factors play a part in pushing the latent delinquent into acts characterized as pathologic delinquency.

The pathologic development that leads to delinquency begins early. Blos describes it as starting in infancy with failure to build up a basic trust in the world; without trust the child is unable to establish confidence in himself. Instead, a sadomasochistic bond develops between mother and child whereby the child learns to control, rather than master, his environment. His ability to control eventually gives him a sense of his own omnipotence. So long as he can maintain the fiction of his omnipotence, he can get along without a sense of inner worth; however, he is in constant need of reaffirming his power over his environment. Any time that the environment seems to control him he becomes overwhelmed by the terror of his utter lack of inner worth. A little child with this early pathologic developmental problem finds it easier to dominate successfully in a household where parents are separated and he only needs to control his mother, a mother whose pattern is a masochistic acceptance of her child's sadistic impulses. This is one reason why the correlation is high between pathologic delinquency and broken homes.

If such a child has an opportunity to build a satisfactory relation with age-mates during the middle years, it is possible that to some extent the pathologic early identity can be modified, but if the child fails here too and jumps from a traumatized early childhood into puberty, the stage is set for delinquency. His need to control dates from infancy; his inability to distinguish fantasy from reality is preschool development carried unmodified into puberty. So in adolescence he attempts to exercise his compelling urge to demonstrate that he can dominate his environment by acting out his fantasies.

Delinquent behavior stands in marked contrast to neurotic behavior (Sperling, 1961). The neurotic is unable to face problems of his own inadequacy; therefore he invents a compromise. For example, the neurotic child, afraid that he cannot successfully compete in school, develops psychosomatic ailments that keep him home, while the delinquent just goes to the movies instead of going to school and, if necessary, steals the money for the movies. Neurotics develop symptoms which cause them discomfort but nevertheless help them avoid the more terrifying consequences of facing their sense of inadequacy. Delinquents skip the compromise. Their aggressive acts are not against themselves but against the outside world; they are a primitive attempt to prove omnipotence. Neurotics cause themselves suffering; delinquents cause others to suffer. The delinquent has been sadistic since early childhood. As long as his environment (his mother) responded with masochistic acceptance, the child functioned; when he grows older and stronger and continues the same tactics on the larger world, his acts are called delinquent. Neurotics are more amenable to treatment than delinquents (Blos, 1961). They can be helped to gain insight into their problems; the delinquent, on the other hand, whose trauma dates back to preverbal experiences, cannot be reached through verbal techniques.

While events during adolescence are of vital importance in ultimate maturation, no community programs for teen-agers are going to solve the basic problems of delinquency. This does not mean these programs are not of great value for the bulk of our adolescents who have developed relatively normally, but it is wishful thinking to assume that a pathologic delinquent can be made into a good citizen by providing him with wholesome activities during his teens. Successful treatment of delinquency in adolescence involves years of intense psychologic and social rehabilitation (Redl, 1951). The earlier in life latent delinquency can be recognized, the greater is the chance that delinquency can be rechanneled. Obviously prevention of delinquency is best begun in infancy.

BIBLIOGRAPHY

Blos, Peter: Delinquency, in Lorand Sandor and Henry I. Schneer (eds.), "Adolescents: Psychoanalytic Approach to Problems and Therapy," p. 132, Paul B. Hoeber, Inc., New York, 1961.

———: "The Adolescent Personality: A Study of Individual Behavior," Appleton-Century-Crofts, Inc., New York, 1941.

Deisher, Robert W., and Jay F. O'Leary: Early Medical Care of Delinquent Children, *Pediatrics,* **25**:329, 1960.

Deutch, Helene: "The Psychology of Women," Grune & Stratton, Inc., New York, 1944.

Fraiberg, Selma H.: Homosexual Conflicts, in Lorand Sandor and Henry I. Schneer (eds.), "Adolescents: Psychoanalytic Approach to Problems and Therapy," p. 78, Paul B. Hoeber, Inc., New York, 1961.

Kestenberg, Judith S.: Menarche, in Lorand Sandor and Henry I. Schneer (eds.), "Adolescents: Psychoanalytic Approach to Problems and Therapy," p. 19, Paul B. Hoeber, Inc., New York, 1961.

Mead, Margaret: "From the South Seas," William Morrow and Company, Inc., New York, 1939.

Noshpitz, Joseph D.: The Antisocial or Asocial Adolescent, *Pediat. Clin. North America,* **7**:97, 1960.

"Occupational Outlook Handbook," bulletin 1450, Bureau of Labor Statistics, U.S. Department of Labor, Washington, D.C. Published annually.

REDL, FRITZ, and DAVID WINEMAN: "Children Who Hate," The Free Press of Glencoe, New York, 1951.

ROTH, ARTHUR: The Teen Age Clinic, *J. Am. Dietet. A.*, **36**:27, 1960.

SALINGER, J. D.: "The Catcher in the Rye," Little, Brown and Company, Boston, 1951.

SPERLING, MELITTA: Psychosomatic Disorders, in Lorand Sandor and Henry J. Schneer (eds.), "Adolescents: Psychoanalytic Approach to Problems and Therapy," p. 202, Paul B. Hoeber, Inc., New York, 1961.

STONE, L. JOSEPH, and JOSEPH CHURCH: "Childhood and Adolescence: A Psychology of the Growing Person," Random House, Inc., New York, 1957.

WHITEHEAD, FLOY E.: How Nutrition Education Can Affect Adolescent's Food Choices, *J. Am. Dietet. A.*, **37**:348, 1960.

WILLIAMS, MURRAY: A Clinic for Adolescents: Survey of 750 Patients, *M. J. Australia*, **2**:201, 1959.

"The Adolescent in Your Family," publication 347, U.S. Children's Bureau, Washington, D.C., 1955.

41

Age-portrait Summaries

In monitoring the development of children, one must know what to expect and what to accept at each age. This knowledge serves two purposes: first, to provide the background with which to help parents understand the ways of children and thus to provide a milieu conducive to optimal development and, second, to provide a means of detecting aberrations from normal development. While individual differences between children are marked, nevertheless there is a limit beyond which deviant behavior must be considered pathologic.

Three aspects of development must be kept in mind in appraising the progress of a given child:

1. Behavior normal at one stage of development becomes pathologic if it persists beyond the time when it should be abandoned for a more mature form of behavior, e.g., the palmar grasp should be replaced by a prehensile grip.

2. New forms of behavior emerge as the organism matures. Failure of expected behavior to appear suggests trouble; e.g., inflected jargon should appear in late infancy.

3. Some behavior patterns are pathologic at any age and whenever detected call for investigation, e.g., tics, psychosomatic illness, failure of weight gain.

Since individual differences within the limits of normal are large, it takes clinical judgment, as well as comparison with standardized norms, to determine the significance of the behavior of any one child. The norms are reference points of average behavior. The child who deviates from them needs to be appraised for his degree of normality but not necessarily labeled as abnormal. For instance, while the norms may indicate 15 months as the time for the transition from sucking to drinking from a cup, it is essential to look at the whole past history of a given child to determine whether or not this is *his* expected transition point. The avid sucker (p. 374) will not be ready for this maturation step at this age, and this can be predicted early in infancy. On the other hand failure to drink from the cup may indicate not that the child is an avid sucker but that he has been deprived of maternal warmth and therefore has not built up sufficient basic trust to be ready for this maturation step at a time when he should be. Distinguishing between two such basically different reasons for the same behavior is part of the art of pediatric care.

The factors responsible for tempo of development are genetic constitution, organic adequacy, and ego development. Genetic constitution in large measure must be accepted and understood. A child's ultimate capacity may be quite normal, but his tempo may vary from the average (e.g., the avid sucker described above). If permitted to mature at his own genetically determined rate, unhampered by anxiety because of his deviant tempo, he will reach full maturity. On the other hand a slow tempo may reflect a true genetic inadequacy. Such a child can never be expected to reach average performance. The earlier in life one can be sure of this, the more adequately can plans be laid for as much development as the individual's potential warrants. Superior genetic endowment may be reflected in a rapid tempo. Here too caution is essential. Some children travel faster but not necessarily farther than others.

Organic inadequacy is somewhat more easily diagnosed than genetic competency, especially if it is looked for. At times organic problems can be remedied, e.g., by a hearing aid, better nutrition, cure of a chronic infection, surgical treatment. In other cases present knowledge is not sufficient to restore normal function, and, like the genetically inadequate individual, the organically inadequate must be accepted as he is and his life so arranged that the handicap is compensated for as much as possible and not compounded by expecting from him behavior and accomplishment of which he is incapable.

Ego development can also influence the progress of total development. Some problems in ego development are minor, transient, and remedial. The preschooler who suddenly begins beating up his classmates without provocation may possibly be reacting to a castration fear. Should this be the case, the problem can be explained to intelligent parents and solved without permanent damage. Suddenly appearing aberrant behavior is in general more amenable to treatment than long-continuing pathologic behavior. Here, again, it is essential to distinguish expected from abnormal behavior. Tantrums, though unpleasant, must be expected from time to time in the toddler, but normally they fade by the time the school years are reached.

When the failure in ego development is long-continued, it is often not difficult to appraise the situation and understand the cause of the deviant behavior; however, remedial measures are fraught with difficulty, since all too often they involve the entire personality of the caretaking person. At times, however, even problems that appear monumental do respond to an intelligent and sympathetic approach.

In the present chapter developmental material is summarized for handy reference in thumbnail sketches of children at key ages. It must be reemphasized that these norms are those of average performance and that the normality of any given child can be determined only by clinical judgment of his entire behavior in the light of his own life history.

I. THE PREMATURE

A—General Appearance

1. Tiny.
2. Limp.
3. Loose.
4. Scrawny.
5. Distant.

B—Dominant Developmental Thrust

1. Physiologic maturation.

C—Physiologic Status

1. The premature of 28 weeks' gestation (1–2 lb):
   a. Poor muscle tone.
   b. Movements sporadic, not well-sustained.
   c. Myoclonic twitching.
   d. Moro and grasp reflexes absent.
   e. Tonic neck and tendon reflexes present.
   f. Body temperature labile.
   g. Breathing irregular.
   h. Sucking and swallowing reflexes weak or absent.
   i. Cry weak, often soundless; fades rather than stops.
2. The premature of 32 weeks' gestation (3–4 lb):
   a. Muscle tone fair.
   b. Movements more purposeful but not well sustained.
   c. Moro and grasp reflexes present.
   d. Sucking and swallowing reflex present but not adequate to maintain nutrition.
   e. Cry thin and high-pitched and may stop before needs are satisfied.

D—Feeding

1. Not interested.
2. Appetite no guide to nutritional requirements.

E—Sleep

1. Periods of sleep and wakefulness fade into each other.

F—Problems

1. Establishment of respiration.
2. Maintenance of homeostasis.
3. Avoidance of infection and environmental stress.

G—Environmental Needs

1. An incubator with controlled temperature, humidity, and oxygen.
2. A vigilant trained nurse to care for him, remove mucus if necessary, turn him, feed him.
3. A doctor alert to his needs to prescribe food and fluids and institute any necessary remedial measures.

H—Parental Attitudes

1. The premature is oblivious of his parents and has no need of them.
2. The parents, however, suffer from anxiety, sometimes guilt, and need sympathetic support throughout the incubator stage of their premature infant.

I—Danger Signals

1. Physiologic, and may indicate an organism too immature for independent existence or one suffering from insurmountable organic maldevelopment, signs of which are:
   a. Cyanosis, apnea, respiratory distress.
   b. Pallor.
   c. Apathy.
   d. Convulsions.

J—Success in Handling the Premature Results in:

1. Physiologic maturation.
2. Gain in weight.
3. Relief of parental anxiety.

K—Failure in Care of the Premature Results in:

1. Death of the infant

II. THE FULL–TERM NEONATE

A—General Appearance

1. Small.
2. Plump.
3. Taut.
4. Vigorous.
5. Noisy.
6. Detached.

B—Dominant Developmental Thrust

1. Establishment of organic independence.
2. Behavior, however, reflects fetal orientation.

C—Physiologic Status

1. Precarious equilibrium:
   a. Can function adequately if not subject to organic stress.
   b. Temperature regulation unsteady.
   c. Peristalsis and swallowing unstable; may reverse direction.
   d. Respiration may be irregular; often noisy, the infant grunts, snores, coughs, sneezes.
   e. Hiccups after "burping."

D—Instinctive Behavior

1. Cry elicited by any discomfort. It is lusty, staccato, rhythmic, with rapid tempo. It ceases when discomfort is removed. The cry is accompanied by all-over body activity.

2. Sucking vigorous when the infant is hungry, preceded by rooting movements. The infant may stop sucking, rest, and even sleep for brief periods during a feeding.
3. Sucking elicited only when hungry.

E—Posture and Neuromuscular Status

1. Muscle tone is good.
2. Asymetric body position maintained:
    a. In supine position head is held on one side with arm on that side extended, the other flexed.
    b. In prone position head is held on side, arms flexed, close to head, legs flexed in kneeling position, pelvis raised.
3. Hands held tight-fisted.
4. Head sags.
5. Moro reflex present and strong.
6. Clonus easily elicited.
7. Grasp reflex strong.

F—Visual, Auditory, Tactile Senses

1. Blinks at bright light.
2. Gaze vague and staring, though may fix momentarily on moving object.
3. Eye movements not coordinated.
4. Soft sounds, pleasant warmth, gentle motion, promote relaxation.

G—Feeding

1. Definitely feels hunger and satiation.
2. Indicates desire for food by crying and rooting movements.

H—Sleep

1. Definitely sleeps and wakes up, but without any relation to day and night.

I—Reactions to Environment

1. Reactions are global.
2. Displeasure produces cry and activity of whole body. The neonate dislikes hunger, bright lights, loud noises, bitter tastes, cold, free space, and agitated people.
3. Pleasure produces relaxation. The neonate enjoys freedom from bodily discomfort, gentle rocking, soft soothing sounds, a snugly wrapped blanket, warmth, and calm people.

J—Environmental Needs

1. Freedom from organic stress.
2. Freedom from human tensions.
3. Satisfaction of needs as they arise.
4. Neonate indifferent to individuality of person who cares for him but sensitive to emotional climate.

K—Parental Attitudes

1. The mother in the postpartum period is almost always in a state of emotional instability and needs understanding sympathetic council.
2. The father of a newborn needs intellectual understanding of his wife's wayward emotions.

L—Danger Signals

1. Excessive crying.
2. Failure in weight gain after first 4–5 days.
3. Serious danger signals of organic origin are cyanosis, pallor, apathy, convulsions.
4. Danger signals which may be organic or may be reactions to adult tensions are referable chiefly to the gastrointestinal tract: anorexia, failure to suck, vomiting, diarrhea.

M—Success in Handling the Newborn Is Manifested by:

1. A vigorous infant who sleeps soundly, waking when he has needs, whose cry is lusty but ceases when his needs are met.
2. A steady weight gain after the first 4–5 days.
3. Parents who accept their responsibilities without undue turmoil.

N—Failure in Handling the Newborn Is Manifested by:

1. A crying fretful infant.
2. Poor weight gain.
3. Agitated parents.

III. THE INFANT AT ONE MONTH

A—General Appearance

1. Plump.
2. Vigorous.
3. Noisy.
4. Self-absorbed.

B—Dominant Developmental Thrust

1. Establishment of contact with environment. Fetal orientation is giving way to acceptance of independent existence.

C—Physiologic Status

1. Equilibrium still precarious and cannot withstand stress.
2. Gain of 1 lb over birth weight.

D—Instinctive Behavior

1. Cry lusty. It is still staccato and rhythmic, but tempo a little slower than at birth. It is still elicited by any discomfort and terminated by satisfaction.
2. Sucking when hungry still preceded by rooting movements; it now remains vigorous until hunger is appeased and is no longer interrupted by short cat naps.
3. Sucking desire present when not hungry—will accept pacifier.
4. Smile—rudimentary smile has usually made its appearance and consists of facial expression only.

E—Posture and Neuromuscular Status

1. Asymmetric position predominates.
2. Flexion of extremities not as tight as at birth.
3. Hands fisted, though not as tight as in newborn.

4. Head sags when held in sitting position.
5. Moro reflex, clonus, involuntary grasp still present.

F—Visual, Auditory, Tactile Senses

1. Eye movements coordinated most of the time.
2. Tears have appeared.
3. Gaze vague, but infant will cease body activity to look at a near object and attempt to keep it within range of vision.
4. Listens to soft sounds and will stop bodily activity apparently to concentrate on sound.

G—Language

1. Comfort sounds during sucking.

H—Feeding

1. Hunger constitutes powerful demand for attention.
2. Periodicity of need for food becoming regularized.
3. Enjoys sensation of warmth and body contact while eating.

I—Sleep

1. Diurnal pattern beginning to emerge.

J—Reactions to Environment

1. Reactions are still global.
2. Displeasure is expressed by crying and thrashing of extremities. Dislikes are similar to those at birth except that threshold of tolerance for light, sound, and motion is slightly greater. However, awareness of, and intolerance for, agitated people is more pronounced. He is also beginning to accept the sensation of free space and no longer requires snug wrapping except for sleep.
3. Pleasure is more pronounced. It is expressed by cessation of bodily activity, sometimes by a tentative smile. The infant responds with pleasure to gentle stimulation of any of his sensory receptors, especially those of sound, motion, warmth.
4. He is oblivious to the individuality of the people who care for him but firm in his approval of any relaxed gentle arms and voice.

K—Environmental Needs

1. Freedom from organic stress.
2. A relaxed, calm, loving, and unhurried person to take care of his needs more or less as they arise.

L—Parental Attitudes

1. Parents have stabilized somewhat, but they are apt to be still in a transitional stage and easily upset by infant behavior they do not understand.
2. Crying is universally upsetting and often creates a vicious circle—the more the child cries, the more the parents are distraught; their agitation in turn further upsets the child, who then cries more.
3. Parents need help in understanding the ways of babies; some need much more help than others.

M—Danger Signals

1. Failure to gain weight.

2. Excessive crying.
3. Apathy.

IV. THREE MONTHS OLD

A—General Appearance

1. Chubby.
2. Friendly.
3. Cuddly.

B—Dominant Developmental Thrust

1. The smile is the outstanding achievement.
2. The infant is beginning to respond socially to his environment.
3. Basic trust (or mistrust) is becoming established.

C—Physiologic Status

1. Stability has increased.
2. Peristalsis is usually in right direction and a little slower than earlier (less "spitting up," stools less frequent and slightly firmer).
3. Gain in weight rapid.

D—Instinctive Behavior

1. Smile is well developed and includes whole body activity. The baby "smiles with his toes."
2. Chuckle and laugh frequently accompany smile.
3. Sucking is strong and vigorous and is no longer preceded by rooting movements.
4. Sucks and "mouths" fingers and anything held in hands.
5. Crying has decreased; the infant can wait a minute to have his needs satisfied, especially if he sees or hears his mother.
6. Cry is less staccato than at birth; variations in pitch and inflection can be heard.

E—Posture and Locomotion

1. Symmetrical body position predominates.
2. Head is held in midline when in supine position.
3. Head is fairly steady on shoulders when baby is held in sitting position.
4. Moro reflex is fading if not gone.
5. On verge of rolling over.

F—Manipulation

1. Hands open or only loosely fisted.
2. Reflex grasp weak.
3. Holds toy actively when put in hand, but does not yet reach for it.
4. Hands clutch each other.
5. May pull blanket or dress over face.

G—Visual, Auditory, Tactile Senses

1. Eyes move coordinately.
2. Likes large bright objects.
3. Looks with interest at people and objects.
4. Looks at toy in hand—regard shifts from hand to toy.

5. Expression is alert.
6. Pays attention to moving object; follows by turning head.
7. Listens to sounds.

H—Language

1. Coos, gurgles.
2. Vocalizes vowel sounds.

I—Feeding

1. Shows excitement at sight of food.
2. Enjoys spoon-fed food, though with considerable spluttering.
3. Wants to be held when sucking milk.

J—Sleep

1. Diurnal pattern established.

K—Social Contact

1. Reactions still global.
2. Shows excitement by breathing heavily and activating whole body.
3. While originally an instinctive pattern, smile now used to beguile adults.

L—Environmental Needs

1. Freedom from organic stress.
2. Protection from infection.
3. Freedom from human tension.
4. Warm, tender care in response to his needs.

M—Parental Attitudes

1. The baby's outgoing friendliness is reflected in parental pleasure in his activities.
2. The baby's smiling responsiveness facilitates parental attitudes conducive to the establishment of basic trust.

N—Danger Signals

1. Failure to gain weight.
2. Lack of smile.
3. Excessive crying.
4. Apathy.

V. SEVEN MONTHS OLD

A—General Appearance

1. Chubby.
2. Friendly in familiar situation.
3. Constantly wet around the chin.
4. Drools and sucks on everything.

B—Dominant Developmental Thrust

1. The ability to distinguish the familiar from the strange, which brings with it anxiety.

C—Health

1. Weight gain in his own channel of growth.
2. Lower incisors may be through.

D—Instinctive Behavior

1. Clinging has emerged. Whenever the infant is distressed or fearful, he wishes to hang on tight to his mother if she is present.
2. Clinging can be transferred to a less familiar person if the mother is not available.
3. Clinging can also be transferred to a toy or blanket. Such an object can be used by the baby to give him security.
4. Cry is elicited more often by anxiety than by physiologic discomfort. It is loud, rhythmic, slower in tempo; prespeech sounds can be detected.
5. Smile used a great deal.
6. Sucking vigorous; enjoys sucking milk but also sucks fingers and anything he can carry to mouth.

E—Posture and Locomotion

1. Head is now completely steady on the shoulders.
2. Sits erect for few minutes, leans forward on hands.
3. Sits propped for half hour or so.
4. Bounces actively.
5. When held erect, carries large part of weight on feet.

F—Manipulation

1. Reaches for object with both hands.
2. Grabs small object with palmar grasp.
3. Holds one object, grabs for second one.
4. Shakes rattle, bangs toy.
5. Reaches for toy out of range.
6. Drops toy; unable to release voluntarily.
7. Plays with feet, puts toes in mouth.
8. Chews on everything, drools constantly.

G—Language

1. Coos, gurgles, laughs.
2. Polysyllabic vowel sounds.
3. Listens attentively to sounds.

H—Eating

1. Has taste preferences—will spit out food he does not like.
2. Wants to help feed himself.
3. Pats bottle.
4. May dive into bowl of food with both hands.
5. May take few sips of water or juice from cup.
6. Chews food put into mouth with fingers, but may object to lumps in spoon-fed food.

I—Sleep

1. Long night's sleep with one, two, or three daytime naps.

J—Play

1. Sensorimotor play has made its appearance.
2. All sensory equipment used to bring feelings to the infant. He looks, listens, feels, tastes, smells everything within range. Mouth, lips, tongue contribute sensations of touch as well as of taste.
3. Is more interested in large objects than small ones.

K—Social Contact

1. In familiar situation is friendly, smiles, laughs.
2. Shows anxiety in strange situations.

L—Environmental Needs

1. Acceptance of need to cling.
2. Avoidance of long separation from mother or other equally familiar person.

M—Parental Attitudes

1. Mother may feel guilt, embarrassment, irritation at infant's refusal to accept attentions from well-meaning friends or relatives. She needs intellectual understanding that the infant's anxiety in strange situations is evidence of a forward step in development. Refusal to let the child cling makes it difficult for him to maintain his trust in his world.

VI. NINE MONTHS OLD

A—General Appearance

1. Mobile on all fours.
2. Wary of strangers.
3. Cheerful, friendly in familiar situation.

B—Dominant Developmental Thrust

1. Index finger approach initiates probing of mysteries of the world.
2. Glimmering independence manifest by voluntarily creeping away from mother.
3. Reaffirmation of trust by clinging to mother.

C—Health

1. Susceptible to infection.
2. Weight gain in his own channel of growth.

D—Instinctive Behavior

1. Clinging very prominent.
2. Crying and smiling still important tools.
3. Sucking vigorous.
4. Rudimentary following as soon as able to creep.

E—Posture and Locomotion

1. Sits indefinitely.
2. Turns over.
3. Creeps—has mustered courage to creep away from mother but also uses creeping ability to seek mother when distressed.
4. Pulls up to stand at rail.
5. Desire to stand irrepressible; objects to lying down long enough to have diaper changed.

F—Manipulation

1. Reaches with one hand.
2. Grasps small object with prehensile grip.
3. Crude release evident.

4. Maturation has extended to distal areas—fingertips, tongue tip, and toes now under control.
5. Approaches objects with outstretched index finger and also with tongue.
6. Heightened interest in small objects, finds every crumb—usually puts it into mouth.
7. Interested in texture, scratches sheet with index finger, feels blanket.
8. Will play with stool if has the opportunity.
9. Interested in genitals and feels them whenever they are uncovered.

I—Play

1. Sensorimotor play occupies most of waking hours.

G—Language

1. Imitates variety of sounds.
2. Uses vowel and consonant combination—"Dada."
3. Comprehends "Bye bye."
4. Prespeech sounds in cry.
5. No true words as yet.

H—Eating

1. Holds own bottle. Some 9-month-olds prefer to lie on back and hold own bottle; others insist on being held to take bottle.
2. Wants to feed self with hands.
3. Interested in chewing.
4. Interested in cup, for water or juice.

J—Social Contact

1. Friendly, active, investigative in familiar situation.
2. Glimmering of independence evidenced by voluntarily separating him-himself from mother—desire to act *his* way.
3. Sensitive to individuality of people; intolerant of strangers.

K—Environmental Needs

1. Acceptance of desire for independence.
2. Provision of safe place where he can explore with minimum of restrictions.
3. Encouragement of desire to feed himself.
4. Acceptance of frequent need for reassurance.
5. Acceptance of interest in stools and in genitals.

L—Parental Attitudes

1. Mobility of infant creates problems of discipline.
2. Familiar mother substitute desirable.

VII. THE YEARLING

A—General Appearance

1. Busy, cheerful in familiar situation.
2. Investigative.

B—Dominant Developmental Thrust

1. The desire to be a biped, which brings with it the urge to go away and the need to run back to security.

C—Health

1. Susceptible to infection.
2. Tripled birth weight.

D—Instinctive Behavior

1. Clinging still prominent.
2. Following is emerging.
3. Sucking is fading.
4. Crying a less frequent tool.
5. Smiling and laughing easily elicited.

E—Posture and Locomotion

1. Wants to be constantly on his feet.
2. Cruises around with one-hand support.
3. Reverts to creeping when support not available.
4. Cannot abide supine position when awake.

F—Manipulation

1. Accurate one-hand grasp.
2. Grasps two small objects at same time.
3. Can release voluntarily.
4. Uses good prehensile grip.
5. Picks up minute objects.
6. Still explores with outstretched index finger.

G—Language

1. Inflected jargon.
2. One or two single words.
3. Understands simple verbal request: "Give it to me."
4. Understands simple gestures: "Come."

H—Eating

1. Anticipation on sight of food.
2. Many also associate sounds with food.
3. Has definite food preferences.
4. Eats spoon-fed food well.
5. Wants to feed self with fingers.
6. Chews soft lumps in food.
7. Enjoys sucking and may insist on holding his own bottle.
8. Prefers water or juice from cup and takes some swallows of milk from cup.

I—Sleep

1. Enjoys bedtime rituals.

J—Play

1. Sensorimotor play.
2. Beginning to appreciate inherent discipline of things.
3. Accepts some mother-applied discipline.

K—Social Contact

1. In familiar situation is busy cruising around, pulling, poking, patting anything within reach.
2. Desirous of an adult finger to hold on to while venturing into free space.

3. Smiles, laughs, enjoys simple games such as pat-a-cake.
4. Enjoys gentle roughhousing.
5. Fearful in strange situation or with strange people and wants to cling to mother.
6. May be devoted to "security" blanket or toy.

L—Environmental Needs

1. Ample safe place for cruising and manipulation.
2. Freedom from overprotection.
3. Acceptance of growing independence.
4. Freedom from adult tension.
5. Consistent firm and friendly discipline.
6. Avoidance of long separation from mother.

M—Parental Attitudes

1. Discipline problems increasing.

VIII. FIFTEEN MONTHS OLD

A—General Appearance

1. Active.
2. Clumsy.
3. Distractible.

B—Dominant Developmental Thrust

1. Stubborn—the age of "No." The semantic accomplishment of the abstract negation ushers in the concept that *I* can refuse, part of autonomy which will flower in the next stage.

C—Health

1. Susceptible to infection, but not usually much exposed.
2. Growth has slowed down.

D—Instinctive Patterns

1. Following prominent.
2. Sucking is fading.
3. Crying seldom used.
4. Smiling and laughing still prominent.

E—Posture and Locomotion

1. Walks alone, falls frequently, often by just collapsing.
2. Creeps upstairs.
3. Backs into small chair to seat himself.
4. Experiments with walking backward and sideways.
5. Runs with many falls.

F—Manipulation

1. Hands ever busy; grabs, pulls, pokes.
2. Index finger approach still evident.
3. Can build tower of two, sometimes three blocks.
4. Can put small objects into container and take them out.
5. Scribbles with pencil; may imitate strokes.

G—Language

1. Ten to fifteen single words (nouns).
2. Concept of simple abstractions.
3. Concept of negation. Understands "No."
4. May also use semantic head-shaking gestures for "No."
5. Uses "No" to excess verbally, although may often do what is asked of him to the accompaniment of vigorous "No."

H—Eating

1. Wants to feed self, except when unusually tired.
2. Drinks water and juice from cup.
3. Drinks some milk from cup, but may want bottle, especially when sleepy.
4. Chews soft lumps in food.
5. Amount of food consumed has decreased.

I—Sleep

1. May object to going to bed.
2. Occasionally wakes during night.

J—Play

1. Sensorimotor play.
2. Accepting some discipline.
3. Imitation beginning to appear.

K—Social Contact

1. Trots around constantly.
2. Investigates everything.
3. Enjoys short trips away from home.
4. Likes other children around but does not play *with* them.
5. Fearful in strange situations.

L—Environmental Needs

1. Consistent gentle discipline.
2. Ample opportunity to exercise independence.
3. Freedom from overprotection.
4. Freedom from adult tensions.
5. Avoidance of long separations from mother.

M—Parental Attitudes

1. Mother needs encouragement to get away from home occasionally.
2. Importance of familiar mother substitute needs stressing.

IX. THE TODDLER

A—General Appearance and Characteristics

1. Clumsy.
2. Incessantly active.
3. Imitative.
4. Talkative.
5. Distractible.
6. Home-bound.

B—Dominant Developmental Thrust

1. "Me do it"—the establishment of autonomy.
2. Sphincter control—part of autonomy.
3. While autonomy is dominant, the toddler needs reaffirmation of his basic trust.

C—Health

1. Physiologically his body is well stabilized.
2. Succumbs to frequent infections.
3. Gain in weight is slow but steady.

D—Instinctive Patterns

1. Following is at its zenith. The toddler must "go see Mommy" many, many times a day. If distressed, his need is urgent.
2. Separation from mother (or some equally familiar person) may have serious repercussions. If hospitalized, mother or her substitute should accompany child.

E—Locomotion and Manipulation

1. Has mastered biped position.
2. Walks, runs, jumps, sidles backward and sideways.
3. Has trouble decelerating in time to turn corners.
4. Bumps into objects, falls frequently.
5. Goes up and down stairs alone, in the beginning of toddlerhood with one foot at a time, later by alternating feet.
6. Can learn to ride a tricycle.
7. Can make tower of several blocks, three blocks in beginning of period, eight to ten toward the end.
8. Can line blocks horizontally to make a train.
9. Likes to pull things around on a string.

F—Behavior

1. Ceaseless activity.
2. Short attention span—flits from one thing to another.
3. Easily frustrated when he attempts the impossible.
4. Frustrations leading to:
    a. Outbursts of temper.
    b. Comfort habits, sucking, rocking, banging.
5. Lack of concern about the feelings of others.

G—Language

1. Speech progresses from single words to full sentences of his native tongue with correct syntax; use of pronouns and plurals. Jargon is abandoned.
2. Talks incessantly; verbalizes whatever occurs to him—"verbal diarrhea."
3. Plays with sounds and rhythms.
4. Uses speech to conceptualize world to himself.
5. Literal.
6. Speech as a means of communication is rudimentary.
7. Enjoys simple stories, repeated with exactly the same words and gestures.
8. Likes to look at books, can turn pages, often several at a time, and name objects in pictures.
9. Scribbles; toward end of period can copy cross and circle.

10. Enjoys songs; some can carry tune by end of period.
11. Paints; loves color and form, but painting reflects feelings and is not a copy of reality.

H—Eating

1. Abandons bottle. Some toddlers enjoy a bottle at bedtime well beyond second birthday; others give it up completely in late infancy.
2. Feeds himself and resents any help with the ever recurrent theme of the age, "Me do it"; he occasionally, however, if unusually tired, may hand the spoon to the adult saying, "You feed me."
3. Dining pleasures consist of getting the food into the mouth; conversation and companionship at meals more often than not a distraction.
4. Table manners are rudimentary. Frequently uses fingers instead of conventional table tools.
5. A "constructive mess" at the dining table is to be tolerated; a "destructive mess," to be stopped.
6. Food consumption small.

I—Sphincter Control

1. Physiologically voluntary control of sphincters develops early in toddlerhood.
2. "Me do it my way" is nowhere more obvious than in the child's final acceptance of the culturally approved place for elimination. He is interested not only in the act of elimination but also in the products and will play happily with urine or stools if he has the opportunity.
3. In relation to control of his anal sphincter the child establishes a feeling tone toward "giving freely" and "holding tight" which may have lifelong ramifications.

J—Sleep

1. Needs 12-hour-night's sleep.
2. Almost all toddlers need a regular daytime nap.
3. Hates to stop playing to go to bed; may be expert in fighting sleep.

K—Play

1. Almost everything a toddler does in his waking hours is a form of play, locomotion, manipulation, language, even eating.
2. Sensorimotor play still prominent—experiments with all his sensorimotor equipment to discover the feelings he can obtain from the world about him.
3. Imitative play has appeared—copies gestures and actions, not only of people, but of animals and even of inanimate objects, e.g., chugs like a train.
4. Likes company during play, but play is parallel, not cooperative.

L—Environmental Needs

1. Adequate medical and nursing care for his frequent infections.
2. Immunizations against preventable diseases.
3. Ample safe opportunity for a variety of experiences.
4. Constant, almost minute-by-minute supervision.
5. Consistent, firm, and gentle discipline.

6. Routines are essential. The toddler does best when he knows that one thing follows another in an orderly and expected way. He is upset by unpredictability.

M—Parental Attitudes

1. Toddlers are wearing.
2. Their ceaseless activity, constant talking, utter lack of appreciation of the dangerous require the constant presence of an adult.
3. The mother of a toddler gets tired, jumpy, nervous and is in great need of some adult companionship.
4. Relatively few young mothers of one or more little children can run a home and take care of the youngsters without some free time for adult activity. When they try to do it, their inevitable irritations are taken out on the children.

N—Danger Signals

1. Excessive use of:
    a. Temper tantrums.
    b. Comfort habits.
2. Failure in toilet training.
3. Failure in speech development.
4. Failure to conform to *reasonable* discipline.

X. THE PRESCHOOLER

A—General Appearance

1. Slender, graceful, lithe.
2. Active and talkative.
3. Tentative independence from home.
4. Imaginative.

B—Dominant Developmental Thrust

1. Having discovered during the toddler years the uniqueness of his own self, is now absorbed in sharpening his focus on what kind of a person he is.
2. Interested in his gender role, his abilities, his feelings, his thoughts, his fantasies. Like the toddler, is absorbed with himself (egocentric) and has little understanding of the feelings of others.

C—Health

1. Extremely susceptible to infection, especially respiratory infection.
2. Weight gain slow and steady.

D—Locomotion and Manipulation

1. His body is now under his control.
2. He is a biped; his hands are good prehensile tools.
3. He is capable of learning many manual skills.
4. Fine motor coordination not as adequate as that of large muscles.

E—Language

1. Can use native language competently with correct grammar, syntax, and pronunciation.

2. Still thinks out loud, but less than the toddler.
3. Plays with sounds and rhythms.
4. Can carry a tune and loves songs and singing.
5. Interested in stories and pictures.
6. Enjoys looking at books, turns pages competently, seldom tears.

F—Eating

1. Has mastered the art of getting food into his mouth.
2. Drinks completely from cup or glass.
3. Chews easily, eats what the family eats.
4. Table manners reasonably acceptable, seldom spills.
5. Interested in companionship at mealtimes.
6. Wants to participate as a member of the group around dining table.
7. Loves picnics, tea parties.
8. Actual food consumption is small.

G—Sphincter Control

1. Completely established, day and night.

H—Sleep

1. Sleep fighting frequent.

I—Play

1. Imitative dramatic play, in which he acts out the life about him.
2. Symbolic play, a technique of unburdening feelings that produce guilt.
3. Rich fantasy life. Has difficulty distinguishing between fantasy and reality.
4. Imaginary companions are frequent.
5. Plays cooperatively with other children.

J—Genital Interest

1. Interested in where babies come from.
2. Interested in differences between boys and girls.
3. Castration fears may occur.
4. Oedipal situations may arise.

K—Environmental Needs

1. Health supervision; adequate immunizations.
    a. Good medical and nursing care for frequent infections.
    b. Good diet, adequate sleep.
2. Routines—an ordered world. The preschool child has difficulty in coping with unpredictability. This is evident in all aspects of his life; he enjoys the same story repeated in exactly the same way; he wants juice to come after his nap; he wants to sleep after evening rituals.
3. Rich opportunity for experiences.
4. Consistent discipline.
5. Good nursery school.
6. Opportunity for gradual separation from home.

L—Parental Attitudes

1. The mother relaxes during the child's preschool years.
2. The child is more responsible, less dependent on mother.
3. The child goes to nursery school, spends time at friends' houses.

4. Mother has opportunity to take a "private breath."
5. Some parents have difficulty accepting the preschooler's normal interest in his genitals and need an intellectual understanding of this phase of development.

M—Danger Signals

1. Persistence of infantile patterns:
   a. Bed wetting.
   b. Comfort habits indulged in so excessively that they interfere with play.
   c. Excessive tantrums.
2. Overdependence on mother.
3. Inability to take on responsibility for self.
4. Failure in language development.

XI. SCHOOL–AGE CHILD

A—General Appearance

1. Strong, sturdy.
2. Dirty and disorderly.
3. Gang-oriented.
4. Independent.

B—Dominant Developmental Thrust

1. Independence from home achieved by identification with peers.
2. Intellectual curiosity.
3. Egocentricity beginning to give way to world-centered orientation: "How *I* feel" maturing into "What *it* is."
4. Still unconcerned for the most part about welfare of adults but developing real concern for welfare of a buddy.

C—Health

1. Usually good, susceptibility to infection has abated.
2. Growth is steady.

D—Locomotion and Manipulation

1. Has neuromuscular coordination sufficient to learn any skill he puts his mind to.

E—Language

1. Semantic meanings of words of more interest than their mere sounds. Enjoys puns, jokes, little moron stories.
2. Reading a useful tool and enjoyable pastime.

F—Eating

1. Companionship essential for dining pleasures; wants to talk and participate in group.
2. Enjoys family dinner table when conversation is at his level.
3. Loves eating with peers on picnics, in a hut, at tea parties.
4. Capable of acceptable table manners, but often enjoys flaunting parental standards.

5. After school snacks a necessity.
6. Usually accepts family food patterns.

G—Sleep

1. Seldom consciously fights sleep.
2. May need firm discipline to get to bed at prescribed hours.

H—Play

1. Oriented to peer group.
2. Enjoys organized games with rigid rules.
3. Ritual keynote of much of play.
4. Athletic skills.
5. Collections.

I—Schools, Learning

1. Insatiable curiosity to learn, fostered by good school, interested parents, rich opportunity for varied experience.

J—Parental Attitudes

1. Understanding of need to break dependence on family.
2. Encouragement of a buddy friendship.
3. Acceptance of peer group mores.
4. Interest and encouragement of intellectual curiosity.
5. Willingness to see the child stand alone on his own feet, neither pushing him out nor holding him down, and at the same time the moral fortitude to apply consistent firm and reasonable discipline when needed.
6. May need help in understanding and accepting growth patterns of fringe children.

K—Danger Signals

1. Failure to establish independence.
2. Being the goody-goody teacher's pet.
3. Loneliness.
4. Psychosomatic illness.
5. Antisocial behavior.

XII. PUBERTY—EARLY ADOLESCENCE

Common Characteristics of Both Sexes

A—General

1. Rebellion against home.
2. Vacillation between considerable maturity and babyishness.
3. Absorption with close friend of same age and sex.
4. Moodiness.
5. Sloppiness and disorder.

B—Dominant Developmental Thrust

1. Establishment of independence of self: "Who am I?" "What kind of a person am I?"

C—Health

1. Rapid growth.
2. Body-conscious.
3. Appearance of sexual maturity.
4. Skin problems.
5. Fringe children need help to accept their own body patterns.

D—Eating

1. Constantly hungry.
2. Companionship at meals and at after-school snacks provides dining pleasure.

E—Sleep

1. Actually needs more sleep than during younger years.
2. Sleepy at getting up time.
3. Wants to sit up at night as sign of increasing maturity.
4. Clash between physiology and culture.

F—Parental Attitudes

1. Acceptance of increasing maturity.
2. Loosening of reins but not complete abolition of home authority.
3. Adequate education concerning body changes:
    a. Nutritional requirements.
    b. Sleep requirements.
    c. Sexual changes.
    d. Sexual changes in opposite sex.
4. Encouragement of independence and the responsibilities it entails.

Special Characteristics of Boys in Puberty

A—General

1. Boisterous.
2. Clumsy.
3. Secretive; "clams up" at home.
4. Aggressive.
5. Dirty (cannot get him near the bathroom).

B—Health

1. Boys in puberty gain more weight and height than girls.
2. Size outstrips strength.

C Social Contact

1. Out of house more and more.
2. Much talk with boy companions about sex.

Special Characteristics of Girls in Puberty

A—General

1. Vague.
2. Diffuse.

3. Talkative, but not communicative.
4. Giggly.

B—Social Contact
1. Crush on older woman.
2. Interested in romantic love.
3. Playacting.

XIII. LATE ADOLESCENCE

Common Characteristics in Both Sexes

A—General
1. Rebellious.
2. Concerned with personal appearance (cannot get them *out* of the bathroom).
3. Moody.
4. Interest in opposite sex.

B—Dominant Developmental Thrust
1. Establishment of ego identity "Where I fit in this world."
2. Ambiguity of society toward adolescent helps to compound the problems.

C—Health
1. Growth has subsided.
2. Full stature almost attained.

D—Eating
1. Food requirements approaching adult level.
2. Companionship provides dining pleasure.

E—Sleep
1. Sleep requirements approaching adult level.

F—Social Contact
1. Intimate relation with buddy fades.
2. Greater interest in opposite sex.

G—Environmental Needs
1. Acceptance by society, in job, in college.

H—Parental Attitudes
1. Respect for opinion.
2. Acceptance of maturity.

Special Characteristics of Boys in Late Adolescence

A—General
1. Sexual problems prominent and demanding.
2. Interested in plans for career.
3. Less interested than girls in mate seeking.

Special Characteristics of Girls in Late Adolescence

A—General

1. Interest in boys, directed toward mate seeking.
2. Absorbed in fantasies of romantic love.
3. Less interested than boys in plans for career.
4. Sexual problems less demanding than in boys.

Section VIII

SOCIOLOGICAL CONSIDERATIONS

42

The Family

The family is the little child's cosmos; for him everything beyond home is outer space. Even when he goes outside the four walls of home, he takes his home orientation with him, through his close association with those who accompany him. It is during these early home-bound years that the child's awareness of himself as a person emerges. These earliest feelings color his lifelong attitude about himself and about the whole world. Concern about the child's emerging personality directs attention toward the family and toward those people who create the climate within the home (Erikson, 1963).

The United States is undergoing a cultural metamorphosis which is having a profound effect upon family life and upon the mother of today. Today's family stands in marked contrast to that characteristic of earlier society, when the extended, rather than the nuclear, family was the rule and when more services were performed within the family. The family then included not only its biologic core but many additional adults—grandparents, grown children, unmarried relatives of either spouse, hired employees. Household tasks—cooking, sewing, laundry, cleaning—were performed within the home without the aid of automation. There were no preschools; education of young children was considered solely the responsibility of the home; while some commercial recreation was available, there was far less than at present. Since income for these big households was produced by the male members, whose job opportunities were more likely to remain geographically fixed than is the case today, families remained in the same area, often for generations. Domesticity was the career to which almost all women, both married and unmarried, devoted their lives.

Urbanization, automation, family mobility, birth and fertility rates, and the employment of women outside the home have been cataclysmic in their effect upon the family life of today. It is beyond the scope of this book, however, to discuss all the multitudinous factors that have influenced the way people work and live in the United States.

The household of today has become denuded of adults other than husband and wife. The increased opportunities for women in the labor market have meant that the superfluous women of the old large families have found independent life more agreeable than life under the aegis of some magnanimous householder. Grown children, especially girls, no longer live at home; maiden aunts who in years past never considered working have discovered they have marketable skills; older women are wanted by industry. Even household help has all but vanished.

The middle class family of today, consisting of husband, wife, and their children, lives in a city (only 10 per cent of families in the United States were rural in 1960). The home is equipped with numerous laborsaving devices, and in addition a large share of the goods and services consumed by the family are produced outside the home—foods, clothes, laundry, education, recreation. The husband provides the main income and is often faced with geographic moves to ensure his advancement. The wife manages the home without the assistance of other women and at times in her life may have an outside job as well (Glick, 1957).

THE MIDDLE CLASS MOTHER IN THE UNITED STATES TODAY

Before children arrive or after they are grown, the management of the home is but a part-time job in our automated society. Child rearing, however, is no part-time occupation. Much of the job cannot be done by machines. There are no gadgets for changing diapers, for answering questions, for reading *The Three Bears*, for playing parchesi. It is true that prepared baby food, diaper service, automatic washers reduce the added household work that comes along with children. Television might be considered a mechanical device for "keeping children quiet." Nevertheless, in spite of these aids, one lone woman with several young children is fully occupied from early morning to late evening. Child rearing remains the one essentially feminine occupation. It does not, however, last a lifetime.

Child rearing is a full-time job (and more!) for perhaps 10 to 15 years, a part-time job possibly another 5 to 10 years. At the most, 25 years of a woman's life can be spent in raising a family, and for many women it is hardly more than 15 years. These years are carved out of the middle of life. A woman's life, therefore, is broken up into discontinuous epochs. Men are not faced with these upheavals, nor were women in the days when domesticity was the lifetime feminine occupation.

Women have attempted various ways of carving out for themselves satisfying lives. In the early part of the century the feminists waged a battle for the admission of women into careers and work outside the home. In their desire to create more opportunities for women the feminists aimed at the elimination of any distinction between men and women. In the long run many of their ideals failed to catch the imagination of women who found it impossible to live either as men or as neuter gender creatures (Erickson, 1964).

Since the end of World War II there has been a swing of the pendulum away from the goals of the feminists. What Friedan has aptly named the *feminine mystique* seems to have taken hold. The ideal feminine image of the mystique has become a woman who closes the door on the outside world and devotes her life exclusively to her husband, children, and home.

The crux of the problem for women in the United States revolves around the fact that the time-honored domestic role of women as a full-time occupation for life has all but evaporated. A second problem, really a corollary of the first and due to the exodus of other women from the home, is that during the child-rearing era the domestic role suddenly becomes so overwhelming that a sizable number of mothers of today are unable to cope adequately with the demands made upon them. Their failures produce a tense, disturbed family climate not conducive to the welfare of their children.

Women in our society must ultimately accept the fact that automation has come to stay and with it the dissolution of a lifetime of productive domesticity. They must also accept the fact that child rearing is an epoch of life and not a lifetime career.

The pediatrician (or other professional) who would help mothers with their children needs an awareness of some of the problems that face women in the United States.

EPOCHS IN A MOTHER'S LIFE

The First Epoch—Education and Marriage

In the United States the girl's education is similar to that of the boys she knows, often in the same school and in the same classes. But unlike the boy, who thinks in terms of a lifelong working career, the girl's attention is most often directed toward an entry job which she intends to hold only for a short time. Relatively few girls since World War II have planned at the outset for careers in the outside world.

Almost every girl hopes to get married and have a family, but her education is not directed toward this goal. She either acquires a general cultural background or learns some skills with which she can earn her living for a few years. Not infrequently she has some ambivalence about her sex role.

It is possible that the neuter-gender quality of her early education and the emphasis on economic independence push girls into a frantic scramble to attain marriage in order to establish their feminine identity. It may push them, too, into an acceptance of the feminine mystique. Whatever the reasons, and doubtless they are complicated, American girls direct their energies toward marriage most successfully. They marry earlier than in past generations, often before their schooling has been completed. Few fail to achieve matrimony. In fact many marry several times; if a first marriage does not work out well, it is terminated and another one tried.

Marriage itself seldom interferes with a young woman's basic pattern of life. She and her husband continue to work at their respective jobs. They set up housekeeping in a small automated apartment that can readily be managed after working hours.

The wife's job may well be an economic necessity in the early years of the marriage, but neither she nor her husband are as concerned with her advancement on the job as they are with the husband's progress. The wife works to help her husband, not to advance herself (Kluckhohn, 1949).

In this first epoch of her grownup life, the girl has a sense of freedom and independence; her ability to achieve marriage establishes confidence in herself as a woman, and she adjusts to life without undue turmoil.

The Second Epoch—Child Rearing

Then come children, and the second epoch begins. About 80 per cent of middle-income women quit their jobs and stay home when the first baby is born. The majority of young mothers have hardly a grain of training for the job of this part of their lives. Our society still assumes that because an individual is female, she automatically knows how to run a household, feed a family, raise children.

Not only is little effort made in our educational system to train women for the jobs that will occupy significant years of their lives, but there is positive pressure against such courses in high school and in many colleges. Reisman maintains that college courses in child development or in nutrition are but trade courses and detract from a woman's capacity for creative expression. It would seem easier to live creatively with some knowledge of the medium in which one is to work. A little academic knowledge can contribute as much, if not more, to a woman's capacity for mature self-expression as a profound knowledge of modern poetry, French literature, or medieval history which, for years, she will have little time to think about. This point of view is not meant to imply that cultural knowledge is not most desirable for any mature human being but only to upgrade the significance of training for one of the most important jobs of a woman's life.

Life in the second epoch is so different from that of the first that many a young mother is overwhelmed by the demands made upon her.

The Mother Who Stays Home

The young mother who stays at home, as most middle-income mothers do, suddenly finds her old free way of life gone and a completely new pattern thrust upon her. The young family lives by itself with no members other than husband, wife, and children. The mother is apt to be isolated in a small apartment in a community in which she is a relative newcomer. She has one baby and soon several more. She has no domestic help (or at best very little). Her husband is out of the house all day every workday and not infrequently many evenings and weekends as well. The mother is immobilized, because she can go nowhere without taking the children. If the young family lives in a housing development, the mother may have some coffee klatches with other young mothers, but these contacts are, more often than not, transient and casual; she has no intimate friends.

In addition to her isolation, she is extremely busy. While doubtless she has many mechanical gadgets, nevertheless her time from the 6 A.M. feeding to the dinner dishes is so fully occupied that she seldom has time to read a book, to play the piano, or even to think about anything but the next task ahead of her. Many a young mother discovers that the only time to get the ironing done is after the children are bedded down for the night. Mechanical gadgets help; in fact, the job would be virtually impossible without them. As one young Vassar graduate remarked as she viewed her brand-new washing machine: "Yes, it is very nice, and I surely do need it, but its not very companionable! You know, I believe the river bank had its compensations."

The young husband often pitches in after his day's work, helps with housework, does the shopping, takes clothes to the laundromat, or feeds and tends the children while his wife does some of the out-of-the-house chores. However, some mothers may feel as one did. "No, indeed, I don't let Harry do the marketing," she said. "You don't know how I look forward to those weekly hours in the supermarket, where I can at least *see* somebody my size."

The mothers who stay at home and make the grade in this epoch of their lives have one prime qualification: they are reasonably mature, self-confident women. They have made a good marriage, and though life may be difficult, they do not find it impossible to accept their role as wife and mother with satisfaction. Some are a real help to their husbands, finding time to keep abreast of their activities, supporting their interests, furthering their careers. Some few women manage, in addition, to pursue activities of their own in their few spare moments—in the arts, in community service.

The second epoch of life for many young mothers is all too frequently a time of great turmoil. Such a woman yearns for adult companionship and some relief from her overburdening duties. Her husband is the only person to whom she can turn.

He is pressed with the economic necessity of paying the bills. Mechanical gadgets come high. He is unaware of his wife's needs, though he may be painfully aware that she is not the helpmate he has been led to believe was her goal in life. He may be amazed at the changes in her. The girl who was so gay, competent, and charming during her "independent life" has turned into a "pain in the neck." At first he probably tries to be patient and understanding. He may try to supplement his income with an extra job to supply his wife with more mechanical appliances, but this may increase his time away from home. Sometimes his extracurricular activities become motivated as much by reluctance to face the turmoil at home as by economic necessity. Suspicion of this on the part of the wife is not conducive to relieving her problems.

The result is that an appalling number of our young middle-class mothers are lonely, overworked, and dissatisfied with life. Their ideal of the fully feminine role has been found wanting. This is not what they bargained for. This is not the goal they saw for themselves as they grew up, as they studied Byzantine art in college. These young women have been unable to achieve a self-image they find comfortable to live with. Some may have hung on to infantile patterns because of inadequacies in their own maturing years; and while they might have made a go of life under less trying circumstances, they are incapable of coping with problems they face (Pavenstedt, 1961; Fisher and Mendell, 1956).

These dissatisfied mothers become tense, anxious, jittery. They are irritable and inconsistent in their handling of their children. They spank and yell and punish, but their children behave more and more like obnoxious brats. The worse the children behave, the more the mother's horizon is limited. There are few places she can go where she will not be embarrassed by unpredictable child behavior.

To one young mother whose two little girls were, to put it mildly, uncooperative in the physician's office the suggestion was made that she bring her children into the playroom occasionally just to have a nice time and become more accustomed to the place. She replied: "Oh, doctor, I would *love* to come! It would give me some place to go." Such is the environment in which quite a sizable number of children in the United States are coming to maturity.

Mothers Who Work

Not all mothers stay at home even when their children are babies. Approximately 20 per cent of mothers of children under 6 have full-time paid jobs, and 41 per cent of mothers of children between 6 and 17 years old work away from home. Among these working mothers are many women who are widowed, divorced, or separated from their husbands and whose work is a necessity for economic survival. However, the increase in the number of working mothers during the past decade has been greatest among women living with husbands whose income is above subsistence level. For these women there is a choice of whether to work outside the home or not.

What motivates the mother to take a job? For many it is the desire for a higher standard of living than the husband's unaided income can supply. The vision of the good things of life that could be theirs with a little more money—a home of their own, a new car, a boat, a vacation, music lessons for the children, college education—these and many like things are worth working for.

Other young mothers find life at home with young children not to their liking; they resent the long hours, the isolation, the lack of companionship, and the incessant demands of their children. In addition, they have become disillusioned about their role as superfemales. They are eager to return to the "peace and quiet" of an office and to a job that offers some self-expression. They are glad to turn over the care of their children to someone else.

This does not mean that there may not be economic motives too. Since society is more sympathetic with economic needs than with the personal needs of a mother, these women, when quizzed, usually say that their job away from home is necessary for the family to maintain an adequate standard of living. Such a statement also gives solace to the mother herself. It is difficult for many a young woman in our present society to admit, even to herself, that her femininity is not strong enough to keep her content in the domestic role.

Ideally and in the abstract, perhaps children profit most if the mother stays at home during her children's early homebound years. But ideals and abstractions exist more on paper than in the hurly-burly of daily living. Not all women can be lumped together into one heap because they have the common property of fertility. Some women do best as full-time mothers at home; others make better mothers (and better human beings) when they combine the responsibilities of motherhood with those of an outside job. In the last analysis what is best for children is a mother who is sufficiently content with herself that she can be relaxed, free from tension, warm, and giving to her children. If she can create these qualities and remain at home 24 hours every day, this is wonderful, but if she needs to have outside activity to give her self-confidence, her children may be better off with quantitatively less of her time but qualitatively more valuable time when they have it.

The decision is an important one, and many a woman needs help in making the choice right for her. If she feels guilty about her choice, this interferes with the adequate performance of her duties both at home and on the job. She may feel guilty if she goes off to work and leaves her children for others to care for; she may feel guilty if she stays at home, because she feels she is depriving her family of material goods her earned income could supply.

The successful working mother is relatively free from guilt about her job. She is content with her conviction that the rewards of her job are greater than its liabilities. She gets satisfaction from the work she does; this does not mean she enjoys every minute of it—no life is all sweetness—but the work she does, the friends she makes, the clothes she *must* buy to appear at the office, the hairdos that are mandatory all contribute to a sense of self-esteem that is satisfying.

When she comes home she is content with herself; she looks forward eagerly to participation in family activities. Her hours before and after work are relaxed times for chores, for talk and play, and for that much overworked thing called *togetherness*. When vacation comes along such a woman looks forward eagerly to full time with children and husband. She feels she would always like to see more of her family than her life permits—in contrast to the overburdened home-bound mother who longs for a vacation *away* from her children.

On the other hand, the mother who feels guilty about leaving her children may be so jealous of whoever replaces her that she smothers the children with lavish attention in an effort to make them love her best—an effort that seldom accomplishes its goal.

Not only is the mother's attitude toward her job important, but so too is that of her husband. It is essential for family well-being that the man of the house accept his wife's outside employment and support her interests. In such an atmosphere both husband and wife build up each other's self-esteem, which is the most significant way each can help the other careerwise.

Aside from the emotional climate in which a mother works away from home, there are practical aspects which need consideration. No matter what a mother does, the responsibility for the home and children are hers. It is she who must see that the domestic work is done. If children are high school age, this is not too difficult. Mechanical gadgets and prepared foods reduce domestic chores to such an extent that she may quite well cope with them in the time not spent on her job.

Younger children present more of a problem. School-age youngsters need supervision after school hours. This is often not an insurmountable problem. Sometimes just the telephone is adequate. A youngster who checks in with his mother by phone as soon as he gets home from school may quite well manage for an hour or so until mother gets home. Many arrangements are satisfactory for the relatively brief interim between school and mother's return. In fact the ease with which adequate after-school care can be accomplished is reflected in the exodus of mothers from home to job as soon as their children reach school age.

Arranging satisfactory care for infants and preschool children while mother works is more difficult. Such youngsters not only need constant supervision, but they need a quality of care not always easy to find. All little children need some one person who is intelligent, careful, loving, and warm. Frequent changes of substitute mothers, either in the home or in a nursery, make it difficult for a youngster to develop security. Care from an indifferent, chilly, overstern, or overprotective person also is difficult for a child to cope with.

If good substitute care can be arranged, a little child can relate adequately to this person as well as to his mother, just as the child of a past generation could relate to members of the extended family. The quality of the care given by the substitute mother is crucial. It is quite possible that the quality of the care is better than the child would receive if his mother stayed at home and vented on him the frustrations stemming from her own unsatisfactory life at home.

Another practical aspect of the problem of the working mother has to do with her physical stamina. The successful working mother must assume responsibility for two jobs. The woman who is tired after her day's work and would like, when she comes home at night, to kick off her shoes, rest, and relax is not going to succeed as a mother. She must have vim and vigor left over in the evening. Ideally, she should have the constitution of an ox!

The further she falls from oxlike physical qualities, the more she must plan to replace her services at home. No woman can expect to carry the load of a demanding office job and do all the chores at home. Some women try to do it. They do the laundry before they leave in the mornings, iron until midnight, clean house over the weekends. The result is a tired out, frazzled, irritable creature with no time or energy for the important part of her home responsibilities: play, talk, companionship. For a mother's job to be an economic asset to her family she must make enough money to replace her services adequately at home, and the frailer she is, the more help she needs to run her home smoothly. Her home job can be simplified with good planning and with mechanical gadgets, but it cannot be simplified out of existence.

Much has been written on the evil effects of mother's outside employment on the well-being of children. Many of the earlier studies compared groups of children of working and nonworking mothers, with no attempt to make the groups comparable with respect to factors other than the employment of their mothers. Children living in a family with a stormy marriage that finally ends in divorce can hardly be compared with children of a tranquil marriage. The divorced woman may become a working mother after the termination of her marriage, but the significant disturbing factors in the lives of her children are more apt to be the turmoil before and after the divorce than the fact that the mother becomes a jobholder.

It is now fairly clear that the quality of the care the child receives and the personalities of his parents are more significant variables for his ultimate well-being than the fact of his mother's employment. More recent studies have attempted to control some of these variables. Herzog has reviewed a large number of studies on the effect of mother's employment on children (there are 63 references in her bibliography). She comes to the conclusion that "The mother's working, in itself, is only one among many factors impinging on children and may well be a secondary factor." Stalz reviewed six studies on the relationship of delinquency and maternal employment and came to the conclusion that the correlation was negligible. These conclusions are in harmony with the author's own clinical (and unstatistical) impression from observations of families who bring their children to the pediatrician, namely, that there is no correlation between behavior disorders in children and the fact of the mother's employment.

Mothers who stay at home but who are tense, lonely, unhappy in their home job are prone to have children who reflect this home climate. On the other hand, parents who accept the mother's employment as good for the whole family and make the necessary arrangements for adequate substitute care have children who take this modern phenomenon in stride. Said one little girl as she passed the cookies at a party: "In our family, Daddy makes the bread and butter and Mommy makes the jelly."

The Third Epoch—After the Children Are Grown

Ultimately children grow up and leave home, and their mother, if she has remained at home, is left unemployed. The job of the home of today is that of rearing children; housework in an automated home is far from a full-time occupation. Empty-handed women feel useless, unwanted, unneeded. They become a burden to themselves and often to their husbands.

The older woman must embark on the third epoch of her life. She must find an occupation that absorbs her interests, gives her purpose and usefulness in life, and maintains her self-respect. She may find fulfillment in community service, she may devote herself to some creative art, or she may prefer a paid job.

The woman who has remained at home during all the years of her children's maturing is handicapped, not only by lack of marketable skills, but by lack of experience in the rigors of a 9-to-5 job. She is further handicapped if she has not finished her formal education. However, industry clamors for workers, and many concerns are willing to retrain older women. A few colleges are offering special classes for women who married before graduation. Some women at the age of 40 or thereabouts find it difficult to start at the bottom. It seems to them undignified to be classed, jobwise, with the fresh young things just out of school and yet be unable to compete with them in youth and beauty. In addition the jobs they find are often dull and not too well paid.

The transition to the third epoch is not easy, and yet women are managing to do it. With every year that passes more older women are entering the labor market. Those women who completed their training before their children were born and went back to work when their children entered school or those who never completely stopped their outside work during their childbearing era have the advantage of years of experience and the job advancement that accompanies improved skills.

It is possible that in the years ahead young girls will see more clearly than at present the long pattern of life. Some halfway point may be found between the masculine-oriented feminist and the superfeminine image, neither of which have provided the good life for many women. Early education can be directed not only toward an entry job but toward the long future. Ideally the childbearing years can provide useful experience to enrich the jobholding years to come. There are numerous occupations that provide stimulating opportunities for the woman who has led a rich life during her childbearing epoch—teaching, nursing, social work, pediatrics, to say nothing of all the arts which flower with human understanding. These professions require academic training which the wise girl of tomorrow may acquire before she raises a family; then her postgraduate education with her own children can give her a rich background with which to contribute to society and to herself in her mature years.

THE FATHER IN MIDDLE-CLASS SOCIETY

The effect of the metamorphosis in family life on a man is nowhere near as catastrophic as on his wife; nevertheless he has not been unscathed.

The man's life is not divided into discontinuous epochs, as is the woman's. The middle-class boy expects to work from the time he finishes school until he retires. His education is directed toward this end; his early jobs are selected with a view to advancement. His family moves when necessary for his job opportunities.

The changes in the man's role lie in psychologic and emotional realms. The old extended family supported, often solely, by the income of its male head owed allegiance and obedience to the man of the house. Father was boss. He made the decisions; he directed family operations. Mother, children, other family members did as they were told. There are, however, not many Clarence Days left.

A woman who has earned her own living before marriage and during her early married life has acquired a degree of independence which makes knuckling under as an obedient subordinate to her husband less than attractive. She does not consider herself a chattel and does not act as though she were. She makes decisions, manages the home, raises the children without directions. Marriage has become a more cooperative venture than when the father, through control of the purse strings, dominated family life.

Not only has the father lost his authoritarian position in the family, but he must also assist in hitherto exclusively feminine occupations. Now that domestic help has virtually disappeared, his single-handed wife needs his help at home, especially when there are several children. His role, like his wife's, has changed as family patterns have changed. The days are over when a man can assume that his domestic role is fulfilled by supplying the income to run his family. For some years, when his children are small, he may have this to do, but in addition he must pinch-hit for all the members of the extended family of days of yore who not only helped with domestic chores but provided companionship and a measure of freedom from constant child care.

Sometimes when his wife holds a job, a man's feeling of competence is threatened. He thinks he is something less than he should be, because the family needs his wife's income. His sense of inadequacy can be greatly increased if his wife acts abused because she must work and blames him for his inability to provide an adequate income. The more his self-esteem is undermined, the more likely he is to compensate by disparaging his wife's job accomplishments and to complain over any inadequacies in her management of the home. Thus husband and wife work against each other, each undermining the self-confidence of the other. Before long both tend to accept the low opinion each has for the other, and the marriage is headed for the rocks.

The old picture of the masculine man is fading and a new one emerging. A man can still be a virile man even though he does not rule with an iron hand, accepts his wife's financial aid, and does not disdain to change a soiled diaper. Masculinity is expressed as power and strength, but not necessarily dictatorial power or brute strength. A virile man has strength to face life, to shoulder responsibilities, domestic as well as economic; he is able to support his wife's efforts to run their home, to approve of her and demonstrate that he needs and wants her.

A woman expresses her femininity in today's world by admiration and support of her man; she has a desire to make life good for him in all ways at her command. Both husband and wife are better equipped to carry out these mutually supportive roles when each has a life that creates self-respect.

The qualities of maleness and femaleness have not been wiped out in our modern world, though they have been modified as the paternalistic society of a past era has ebbed and greater cooperation between the sexes has taken its place.

BIBLIOGRAPHY

Bell, Norman, Ezra Ward, and V. Vegel (eds.): "The Family," The Free Press of Glencoe, New York, 1960.

Benedict, Ruth: "The Chrysanthemum and the Sword," Houghton Mifflin Company, Boston, 1946.

Day, Clarence: "Life with Father," Alfred A. Knopf, Inc., New York, 1935.

Erikson, Erik H.: "Childhood and Society," 2d ed., W. W. Norton & Company, Inc., New York, 1963.

———: The Woman in America, *Daedalus,* p. 582, Spring, 1964.

[1] Fisher, Seymour, and David Mendell: The Communication of Neurotic Patterns over Two or Three Generations, *Psychiatry,* **19**:41, 1956. (See also Bell, Norman.)

Freidan, Betty: "The Feminine Mystique," W. W. Norton & Company, Inc., New York, 1963.

Glick, Paul C.: "American Families," John Wiley & Sons, Inc., New York, 1957.

"1960 Handbook on Women Workers," U.S. Department of Labor, Women's Bureau Bulletin 275, 1960.

Herzog, Elizabeth: "Children of Working Mothers," U.S. Department of Health, Education and Welfare, Children's Bureau Publication 382, 1960.

"Historical Statistics of the U.S.: Colonial Times to 1957," U.S. Department of Commerce, Bureau of the Census, Washington, D.C., 1960.

Kardiner, A.: "The Psychological Frontiers of Society," Columbia University Press, New York, 1945.

[1] These articles have been published in Norman Bell, Ezra Wand, and V. Veel (eds.), "The Family," The Free Press of Glencoe, New York, 1960.

[1] KLUCKHOHN, CLYDE: Variations in the Human Family, in "The Family in a Democratic Society," p. 3, Columbia University Press, New York, 1949.

[1] MACCABY, ELEANOR E.: Effects upon Children of Their Mothers' Outside Employment, in "Work in the Lives of Married Women," p. 150, Columbia University Press, New York, 1958.

"Manpower—Challenge of the 60s," U.S. Department of Labor, Washington, D.C.

"Marital and Family Characteristics of Workers, 1960," U.S. Department of Labor, Special Labor Force Report, *Monthly Labor Review*, no. 13, April, 1961.

"Mobility of the Population of the United States," U.S. Department of Commerce, Bureau of the Census, no. 104, 1960, p. 20.

PAVENSTEDT, ELEANOR: A Study of Immature Mothers and Their Children, in Gerald Capalon (ed.), "Prevention of Mental Disorders in Children," p. 192, Basic Books, Inc., Publishers, New York, 1961.

"Population, Differential Fertility, 1940 and 1910," U.S. Department of Commerce, Bureau of the Census, series P-20, no. 105, 1961.

"Population and Labor Force Projection for the United States 1960–1975," U.S. Department of Labor, Bureau of Labor Statistics, Bulletin 1242.

REISMAN, DAVID: "Some Continuities and Discontinuities in the Education of Women," lecture delivered at Bennington College, June 7, 1956.

STALZ, LOIS MARK: Effects of Maternal Employment on Children: Evidence from Research, *Child Development*, **31**:749, 1960.

"Womanpower," National Manpower Council, Columbia University Press, New York, 1957.

"Work in the Lives of Married Women," National Manpower Council, Columbia University Press, New York, 1958.

Index

Abstraction, categories, 468
further, 469
negation as first, 467
Accidents, death from, 26
incidence of, 14
Achromatopsia (*see* Color blindness)
Acid, linoleic, 328
Acne, 251–253
emotional aspects, 253
physiology of, 252
and puberty, 251–252
and sebum formation, 251
treatment, 252
Acromegaly and PGH, 225
Active immunity, 298
Adenoids (*see* Tonsils and adenoids)
Adipose tissue, 229–234
and body build, 232
and diet, 232
and exercise, 232
and health, 232
life cycle of, 230
in newborn, 535
and tempo of growth, 232
(*See also* Obesity)
Adolescence, 573–590
age portraits, 614–615
breaking family tie, 584
crushes, 581
dining, 381
driving car, 404
independence, urge for, 584
internal forces, 575
maternal love, 445
prolongation of, 574
and puberty, 573
reducing regimes, 382
skills, 404
sleep, 317–318
in various cultures, 573
(*See also* Puberty)
Adrenal glands, 223
Adult, mature, definition, 351
sensitivity in, 495
Aesthetic pleasure, relation to sensorimotor play, 493
Afferent stimuli, 505
Agammaglobulinemia, 295
Age portrait summaries, 592–615
Aggression in boys, relation to castration fear, 428
Aldosterone, 223
Alleles, definition, 37
Allergic reactions, from absorption of whole proteins, 325
diets for potentially allergic infant, 304
Alphabet, 476
Amblyopia, 281
Amino acids, 324
in dietary protein (FAO), 325
essential, 324, 325
Anal stage, 409, 552
Androgens, 202, 223
Androgyny, 92
Anemia in infancy, 174
hematocrit, 183
and iron stores, 334
and maternal hemoglobin, 179
milk intake, excessive, 374
and placental transfusion, 179
and poor diet, 312
Anger in little child, 495
expressions of, 496
play as tool to cope with, 496
Animals, language of, 451–456
Anisometropia, 279
Anorexia nervosa, 384
Antibodies, definition, 291
and gamma globulin, 292
nature of, 291
site of formation, 293
transfer through placenta, 65, 292
Antidiuretic hormone, 225
Antisocial behavior in school-age child, 571
Anxiety at bedtime, 316
and clinging, 395
Apgar tests, 77
Aphasia, 267
education, 271
failure to talk, 481
tests for, 271
types, 269
(*See also* Deafness)
Apocrine sweat, 243
distribution, 256
formation in fetus, 246
maturation at puberty, 256
response to emotional stimuli, 256
Appendix, 192
Appetite, 367
and growth rate, 376
relation to dining, 367

Artificial immunity (*see* Immunity, artificial)
Atherosclerosis, 166
in infancy, 169
relation to cholesterol, 169
Atopy, 303
Audiogram, interpreting, 271
(*See also* Deafness, tests for)
Auditory apparatus, 266–273
development, 266
Auditory sensation, hearing behavior, 267
impairment, 267
Autism, 267
and failure to talk, 481
Automobile driving, 404
Autonomy, and childish love, 423
and defecation, 411–412
and dining, 377
and personality, 356
and products of elimination, 407
and sensation, 512
versus shame, 356
and skills, 403
and sphincter control, 356
and walking, 400
Autosomes, aberration of, 48
nomenclature, 39

Babbling, delayed in deprived child, 515
as stage of language learning, 465
Babinski sign, 388
Bad behavior, 498
Baldness, 254
Barr body, 45
Basal metabolism, 157
Basic trust, and antisocial behavior, 571
and clinging, 395
and crying, 390
and deprived child, 515
description of, 356
and eating, 370
and following, 397
and genital sensation, 423
and locomotion, 398
and maternal love, 443
and sensation, 512
Bats, use of sound, 455
Bedtime rituals, 316
Behavior, aberrations of, 17
bad,498
essential for survival, 348
instinctive, 348, 388–397
motor (*see* Motor behavior)
and will, 431, 496
(*See also* Delinquency; Discipline)
Between-meal snacks, for adolescent, 382
for preschooler, 378
Big children, 131

Birth, before, 56–70
injuries at, 78
normal, 73–74
Birth cry, 462
Biting, 373
Bladder, development of, 213
size, 415
training, 414
Blanket toting, 395
Blindness, 518–521
(*See also* Visual sensation)
Blood, elements in, 172–183
life patterns, 177–178
of neonate, 176
(*See also* Formed elements in blood)
Blood corpuscles, first appearance, 161
Blood islands, 172
Blood pressure, 168–169
Body constitution, 232
Body weight, ratio to brain weight, 140
Body temperature, sex difference, 168
Bone, and cartilage, 234
development of, 234
kinds of, 234
ossification in hand and wrist, 117
Bone marrow, hematopoiesis, 173
Bottle feeding, 369
Bowman's capsule, 213
Boys, aggression in, relation to castration fear, 428
Brain-damaged child, crying in, 464
Brain weight, ratio to body weight, 140
Breakfast for adolescent, 382
Breast, of newborn, 536
in pregnancy and lactation, 207
at puberty, in boy, 206
in girl, 206
Breast feeding, 369
Buddy love, 432–434
Buddy relation, 566

Calcium, absorption and excretion, 332
dietary sources, 332
functions of, 332
and vitamin D, 332
Calcium-phosphorus ratio in human milk, 226
Calories, during illness, 324
life pattern, 323
(*See also* Obesity)
Carbohydrates, 327
excessive, 339
main sources in human dietary, 327
Cardiovascular system, 160–170
and cholesterol, 169, 170
congenital abnormalities, 161
death from, 28
development before birth, 161
functions of, 160

Cardiovascular system, phylogenesis of, 160
surgical repair of, 166
Carnivorous animals, 320
Cartilage and bone, 234
Castration fear, and birth of new baby, 432
in boys, 428
in girls, 428
and menstruation, 435
Cell multiplication, after birth, 69
before birth, 56
Cells, Kupffer, 196
Leydig, 199, 210
Cerebral palsy, relation to speech, 485
Chewing, 372
Chickenpox in mother, effect on fetus, 65
Child without hands, 521
thalidomide, effect of, 66
Child rearing, epoch in life, 622
mother who stays home, 622
mother who works, 624
the one essentially feminine occupation, 620
not career for life, 620
Child's word for feces, 409
Childbirth, natural, 76
Cholesterol, and atherosclerosis, 169
life pattern, 169
in nutrition, 328
uses in body, 328
Chorion, 161
Chromosomes, human, aberrations, 46
mosaicism, 48
nomenclature, 39
Chvostek's sign, 388
Circulation, extraembryonic, 161
fetal, 162
through placenta, 58
portal, 162, 195, 196
postnatal, 164
Cleft lip and cleft palate, relation to speech, 484
Climacteric, female, 205
male, 211
Clinging, infant's need for, 395
mother's need for, 395
relation to anxiety, 395
transference to object, 395
Clonus, 387
Cognition, 504–524
Coitus, interest in puberty, of boy, 437
of girl, 436
Colic, nature of, 193–194
pain in, 262
Colitis, ulcerative, 193
Collagen diseases, 229
Color blindness, and child's sense of adequacy, 521
physiology of, 276
Color vision, development of, 276
Comfort sounds, 464
Communication, 451–488
autonomous reactions, 451
danger signals, 480
of emotion, 451
kinds of, 451
kinesthetic, 451
phatic, 451–454
acceptance of gender, 427
reading and writing, 475–478
symbolic language, 454
(*See also* Language; Speech)
Competence and motor skills, 404
Conformity of school-age child, 500, 566
Congenital malformations, from drugs administered to mother, 66
of heart, 164
incidence, 61
intrauterine conditions, 63
maternal conditions, age, 63
antibodies, 65
diet, 63–64
emotions, 68
health, 65
smoking, 65
vaccinations, 65
mortality, 26
physical agents, 68
of urinary tract, 214
Connective and supportive tissue, adipose, 229–234
bone, 234
cartilage, 234
common origins, 228
fibroelastic, 229
Consonants, 458
Constipation, emotional causes, 413
in infancy, 413
organic causes, 413
after voluntary control, 413
before voluntary control, 413
(*See also* Toilet training)
Cooking techniques and nutritional value of foods, 341
Corpus luteum, 202
Cortex, 261
Cortisol, 223
Crawling, 398
Cretinism, 222
Critical stages in development, in fetus, 62, 70
in loving, 420
Cross-sectional studies, 86
Crying, age pattern, 390–392
in brain-damaged child, 464
in deprived child, 515
early vocalizations in, 464
excessive, 540

Crying, instinctual response, 390
  in normal child, 464
  in rejected child, 392
Cryptorchism, 199, 216
Cultural concepts through languages, 474
Cystic fibrosis of pancreas, relation to eccrine sweat, 256
Cystourethroscopic examinations, 216

Danger signals, antisocial behavior, 571
  in communication skills, 480
  neurotic symptoms, 571
  school failure, 570
  in toddlerhood, 556
  (*See also* Age portrait summaries)
Deafness, causes, 268, 269
  failure to talk, 481
  in infant, 545
  Jack of jargon, 465
  reading difficulty, 518
  significance of inability to hear, 517
  speech difficulty, 518
  tests for, 269
  tone, 521
Death, and age, 20–29
  by cause, 26
  of child, 26
  fetal, 22, 23
  of infant, 23
  by organ system, 27
  relation to X-Y chromosomes, 45
  and sex, 18–20
Death rate, century ago, 3
  in four countries of Americas, 9, 27
  in United States, 21, 22, 26, 27
Decibel, 272
Defecation, and autonomy, 411–412
  in infancy, 193
  physiology of, 407
  stages in sphincter control, 409
  (*See also* Toilet training)
Defects, inherent, death from, 27
Delinquency, classification of, 588
  definition, 588
  correlation with broken homes, 589
Deoxycorticosterone, 223
Deoxyribonucleic acid (*see* DNA)
Dermis, 257
Despair versus integrity, 361
Development, aberrations in fetus, 61
  appraisal, 405
  critical stages in, 62, 70
Developmental quotient, 405
Diet, for all ages, 339
  for allergic infants, 304
  carnivorous, 320
  herbivorous, 320
Diet, maternal, effect on fetus, 63–64
  omnivorous, 321
  poor, and anemia in infancy, 312
Dining, 366–384
  in adolescence, 381
  in adult, 366, 382
  and appetite, 367
  and autonomy, 377
  family (*see* Family dinner table)
  definition, 365
  in infancy, early, 365, 367
    late, 365
  in preschool child, 377
  in school-age child, 366, 379
  in toddler, 366, 376, 552
  and weaning, 375
  (*See also* Eating through life)
Dinosaur, brain size, 140
Disability, from illness, acute, 11
    chronic, 15
  incidence, 11, 12, 15
Discipline, adaptation to reality, 491
  beginnings of, 490
  getting out of hand, 497
  and infant's eating, 374
  and maternal love, 444
  and mother, 491
  from objects, 491
  from people, 491
  and play, 490
  in toddlerhood, need for, 492
Disease, collagen, 229
  infectious, incidence in United States, 13
  maternal, effect on fetus, 64
  mortality, in underdeveloped areas, 19
    in United States, 25
Distance senses, 259
  hearing, 266–273
  vision, 273–284
Diverticulum, Meckel's, 193
DNA (deoxyribonucleic acid), replication, 40
  structure, 39
Dolphin, brain size, 140
  language of, 456
  use of sound, 455
Domesticity as career, 618
Dramatic play (*see* Symbolic dramatic play)
Dreaming, 312
Driving, automobile, 404
Drugs, during labor, 74–75
  placental transmission, 66, 67
Ductus arteriosus, 164
Dyslexia, causes, 485
  incidence, 485
  secondary complications, 485
Dysuria, 216

Ear (*see* Auditory apparatus)
Eating through life, 365–384
  with family, 377
  too little, 384
  too much, 383
  (*See also* Dining)
Eccrine sweat, change with acclimatization, 256
  composition of, 256
  development of, 254
  distribution of, emotional sweat, 255
    thermal sweat, 255
  formation in fetus, 246
  relation to cystic fibrosis of pancreas, 256
  sex differences, 255
  stimulated, by emotion, 255
    by temperature, 255
Echolation in bats, 455
Ectoderm, 57–59
Ectomorph, description, 92
  early differentiation, 58
  and food intake, 384
Ego, raw materials, 8
Ego identity, Erikson's, definition, 355
    in puberty, 359
    satisfaction with, 349
Egocentric sensation, 505
  of body touch, 509
  in infancy, 511
  of sound, 507
  of taste and smell, 508
  of vision, 508
  (*See also* Love)
Elimination, 407–417
  products of, 408
  (*See also* Toilet training)
Embryo, growth to fetus, 59
  independence in, 58, 70
  qualities of, 62
Emotion, communication of, 451
  maternal, effect on fetus, 68
  and sound, 455
Endocrines, 221–227
  adrenal, 223
  growth, 85
  immaturity in neonate, 221
  sex, female, 202–204
    male, 210
  thyroid, 222, 223
Endoderm, 57–59
Endomorph, description, 90
  early differentiation, 58
  good cook, 383
  growth of, 92
  relation to obesity, 383
Energy, individual differences, 323
  life patterns, 323
  needs for, 322
Enuresis, 415–417
Enuresis, and bladder size, 416
  and emotional stress, 417
  family incidence, 416
Eosinophils, function, 175
  in hypersensitive state, 303
  life pattern, 182
Epidermis, 248–250
  bacterial resistance, 250
  function of, 249
  protection, 243
  structure of, 248
Epinephrine, 223
Erikson's egoepigenesis, 355–361
Erythroblastosis foetalis, cause, 66
  diagnosis and treatment before birth, 67
Erythrocytes, 172–175
  formation, 174
  life patterns, 177, 179
  sex differences, 180
Estrogen, 202, 203
Euthenic pediatrics, 6
Evolution, behavior in, modifications of, 348
  and heredity, 33
  man's place, 347
  of pediatrics, 3
  structural modifications, 348
Ex-baby, 432
Exercise, and physical fitness, 239
  sex difference at puberty, 157
External reality, 349
Exteroceptive sensation, 259
Extraembryonic circulation, 161
Eye (*see* Visual apparatus)

Family, 618–631
  cultural metamorphosis, 618
  of past generations, 618
  of today, 620
Family dinner table, and adolescent, 381
  conversation, 378, 379
  and preschooler, 378
  and school-age child, 379
  and toddler, 377
FAO (Food and Agriculture Organization of the United Nations), 325
Fat, 327–329
  in diet, 328
  infant's ability to digest, 329
  saturated, 328
  sources, 328
  unsaturated, 328
Father, in middle-class society, 629
  paternal love, 448, 449
Feces, child's word for, 409
  impaction, 413
  in infancy, 188
  infant's interest in, 408

Feces, mother's attitude toward, 408
toddler's attitude toward, 409
(*See also* Constipation; Stools; Toilet Training)
Feeding, bottle, 369
breast, 369
Feelings, bad, accepted and controlled, 496
raw material of ego development, 8
Female sex function, 208, 209
Female sex organs, early differentiation, 198
in infancy, 201
at puberty, 202
Fetal membranes, 56
Fetus, circulation, 162
death of, 22, 23
development, aberrations in, 61
stages in, 62, 70
effect of mother's diseases, 65
gonads in, 198
growth in life span, 69
heart in, 58
independence, 70
individuality, 59
mother's conditions affecting, 63–68
need for iodine, 334
nutrition of, 61–63
posture of, 236
protection of, 64
sweat formation in, 246
Fever, and activity, 324
caloric need, 324
in infection, 290
Fibroelastic tissue, 229
Fifteen-month-old infant, 548
Fingerprint patterns of fetus, 245
Fluorine in drinking water, 336
relation to teeth, 336
Focal attention, 147
Follicle graafian, 202
Following, 396
Food and Agriculture Organization of the United Nations (FAO), 325
Foramen ovale, 163, 164
Formed elements in blood, 172–183
classification, 172
life patterns, 177, 178
origin, 172
Fringe children, 128–132
Functions, human (*see* Human dimensions of function)

Galactose, 327
Games of school-age child, 500
Gametes, formation of, 44
Gammaglobulin, types, 292
(*See also* Antibodies)
Gangs of school-age children, 500
Gastrointestinal tract, 185–197
death from disease of, 27
development of, 188–193
diseases of, 14
in early infancy, 185–188
gastric juice, 191
bactericidal properties of, 289
psychosomatic disorders, 193
Gender, child's acceptance, 425
and personality, 357
Generativity versus stagnation, 360
Genetic counseling, 49
Genetic material, ancestral origin, 34, 35
continuity of, 34
defective, 42
function of, 40
influence on growth, 85
inviolability of, 38
properties, 40
Genetic pool, 52
Genital phase, and parents, 427
in preschooler, 357, 561
relation to new baby, 432
Genital sensation, in boy in puberty, 437
in infancy, 423
Genital trauma, 429
Germ plasm, 198
Giantism, relation to PGH, 225
Girls and castration fear, 428
Glands (*see* specific glands, e.g., Adrenal glands)
Glomeruli, 213
Glucagon, 226
Gonads in fetus, 198
Graafian follicle, development of, 202
Grammar, in language development, 469
structure, 460
Granulocytes, 172, 175
life patterns, 179, 180, 182
Grasp reflex, 387
Grief due to separation, 516
Growth, assessment of, after first year, 110
in first year, 107
of premature babies, 108
of twins, 109
change in shape with, 120–123
influences on, climate, 96
emotion, 95
endocrines, 85
environment, 94
genes, 85, 88
nutrition, 94
physical health, 95
season, 97
socioeconomic level, 96
intellectual, 568
of organ systems, blood, 126
endocrine, 126
gastrointestinal, 127

Growth, of organ systems, heart, 126
liver, 127
respiratory, 126
urinary, 126
patterns of, animal, 83, 84
human, 84, 85
profiles of, 105
rate of, and appetite, 376
tempo of, 115
of tissues, adipose, 125
bone, 125
lymph, 125
muscle, 124
neural, 125
Growth charts, 102–107
Growth data, use of, to assess health, 113
to explain to child, 114
to interpret to parents, 113
Growth failure, causes of, 113
inadequate protein, 325
Growth potential, correlated, with body build, 90
with sex, 89
with size at birth, 89
with speed of maturing, 90
Guilt versus initiative, 357
Gynecomastia, 206

Hair, baldness, 254
to beautify, 244
development of, 253
hirsutism, 254
at puberty, 253
Handicapping condition, 15, 16
Hands, control, 400
index finger approach, 402
lack of, 521
at play, 400
prehensile grip, 402
sensory powers in, 259, 261
Head control, 398
Health, maternal, effect on fetus, 65
Hearing, 266–273
behavior, 267
after birth, 267
development of organs for, 266
Hearing impairment (*see* Deafness)
Heart, congenital malformation of, 164
in fetus, 58
(*See also* Cardiovascular system)
Height prediction, 112
Hemangioma in newborn, 535
Hematocrit, 183, 177
Hematopoiesis, 173
Hemoglobin, factors influencing, 180
formation, 174, 179
life patterns, 177, 179
sex differences, 180
Hemogram, 183
Herbivorous animals, 320
Heredity, 33–55
basic tenets, 36
and evolution, 33
Hersprung's disease, 413
Hirsutism, 254
Homeostasis, 242
Homunculus, 4
Hormone control of human milk, 257
Hospitalization and separation anxiety, 516, 543
Human dimensions of function, 361, 362
in adolescence, 573
and autonomy, 423
and dining, 365
of sensation, 507
of sound, 508
of vision, 508
Humanness, before birth, 353
development after birth, 354
qualities of, 349
theories of, 353
Hunger, 366
Hydrocele in newborn, 536
Hyperopia, age trends, 279
and strabismus, 281
Hypersensitivity, 301–304
allergic infant, 304
atopy, 303
comparison with immunity, 302
emotional states, 304
iatrogenic reactions, 303
reaction types, 302
target area, 303
Hypertension, in infancy, 169
pulmonary, 166
Hypogammaglobulinemia, 295
Hypoglycemia in early childhood, 226
Hypophysis, 224
anterior lobe, 224
hormones acting on target glands, 225
pituitary growth hormone, 225
posterior lobe, 225
Hypospadias, 200, 216
Hypothalamus, 224
Hypothermia in pregnant women, effect on fetus, 68
Hypoxia in pregnant women, effect on fetus, 68

Identity versus identity diffusion, 359
Illness, incidence of, 11–17
acute, 11, 12
chronic, 12, 15
gastrointestinal, 14
infectious and parasitic, 13
respiratory, 11
(*See also* Disease)

Imaginary companions, 559
Imaginative make-believe, form of play, 493–496
Immunity, 287–301
artificial, 297
active, 298
recommended schedule, 300
types of antigens, 298
passive, 297
available procedures, 298
of infant at birth, 297
placental transmission, 65
comparison with hypersensitivity, 302
natural, 296
nonspecific factors influencing, 301
Inborn errors of metabolism, 42
Independence, in adolescence, 584
autonomy and, 356
critical stages, 70
eating and, 373
in embryo, 58, 70
in fetus, 70
maternal love and, 444
in neonate, 70
walking and, 399
Infant, 535–549
age portraits, 536–548
allergic, diet for, 304
basic trust, 356
blood picture, 176–178
(*See also* Anemia in infancy)
danger signs, 549
deafness, 545
death, 23
defecation, 193
descriptions, fifteen months, 548
newborn, 535
nine months, 545
one month, 538
seven months, 545
three months, 541
yearling, 547
dining, 365, 367
discipline, 374
egocentric sensation in, 511
endocrines, 221
genital sensation, 423
growth of, 107
hypertension in, 169
immunity, 292
low birth weight of, 527
motor skills, 400
obesity in, 230
play, 490
posture, 238
premature (*see* Premature infant)
recapitulation, 546
sexuality, 420
sleep, 314, 536
Infant, urine, 214
vocalization, 462
Infection, fever in, 290
in illness, 13
Inflammation, local, 290
Inherent defects, death from, 27
Initiative versus guilt, 357
Inorganic elements in diet, 332–336
Instinctive behavior, 348, 388–397
Insulin, 226
Integrity versus despair, 361
Integumentary system, 242–257
development, after birth, 247
before birth, 245
functions, cosmetic, 242
expressive, 242
homeostasis, 242
protection, 243
sensory contact, 242
Intellectual growth, 568
Interoceptive sensation, 259
Intestine, lymphoid tissue in, 193
Intimacy versus isolation, 360
Involuntary defecation, 412
Iodine, dietary sources, 334
fetal need, 334
relation to thyroid, 334
Iron, absorption and excretion, 333
and anemia, 334
dietary sources, 334
functions, 333
sex differences, 333
stores at birth, 333
Isolation versus intimacy, 360
Islets of Langerhans, 226

Jargon, imitation of sounds, 465

Keratin, bactericidal properties, 250
in skin, 248
Kidney, development, 213
tubules in, 213
Kinesthetic communication, 451
Kraus-Weber tests for muscle strength, 239
Kupffer cells, 196

Labor, drugs during, 74–75
normal, process of, 73
pain of, 74
Lacrimal gland, 274
(*See also* Tears)
Lactation, hormone and neural control, 207
sensations of, 207
(*See also* Breast)
Lactose, 327
infant's special ability to use, 327
source of galactose, 327

Langerhans, islets of, 226
Language, of animals, 451–456
of dolphins, 456
kinesthetic, 452
of primates, 452
vocal, 452
as child's tool, 471
components of, 456
crystallization of cultural concepts, 474
melody of, 466
optimal development of, 479
second, learning of, 475
stages, in understanding, 462–470
auditory expressive, 467
auditory receptive, 467
inner, 466
in use of, egocentric, 472
imaginative, 473
intelligent, 472
tempo of learning, 470
(*See also* Communication; Speech)
Lanugo, 245
Latency period, 358, 434
Learning, 504–524
Leukocytes, 172, 175, 176
granular, 289
life patterns, 179, 180, 182
Leydig cells, 199, 210
Linoleic acid, 328
Lipids, 327
(*See also* Cholesterol)
Little children, 128–130
Liver, 194–197
circulation prior to birth, 161
development, 196
functions of, 194
hematopoiesis in fetus, 173
immaturity at birth, 196
Kupffer cells, 196
unit of structure, 195
Loading test for detection of defective genes, 43
Local inflammation, 290
Locomotion, crawling, 398
walking, 399
Longevity, 28
Longitudinal studies, 86, 88
Love, 419–449
ability and need, 419
baby, 420–423
and basic trust, 443
buddy, 432–434
childish, 423–429
development, 419
discipline, relation to, 497
erotic, 440
maternal, 442–447
maturation of, 439
mature, 441
Love, oedipal, 429–431
paternal, 448, 449
pubertal, 434–439
Low-birth-weight infant, 527–534
age portrait, 594
definition, 527
description, 530–532
mortality, 528
neonatal care, 528
parents, 533
(*See also* Premature infant)
Lust, 441
Lymphocytes, 172, 175, 176
age trends, 176, 179, 180, 182
formation, 176
relation to thymus, 176
Lymphoid tissue, in antibody formation, 292
growth, 125
in intestine, 193
life cycle, 304
response to infection, 304
Lyon hypothesis, 45

Macrophages, 290
Macula of eye, 275
Make-believe, form of play, 493–496
Male sex function, 211, 212
Malformations, congenital (*see* Congenital malformations)
Mammary glands, 205
development before birth, 205
gynecomastia, 206
during lactation, 207
in pregnancy, 207
in puberty of girl, 206
"witches' milk," 205
Man's early concept of himself, 352
Masochism in girls, in preschool child, 428
during puberty, 435, 582
Masturbation at puberty, in boy, 211, 437–439
in girl, 436
Mature adult, definition, 351
Maturing children, 132
Measles (rubeola) in mother, effect on fetus, 65
vaccination of pregnant woman, effect on fetus, 65
Meckel's diverticulum, 193
Meconium, 185, 536
Melanin in skin, 248
Melody of native language, 466
Memory, 146
Menarche, age of, influence of nutrition, 97, 98
and maximum growth, 87
secular trend in, 98
(*See also* Menstruation)

Menopause, 205
Menstruation, girl's attitude toward, 435
  physiology of, 202, 203
Mental deviants, 351
Mental retardation, 148, 151
  causes, 150
  definition, 149
  failure to talk, 481
  incidence, 149
Mesoderm, 57–59
Mesomorph, description of, 90
  early differentiation, 58
  growth of, 92
Mesonephros, 213
Metabolism, basal, 157
  inborn errors of, 42
Metanephros, 213
Milk, human, calcium-phosphorus ratio in, 226
  hormone control, 257
  neural control, 207
  relative to parathyroids, 226
  (*See also* Lactation)
Misbehavior, chronic, 497
  cues in handling, 499
Monocytes, 172
Morbidity (*see* Illness)
Moro reflex, description, 387
  in premature infant, 533
Mortality (*see* Death)
Mosaicism, 48
Mother, attitudes of, toward appetite of infant, 376
    during labor, 76
    during pregnancy, 75
  conditions affecting fetus, 63–68
  cultural metamorphosis, 618
  deprivation of, 515, 516
    in one-month-old infant, 541
  and discipline, 491
  epochs in life of, 621
    child rearing, 622
    after children are grown, 628
    education and marriage, 621
  and infant's cry, 390
  love, 442–447
  qualities of, 369
  of today, 550, 620
Motor behavior, 386–406
  at birth, 386
  classification, 386
  in deprived child, 515
  instinctive, 388
  involuntary, 386
  reflex, 386
  and sensory impairment, 405
  voluntary, 397
Mouth breathing, 305
Mumps in mother, effect on fetus, 65
Muscle, and body build, 235
  development, 235
  and exercise, 157
  strength of, Kraus-Weber tests for, 239
  tissue of, 124
Mutation, definition, 42
  effect of radiation, 42
  frequencies of, 42
  gene changes responsible for, 42
  spontaneous, 42
Myelination of nerve pathways, 144, 145
Myopia, age trends, 279
  relation to length of eyeball, 278

Naps, 314
Narcolepsy, 312
Natural childbirth, 76
Natural immunity, 296
Negation, first abstraction, 467
Neonatal care of low-birth-weight infant, 528
Neonate, age portrait, 595
  blood of, 176
  description of, 535
  full term, 535–538
  independence in, 70
  parents of, 538
  posture of, 238
  taste in, 189, 264
  (*See also* Infant)
Nephrons, 213, 215
Nervous system, 139–152
  aberrations of development, 148
  at birth, 143
  development prior to birth, 141
  phylogenesis of, 139–141
  postnatal changes, 144
Neural tissue, 125
Neurotic symptoms, 571
Neutrophils, 175, 179, 180, 182
Night terrors, 317
Nine-month-old infant, 545
  age portrait, 602
Nipples, care during lactation, 208
  sucking on, 370
Nocturnal seminal emissions, 211
Norepinephrine, 223
Nourishment, 365
  prior to birth, 367
Nucleotides, structure of, 40
Nursery school, 561
Nutrition, 320–342
  effect on growth, 94
  of fetus, 61–63
  influence on menarche, 97, 98
  in pregnancy, 338

Obesity, and body build, 233
emotional factors, 383
genetic factors, 383
and home dietary, 383
in infants, 230
organic factors, 383
in prepuberty, 231
and thyroid, 222
(*See also* Adipose tissue; Dining)
Oedipal love, 429–431
and maternal love, 445
and new baby, 432
Oedipal phase, 457
Omnivorous animal, 321
One-gene–one-enzyme hypothesis, 41
Optimal posture, 236
Oral phase of development, and baby love, 420
and organ modes, 362
and use of mouth, 464
Organ modes, 362
Organ systems, emergence in fetus, 58
Organic structure, similarity in all mammals, 347
Organs of special sense, 259–286
man's sensory equipment, 259
sensation in development, 284
Orgasm at puberty, in boy, 437
in girl, 436
Ossification in bones of hand and wrist, 117
Ovaries, 201
during childhood, 202
prior to birth, 198
at puberty, 198
Oxytocin, 225

Pacifier, use and abuse, 370, 371
Pancreatic juice, 192
Parathyroids, 225
and relation to milk, 226
Parents, of newborn, 538
of premature infant, 533
of today, 619
Partially seeing child, 520
Passive immunity, 297
Paternal love, 448, 449
Pediatrician, activities of, 5–7
hospital-based, 5
in private practice, 5
Pediatrics, euthenic, 6
evolution of, 3
in United States today, 5
Peer group in school years, 566
Peptic ulcer, 193
Peristalsis, 192
Personality, and autonomy, 356
and gender, 357
PGH (pituitary growth hormone), 225
Phagocytes, 289
granular leukocytes, 289
macrophages, 290
neutrophils, 175
Phatic communication, 451–454
acceptance of gender, 427
Phimosis at birth, 536
Phocomelia, ingestion by pregnant woman, 66
Phonemes, 459
Phonetic teaching of reading, 476
Phonetics, 457
duration, amplitude, pitch, 458
physical quality of sound, 457
Phosphorus-calcium ratio in human milk, 226
Phylogenesis, of cardiovascular system, 160
of immune mechanisms, 287
of nervous system, 139–141
of nourishment, 365
of play, 489
of posture, 228
theories of, 489
(*See also* Evolution)
Pilosebaceous apparatus, 245
Pituitary body (*see* Hypophysis)
Pituitary growth hormone (PGH), 225
Placenta, antibody transfer through, 65, 292
circulation through, 58
function of, 60
protective action of, 64
transfer of drugs through, 66, 67
transfusion through, 175–177
Plasm, germ, 198
Platelets, 172, 176
Play, 489–503
as amusement, 489
definition, 490
and discipline, 490
imaginative make-believe, 493
imitative, 491
necessity of, 490
phylogenesis of, 489
practice, 491
versus recreation, 502
sensorimotor, 490
symbolic dramatic, 495
as tool to cope with anger, 496
Pleasure, aesthetic, relation to sensorimotor play, 493
Poliomyelitis, in mother, effect on fetus, 65
vaccination against, in mother, effect on fetus, 65
Portal circulation, 195, 196
prior to birth, 162
Posture, and exercise, 239

Posture, fetal, 236
head control, 398
in infant, 238
and locomotion, 398
mechanics of, 236
neonatal, 238
optimal, 236
phylogenesis, 228
in preschool child, 238
in puberty, 239
in school-age child, 239
sitting, 398
Pregnancy, breast in, 207
dangers of excess weight gain, 336
mammary glands in, 207
nutritional requirements, 338
pubescent girls' interest in, 430
Premature infant, 527–534
age portrait, 594
definition, 527
growth of, 108
parents of, 533
sleep, 536
28 weeks gestation, 530
32 weeks gestation, 532
value of placental transfusion, 179
(*See also* Low-birth-weight infant)
Preschool child, 558–562
age portrait, 609
companionship, 378
dining, 377
gender acceptance, 357, 425
general behavior, 559
genital interest, 428
genital phase, 357, 561
initiative versus guilt, 357
nursery school, 561
oedipal phase, 427
physical health, 558
posture, 238
sexuality in, 429
Primates, brain size, 140
language of, 452
Progesterone, 202–204
Pronephros, 213
Pronouns in language development, 469
Proprioceptive sensation, 259
Prosthesis for child amputee, 521
Protein, 324–326
biologic value scored by FAO, 325
need for growth, 325
Proximity senses, 259
smell, 264
tactation, 260
taste, 263
Ptyalin, 185
Puberty, 434–439
acne, 251–252
and adolescence, 573
Puberty, apocrine sweat, 256
blood picture, 177
blood pressure, 168
body changes, 575–577
breast development, 206
capacity for exercise, 157
definition, 573
ego-identity, 359
growth during, 121, 122
hair at, 253
heart rate, 167
interest in sex, 436, 437
masturbation, 436–439
menarche, 582
posture, 239
psychic development, in boys, 583
in girls, 579
(*See also* Adolescence)
Pulmonary hypertension, 166
Pulse rate, effect of age and sex, 166–168
Pyuria, 216

Questions asked, by preschooler, 427
in puberty, by boy, 437
by girl, 436
by school-age child, 568
by toddler, 473

Radiation, effect on mutation, 42
Rapidly maturing children, 132
Ratio of brain weight to body weight, 140
Reading and writing, 475–478
difficulty due to deafness, 518
failure, 485
(*See also* Dyslexia)
readiness, 478
teaching, look-and-say, 477
phonetic, 476
Reality, external, 349
Recreation versus play, 502
Reducing regimes in adolescent girls, 382
Reflex, grasp, 387
moro (*see* Moro reflex)
seeking, 387
tendon, 388
tonic neck, 387
Refraction, changes with age, 278
Relativity, child's concept of, 514
Reproductive system, 198–212
at birth, 201
development prior to birth, 198
in female, 201–209
in male, 209–212
sex and death, 18
(*See also* Sexuality)
Resentment and castration fear in girls, 428

Respiratory system, 153–159
  bactericidal properties of, 289
  diseases of, death from, 27
    incidence of, 11, 13
  efficiency of, 155
  onset of function at birth, 154
  rate of, by age and sex, 154
Resuscitation of newborn, 77
Retardation, mental (*see* Mental retardation)
Reticuloendothelium, 173, 290
Retina, at birth, 273
  formation in embryo, 273
  macula, 275
  periphery of, 276
Ribonucleic acid (RNA), 41, 57
Ritualism, at bedtime, 316, 317
  during school years, function of, 502
    in ideas, 501
    in language, 500
    in play, 500
RNA (ribonucleic acid), 41, 57
Rubella in mother, effect on fetus, 64
Rubeola in mother, effect on fetus, 65

Salivary glands, bactericidal properties of, 289
  development of, 191
  secretion, composition of, 191
Satiety, 366
Saturated fat, 328
School, nursery, 561
School-age child, 562–572
  age portrait, 611
  antisocial behavior, 571
  buddy love, 432
  clubs, 501
  collections, 501
  conformity, 500, 566
  danger signs, 569
  dining, 366, 379
  discipline, 567
  failure as danger signal, 570
  independence, 564
  initiative versus shame, 357
  intellectual growth, 568
  moral values, 569
  and parents, 567, 568
  and peer group, 566
  personality development, 564
  physical health, 562
  play, 500
  posture, 239
  problems in school, 570
    due to myopia, 280
    reading failure, 485
  and siblings, 567
Sebaceous glands, and acne, 251
Sebaceous glands, activity of, 251
  development before birth, 244
  postnatal changes, 250
Second language, learning of, 475
Secular trend in growth, 95
Sedimentation rate, 174, 183
Seeking reflex, 387
Seminal emissions, nocturnal, 211
Sensation, 504–524
  exteroceptive, 259
  in hands, 259, 261
  interoceptive, 259
  proprioceptive, 259
Sensitivity in adult, 495
Sensorimotor play, 490
Sensory deprivation, and growth of ego, 516
  from maternal inadequacy, 515
  from organic inadequacy, 516
    blindness, 518
      color, 521
      partial, 520
    deafness, 517
      tone, 521
  primitive level, 505
Sensory equipment of man, cortex, 261
  exteroceptive, 259
  formation in fetus, 246
  interoceptive, 259
  proprioceptive, 259
Sensory experience of man, and autonomy, 512
  egocentric sensation, 505
  in infancy, 422, 510
  primitive level of awareness, 504
  prior to birth, 509
  from various receptors, 507
  world-centered perception, 506
  during school years, 512
Sensory pleasures through life, 493
Sentences, first, 467
Separation anxiety, at bedtime, 317
  and grief, 516
  and hospitalization, 516, 543
  in seven-month-old infant, 542
  in toddler, 516, 543, 555
Seven-month-old infant, 543–545
  age portrait, 600
Sex education in puberty, in boy, 437
  in girl, 425
  concerning opposite sex, 436, 437
Sex glands, female, 202–204
  male, 210
Sexuality, 419–449
  in infant, 420
  maturation of, 440, 441
  in preschooler, 429
  at puberty, in boy, 210
    in girl, 206

Sexuality, in toddler, 427
union, desire for, 440
(*See also* Reproductive system)
Shame versus autonomy, 356
Sinus arrhythmia, 166
Skeletal age, 116–119
Skin, dermis, 257
development of, after birth, 247–248
before birth, 245–247
epidermis (*see* Epidermis)
keratin in, 248
melanin in, 248
Sleep, 311–318
arousal stimuli, 311
center of, 311
deprivation, 311
dreaming, 312
"fighting," 315
life patterns, 313, 314
in adolescence, 317–318
in early years, 315
in infancy, 314, 536
in middle years, 317
in premature infant, 536
optimal amount, 312
Slow maturing children, 132
Smallpox vaccination of mother, effect on fetus, 65
Smell, development of organ of, 264
in neonate, 264
phylogenesis, 264
sensation of, 508
Smiling, 392–395
age of, 541
in deprived child, 515
Smoking, maternal, effect on fetus, 65
Snacks (*see* Between-meal snacks)
Socioeconomic level, effect on growth, 96
Somatypes, 90
Sonar in dolphins, 455
Sound, and background awareness, 507
bats use of, 455
comfort, 464
distance sense, 507
dolphins use of, 455
and emotion, 455
imitation of, jargon, 465
lead sense, 507
and orientation in space, 455
phatic quality of, 272
physical properties of, 272
and symbolic language, 454
into symbols, 466
temporal sense, 508
Spankings and deprivation, 498
Speech, center of, 454
defects, 481–483
development of oral stages, 462
difficulty due to deafness, 518
Speech, failure of, deprivation of contact with, 461
organic, 481
human, 460
learning of, medieval experiments in, 461
relation to cerebral palsy, 485
(*See also* Communication; Language)
Sphincter control, and autonomy, 356
significance of, 411
stages in, 409, 410
Spleen, hematopoiesis in fetus, 173
Spoiled child and quality of maternal love, 445
Spoon, introduction of, 371
Squint (*see* Strabismus)
Stagnation versus generativity, 360
Stepping reflex, 388
Stomach, size in early months, 187
Stools, as gift, 409
meaning to child, 409
physiology, 188, 193
(*See also* Defecation)
Strabismus, and amblyopia, 281
classification, 280
and hyperopia, 281
Structure, organic, similarity in all mammals, 347
Stubbornness, 468, 548
Sucking, avid and lackadaisical, 374
instinctive patterns, 388
on nipple, 370
on pacifier, 370–371
thumb, 370–371, 393
Survival, behavior necessary for, 348
structure necessary for, 347
Swallowing, 188
Sweat, apocrine (*see* Apocrine sweat)
eccrine (*see* Eccrine sweat)
Swimming reflex, 388
Symbolic dramatic play, 495–497
catharsis of tensions, 497
coping with frustration, 496
in primitive society, burning in effigy, 497
residue in adult confined to dreams, 497
Symbolization, use of gesture, 454
use of sound, 454
and vocabulary, 456
Synesthesia, 510

Tactation, nerve endings, 260
nerve tracts, 260
organic structures, after birth, 263
before birth, 262
pain, 261
pressure, 261
sensation from, in hands, 508
in total body, 508
used symbolically, 509

Talk (*see* Communication; Language; Speech)
Tantrums in toddler, 551
Taste, before birth, 263
in neonate, 189, 264
proximity, sense, 508
Tears, bactericidal properties, 288
lacrimal glands, 274
in one-month-old infant, 538
Teeth, 189, 190
chronology of dentition, 189
development, 190
and fluorine in drinking water, 336
Television and nightmares, 317
Temperature, body, sex difference, 168
Tempo of language learning, 470
Tenderness and erotic love, 440
Tendon reflexes, 388
Testes, before birth, 209
during childhood, 210
at puberty, 210
Tetany, 226
Tetragenic drugs, 66, 67
Thalidomide, effect on fetus, 66
Thermoregulation, and eccrine sweat, 243, 255
in full-term newborn, 536
in low-birth-weight infant, 529
Three-month-old infant, 541–543
age portrait, 599
Thrombocytes, 172, 176
Thumb sucking, 370–371, 393
and new baby, 432
and spoon feeding, 371
Thymus, immunologic organ, 294
site of lymphogenesis, 176
Thyroid, before birth, 222
deficiency, in fetal life, 222
postnatal, 222
and obesity, 222
relation to iodine, 331
tests for, 223
Tissue (*see* Connective and supportive tissue)
Toddler, 550–557
age portrait, 606
autonomy versus shame, 356
castration fears, 428
danger signals, 556
dining, 366, 376, 552
discipline, 492
feces, attitude toward, 409
following, 396, 555
gender role, 425
general behavior, 550, 551
handling of, 554
imaginative make-believe, 493
language, 471–473, 552
love, 423
Toddler, mother of, 556
motor activities, 403, 551
physical health, 550
play, 493, 552
sensation and autonomy, 512
separation anxiety, 516, 543, 555
sexuality in, 427
tantrums in, 551
toilet training, 409–413, 552
toting, 395, 535
Toilet training, and birth of sibling, 432
for defecation, 409
difficulties in, 413
for urination, 414
Tone deafness, 521
Tonic neck reflex, 387
Tonsils and adenoids, indication for removal, 306
and hearing, 305
life cycle, 305
mouth breathing, 305
Tonus, 386
Toting, 555
Touch (*see* Tactation)
Toxoplasmosis in mother, effect on fetus, 65
Transfusion of fetus in utero, 66
Trust (*see* Basic trust)
Twins, growth of, 109
Two-month-old infant, 541

Ulcerative colitis, 193
Unconditional maternal love, 442
Unsaturated fat, 328
Urethral meatus, bactericidal properties, 289
Urinary system, 213–219
development of, 213
immaturity in infancy, 214
Urination (*see* Toilet training)
Urine, amount by age, 217
in childhood, 217
"clean catch," 217
of neonate, 216

Vaccinations of mother, effect on fetus, 65
Vagina, bactericidal properties, 289
Variation within genetic limits, 35
Vascular network in skin, 243
formation in fetus, 246
Verbal incontinence, 472
Vernix caseosa, formation, 245
of newborn, 247, 535
Visual apparatus, accommodation, 277, 278
anisometropia, 279
behavior, 282, 283
binocular, 280
before birth, 273

Visual apparatus, color perception, 276
depth perception, 277
hyperopia, 279
light perception, 276
myopia, 278
in neonate, 275, 536
optimal, 275
refraction, 277, 278
sharp, 276
strabismus, 280
testing, 282
(*See also* Retina)
Visual sensation, distance sense, 507
foreground sense, 508
lead sense, 507
spatial sense, 508
(*See also* Blindness)
Vitamins, 329–332
classification, 329
fat-soluble, 330, 331
dietary sources, 330
functions, 330
ingestion and absorption, 330
storage in liver, 330
water-soluble, 331, 332
dietary sources, 331
functions, 331
ingestion and absorption, 331
Vocabulary and symbolization, 456
Voluntary behavior, 397–402
Vowels and consonants, 458

Water, drinking, fluorine in, 336
Weaning and dining, 375
Weight, brain, ratio to body weight, 140
Will, and behavior, 431, 496
and feelings, 431, 496
of mother, effect on child rearing, 354
on fetus, 353
"Witches' milk," 205
Working mother, 624–628
attitude, of husband, 626
of wife, 625
child care, adolescent, 626
school child, 626
young child, 626
effects on children, 627
physical stamina, 626
reasons for work, 624
World-centered perception, 506, 507
during school years, 512
of sound, 507
of tactation in hand, 261, 509
of vision, 508
Writing (*see* Reading and writing)

Yearling, 547–549
age portrait, 603
eating behavior, 547
language, 547
motor skills, 547
walking, 547
weight, 548
Yolk sac, blood islands in, 161
empty of yolk in mammals, 34
vascular channels in, 58

Zygote, 4, 33, 45, 56, 57